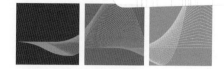

Multiple Sclerosis
for the Non-Neurologist

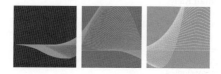

Multiple Sclerosis for the Non-Neurologist

Mary Ann Picone, MD
Medical Director
Multiple Sclerosis Comprehensive Care
Center at Holy Name Medical Center
Teaneck, New Jersey
Adjunct Clinical Associate Professor
Touro College of Osteopathic Medicine
New York, New York

Rock G. Positano, DPM, MSc, MPH, DSc (hon)
Professor and Director of the Non-Surgical Foot and Ankle Service
Joe DiMaggio Sports Medicine Foot and Ankle Center
Sports Medicine Service
Hospital For Special Surgery
Weill Cornell Medical College and New York–Presbyterian Hospital
Department of Medicine, Division of Endocrinology, Diabetes and Metabolism
Department of Cardiothoracic Surgery
Department of Obstetrics and Gynecology
Memorial Sloan Kettering Cancer Center (MSKCC)
Orthopedic Service/Foot and Ankle Division/Department of Surgery
New York College of Podiatric Medicine/Foot Center of New York
Departments of Academic Orthopedic Science/Medicine/Orthopedics
New York, New York

Dexter Sun, MD, PhD
Clinical Professor of Neurology
Weill Cornell Medical College
New York, New York

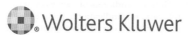

Philadelphia • Baltimore • New York • London
Buenos Aires • Hong Kong • Sydney • Tokyo

Acquisitions Editor: Chris Teja
Product Development Editor: Ariel S. Winter
Editorial Assistant: Jeremiah Kiely
Marketing Manager: Julie Sikora
Production Project Manager: Barton Dudlick
Design Coordinator: Terry Mallon
Artist/Illustrator: Jen Clements
Manufacturing Coordinator: Beth Welsh,
Prepress Vendor: TNQ Technologies

9 8 7 6 5 4 3 2 1

Printed in China

Library of Congress Cataloging-in-Publication Data

Names: Picone, Mary Ann, editor. | Positano, Rock G., editor. | Sun, Dexter, editor.
Title: Multiple sclerosis for the non-neurologist / [edited by] Mary Ann Picone, Rock G. Positano, Dexter Sun.
Description: Philadelphia : Wolters Kluwer, [2020] | Includes bibliographical references and index.
Identifiers: LCCN 2019013826 | ISBN 9781975102517 (pbk.)
Subjects: | MESH: Multiple Sclerosis
Classification: LCC RC377 | NLM WL 360 | DDC 616.8/34–dc23
LC record available at https://lccn.loc.gov/2019013826

This book is dedicated to our MS patients and their families whose courage and spirit have been a constant source of inspiration.

CONTRIBUTORS LIST

George Alexiades, MD
Associate Professor of Clinical Otolaryngology
Department of Otolaryngology
Weill Cornell Medical College
New York, New York

Philip J. Aliotta, MD, MSHA, CHCQM, FACS
Chairman
Department of Urology
Catholic Health System of Western New York
Chief of Urology, Sisters of Charity Hospital and
St. Joseph Campus, Buffalo, New York

Mohini Aras, MD
Assistant Professor
Department of Medicine
Weill Cornell Medical College
New York, New York

Louis J. Aronne, MD, FACP, DABOM
Stanford I. Weill Professor of Metabolic Research
Department of Medicine
Weill Cornell Medical College
Attending Physician
Department of Medicine
New York–Presbyterian Hospital
New York, New York

Andrea Arzt, LSCW
Director of Healthcare Provider Engagement
National Multiple Sclerosis Society
New York, New York

Meghan Beier, PhD
Assistant Professor
Department of Physical Medicine and Rehabilitation
Johns Hopkins University School of Medicine
Baltimore, Maryland

Regina Berkovich, MD, PhD
Assistant Professor of Clinical Neurology
Department of Neurology
University of Southern California
Los Angeles, California

Francois Bethoux, MD
Professor
Department of Medicine
Cleveland Clinic Lerner College of Medicine
Director of Rehabilitation Services
Mellen Center for Multiple Sclerosis Treatment and Research
Cleveland Clinic
Cleveland, Ohio

Jagriti "Jackie" Bhattarai, PhD
National MS Society Postdoctoral Fellow
Department of Physical Medicine and Rehabilitation
Johns Hopkins University School of Medicine
Baltimore, Maryland

Michelle G. Carlson, MD
Professor
Department of Clinical Orthopedic Surgery
Weill Cornell Medical College
Attending Orthopedic Surgeon
Department of Orthopedic Surgery
Hospital for Special Surgery
New York, New York

Tanuja Chitnis, MD
Associate Professor
Department of Neurology
Harvard Medical School
Director, Partners Pediatric Multiple Sclerosis Center
Department of Child Neurology
Massachusetts General Hospital
Boston, Massachusetts

Michael A. Ciaramella, BA
Medical Student
Rutgers-Robert Wood Johnson Medical School
Piscataway, New Jersey

Joseph T. Cooke, MD
Associate Professor of Clinical Medicine
Department of Medicine
Weill Cornell Medical College
Chairman
Department of Medicine
New York–Presbyterian Queens
New York, New York

Danielle E. Currier, DMD
Clinical Instructor in Surgery
Department of Oral & Maxillofacial Surgery
Weill Cornell Medical College
New York, New York

Christopher Der, MD
Assistant Clinical Professor
Department of Anesthesiology
Harbor – UCLA Medical Center
Torrance, California

Joshua S. Dines, MD
Associate Professor
Department of Orthopedic Surgery
Weill Cornell Medical College
Associate Attending Physician
Department of Sports Medicine and Shoulder Service
Hospital for Special Surgery
New York, New York

Alisha N. Dua, MRES
Medical Student
Department of Otolaryngology
Weill Cornell Medical College
New York, New York

Mostafa El Khashab, MD, FACS, IFAANS
Attending Neurological Surgeon
Attending Pediatric Neurological Surgeon
Department of Neurological Surgery
Advanced Neurosurgeons Associates
Rutherford, New Jersey

Brandon J. Erickson, MD
Chief, Shoulder & Elbow Surgery
Phelps Hospital
Department of Orthopedic Surgery
Rothman Orthopedic Institute
New York, New York

Dorothy A. Fink, MD
Assistant Professor of Medicine
Department of Medicine
Weill Cornell Medical College
Assistant Attending Physician
Department of Medicine
Hospital of Special Surgery
New York, New York

Frederick W. Foley, PhD
Professor of Psychology
Department of Ferkauf Graduate School of Psychlogy
Yeshiva University
Bronx, New York
Director of Clinical Psychology
Multiple Sclerosis Comprehensive Care Center
Holy Name Medical Center
Teaneck, New Jersey

Molly Forlines, BA
Research Assistant
Non-Surgical Foot and Ankle Service
Hospital for Special Surgery
New York, New York

Steven Galetta, MD, FAAN
Professor and Chair
Department of Neurology
New York University School Of Medicine
New York, New York

Doria M. Gold, MD
Resident
Department of Neurology
New York University School of Medicine
New York, New York

Tracy B. Grossman, MD, MSc
Fellow
Maternal Fetal Medicine
Department of Obstetrics and Gynecology
Weill Cornell Medical College
New York, New York

Ronald Guberman, DPM, DABPS
Podiatry Residency Program Director
Department of Surgery
Wyckoff Heights Medical Center
Brooklyn, New York

June Halper, MSH, APN-C, MSCN, FAAN
Chief Executive Officer
Consortium of Multiple Sclerosis Centers
Hackensack, New Jersey

Lauren Hooper, BA
Director of Education, Healthcare Relations, and Grants Management
Multiple Sclerosis Association of America
Cherry Hill, New Jersey

Anna-Marie Hosking, BS
Medical Student IV
University of California, Irvine School of Medicine
Irvine, California

Misa Hyakutake, MD
Resident/Future Fellow
Department of Medicine/Department of Geriatrics and Palliative Medicine
Icahn School of Medicine at Mount Sinai
New York, New York

Anthony M. Iuso, OMS-I, BS
Medical Student, OMS-I
Touro College of Osteopathic Medicine
New York, New York
Research Assistant
Department of Clinical Research
Holy Name Medical Center
Teaneck, New Jersey

Joseph L. Jorizzo, MD
Professor of Clinical Dermatology
Department of Dermatology
Weill Cornell Medical College
Professor of Dermatology
Department of Dermatology
New York–Presbyterian Hospital
New York, New York
Professor, Former and Founding Chair
Department of Dermatology
Wake Forest University School of Medicine
Winston Salem, North Carolina

Randy Karim, PT, DPT, NCS, CBIS
Clinical Specialist
Director of Neurologic PT Residency Program
Department of Rehabilitation and Sports Therapy
Mellen Center for MS Treatment and Research
Cleveland Clinic
Cleveland, Ohio

Herbert I. Karpatkin, PT, DSc, NCS, MSCS
Assistant Professor
Department of Physical Therapy
Hunter College, City University of New York
New York, New York

Dale J. Lange, MD
Professor of Neurology
Department of Neurology
Weill Cornell Medical College
Chair and Neurologist In-Chief
Department of Neurology
Hospital for Special Surgery
New York, New York

Richard I. Lappin, MD, PhD
Assistant Professor of Clinical Medicine
Department of Emergency Medicine
Weill Cornell Medical College
Attending Physician
Department of Emergency Medicine
New York–Presbyterian Hospital
New York, New York

John A. Lincoln, MD, PhD
Associate Professor
Department of Neurology
McGovern Medical School - UT Health
Staff Physician
Department of Neurology
Memorial Hermann Hospital
Houston, Texas

Waldemar Majdanski, DPM, FACFAS
Associate Attending Physcian
Department of Podiatry
Wyckoff Medical Center
Brooklyn, New York

Kathy C. Matthews, MD
Fellow
Maternal Fetal Medicine
Department of Obstetrics and Gynecology
Weill Cornell Medical College
New York, New York

Kyle W. Morse, MD
Resident
Department of Orthopedic Surgery
Hospital for Special Surgery
New York, New York

Robert W. Motl, PhD
Professor and Director of Research
Department of Physical Therapy
University of Alabama at Birmingham
Birmingham, Alabama

Nida Naushad, BA
Medical Student
Yale School of Medicine
New Haven, Connecticut

Andrui Nazarian, MD, MS, MSHAM
Clinical Anthesiologist
Department of Anthesiology
Olive View – University of California Los Angeles Medical Center
Sylmar, California

Dorothy E. Northrop, MSW, ACSW
Social Worker
Multiple Sclerosis Comprehensive Care Center
Holy Name Medical Center
Teaneck, New Jersey

Annette F. Okai, MD
Medical Director
Baylor Scott & White Multiple Sclerosis Treatment Center of Dallas
Dallas, Texas

Constantine J. Pella, BS
Research Assistant
Holy Name Medical Center
Teaneck, New Jersey

Tiffany Peng, MD
Resident Physician
Department of Otolaryngology
New York–Presbyterian Hospital of Columbia & Cornell
New York, New York

Carlos A. Pérez, MD
Fellow
Department of Pediatrics – Division of Child and Adolescent Neurology
University of Texas Health Science Center at Houston
Houston, Texas

Mary Ann Picone, MD
Medical Director Multiple Sclerosis Comprehensive Care
Center at Holy Name Medical Center
Teaneck, New Jersey
Adjunct Clinical Associate Professor
Touro College of Osteopathic Medicine
New York, New York

Jeffrey G. Portnoy, MA
PhD Candidate
Ferkauf Graduate School of Psychology
Yeshiva University
Bronx, New York
Neuropsychology Staff
Multiple Sclerosis Center
Holy Name Medical Center
Teaneck, New Jersey

Rock CJay Positano, DPM
Co-Director of the Non-Surgical Foot and Ankle Service
Joe DiMaggio Sports Medicine Foot and Ankle Center
Hospital for Special Surgery
New York, New York
Resident Physician
Department of Podiatry
New York–Presbyterian/Brooklyn Methodist Hospital
Brooklyn, New York

Rock G. Positano, DPM, MSc, MPH, DSc (hon)
Professor and Director of the Non-Surgical Foot and Ankle Service
Joe DiMaggio Sports Medicine Foot and Ankle Center
Sports Medicine Service
Hospital For Special Surgery
Weill Cornell Medical College and New York–Presbyterian Hospital
Department of Medicine, Division of Endocrinology, Diabetes and Metabolism
Department of Cardiothoracic Surgery
Department of Obstetrics and Gynecology
Memorial Sloan Kettering Cancer Center (MSKCC)
Orthopedic Service/Foot and Ankle Division/Department of Surgery
New York College of Podiatric Medicine/Foot Center of New York
Departments of Academic Orthopedic Science/Medicine/Orthopedics
New York, New York

Qibin Qi, PhD
Associate Professor
Department of Epidemiology and Population Health
Albert Einstein College of Medicine
Bronx, New York

Gwendolyn S. Reeve, DMD
Assistant Professor
Department of Surgery
Weill Cornell Medical College
Attending Surgeon
Department of Surgery
New York–Presbyterian Hospital
New York, New York

W. Mark Richardson, BA
Clinical Research Coordinator
Department of Neurology
Hospital for Special Surgery
New York, New York

Marsha E. Rubin, DDS
Assistant Professor
Department of Surgery
Weill Cornell Medical College
Director of Dentistry/ Chief of Dental Medicine
Department of Surgery
New York–Presbyterian Hospital
New York, New York

Janet C. Rucker, MD
Professor
Department of Neurology
New York University School of Medicine
New York, New York

Katherine H. Saunders, MD
Assistant Professor of Clinical Medicine
Comprehensive Weight Control Center
Weill Cornell Medical College
New York, New York

Stephanie L. Silveira, PhD
Postdoctoral Fellow
Department of Physical Therapy
University of Alabama at Birmingham
Birmingham, Alabama

Anthony J. Smith, MD
Associate Attending of Clinical Medicine
Department of Medicine
Weill Cornell Medical College
New York, New York
Division Chief of Pulmonary and Critical Care Medicine
Department of Medicine
New York–Presbyterian Queens
Queens, New York

Catherine Stratton, BA
MPH Candidate
Chronic Disease Epidemiology
Yale School of Public Health
New Haven, Connecticut

Quy Tran, MD
Assistant Clinical Professor
Department of Anesthesiology
David Geffen School of Medicine at UCLA
Los Angeles, California
Attending Physician
Department of Anesthesiology
Harbor - UCLA Medical Center
Torrance, California

Priyank Trivedi, MD
Fellow
Weill Cornell Medical College
Fellow
Department of Pulmonary and Critical Care
New York–Presbyterian Queens
Queens, New York

Yetsa A. Tuakli-Wosornu, MD, MPH
Assistant Clinical Professor
Department of Chronic Disease Epidemiology
Yale School of Public Health
New Haven, Connecticut

Hunter Vincent, DO
Resident Physician
Department of Physical Medicine and Rehabilitation
University of California Davis
Sacramento, California

Karen Yanelli, PT, DPT, Cert-MDT
Owner/Operator
Karren Yanelli, LLC
Physical Therapy Private Practice
New York, New York

Sydney Yee, MD
Anesthesiology Resident
Department of Anesthesia
Harbor – UCLA Medical Center
Torrance, California

Tiffany Yeh, MD
Fellow
Division of Endocrinology, Diabetes, and Metabolism
New York–Presbyterian Hospital – Weill Cornell Medical College
New York, New York

Michele Yeung, MD
Fellow
Department of Endocrinology/Department of Diabetes and Metabolism
New York–Presbyterian Hospital
Weill Cornell Medical College
New York, New York

■■■ PREFACE

"My doctor doesn't understand my MS." It was statements such as this heard from my patients that led to the development of this book. The incidence of MS has increased but fortunately so has the development of effective disease-modifying therapies to decrease relapses and slow disability progression. Patients can discuss many treatment options with their physicians and are living longer, more active lives. Research regarding the immunology and epidemiology of the disease continues to evolve. Therapies used for disease treatment are often associated with adverse effects and potential for drug interaction. This book aims to increase awareness of the problems associated with MS for nonneurologic specialties such as internal medicine, emergency medicine, urology, ophthalmology, dermatology, for example, who often will treat patients with MS. Optimal comprehensive care for patients involves coordination of care among many medical fields, not just neurology. Physiatrists, physical and occupational therapists, podiatrists, residents, fellows, and nurse practitioners working together can help improve quality of life for patients and their families. Chapters in the book are devoted to evaluation of the patient with MS, public health issues associated with the disease, better understanding of MRI findings in MS, issues encountered in surgery and pain management, dental care, and identification of services for patients and their families.

It is my hope that this book will provide a practical and comprehensive guide to wide variety of health care professionals and trainees to increase awareness and recognition of MS, the problems that MS patients face particularly as they are encountered in the various medical and surgical specialties, better understanding of the importance of coordination of care with the ultimate goal of improving patient outcomes. It is meant to be a resource easily accessible for reference in daily office practice.

I would like to acknowledge and thank all the distinguished chapter contributors and the team at Wolters Kluwer for their assistance. I thank my children for their love and support during the writing of this book.

The editors would also like to thank all our colleagues at Holy Name Medical Center, Hospital for Special Surgery, New York–Presbyterian Hospital/Weill Cornell, Yale School of Public Health, Weill Cornell Medical College, Memorial Sloan Kettering Cancer Center, and the New York College of Podiatric Medicine.

In addition the generous support of the Stavros Niarchos Foundation, Weill Family Foundation, Durst Organization, James Family Charitable Foundation, Louis and Rachel Rudin Foundation, Heckscher Foundation, O'Toole Family Fund at JP Morgan, Jim and Linda Robinson Foundation, Thomas H. Lee, Mary Lupo, and Ed Ricci.

I want to also thank the Alfiero and Lucia Palestroni Foundation, George P. Pitkin Foundation, and Larry Inserra for their invaluable support of the Holy Name MS Center.

Mary Ann Picone, MD

■■■ FOREWORD

Multiple Sclerosis (MS) is the most prevalent, nontraumatic neurologic condition among young adults worldwide. Diagnosis is most common in 20- to 50-year-old individuals and far more common in females than males.

The disease is remarkably heterogeneous. For some, the effects of MS are relatively mild and stable. Others experience wide-ranging, progressive symptoms that can affect a constellation of physical and mental functions. For the medical practitioner, optimal management of patients with MS poses several challenges.

Broad variability in the nature and severity of MS symptoms may confound the diagnosis of other, unrelated conditions, challenging physicians across medical specialties, who must determine whether new symptoms are related to the underlying MS or represent a distinct medical problem. Moreover, common symptoms of MS—vision problems, fatigue and weakness, dizziness, bladder problems, and sexual dysfunction—can mimic a host of unrelated medical conditions.

Patients with an established diagnosis of MS also present challenging management problems to the medical specialist—internist, gynecologist, surgeon, etc.,—who is not a neurologist. This comprehensive collection of chapters by prominent specialists from across the spectrum of medical disciplines offers practical insights and sage advice about the differential diagnosis and effective management of patients with this challenging disease.

Peter T. Scardino, MD
Chairman Emeritus
Department of Surgery
Memorial Sloan Kettering Cancer Center
Professor of Surgery
Department of Urology
Weill Medical College of Cornell University

CONTENTS ■ ■ ■

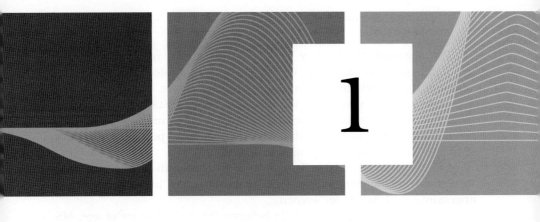

Epidemiology

■ ▨ ▨ Mary Ann Picone, Qibin Qi

Introduction

The etiology of multiple sclerosis (MS) is complex and not fully under-stood, but there have been various environmental and genetic factors associated with increased MS risk.[1] The prevailing thought is that MS is an autoimmune disorder whereby either viral or environmental agents, or both, trigger a T cell–mediated inflammatory attack, causing demyelination in the central nervous system (CNS). This is thought to result from a complex interplay between genes and the environment. The environmental factors most thought to be involved are vitamin D and Epstein-Barr virus (EBV). Obesity, particularly when present early in life, appears to play a role. Cigarette smoking also has been linked.[1] The aim of this chapter is to discuss genetic and environmental risk factors, both infectious and noninfectious, that are associated with MS development.

Demographics

MS is the most common cause of nontraumatic disability in young adults.[1,2] **The exact etiology remains unknown, but it is thought to be associated with genetic factors and environmental exposures with environmental factors playing a role in altering gene expression.**[3] Genes are needed for the development of MS, but the environment plays a predominant role in determining risk. These factors must act at an early age.

The National MS Society Prevalence Initiative, using administrative databases from a variety of sources including Medicare, Medicaid, Veterans Health Administration, and private insurers, estimated nearly 1.1 million people are living with MS in the United States.[4] This is over twice the number reported since the late 1970s. Estimates of prevalence are important for public health initiatives regarding possible preventive strategies and cost to society, among others.

Lifetime risk for MS has a female predominance with an approximately three times greater risk in women than in men, and incidence of MS is approximately 1 in 200 for women.

The peak time for diagnosis is between 20 and 40 years of age. MS is less frequently diagnosed in childhood, and diagnosis tends to decline after 50 years of age.[66] It can begin within the first or second year of life and can also be diagnosed beyond the age of 70 years.[5] Symptoms of the disease may often be present for years before a diagnosis is made. Critical exposure seems to occur before the age of 15 years, according to migration studies. The advent of magnetic resonance imaging (MRI) and improved diagnostic criteria throughout the years has led to earlier diagnosis of the disease.

Individuals of higher socioeconomic background have a greater risk than those of lower socioeconomic background. MS is more common in Caucasian population, whereas less frequent in African American and Asian populations. Studies have shown African American men to have an approximately 40% lower risk than white men.[6] However, MS tends to have a more severe course in African Americans. It is rare in Inuits.

Life expectancy of patients with MS has increased in the recent years, and this can be one explanation for the increase in the prevalence seen.[7] Increased awareness and diagnosis of the disease and improved access to neurologists can also increase incidence. One of the difficulties with ascertaining prevalence and incidence has been the problems encountered in consistency in the methodologies and quality of epidemiological studies which have been done.

A retrospective analysis done in the United States looking at commercially insured patient claims from 2008 to 2012 showed a prevalence of about 150 per 100,000 individuals. Females were three times more likely to have MS than males, and peak prevalence occurred at ages 45 to 49 years. Prevalence was relatively consistent during this time span.[8] Population-based administrative data from British Columbia during the years 1991 to 2008 showed an increase in prevalence by 4.7% per year on average. This could be explained by increased peak prevalence of MS, longer survival rates for MS, and greater life expectancy of women compared with men.[9] Recent data published from a prospective epidemiological Danish study looking at incidence of MS between 1950 to 1959 and 2000 to 2009 revealed an increased incidence of MS over a 60-year period, particularly

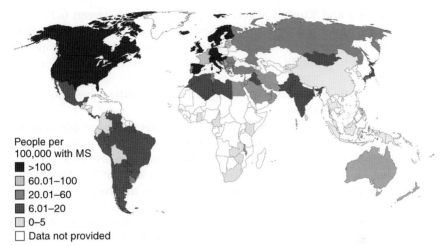

People per
100,000 with MS
■ >100
☐ 60.01–100
■ 20.01–60
■ 6.01–20
☐ 0–5
☐ Data not provided

Figure 1.1. **Worldwide prevalence of multiple sclerosis (MS) in 2013.** Reprinted with permission from Browne P, Chandraratna D, Angood C, et al. Atlas of Multiple Sclerosis 2013: A growing global problem with widespread inequity. *Neurology*. 2014;83(11):1022-1024. doi:10.1212/WNL.0000000000000768. See eBook for color figure.

in women and older age-groups, ages 50 to 64 years. The study analyzed 19,536 cases of MS with onset between 1950 and 2009 that were recorded in the Danish registry. Prevalence of risk factors, smoking and obesity, increased during this time period in Denmark, but in females, hormonal factors seem to have played an even more important role. Increased incidence in females seemed to parallel age at first pregnancy and had a link to fewer pregnancies. For older patients, improved MRI diagnostic ability to distinguish between smaller vascular lesions and MS lesions could also contribute to the increased incidence seen.[10,11] Prevalence of MS in Norway has increased 10-fold over the past 50 years, and female-to-male sex ratio has increased. Changes in lifestyle and improved health services and life expectancy with MS could be contributing factors.[10]

Where in the World Does MS Typically Occur?

MS is most common in the northern parts of North America and Europe (Figure 1.1).[12] Prevalence in these areas is between 0.1% and 0.2% of the population. Incidence is approximately 5 to 6 per 100,000 yearly.[13] Incidence being the risk of contracting the disease, and prevalence the proportion of cases in the population at any one time.

Geographic distribution appears to inversely parallel that of regional ultraviolet radiation with low incidence in subtropical and tropical regions and higher incidence with increasing latitudes both north and south of the equator,[3] with higher incidence in the northern parts of

North America and Europe, where the prevalence is between 0.1% and 0.2% of the population, and the incidence is about 5 to 6 per 100,000 population per year.[14] Because of this observation, it has been proposed that exposure to sunlight and higher vitamin D levels may have a protective effect.[69]

MS is rare in Asia, where the demyelinating disorder more commonly seen is neuromyelitis optica.

Migration effects: MS risk appears to decrease when people migrate from an area of higher incidence to that of lower incidence, particularly before the age of 15 years. When individuals move before their teenage years from an area of high MS prevalence to an area of low MS prevalence, their MS risk becomes similar to the region in which they moved. Children of immigrants from lower MS-prevalent regions born in a higher MS-prevalent region have a risk similar to those in the country of birth. Opposite migration does not appear to increase risk.[3,6]

Environmental Factors (Noninfectious)

Genetic factors are needed for MS to develop, but environmental factors play an important role in determining MS risk, particularly at an early stage in life.

Latitude

In temperate climate regions, MS incidence and prevalence increase with latitude.[6] Latitude appears to be the strongest risk factor for MS. In the northern hemisphere, MS prevalence tends to follow a north-south gradient and in the Southern hemisphere, a south-north gradient. However, this gradient appears to be decreasing. Over the last few decades, relative risk of MS was 2.02 comparing residence in northern US states to southern states for Vietnam veterans.[6]

For earlier born World War II veterans, the risk was 2.64. Recent studies have shown that the prevalence of MS in formerly considered low-risk areas such as South America and regions closer to the equator is increasing.[6] MS prevalence decreases with increasing light exposure.

Month and Place of Birth

Studies from Canada, Australia, and northern Europe[1,6,15] showed latitude-related increased risks for spring births that may reflect lower maternal vitamin D levels in winter pregnancies. During winter months at latitudes >42°N, most ultraviolet B (UVB) radiation is absorbed by the atmosphere with little production of vitamin D in the skin.

High-Salt Diets

Diet has been discussed as a potential risk factor for MS in developed countries. With increased adoption of the western diet and use of more processed food, salt intake has increased, and this can play a role in MS pathogenesis.[16] Salt intake has been shown to participate in modulating the differentiation of human and mouse Th17 cells. Mice fed a high-sodium diet had more aggressive courses of experimental autoimmune encephalomyelitis associated with increased IL-17. Increased sodium intake can boost the induction of IL-17–producing CD4+ helper T cells, which have been shown to be involved in MS pathogenesis. High-salt diets also affect the renin-angiotensin aldosterone system, which potentially can modulate immune responses.

Sodium intake has been associated with increased disease activity in MS.[17] Farez and colleagues found a positive correlation between exacerbation rates and sodium intake.[17] Increased radiological disease activity was also noted.

Diet and Gut Microbiome

Specific gut bacteria seem to be more common in MS patients than in controls, and pro-inflammatory responses in human blood mononuclear cells could be produced by these bacteria and trigger experimental allergic encephalomyelitis, an animal model of MS.[18] Bacteria in the gut have been suggested to interact with myelin antigens to trigger autoimmune responses.[19,20]

The cause-and-effect relationship between dysfunctional gut bacteria and MS is still uncertain. In a case-control study in Canada, authors reported increased risk of MS in persons whose diet was higher in animal fats and lower risk in persons with diet consisting of more vegetables and higher dietary fiber. Eating a high-fiber diet helps to promote microbial diversity particularly species within the firmicutes and bacteroidetes phyla.[18] Low dietary polyunsaturated fatty acids may also be another modifiable risk factor for MS.[21]

Vitamin D

Vitamin D levels can play a role in decreasing MS risk. Exposure to sunlight and greater vitamin D absorption in latitudes closer to the equator may help explain the relatively low prevalence of MS in these areas. The incidence of MS diagnosis appears to be the lowest near the equator and increases with increasing latitude. Migration studies have shown that moving from areas of higher to lower incidence appears to decrease future risk of developing MS, with the change in MS risk being most significant when migration occurs in childhood and early adolescence. These areas of low MS prevalence are noted to be areas with higher sunlight exposure, sunlight being the principal inducer of Vitamin D synthesis. Vitamin D has been shown to have immunomodulatory effects, mediating a shift to a more anti-inflammatory immune response by increasing Th2 and regulatory T cell functionality. In its hormonal form, it has been shown to prevent experimental autoimmune encephalomyelitis, an animal model of MS.[22]

Low vitamin D levels in early life in individuals who bear HLA-DRB1*15, a genetic variant associated with increased MS risk, could allow autoreactive T cells to escape deletion by the thymus.[23] This has prompted the question of whether exposure to sunlight and higher vitamin D levels earlier in life confer a protective effect for MS. A study done by Munger supported this view, showing a strong protective effect of 25-hydroxy vitamin D levels of 100 nmol/L or higher before the age of 20 years.[24] Patients with MS studied prospectively had significantly lower levels of vitamin D during adolescence before disease onset.[24] A cross-sectional study by Laursen suggested that shorter amount of sun exposure during adolescence as well as higher body mass index (BMI) at the age of 20 years were associated with an earlier age of onset of MS.[25] Increased time spent in the sun during childhood has also been shown to be associated with decreased risk of MS.[25] Exposure to sunlight is the major source of vitamin D for many people. Sunscreen use has increased, so there is less UVB absorption. In addition, people with MS are likely to spend more time indoors because of heat sensitivity, as heat can often exacerbate symptoms. UVB radiation converts cutaneous 7 dehydrocholesterol to previtamin D3, which isomerizes to vitamin D3. Vitamin D3 hydroxylizes first to 25 hydroxyvitamin D3 (25(OH)D3) and then to 1,25, dihydroxyvitamin D3, which is the biologically active hormone. At higher latitudes, >42°N, very little vitamin D is absorbed by the skin because most UVB is absorbed by the atmosphere, especially in the winter months.[26] One recent study examining Finnish women of reproductive age showed that women who had deficient levels of vitamin D (i.e., <30 nmol/L) had a 43% higher risk of MS compared with women who had adequate levels of vitamin D (i.e., >50 nmol/L).[27]

Average diet and supplement intake in the United States is <400 IU/d. Studies done in vitamin D–deficient mice treated with vitamin D supplements have shown induction of regulatory T cells. Reduction in risk for developing MS with 25(OH)D levels > 100 nmol/L was stronger before the age of 20 years than at age 20 years or older.

Vitamin D supplementation and increase in blood levels are also beneficial in patients who already have the disease. Serum levels tend to increase by 0.8 to 1 nmol/L for every 1 μg ingested. In a study done by Munger et al examining vitamin D levels and MS risk, among whites, there was a 41% decrease in MS risk for every 50 nmol/L increase in 25 hydroxyvitamin D.[28]

Stress and Trauma

Regarding physical trauma and its association with development of MS, studies have not shown evidence to support a relationship between MS and trauma. The relationship between MS and psychologic or emotional stress, however, is possible.[1] An MRI prospective study done by Mohr et al. looked at life stress and new brain lesion formation. It reported that new MRI lesions increased after a lag of 8 weeks following increase in stress such as family or job conflict or changes in routine but not after major stressful events and that the MRI changes were not associated with clinical changes.[29]

Cigarette Smoking

There have been several prospective epidemiological studies linking smoking with increased risk of MS. Compared with nonsmokers, smokers had 40% to 80% increased risk of MS.[30] A British study using information obtained from The General Practice Database assessed the association between cigarette smoking and progression of MS. This was done using a nested case-control study design, and it was found that the risk of developing secondary progressive MS was over three times higher in smokers than in nonsmokers who had relapsing onset of disease. A Swedish study by Hedstrom et al. investigating the interaction between smoking and HLA genotype showed that smokers carrying HLA-DRB1*15 and lacking HLA-A*02 had a 13-fold increased risk compared with nonsmokers without those genetic factors.[31] Risk of MS with positive HLA genotypes was strongly influenced by smoking status. For those who have the disease, smoking has also been associated with increased risk of progression from relapsing to secondary progressive MS.[30] The mechanism may involve the components of cigarette smoke and lung irritation. Secondhand cigarette smoke exposure has also been observed to increase MS risk. This lung irritation causes increased pro-inflammatory cell activation in the lung.[31] CNS autoreactive aggressive T cells in the lungs can potentially be activated by smoking and then enter the CNS and induce autoimmune responses in genetically susceptible individuals. Earlier age of smoking can increase the risk of more severe MS.[32] Oral tobacco use has not been associated with increased risk of MS. Cigarette smoking can also increase the risk of other autoimmune diseases and respiratory infections. Animal models have suggested that cigarette smoke exposure affected innate and adaptive immunity, natural killer cells and B and T lymphocytes. Free radical nitric oxide may also play a role. Nitric oxide has been shown to block axonal conduction and cause axonal degeneration. Cigarette smoke contains nitric oxide. Smoking increases plasma levels of nitric oxide and may increase nitric oxide levels in the CNS that can contribute to axonal degeneration and progressive disease.[30,32] Oligodendroglia, as compared with astrocytes and microglia, are more vulnerable to the harmful effects of nitric oxide.

Organic Solvents

Organic solvent exposure and nonspecific lung irritation have also been studied to show increased risk of MS in individuals who carry the HLA-DRB1*15 susceptibility gene, and particularly if someone also smokes, the risk is increased by 30-fold.[33,34]

Obesity

Increased rates of obesity in industrialized countries over the last 50 years have also played a role in increased incidence of MS.[35,36]

There does seem to be an association between higher BMI at the age of 20 years and lower age at the onset of MS. Observational studies have shown that obesity in early life can increase the risk of developing MS twofold. One US prospective study showed women with BMI >30 kg/m^2 at age 18 years had over twofold risk of developing MS than leaner women, and a Danish study showed that individuals with a childhood BMI >95th percentile were 70% more likely to develop MS than those with a childhood BMI <85th percentile.[37,38] Richards and colleagues used Mendelian randomization approach to evaluate causality between obesity and MS risk and suggested that early life obesity does seem to be causally related to MS risk.[39] This raises important public health signals for continued strategies to decrease childhood obesity. Vitamin D is stored in fat, so people who are obese have lower serum vitamin D levels than thin people.

Sex Hormones

Estrogens in high levels seem to shift immune response from pro-inflammatory type 1 to noninflammatory type 2. There is decreased risk of relapses during pregnancy when levels are high and increased risk postpartum.

Vaccinations

A nested case-control analysis in two large cohorts of nurses in the United States, in the Nurses' Health Study 1 and Nurses' Health Study II using vaccination records did not reveal any association between hepatitis B vaccination and the development of MS.[40]

Environmental Factors (Infectious)

Hygiene Hypothesis

Hygiene hypothesis proposes that early life infections downregulate allergic and autoimmune disorders and lower incidence of early life infections increases incidence of allergic and autoimmune diseases. Later age of infection in genetically susceptible individuals could increase risk.[3] Higher sibling exposure early in life in Caucasians also is associated with decreased MS risk.[41]

HHV-6

Human herpes virus (HHV) variant A is more commonly reported in MS patients. Interaction of HHV-6 variant A has been postulated to play a role in infecting EBV-positive B cell lines and activating the latent EBV genome.[42]

Parasitic Infections

According to the hygiene hypothesis, in developed countries where there is decreased incidence of early childhood infections, the immune system may not develop normally and can turn on itself. Parasitic worms may play a beneficial role. Several studies in animal and human models have demonstrated the ability of helminths to alter immune responses. Correale and Farez showed evidence of parasitic infection leading to increased production of regulatory cells that inhibit T cell proliferation, suppress interferon gamma production, and produce IL-10 and TGF-B that can lead to decreased inflammatory activity in MS.[43]

EBV

EBV is a double-stranded DNA virus of the herpes family, which is responsible for the highly immunogenic infection of B lymphocytes. Infants are susceptible to the virus as maternal protection subsides. It is a common early life infection, especially in developing countries, often seropositive in children by the age of 3 years, usually transmitted by saliva.[3,42] Once infection occurs, antigen-specific cytotoxic T cells expand in response and persist at high levels. If some of the cells carrying T cell receptors recognize self peptides, autoimmunity could result.[42] The virus remains latent with intermittent reactivation. If exposure, as is often the case in developed countries, is delayed into adolescence or adulthood, infectious mononucleosis can occur in 35% to 50% of cases. There is a low risk of

MS in EBV antibody–negative individuals, but in EBV antibody–positive individuals, particularly if they have had infectious mononucleosis, there is an increased risk. This risk has been noted across racial groups and ethnicities, in whites, blacks, and Hispanics.[44] As so many individuals are infected with EBV and do not develop MS, cofactors such as age at time of infection, genetic susceptibility, or infection with other microbes along with EBV may be required.

CMV

Cytomegalovirus (CMV) is also a common early life infection in low-/ middle-income countries. Early infection is often asymptomatic; however, if delayed into adulthood, particularly in females, can result in birth defects from congenital CMV. A large population-based multiethnic study of incident MS cases conducted by Langer-Gould noted CMV serum positivity at an early age showed inconsistent association between CMV seropositivity in whites and later development of MS; however, it did support the hygiene hypothesis. Higher CMV virus exposure was noted in the Hispanic population studied. Previous studies have shown inverse association between CMV seropositivity and MS.[44]

Breastfeeding

Whether breastfeeding is a modifiable risk factor for MS remains unclear. It can result in vertical transmission of virus such as HIV (human immunodeficiency virus) and CMV, but can also protect against common early childhood infections. Several studies in Europeans and Mexicans has found that breastfeeding, especially for greater than 4 months of age, was associated with lower risk of MS.[45,46]

Genetics of Multiple Sclerosis

MS Risk in Families

It has long been noted that there is an important genetic component in the development of MS. Prior family studies have indicated that MS aggregates in families, with increased family risks ranging from ~300-fold for monozygotic twins[47,48] to 20-40-fold for first-degree relatives (dizygotic twins, nontwin siblings, and parent-offspring pairs)[49] compared with the general population. Prior twin studies have shown relatively higher concordance rates of MS in monozygotic twins (24%-30%) than dizygotic twins (3%-5%), and there was no significant difference in concordance rates between dizygotic twins and nontwin siblings.[48,50] Although shared environment may contribute to familial aggregation of MS, the significant excess risk for monozygotic twins and similar concordance rates between dizygotic twins and nontwin siblings suggested that this aggregation is more likely to be genetically determined.[48] This was further supported by findings from a large population-based study, which showed that the frequency of MS among first-degree nonbiological relatives living with the MS index cases was significantly lower than that among biological relatives and very similar to that of the general population.[51]

As the prevalence of MS is higher in women, it was hypothesized that affected males, compared with affected females, had a stronger genetic predisposition, and thus their offspring would have a higher risk for MS, a phenomenon known as the Carter effect.[52] A previous study of 441 children (45 with definite MS) of an affected father or mother (197 families of interest) from 3598 individuals suggested that fathers with MS are 2.2-fold more likely to transmit MS to their children than mothers with MS.[52] However, another study with a relatively larger sample size, including a total of 8401 offspring (798 had MS) from 3088 nuclear families with one affected parent, indicated that there was equal transmission of MS from affected fathers versus affected mothers (9.41% vs. 9.76%).[12] In addition, the sex ratio among affected offspring was the same between affected fathers and affected mothers.[12] Thus, while whether men or women transmit MS more often to their children needs further investigation, there is a great interest in another parent-of-origin effect imparted by the unaffected mothers of MS patients. The first line of evidence was from a study including 1567 index MS cases with half-siblings which reported that the MS risk was significantly higher for maternal half-siblings (2.35%) than that for paternal half-siblings (1.31%).[53] This maternal parent-of-origin effect in MS was further supported by observations from avuncular pairs that the number of avuncular pairs with MS connected through an unaffected mother was significantly higher compared with those connected through an unaffected father.[54] Although the mechanisms remain unclear, the observed maternal effect in MS might be due to the maternal uterine environment and/or potential gene-environment interactions rather than maternal genetic predisposition.

MS Genetic Loci

Until very recently, MS susceptibility genes have been poorly understood. Many candidate-gene and family-based linkage studies (or genome-wide linkage studies) have demonstrated that the human leukocyte antigen (HLA) is the main genetic susceptibility locus associated with MS.[55] For example, the *HLA DRB1*1501* allele has been associated with a three to four times increased risk of MS.[56] Despite the success of identification of MS-associated *HLA* locus, candidate-gene and family-based linkage studies have failed to identify any other loci beyond the *HLA*.

With rapid improvements in high-throughput single nucleotide polymorphism (SNP) genotyping technology and the development of the HapMap project, the method for identifying susceptibility genes has changed dramatically. Genome-wide association study (GWAS) is currently the most commonly used approach for searching novel loci associated with MS. The largest GWAS for MS to date, conducted by the International Multiple Sclerosis Genetics Consortium (IMSGC), including a total of 80,094 individuals of European ancestry (14,498 MS cases and 24,091 controls in the discovery phase; 14,802 MS cases and 26,703 controls in the replication phase), identified 48 new genetic variants associated MS.[57] To date, more than 100 genetic loci beyond the HLA have been identified through GWAS.[58] The previously identified *HLA* loci have been confirmed by the GWAS and showed the largest genetic effect on MS (odds ratio [OR] = 3.10, $P < 1.0 \times 10^{-320}$), while other non-*HLA* genetic variants showed modest effect on MS (OR = 1.1-1.3). Many of these identified variants are in or near to genes which are involved in the immune system, particularly in T cell–mediated immune mechanisms.[57,58] Yet, the MS genetic loci identified so far only explain a small proportion (~27%) of MS heritability.[59] There are a number of theories unproven as yet which may explain the missing heritability, including rare variants with larger effects, common variants with smaller effects, structural variants, epigenetics, and pathway involvement, gene-gene interactions, and gene-environment interactions.[55,58]

Sex-specific genetic effects have been also analyzed in two GWAS[60,61]; however, only a few genetic loci showed suggestive sex differences in associations with MS. For example, in the IMSGC, SNP rs1800693 in *TNFRSF1A* was associated with MS at the genome-wide significance in women (OR = 1.16; $P = 8.9 \times 10^{-11}$) but not in men (OR = 1.05; $P = 0.14$), while SNP rs2293370 in *TIMMDC1* and SNP rs13333054 near *IRF8* were associated with MS at the genome-wide significance in men (OR = 1.26 and 1.24; $P = 1.4 \times 10^{-8}$ and 2.1×10^{-9}, respectively) but not in women (OR = 1.11 and 1.06; $P = 0.008$ and 0.04, respectively).[60] Given significant differences in prevalence and clinical phenotypes of MS between women and men, future GWAS with larger sample sizes are needed to identify sex-specific genetic loci which may help explain the sex differences in MS risk.

In addition, differences in MS risk have been observed across racial and ethnic groups, which might be, at least partially, due to genetic backgrounds. For example, the frequency of HLA-DRB1*1501 allele was high in Caucasian individuals and low in African and Asian individuals.[55] However, most existing GWAS of MS were largely conducted among individuals of European ancestry,[57] and race-/ethnicity-specific genetic effects for other MS genetic loci have not been well studied. Thus, GWAS in multiple racial and ethnic groups are warranted to identify more population-specific genetic loci which may help explain ethnic differences in MS risk.

Gene-Environment Interactions in MS

Besides genetic variants, gene-environment interactions may play an important role in the development of MS. Of note, several nongenetic risk factors for MS, such as smoking, EBV infection, and low vitamin D levels caused by insufficient sun exposure deficiency, have been reported to interact with MS genes, mostly HLA locus, in relation to MS risk in recent studies.[62] For example, a pooled analysis of 6 datasets suggested that smokers carrying HLA-DRB1*15 and lacking HLA-A*02 had an ~13-fold increased risk for MS (OR = 12.7, 95% CI 10.8-14.9) compared with never smokers without these genetic risk factors.[32] In a pattern of gene-environment interaction similar to that observed with smoking, infectious mononucleosis significantly accentuated the genetic effects of *HLA* on MS risk.[63,64]

There is a great interest in the role of vitamin D, vitamin D–associated genetic variants, and their interactions with MS genetic loci in the development of MS. Genetic variants in *CYP27B1*, a central vitamin D metabolism enzyme gene, have been identified to be associated with increased risk of MS through GWAS.[57] A more recent study using whole genome sequencing data identified a low-frequency coding variation in *CYP2R1*, which has large effects on lower vitamin D levels and increased MS risk.[65] Moreover, two Mendelian randomization analyses demonstrated the significant association between vitamin D–associated genetic variants and MS risk, suggesting a potential causal effect of vitamin D in MS.[66-68] Interestingly, in vitro experiments have provided evidence for a direct biological gene-environment interaction between vitamin D and *HLA-DRB1*,[26] the main MS susceptibility locus, although this interaction has not been well studied in human populations. It has been speculated that vitamin D deficiency in early childhood can reduce the expression of *HLA-DRB1* in the thymus, which might result in loss of central tolerance and then increase the risk of autoimmunity and MS in later life.[26] Thus, it is very important to clarify the role of the interaction between vitamin D and *HLA-DRB1* in the MS etiology, which will help provide new insights into the early prevention of MS.

References

1. Goodin DS. The epidemiology of multiple sclerosis: insights to a causal cascade. *Handb Clin Neurol.* 2016;138:173-206.
2. Noseworthy J, Lucchinetti C, Rodriguez M, Weinshenker B. Multiple sclerosis. *NEJM.* 2000;343:938-952.
3. Asherio A, Munger K. Environmental risk factors for multiple sclerosis. Part 1: the role of infection. *Ann Neurol.* 2007;61:288-299.
4. Wallin M. *The Prevalence of Multiple Sclerosis in the United States.* ECTRIMS; 2017. Abstract P344.

5. Lee JY, Chitnis T. Pediatric multiple sclerosis. *Semin Neurol.* 2016;36(02):148-153. doi:10.1055/s-0036-1579738.

6. Ramagopalan SV, Sadovonik AD. Epidemiology of multiple sclerosis. *Neurol Clin.* 2011;29(2):207-217. doi: 10.1016/j.ncl.2010.12.010.

7. Kingwell E, Marriott JJ, Jette N. Incidence and prevalence of multiple sclerosis in Europe: a systematic review. *BMC Neurol.* 2013;13:128.

8. Dilokthornsakul P, Valuck R, Nair K, Corboy J, Allen R, Campbell J. Multiple sclerosis prevalence in the United States commerically insured population. *Neurology.* 2016;86:1014-1021.

9. Kingwell E, Zhu F, Marrie RA, et al. High Incidence and increasing prevalence of multiple sclerosis in British Columbia, Canada: findings from over two decades (1991–2010). *J Neurol.* 2015;262(10):2352-2363.

10. Koch-Hendriksen N, Thygesen LC, Stnager E, Lauarsen B, Magyari M. Incidence of MSA has increased markedly over six decades in Denmark particularly with late onset and in women. *Neurology.* 2018;90:e1954-e1963.

11. Grytten N, Torkildsen O, Myhr KM. Time trends in the incidence and prevalence of multiple sclerosis in Norway during eight decades. *Acta Neurol Scand.* 2015;132(suppl 199):29-36.

12. Herrera BM, Ramagopalan SV, Orton S, et al. Parental transmission of MS in a population-based Canadian cohort. *Neurology.* 2007;69:1208-1212.

13. Wynn DR, Rodriquez M, OFallon M, et al. A reappraisal of the epidemiology of multiple sclerosis in Olmsted County, Monnesota. *Neurology.* 1990;40:780-786.

14. Goodin DS. *Handbook of Clinical Neurology;* 2016; Vol. 138.

15. Templer DI, Trent NH, Spencer DA, et al. Season of birth in multiple sclerosis. *Acta Neurol Scand.* 1992;85(2):107-109. doi:10.1111/j.1600-0404.1992.tb04007.x.

16. Kleinewietfeld M, Manzel A, Titze J, et al. Sodium chloride drives autoimmune disease by the induction of pathogenic Th17 cells. *Nature.* 2013;496(7446):518-522. doi:10.1038/nature11868.

17. Farez MF, Fiol MP, Gaitlan M, Quintana F, Correale J. Sodium intake is associated with increased disease activity in multiple sclerosis. *J Neurol Neurosurg Psychiatry.* 2015;86:26-31.

18. Joscelyn J, Kasper L. Digesting the emerging role for the gut microbiome in central nervous system demyelination. *Mult Scler.* 2014;20(12):1553-1559.

19. Berer K, Mues M, Koutrolos M, et al. Commensal microbiota and myelin autoantigen cooperate to trigger autoimmune demyelination. *Nature.* 2011;479:538-541

20. Cekanavicuite E, Yoo BB, Runia TF, et al. Gut bacteria from multiple sclerosis patients modulate human T cells and exacerbate symptoms in mouse models. *Proc Natl Acad Sci USA.* 2017;114:10713-10718.

21. Bjornevik K, Chitnis T, Ascherio A, Munger K. Polyunsaturated fatty acids and the risk of multiple sclerosis. *Mult Scler.* 2017;23(14):1830-1838.

22. Hayes CE, Nashold FE, Spach KM, Pedersen LB. The immunological functions of the vitamin D endocrine system. *Cell Mol Biol.* 2003;49:277-300.

23. Nolan D, Castle A, Tschochner M, et al. Contributions of vitamin D response elements and hLA promoters to multiple sclerosis risk. *Neurology.* 2012;79:538-546.

24. Munger KL, Levin LI, Hollis BW, Howard NS, Ascherio A. Serum 25 hydroxyvitamin D levels and risk of multiple sclerosis. *JAMA.* 2006;296:2832-2838.

25. Laursen JH, Søndergaard HB, Sørensen PS, Sellebjerg F, Oturai AB. Association between age at onset of multiple sclerosis and vitamin D level–related factors. *Neurology.* 2016;86(1):88-93. doi:10.1212/WNL.0000000000002075.

26. Handunnetthi L, Ramagopalan SV, Ebers GC. Multiple sclerosis, vitamin D, and HLA-DRB1*15. *Neurology.* 2010;74(23):1905-1910.

27. Munger KL, Hongell K, Åivo J, Soilu-Hänninen M, Surcel H-M, Ascherio A, 25-Hydroxyvitamin D deficiency and risk of MS among women in the Finnish Maternity Cohort. *Neurology.* 2017;89(15):1578-1583. doi:10.1212/ WNL.0000000000004489.
28. Munger KL, Zhang SM, Oreilly E, et al. Vitamin D intake and incidence of multiple sclerosis. *Neurology.* 2004;62:60-65.
29. Mohr DC, Goodkin DE, Bacchetti P, et al. Pychological stress and the subsequent appearance of new brain lesions in MS. *Neurology.* 2003;55:55-61.
30. Hernan MA, Jick SS, Logroscino G, Olek M, Ascherio A, Jick H. Cigarette smoking and the progression of multiple sclerosis. *Brain.* 2005;128(6):1461-1465.
31. Hedstrom AK, Katsoulis M, Hossjer O, et al. The interaction between smoking and HLA genes in multiple sclerosis: replication and refinement. *Eur J Epidemiol.* 2017;32:909-919.
32. Handel AE, Williamson AJ, Disanto G, et al. Smoking and multiple sclerosis: an updated meta-analysis. *PLoS One.* 2011;6(1):e16149. doi:10.1371/journal. pone.0016149.
33. Hedsrrom AK, Hossjer O, Katsoulis M, Kockum I, Olsson T, Alfredsson L. Organic solvents and MS susceptibility. *Neurology.* 2018;91:209.
34. Barragan-Martinez C, Speck-Hernandez CA, Montoya-Ortiz G, Mantilla RD, Anaya M, Rojas-Villarraga A. Organic solvents as risk factor for autoimmune diseases: a systematic review and meta analysis. *PLoS One.* 2012;7:e51506.
35. Franklin G, McDonnell G. Free health care, great data, and new clues on multiple sclerosis. *Neurology.* 2018;90:997-998.
36. Ascherio A, Munger KL. Weighing evidence from Mendelian randomization-early life obesity as a causal factor in multiple sclerosis? *PLoS Med.* 2016;13(6):e1002054.
37. Munger KL, Chitnis T, Ascherio A. Body size and risk of MS in two cohorts of US women. *Neurology.* 2009;73:1543-1550.
38. Hedstrom AK, Olsson T, Alfredsson L. High body mass index before age 20 is associated with increased risk for multiple sclerosis in both men and women. *Mult Scler.* 2012;18:1334-1336.
39. Mokry LE, Ross S, Timpson NJ, Sawcer S, Davey Smith G, Richards BJ. Obesity and multiple sclerosis: a Mendelian randomization study. *PLoS Med.* 2016;13(6):e1002053.
40. Ascherio A, Zhang S, Hernan M, et al. Hepatitis B vaccination and the risk of multiple sclerosis. *NEJM.* 2001;344(5):327-332.
41. Ponsonby AL, van der Mei I, Dwyer T, et al. Exposure to infant siblings during early life and risk of multiple sclerosis. *JAMA.* 2005;293:463-469.
42. Ascherio A, Munger KL, Lennette ET, et al. Epstein-Barr virus antibodies and risk of multiple sclerosis: a prospective study. *JAMA.* 2001;286(24):3083-3088. doi:10.1001/jama.286.24.3083.
43. Correale J, Farez M. Association between parasitic infection and immune responses in multiple sclerosis. *Ann Neurol.* 2007;61(2).
44. Langer-Gould A, Wu J, Lucas R, et al. Epstein-Barrr virus, cytomegalovirus and multiple sclerosis susceptibility. a multiethnic study. *Neurology.* 2017;89:1330-1337.
45. Conradi S, Malzahn U, Paul F, et al. Breastfeeding is associated with lower risk for multiple sclerosis. *Mult Scler.* 2013;19:553-558.
46. Ragnedda G, Leoni S, Parpinel M, et al. Reduced duration of breastfeeding is associated with a higher risk of multiple sclerosis in both Italian and Norwegian adult males; the EnvIMS study. *J Neurol.* 2015;262:1271-1277.

47. Kurtzke JF. Epidemiologic evidence for multiple sclerosis as an infection. *Clin Microbiol Rev.* 1993;6:382-427.
48. Sadovnick AD, Armstrong H, Rice GP, et al. A population-based study of multiple sclerosis in twins: update. *Ann Neurol.* 1993;33:281-285.
49. Sadovnick AD, Baird PA, Ward RH. Multiple sclerosis: updated risks for relatives. *Am J Med Genet.* 1988;29:533-541.
50. Hansen T, Skytthe A, Stenager E, Petersen HC, Bronnum-Hansen H, Kyvik KO. Concordance for multiple sclerosis in Danish twins: an update of a nationwide study. *Mult Scler.* 2005;11:504-510.
51. Ebers GC, Sadovnick AD, Risch NJ. A genetic basis for familial aggregation in multiple sclerosis. Canadian Collaborative Study Group. *Nature.* 1995; 377:150-151.
52. Kantarci OH, Barcellos LF, Atkinson EJ, et al. Men transmit MS more often to their children vs women: the Carter effect. *Neurology.* 2006;67:305-310.
53. Ebers GC, Sadovnick AD, Dyment DA, Yee IM, Willer CJ, Risch N. Parent-of-origin effect in multiple sclerosis: observations in half-siblings. *Lancet.* 2004;363:1773-1774.
54. Herrera BM, Ramagopalan SV, Lincoln MR, et al. Parent-of-origin effects in MS: observations from avuncular pairs. *Neurology.* 2008;71:799-803.
55. Lin R, Charlesworth J, van der Mei I, Taylor BV. The genetics of multiple sclerosis. *Pract Neurol.* 2012;12:279-288.
56. Sawcer S, Ban M, Maranian M, et al; International Multiple Sclerosis Genetics C. A high-density screen for linkage in multiple sclerosis. *Am J Hum Genet.* 2005;77:454-467.
57. International Multiple Sclerosis Genetics C, Beecham AH, Patsopoulos NA, et al. Analysis of immune-related loci identifies 48 new susceptibility variants for multiple sclerosis. *Nat Genet.* 2013;45:1353-1360.
58. Bashinskaya VV, Kulakova OG, Boyko AN, Favorov AV, Favorova OO. A review of genome-wide association studies for multiple sclerosis: classical and hypothesis-driven approaches. *Hum Genet.* 2015;134:1143-1162.
59. Lill CM. Recent advances and future challenges in the genetics of multiple sclerosis. *Front Neurol.* 2014;5:130.
60. International Multiple Sclerosis Genetics C, Wellcome Trust Case Control C, Sawcer S, et al. Genetic risk and a primary role for cell-mediated immune mechanisms in multiple sclerosis. *Nature.* 2011;476:214-219.
61. Baranzini SE, Wang J, Gibson RA, et al. Genome-wide association analysis of susceptibility and clinical phenotype in multiple sclerosis. *Hum Mol Genet.* 2009;18:767-778.
62. Olsson T, Barcellos LF, Alfredsson L. Interactions between genetic, lifestyle and environmental risk factors for multiple sclerosis. *Nat Rev Neurol.* 2017;13:25-36.
63. Sundqvist E, Sundstrom P, Linden M, et al. Epstein-Barr virus and multiple sclerosis: interaction with HLA. *Genes Immun.* 2012;13:14-20.
64. Nielsen TR, Rostgaard K, Askling J, et al. Effects of infectious mononucleosis and HLA-DRB1*15 in multiple sclerosis. *Mult Scler.* 2009;15:431-436.
65. Manousaki D, Dudding T, Haworth S, et al. Low-frequency synonymous coding variation in CYP2R1 has large effects on vitamin D levels and risk of multiple sclerosis. *Am J Hum Genet.* 2017;101:227-238.
66. Mokry LE, Ross S, Ahmad OS, et al. Vitamin D and risk of multiple sclerosis: a Mendelian randomization study. *PLoS Med.* 2015;12:e1001866.
67. Rhead B, Baarnhielm M, Gianfrancesco M, et al. Mendelian randomization shows a causal effect of low vitamin D on multiple sclerosis risk. *Neurol Genet.* 2016;2:e97.
68. Islam T, Gauderman WJ, Cozen W, Mack TM. Childhood sun exposure influences risk of multiple sclerosis in monozygotic twins. *Neurology.* 2007;69:381-388.

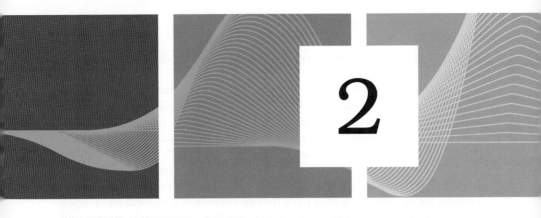

Immunology of Multiple Sclerosis

■ ■ ■ Regina Berkovich

Introduction

This author proposes to approach the subject of immunology of multiple sclerosis (MS) from the standpoint of available acute and disease-modifying therapies (DMTs) and currently known immunologic targets for them.

This seems to be a sound approach because historically this vision point has helped to shape and direct our knowledge on MS immunology and has developed and enriched the field over the years.

Another good reason to adopt this approach is its immediate applicability. By engaging this view, we learn not only MS immunology but also how various different medications work. And we not only learn how they work (in other words, mechanism of action or MoA of DMTs) but also come very close to understanding their potential efficacy, risks, and side effects. This strategic approach will serve well in understanding emerging MS therapies.

Unlike many other diseases of the immune system, such as lupus, psoriasis, or rheumatoid arthritis, MS has a single target, and that is myelin. Therefore, we do not expect to see multiple different tissues involved—the

17

immune system and central nervous system (CNS) are the fields where the events take place.

Contrary to many patients' beliefs, MS is not a disease of a "weak" immune system; it is a disease of a mistaken immune system. In fact, immune reactions in MS can prove to be very strong, leading to remarkable CNS inflammatory reactions and subsequent damage. But the initial "intentions" of the activated immune system are "good"; it intends to "protect" the human, the host. There is a hypothesis of strong initial inflammatory reaction, which leads to cascades of delayed events in the immune system; for example, one may have had an episode of acute infection, such as, for example, mononucleosis, which made a particularly strong and lasting impression on the immune system, and ever since that episode the immune system gets itself activated trying to find the offending agent, virus or bacteria, for weeks, months, or even years and decades after this particular infection is over. The overzealous protective efforts may get so intense that even mere resemblance to the offending antigen (e.g., the encounter of biochemical structures similar to the structures of relevant viral molecules) may be sufficient to trigger a very strong and destructive immune reaction. The most acute form of inflammation in MS clinically presents itself as a relapse or exacerbation.

Particular environmental factors may predispose to ongoing immune reactions to produce the disease. In addition to the aforementioned infectious exposure, lower levels of vitamin D, increased salt intake, genetic predisposition, obesity, and tobacco exposure seem to contribute to the process.

Initially intended as a protective mechanism, reactive inflammation fails to curb itself to a reasonable or adequate intensity, and chronic progressive disease develops.

As mentioned earlier, the singular target in MS is myelin represented specifically in the CNS, and MS is one of the most prominent CNS demyelinating conditions.

As the term suggests, demyelination is the key component of this disease. As you recall, myelin is a layer of "insulation" surrounding the central nerve fiber or axon. Every fragment of myelin is built by several layers of a single oligodendrocyte, a CNS cell that rolls its own body and membranes around the axon multiple times, thus creating the myelin. It is remarkable that myelin of the CNS is principally different from that of the peripheral nervous system; the latter is built by Schwann cells and the peripheral myelin is not a target for MS. Therefore, peripheral neuropathies are rarely seen in patients with MS, unless those are comorbid or in other words independently developed. As a side note: remember that the only "nerve" directly involved in MS is the optic nerve, but it is not a peripheral nerve per se; it is in fact a "continuation" or "processes" of the brain.

Destruction of myelin is a result of inflammation, which can be acute, subacute, and/or chronic. The three conditions can overlap and coexist. Acute inflammation tends to coincide with the first event of MS or subsequent MS relapses (acute exacerbation) and/or new, active, or enlarged MS lesion formation. Events leading to inflammation targeting myelin usually start outside of the CNS and where the main representation of immune system tends to be, in hematolymphatic system. Mature activated lymphocytes in their search of a potential target encounter the blood-brain barrier (BBB) and gain an increasingly strong ability to cross it; subsequently, they enter the CNS. Activation of the lymphocytes and increased permeability of the BBB result from antigen presentation by the antigen-presenting cells, increased production of proinflammatory cytokines, involvement of the complement cascade, and increased differentiation of activated aggressive lymphocytes.

Thus, the activation of the immune process is initiated systematically, resulting in migration of activated immune cells into the CNS where they get reactivated and their interactions result in parenchymal inflammation; the acute inflammation in MS may be focal, multifocal, or diffuse and is characterized by infiltration of activated lymphocytes, macrophages, and microglia, with involvement of cortex, white matter, and deep gray matter with myelin destruction; axonal, neuronal, and synaptic loss; astroglial reaction; remyelination; and synaptic rearrangement.

Indeed, the experimental studies on the intimate mechanisms of action of the approved or developing drugs for relapsing-remitting MS (RRMS) provide a strong foundation for understanding the immunology of MS. Deregulated immune response, including inflammatory cells (e.g., T cells, B cells, macrophages) and immune mediators (e.g., cytokines, chemokines, matrix metalloproteinases, complement), contributes to the expansion of autoreactive T cells; proinflammatory shifts promote BBB lymphocyte and monocyte extravasation. It was found that activation of B cells of patients with MS may contribute to increased BBB permeability. Regulatory T cells (Tregs) normally control the intensity of an immune response; however, their regulatory function in patients with MS is dramatically impaired. Remarkably, the immunomodulatory role of Tregs and their suppressive capacity are more affected in the early stages of the disease. Consistent with this, there are differences in function and expression of FOXP3 (a master regulator in the development and function of regulatory T cells). Disease exacerbation of MS is also associated with loss of the differentiated autoregulatory CD8+ T cells. The regulatory cell dysfunction in patients with RRMS is especially profound during MS exacerbations as compared with the remission periods or in healthy controls. It was observed that, for example, proinflammatory Th17 cell expansion in patients with MS is counterbalanced by an expanded CD39+ regulatory T cell population during remission but not during relapse. Regulatory B cell (Bregs) subsets were found to be higher during relapse as compared with patients with non–clinically active MS. There is a growing body of evidence that antibodies play an important role in the pathobiology of MS and MS relapse; IgG antibodies purified from a patient with MS and transferred to mice with experimental autoimmune encephalomyelitis caused a dramatic clinical improvement during relapse after selective IgG removal, whereas passive transfer of patient's IgG exacerbated motor deficits in animals. These data provide evidence for a previously unknown mechanism involved in immune regulation in acute MS.

Destruction of myelin leads to exposure and increased vulnerability of the axons. According to the data by Bruce Trapp, the number of transected axons increases with the level of activity in MS lesions, and in active MS lesions can be more than 11,000. Transected axons indicate permanent damage. Conglomerates of transected axons form permanent CNS lesions, which subsequently advance the brain tissue volume loss.

Brain tissue loss is the strongest morphologic correlate with MS disability progression. Therefore, the famous sentence "time is brain" so actively and successfully used in stroke neurology has its specific relevance to MS as well, with the only difference that, in stroke, time means minutes and hours and in MS, time means weeks and months. The sentiment, however, is the same: Do not delay the start of treatment.

As mentioned earlier, the knowledge on MS immunology grew together with the continuous and ongoing introduction of different DMTs for MS treatment. The mechanism of action of different treatments for MS targets specific "key players" as discussed earlier.

Let us review the **targets**.

Blood-Brain Barrier

As we remember, increased permeability of the BBB allows activated aggressive lymphocytes to travel from the bloodstream and into the CNS (brain, spinal cord, or optic nerves).

High-dose systemic steroids and **adrenocorticotrophic hormone,** two Food and Drug Administration (FDA)-approved options for immediate treatment of MS relapse, are known to dramatically reduce the BBB permeability among their other direct and indirect anti-inflammatory functions, helping them to significantly shorten prolongation of disturbing symptoms associated with MS exacerbation.

While we are on this relevant subject, let us discuss specifically the specifics of MS relapse treatment.

Relapses (exacerbations, attacks, or flares) are a hallmark of MS and are often associated with significant functional impairment and decreased health-related quality of life. For the vast majority of patients with MS, relapses are the central concern and provoke most of the fears and uncertainty associated with the disease. The unpredictability of MS exacerbations only adds to the notoriety of this entity.

The generally accepted definition of an MS exacerbation is a new or worsening neurologic deficit lasting 24 hours or more, in the absence of fever or infection.

The symptoms associated with MS relapse represent activation of any demyelinating lesion or lesions located in any segment of the CNS; therefore, there may be a broad variety of different signs (which may or may not replicate previously experienced episodes).

In general, the most commonly seen symptom complexes are related to new or worsened inflammatory processes involving the optic nerves, spinal cord, cerebellum, and/or cerebrum. Thus, the symptoms may present alone or as a combination of visual disturbances, motor and sensory impairments, balance issues, and cognitive deficits.

It is important to rule out symptoms that mimic exacerbations but that do not represent new damage to the nervous system. These pseudoexacerbations are caused by an uncovering of older symptoms due to Uhthoff phenomenon (overheating shortens the duration of action potentials, leading to electrochemical transmission failure along demyelinated axons); common causes include fever, infections (most commonly seen urinary tract and upper respiratory infections), and exposure to significant temperature extremes.

Usually the natural course of most of MS exacerbations completes itself with a period of repair leading to clinical remission and, sometimes, especially early in the disease course, to a complete recovery; however, the residual deficit after an MS relapse may persist and contribute to the stepwise progression of disability.

There are many reasons to treat an MS relapse:

1. Treatment of MS relapses is important because it may help to shorten and lessen the disability associated with it.
2. Successful treatment of MS relapse has another important psychological aspect: it helps to establish good physician-patient relationship and to develop in patients with MS a feeling of trust that they may be able to take control over their disease.

The history of acute relapse treatment in MS reflects well the history of what we know about MS and how the knowledge evolved. In the early 20th century, the treatment of choice for an acute MS relapse was bed rest. In 1978, the first medication for MS relapse treatment was approved—adrenocorticotropic hormone, or ACTH.

The presumption that the efficacy of ACTH gel results solely from its corticotropic effects later led to the acceptance of high-dose corticosteroids for MS exacerbation treatment. However, more recent data in other disease states (e.g., nephrotic syndrome, opsoclonus-myoclonus, and infantile spasms) provide clinical evidence that steroidogenic actions fail to fully explain the efficacy of ACTH gel in these conditions. In addition, research into melanocortin peptides and their receptors argues against the long-standing belief that the beneficial effect of ACTH depends solely on its ability to stimulate the release of endogenous corticosteroids and suggests that further exploration of how best to use ACTH in MS should be considered. The melanocortin system has many diverse functions in the human body, including melanogenesis, glucocorticoid production, control of food intake and energy expenditure, control of sexual function, behavioral effects, attention, memory, learning, and, important for MS, neuroprotection, immune modulation, and anti-inflammatory effects. The description of the melanocortin system and the recognition of the other proposed mechanisms of action of ACTH may help to explain the renewed interest in ACTH.

As mentioned previously, in the 1980s focus shifted to intravenous methylprednisolone (IVMP) as the preferred treatment option for MS relapse.

Low dosages of systemic steroids were found to be ineffective in MS, and the dosages from 500 mg to 1 g of IVMP per day became widely accepted and the preferred regimen.

Ever since ACTH and corticosteroids have been used to treat MS relapses, it was observed that some cases may not respond to these treatment options.

Several alternatives, including plasmapheresis, cyclophosphamide, or intravenous immunoglobulin were attempted, but it seems that only the plasmapheresis option is supported by strong evidence. In 2011, American Academy of Neurology guidelines recommended **plasmapheresis** for severe MS exacerbations not responding to the first-line treatments.

Summary and Practical Recommendations

Adequate diagnosis of MS relapses is essential.

Mild exacerbations may not require steroid treatment.

There is a general consensus that moderate to severe MS exacerbations with disabling symptoms should be treated using high-dose systemic steroids (intravenous or oral).

- Patients suspected to have a possible relapse should be evaluated within a week (or 5 working days) of the new or worsening symptom onset;
- If MS relapse is confirmed, start the treatment as soon as possible;
- IVMP 1 g per day for 3 to 5 days is generally recommended as a first choice.

Although not FDA approved, oral administration of high-dose MP may be suggested.

Patients with MS relapse, who did not respond or did not tolerate the MP, may be offered another FDA-approved option—ACTH. Given as ACTH gel, it should be administered either intramuscularly or subcutaneously (SQ) 80 units a day for at least 5 days and up to 10 to 15 days.

For patients with disabling MS relapse symptoms not responding to either systemic steroids or ACTH, plasmapheresis should be considered as an every other day procedure to a total of up to seven exchanges.

Historically, MS relapse therapies were first introduced for MS treatment back in the 1970s. At that time, the general understanding was that RRMS is immunologically active mostly during relapses and remissions are the opposite state, not or much less associated with inflammation. This view, however, failed to explain the polyphasic nature of MS, with acute exacerbations being born within the time of seemingly peaceful remissions.

The growing need for relapse prevention presented itself. The new disease-modification approach arrived.

Indeed, the DMTs are medications that modify the course of a chronic progressive disease such as MS, ideally improving its long-term prognosis as compared with the natural history of untreated MS.

The very first DMT introduced back in 1993, interferon **(IFN)-beta-1B** or **Betaseron** (SQ every other day), along with other **beta-IFN-1As,** such as **Avonex, Rebif,** and **Plegridy**, modulate the immune system in MS and as a part of their anti-inflammatory action regulate and eventually normalize permeability of the BBB. These have been associated with significant reduction of MS relapses and also with reduction of new and active magnetic resonance imaging (MRI) lesions.

The class of **beta-IFNs** were developed after the initial unsuccessful attempts to study gamma-IFNs for MS treatment. The theory stemmed from the known antiviral properties of the IFNs and understanding of the potential role of infectious (likely viral ones) in the triggering of MS debut. However, the gamma-IFNs proved to be harmful and in fact were shown to exacerbate MS. In contrast, the beta-IFNs, which were studied next, had shown strong anti-inflammatory effects in MS, believed to be caused at least partly by regulating the BBB permeability and partly by peripheral and central direct and indirect shifts in immune system with results favoring a less inflammatory state. Betaseron became historically the very first DMT for MS approved and broadly used. Its extensive clinical research has shown positive results in both clinical and MRI metrics. The participants of the very first pivotal study of Betaseron in MS DMT were evaluated 21 years later and were found to have a significantly higher chance of being alive two decades later as compared with their placebo counterparts.

The most common side effects of the beta-IFNs are, predictably, flulike symptoms, well-known symptoms associated with inner IFN production that we all have a chance to experience during flu seasons as sufferers from upper respiratory viral infections. Importantly, in patients with MS with other autoimmune conditions, such as lupus, autoimmune thyroiditis, or neuromyelitis optica, the beta-IFN treatment results may not be positive because of their alternative immune reactions with more antibody-driven and interleukin 17 immunity tendencies, and therefore in such individuals IFNs should be avoided. Finally, it needs to be stated that, even though the decreased permeability of the BBB seems to play an important role in the MoA of beta IFNs, the action is rather regulatory and not absolute, and therefore, although significant clinical and MRI results are achieved, no CNS opportunistic infections were ever observed or reported. The beta-IFNs are considered truly immunomodulatory DMTs with a favorable safety profile of variable tolerability.

Another great example of MS medication classically being associated with the function of the BBB is one of the very robust and potent DMTs, **natalizumab or Tysabri** (intravenously [IV] every 4 wk). It blocks the adhesion molecule on the surface of the lymphocytes, preventing their trafficking through the BBB and into the CNS. This results in the unique opportunity of significant reduction of CNS inflammation, which translates into a dramatic reduction of relapse frequency, stopping or significantly slowing the disability progression and strong MRI results demonstrating a significant reduction in active and newly developed MS lesions. The action of cell redistribution is so powerful that even minimally physiologically necessary number of lymphocytes do not seem to be able to cross the BBB, which, unfortunately, predisposes some patients to opportunistic brain infection, such as progressive multifocal leukoencephalopathy (PML). The overall estimated risk of PML in patients administered Tysabri is relatively small, between 1:10,000 and 1:1000. However, prolonged use of Tysabri, previous use of immunosupressants, and exposure to the JC virus (JCV) are the three factors that are known to increase the risk of PML so that in worst circumstances it can approach roughly 1%. Patients with MS who have never been previously exposed to natalizumab are in the spectrum of significantly lower risk of PML, even though some of them may have been previously exposed to the JCV (in fact, more than half of adult population has been previously exposed to the JCV, which in individuals with preserved immune system does not cause a disease). If, in addition, these natalizumab-naive patients never had previously been treated with immunosuppressants such as chemotherapy, then such individuals have one single risk factor of the three known and their PML risk is still relatively low. Importantly, simple discontinuation of natalizumab results in restoration of the BBB permeability within few weeks (around 50-60 d); this can be significantly speeded up by administering of plasmapheresis, which can rapidly remove natalizumab from the system. This reversibility of the immunologic effect of natalizumab and the absence of associated lymphopenia seem to support the opinion that natalizumab is an immunomodulatory drug rather than an immunosuppressive one, although the fact of associated opportunistic infection such as PML tends to suggest the opposite viewpoint maintaining its potentially immunosuppressive character.

Importantly, following discontinuation of Tysabri the restoration of the baseline BBB permeability may be associated with the prompt return of aggressive lymphocytes increasingly trafficking into the CNS and with the return of MS activity, sometimes referred to as "MS rebound." If discontinuation of natalizumab (Tysabri) seems to be necessary, the prescriber needs to have a sound "exit strategy" to assure firm control over otherwise potentially serious possibility of returned MS activity.

Another way of decreasing trafficking of aggressive lymphocytes into the CNS is to minimize their presence in the circulating blood by capturing those cells in lymphoid organs such as lymph nodes. The medications doing just that are the **S1P receptor modulators** such as **fingolimod (Gilenya**, oral once a day) and siponimod. The S1P receptor is needed to establish free exit of lymphocytes from the lymph nodes; once it is blocked, the cells end up being sequestered inside of the lymphoid tissues, and their presence in the peripheral blood drops dramatically. In fact, one may expect to see the mere three-digit numbers of circulating lymphocytes as assessed by the absolute lymphocyte counts (ALCs) of the complete blood count test. In spite this seemingly severe lymphopenia, the patient is not expected to experience frequent or unusually severe infections (one should monitor for oneself nevertheless); it has been proposed that the factual ALC number does not represent the true state of immune surveillance and may in fact be so-called pseudolymphopenia. Nevertheless, rare cases of opportunistic infections uniquely associated with fingolimod have been reported, including coccideomycosis and PML. It appears that two possible risk factors here are the patient's advanced age and length of fingolimod exposure; remarkably, the level of lymphocytes and degree of lymphopenia are not among the risk factors.

Higher or lower selectivity of S1P receptor inhibition in different existing and upcoming DMTs of this class may call for less or more laborious screening pretreatment tests, which include electrocardiography, eye examination to rule out macular edema, laboratory tests, and observation following the administration of the first dose. Furthermore, it is important to keep in mind that those individuals not immune to the varicella zoster virus need to be vaccinated to prevent serious systemic zoster infections. Fingolimod is classified as an immunomodulatory drug by the FDA, and indeed, once discontinued, the status quo of the immune system gets restored within 6 to 8 weeks back to the pretreatment baseline levels. This supports the notion that lymphocytes indeed get released from the lymph nodes where they were previously sequestered and do not merely get reproduced, which would have required a significantly longer time.

Myelin

Myelin itself is undoubtedly a key player in MS pathology. One DMT that developed out of the copolymer strikingly resembling the myelin basic protein structure is called glatiramer acetate (GA) or Copaxone (SQ every day or three times a week).

An interesting fact is that initially the molecule was introduced with the hope to help create a better animal model for MS. It was expected to induce MS-like disease in rodents. It is remarkable that, in fact, animals seem to be much better protected by nature from MS-like conditions, and therefore, researchers are always looking into better ways to model MS in animals. Thus, the copolymer was hoped to induce more robust MS-like events in animals by being structurally close to myelin. Instead, it repeatedly showed the opposite action. Not only was it not inducing the expected demyelination but in fact it was preventing it from developing and was treating the existing one. After several more years of laborious research and development GA was born and approved. It is assumed that its MoA modulates the immune system via series of different events in the periphery and in the CNS resulting in a more anti-inflammatory immune climate. The resemblance to the myelin basic protein may play a role in what has been hypothesized as possible vaccinelike effects. As we see, however, the BBB function does not seem to have a major role here. Because of this we may need to be aware of a few things: less robust effects with less impressive MRI results and also no risk of PML or other opportunistic infections.

Free Radicals

Dimethyl fumarate (DMF) (Tecfidera, oral twice a day) is believed to work by regulating the free radical formation that is involved in inflammatory reactions, and by doing so the DMF creates a less inflammatory environment in the systems, including the CNS. The medication does not seem to be active on the level of the BBB, and therefore, immediate robust clinical and MRI effects should not be expected; however, an early start and monitored response may place this DMT among good options for the first-line and early second-line use. Some individuals may run into a problem of lymphopenia, and because it is impossible to predict who is more likely to be prone to it, the ALC levels of every patient administered Tecfidera needs to be checked at least every 6 months, with discontinuation recommended with an ALC below 500 cells. Neglect to follow this recommendation may predispose lymphopenic patients to opportunistic infections, including PML.

Common side effects include flushing episodes and gastrointestinal symptoms, which may create certain tolerability and compliance issues, but once persevered tend to dissipate with time.

Overall, all three oral therapies can be used as first-line or second-line agents.

These three drugs do not have similar mechanisms and associated risks; the only thing they have in common is that all three are oral drugs. The three should be approached differently.

Cells

In previous sections, as we discussed the role of the BBB permeability, the phenomenon of sequestration, and the shifts in immunologic states we already mentioned the lymphocytes. Now we will see how the immune status can get affected by direct targeting of lymphocytes and their reproductive mechanisms.

Let us start with the DMT that causes a less dramatic impact on the cell counts and is associated with no or very rare absolute lymphopenia. **Teriflunomide (Aubagio**, oral daily) blocks a specific mitochondrial enzyme dehydroorotatedehydrogenase, which is involved in the reproduction of fast-developing activated lymphocytes, which account for less than 15% of functional lymphocytes. One therefore expects to see not more than 15% of ALC drop, which indeed is a fact. The ALC in a patient administered Aubagio in general is expected to remain within the normal range. The cases of lymphopenia are extremely rare. The opportunistic infections uniquely associated with Aubagio have not been reported. The common infection rate is close to that of the placebo group. No specific cancer signal was observed. The medication was classified by the FDA as an immunomodulatory drug. Teriflunomide demonstrates a clinical and MRI efficacy comparable with that of the high-dose high-frequency injectable IFNs, arguably the stronger ones in their class, as it has been compared head-to-head with Rebif. It has the convenience of oral administration, good tolerability, and compliance. In addition, it is the only oral DMT at this point demonstrating reproducible effects in preventing disability progression in two independent clinical trials. It can be rapidly eliminated from the system by administration of activated charcoal or cholestiramin orally for 11 days, a useful property for the patients desiring to get pregnant.

B Lymphocyte Depletion

Here we will discuss ocrelizumab (Ocrevus), which is FDA approved for RRMS and primary progressive MS, and rituximab (Rituxan), which is used off-label. Both are used IV roughly every 6 months continuously.

The theory behind the use of the B cell depletion is the increasingly recognized role of B lymphocytes in MS pathology. They not only serve as antigen-presenting cells but also act as active producers of immunoglobulins and play an important role in various humoral immune reactions getting more recognized in the MS process. The medications are clearly classified by the FDA as immunosuppressive drugs. Indeed, once the drug is discontinued, it may require many months and even (in the case of ocrelizumab) longer than a year to see the resurgence of newly developed B cells. Removing the important player of MS pathology—B lymphocytes—results in significant clinical and MRI results, affording these DMTs the well-deserved place among high-efficacy MS medications. It comes as no surprise that high efficacy frequently associates with higher risks. In this particular class, to understand the specific risks we need to look closer into the fundamental role of B lymphocytes in the immune defense. As mentioned previously, they develop into antibody-producing cells. Depletion of B cells leads to decreased antibody production, which may result in deficiencies in anti-infectious and anticancerogenic surveillance activities.

Depletion Followed by Reproduction

We discussed previously that MS is a disease of mistaken immune system. Clearly, the natural reaction would be to attempt to fix the mistake. And many DMTs we discussed earlier attempt to fix the errors of the immune system on variably peripheral levels by blocking the immediate results of the pathological immune reactions. The DMTs we are about to review now tend to attempt to get closer to the root of the problem, to the very production of the immune cells. In a nutshell, the idea is to reprogram the immune system from the very level of bone marrow cell differentiation. Alemtuzumab (Lemtrada, IV, +_two courses 12 mo apart) is the only currently approved DMT of this class. Designed to recognize and destroy the mature circulating T and B lymphocytes predominantly, it causes profound acute lymphopenia, which by itself dramatically stimulates the bone marrow into urgent production of new lymphocytes. The newly reproduced lymphocytes then get destroyed again by the second course of treatment 12 months later, and the process of reproduction repeats itself. Most patients with MS were shown to get into long-term remission induced just by the two initial treatment courses. This DMT, clearly recognized by the FDA as an immunosupressive drug, is among, if not the, strongest MS medication. The associated risks are direct results of the unique MoA. The above-mentioned cell reproduction starts with the resurgence of much faster reproduced B cells, which may predispose patients to the development of certain antibody-driven autoimmune complications, such as Grave disease, idiopathic thrombocytopenia, and more rare autoimmune nephropathies. Although these potential complications are treatable, they should be diagnosed as early as possible. The monitoring requires monthly blood and urine tests for 4 years following the last Lemtrada infusion (REMS program). Even though this drug is approved in the European Union as a first-line DMT (given its great and proven promise of long-lasting MS remission), in the United States it is generally recommended after two tried and failed DMTs. Probably because the lymphopenia caused by alemtuzumab is not long lasting, it has not been associated with PML and there is no specific cancer signal.

Summary

We reviewed several pharmacologic targets and a majority of available specific DMTs (Table 2.1).

We discussed the **beta-IFNs** and **glatiramer acetate**, which are frequently combined into one section as **injectable DMTs**. Indeed, they all need to be injected, as their molecules are fragile and get destroyed in the gastric tract. Another common feature is that they all are **immunomodulatory** and as such are not associated with opportunistic infections or

TABLE 2.1
DISEASE-MODIFYING THERAPIES AND ADVERSE EVENTS AND TARGETS OF ACTION

Product	Teriflunomide	Fingolimod	Dimethyl Fumarate (DMF)	IFNβ-1a, IFNβ-1b, PEG IFNβ-1a	Glatiramer Acetate
Brief MoA	Immunomodulatory agent ■ Inhibits DHODH enzyme ■ Reduces number of activated T and B lymphocytes in CNS	■ S1P receptor modulator ■ High affinity for SIP 1, 3, 4, 5 ■ Blocks capacity of lymphocytes to egress from lymph nodes, reducing number of lymphocytes in peripheral blood, which may reduce lymphocyte migration into CNS	■ DMF activates Nrf2 pathway, which is involved in cellular response to oxidative stress	■ Affects antigen presentation to drive T helper cells into an anti-inflammatory state, increase activity of regulatory T and B lymphocytes, and reduce the abilities of B cells to act as antigen-presenting cells	■ Modifies immune processes believed to be responsible for the pathogenesis of MS. Studies in animals and in vitro systems show induction and activation of specific suppressor T cells in the periphery
PML Warning	No	Yes	Yes	No	No
Contraception	Required	Required	Required	Required	Required
Side Effects	Headache, ↑ALT, diarrhea, hair thinning, and nausea	Headache, ↑LFTs, diarrhea, cough, influenza, sinusitis, back pain, abdominal pain, and pain in extremity, macular edema	Flushing, abdominal pain, diarrhea, and nausea	Flulike symptoms, injection site reactions, ↑LFTs, thrombotic microangiopathy seizures, depression	Injection site reactions, chest pain, rash, dyspnea, vasodilatation, urticaria, hypersensitivity, lipoatrophy

(Continued)

TABLE 2.1
DISEASE-MODIFYING THERAPIES AND ADVERSE EVENTS AND TARGETS OF ACTION (CONTINUED)

Monitoring				
■ Before starting: CBC, LFT, TB test, blood pressure ■ After starting: monthly LFT × 6 mo, periodic BP monitoring	■ Monitor ECG before and for 6 h after starting first dose in a setting that can readily manage symptomatic bradycardia ■ Others: monitor heart rate, CBC, pulmonary function test, liver enzymes, and BP	■ Before starting: CBC, LFTs ■ After starting: CBC, LFTs at 6 mo, then every 6-12 mo, and as clinically indicated. Obtain LFTs as clinically indicated ■ Consider interrupting treatment in patients with lymphocyte counts <500, persisting more than 6 mo ■ Discontinue treatment if there is clinically significant liver injury	■ CBC, LFTs at 1, 3, 6 mo ■ Thyroid function tests	No laboratory monitoring required

ALT, alanintransferase; BP, blood pressure; CBC, complete blood count; CNS, central nervous system; DHODH, dehydroorotatedehydrogenase; ECG, electrocardiography; IFN, interferon; LFT, liver functional tests; MoA, mechanism of action; MS, multiple sclerosis; PEG, polyethylene glycol; PML, progressive multifocal leukoencephalopathy; TB, tuberculosis.

cancer signals. The injectables (beta-IFNs and glatiramer acetate) have been around since 1990s, are well known, and tend to be viewed as safe. A careful physician needs to reassess their efficacy on a regular basis, using clinical and MRI parameters, as not every patient with MS will respond to them even after a period of initial success (but this, admittedly, is relevant to all DMTs). Injectables are commonly used as a first-line DMT and at times as a second-line DMT, although the later becomes less common in the light of newer DMTs.

Furthermore, we discussed **oral DMTs**, specifically **fingolimod, teriflunomide**, and **dimethyl fumarate**.

A good exercise to check your understanding of one important issue with different DMTs is self-assessment on potential lymphopenia.

Let us look into this.

- Recall that lymphopenia is rare with immunomodulatory DMTs such as injectables and teriflunomide. In a majority of patients, the ALC remains within normal limits.
- Recall that lymphopenia is very dramatic and common with fingolimod, because this is exactly how this drug works—by shifting the lymphocytes from the circulating blood into the lymph nodes, an action known as sequestration. A low ALC should not be expected in the setting of fingolimod use (and the drug should not be associated with an increased risk of infections) and is being viewed by many experts as pseudo lymphopenia.
- Finally, recall that the ALC numbers seen in the setting of DMF use actually represent the real numbers, and therefore, if lymphopenia is seen, it is for real and the DMF needs to be discontinued if the ALC drops below 500 cells.

Finally, we discussed the **infusible DMTs natalizumab, ocrelizumab**, and **alemtuzumab**, which, despite having strikingly different MoAs and risk profiles, all are recognized as **high-efficacy DMTs.**

They tend to be used earlier in patients with MS with unfavorable prognostic indicators, such as highly active clinical course of MS; frequent and severe relapses; faster disability accumulation including early presentation of motor, cerebellar, and sphincter deficits; male patients; and patients of ethnic minority for MS (African Americans, Asians, Hispanics).

It is important to remember that both ocrelizumab and alemtuzumab are immunosuppressive agents. Therefore, if the plan is to use natalizumab at some point, it should be positioned before any immunosupressive drugs to minimize the potential PML risks.

Although infusible DMTs can be used as a first-line agent in cases of highly active MS, they are frequently used as second- and third-line agents in those patients with MS who tried and failed other less risky DMTs.

Bibliography

1. Noseworthy JH, Lucchinetti C, Rodriguez M, et al. Multiple sclerosis. *N Engl J Med.* 2000;343:938-952.
2. Giovannoni G, Butzkueven H, Dhib-Jalbut S, et al. Brain health: time matters in multiple sclerosis. *Mult Scler Relat Disord.* 2016;9(suppl 1):S5-S48.
3. Arnason B, Berkovich R, Catania A, et al. Therapeutic mechanisms of action of adrenocorticotropic hormone (ACTH) and other melanocortin peptides for the clinical management of patients with MS. *Mult Scler.* 2012. (in press).
4. Barnes D, Hughes RAC, Morris RW, et al. Randomised trial of oral and intravenous methylprednisolone in acute relapses of multiple sclerosis. *Lancet.* 1997;349:902-906.
5. Barnes M, Bateman D, Cleland P, et al. Intravenous methylprednisolone for multiple sclerosis in relapse. *J Neurol Neurosurg Psychiatry.* 1985;48:157-159.
6. Beck RW, Cleary PA, Anderson MM, et al. A randomized, controlled trial of corticosteroids in the treatment of acute optic neuritis. *N Engl J Med.* 1992;9:581-588.
7. Berkovich R, Subhani D, Steinman L. Autoimmune comorbid conditions in multiple sclerosis. *US Neurol,* 2011;7(2):132-138.
8. Berkovich R. Treatment of acute MS relapses. *Neurotherapeutics.* 2013;10(1):97-105.
9. Merkel B, Butzkueven H, Traboulsee AL, et al. Timing of high-efficacy therapy in relapsing–remitting multiple sclerosis: a systematic review. *Autoimmun Rev.* 2017;16:658-665.
10. Giovannoni G, Southam E, Waubant E. Systematic review of disease-modifying therapies to assess unmet needs in multiple sclerosis: tolerability and adherence. *Mult Scler.* 2012;18:932-946.
11. Comi G. Induction vs. escalating therapy in multiple sclerosis: practical implications. *Neurol Sci.* 2008;29(suppl 2):S253-S255.
12. Fenu G, Lorefice L, Frau F, et al. Induction and escalation therapies in multiple sclerosis. *Antiinflamm Antiallergy Agents Med Chem.* 2015;14:26-34.
13. Rush CA, MacLean HJ, Freedman MS. Aggressive multiple sclerosis: proposed definition and treatment algorithm. *Nat Rev Neurol.* 2015;11:379-389.
14. Biogen Press Release on 2 March, 2018. Available at http://newsroom.biogen.com/press-release/autoimmune-diseases/biogen%C2%A0and-abbvie-announce%C2%A0-voluntary%C2%A0worldwide-withdrawal-marketi. Last accessed March 5, 2018.
15. Gajofatto A, Benedetti MD. Treatment strategies for multiple sclerosis: when to start, when to change, when to stop? *World J Clin Cases.* 2015;3:545-555.
16. McGraw CA, Lublin FD. Interferon beta and glatiramer acetate therapy. *Neurotherapeutics.* 2013;10:2-18.
17. Filippini G, Del Giovane C, Clerico M, et al. Treatment with disease-modifying drugs for people with a first clinical attack suggestive of multiple sclerosis. *Cochrane Database Syst Rev.* 2017;4:CD012200.
18. Metz LM, Li DKB, Traboulsee AL, et al. Trial of minocycline in a clinically isolated syndrome of multiple sclerosis. *N Engl J Med.* 2017;376:2122-2133.
19. Miller AE, Wolinsky JS, Kappos L, et al. Oral teriflunomide for patients with a first clinical episode suggestive of multiple sclerosis (TOPIC): a randomised, double-blind, placebo-controlled, phase 3 trial. *Lancet Neurol.* 2014;13:977-986.
20. Burness CB, Deeks ED. Dimethyl fumarate: a review of its use in patients with relapsing–remitting multiple sclerosis. *CNS Drugs.* 2014;28:373-387.

21. Schulze-Topphoff U, Varrin-Doyer M, Pekarek K, et al. Dimethyl fumarate treatment induces adaptive and innate immune modulation independent of Nrf2. *Proc Natl Acad Sci USA.* 2016;113:4777-4782.
22. Fox RJ, Miller DH, Phillips JT, et al. Placebo-controlled phase 3 study of oral BG-12 or glatiramer in multiple sclerosis. *N Engl J Med.* 2012;367:1087-1097.
23. Bar-Or A, Pachner A, Menguy-Vacheron F, et al. Teriflunomide and its mechanism of action in multiple sclerosis. *Drugs.* 2014;74:659-674.
24. Vermersch P, Czlonkowska A, Grimaldi LM, et al. Teriflunomide versus subcutaneous interferon beta-1a in patients with relapsing multiple sclerosis: a randomised, controlled phase 3 trial. *Mult Scler.* 2014;20:705-716.
25. D'Amico E, Zanghi A, Leone C, et al. Treatment-related progressive multifocal leukoencephalopathy in multiple sclerosis: a comprehensive review of current evidence and future needs. *Drug Saf.* 2016;39:1163-1174.
26. Gold R, Kappos L, Arnold DL, et al. Placebo-controlled phase 3 study of oral BG-12 for relapsing multiple sclerosis. *N Engl J Med.* 2012;367:1098-1107.
27. Kappos L, De Stefano N, Freedman MS, et al. Inclusion of brain volume loss in a revised measure of 'no evidence of disease activity' (NEDA-4) in relapsing–remitting multiple sclerosis. *Mult Scler.* 2016;22:1297-1305.
28. Matta AP, Nascimento OJ, Ferreira AC, et al. No evidence of disease activity in multiple sclerosis patients. *Expert Rev Neurother.* 2016;16:1279-1284.
29. Nixon R, Bergvall N, Tomic D, et al. No evidence of disease activity: indirect comparisons of oral therapies for the treatment of relapsing–remitting multiple sclerosis. *Adv Ther.* 2014;31:1134-1154.
30. Alroughani R, Deleu D, El Salem K, et al. A regional consensus recommendation on brain atrophy as an outcome measure in multiple sclerosis. *BMC Neurol.* 2016;16:240.
31. Sormani MP, De Stefano N. Defining and scoring response to IFN-[beta] in multiple sclerosis. *Nat Rev Neurol.* 2013;9:504-512.
32. Belachew S, Phan-Ba R, Bartholome E, et al. Natalizumab induces a rapid improvement of disability status and ambulation after failure of previous therapy in relapsing–remitting multiple sclerosis. *Eur J Neurol.* 2011;18:240-245.
33. Castillo-Trivino T, Mowry EM, Gajofatto A, et al. Switching multiple sclerosis patients with breakthrough disease to second-line therapy. *PLoS One.* 2011;6:e16664.
34. Cohen JA, Coles AJ, Arnold DL, et al. Alemtuzumab versus interferon beta 1a as first-line treatment for patients with relapsing–remitting multiple sclerosis: a randomised controlled phase 3 trial. *Lancet.* 2012;380:1819-1828.
35. Cohen JA, Khatri B, Barkhof F, et al. Long-term (up to 4.5 years) treatment with fingolimod in multiple sclerosis: results from the extension of the randomised TRANSFORMS study. *J Neurol Neurosurg Psychiatry.* 2016;87:468-475.
36. Hauser SL, Bar-Or A, Comi G, et al. Ocrelizumab versus interferon beta-1a in relapsing multiple sclerosis. *N Engl J Med.* 2017;376:221-234.
37. Putzki N, Kollia K, Woods S, et al. Natalizumab is effective as second line therapy in the treatment of relapsing remitting multiple sclerosis. *Eur J Neurol.* 2009;16:424-426.
38. Ziemssen T, De Stefano N, Pia Sormani M, et al. Optimizing therapy early in multiple sclerosis: an evidence-based view. *Mult Scler Relat Disord.* 2015;4:460-469.
39. Polman CH, O'Connor PW, Havrdova E, et al. A randomized, placebo-controlled trial of natalizumab for relapsing multiple sclerosis. *N Engl J Med.* 2006;354:899-910.

40. Kalincik T, Horakova D, Spelman T, et al. Switch to natalizumab versus fingolimod in active relapsing–remitting multiple sclerosis. *Ann Neurol.* 2015;77:425-435.
41. O'Connor PW, Goodman A, Kappos L, et al. Disease activity return during natalizumab treatment interruption in patients with multiple sclerosis. *Neurology.* 2011;76:1858-1865.
42. Giovannoni G, Marta M, Davis A, et al. Switching patients at high risk of PML from natalizumab to another disease-modifying therapy. *Pract Neurol.* 2016;16:389-393.
43. Tuohy O, Costelloe L, Bjornson I, et al. Alemtuzumab treatment of multiple sclerosis: long-term safety and efficacy. *J Neurol Neurosurg Psychiatr.* 2015;86:208-215.
44. Willis MD, Harding KE, Pickersgill TP, et al. Alemtuzumab for multiple sclerosis: long term follow-up in a multi-centre cohort. *Mult Scler.* 2016;22:1215-1223.
45. Montalban X, Hauser SL, Kappos L, et al. Ocrelizumab versus placebo in primary progressive multiple sclerosis. *N Engl J Med.* 2017;376:209-220.
46. Menge T, Dubey D, Warnke C, et al. Ocrelizumab for the treatment of relapsing–remitting multiple sclerosis. *Expert Rev Neurother.* 2016;16:1131-1139.
47. Chen DR, Cohen PL. Living life without B cells: is repeated B-cell depletion a safe and effective long-term treatment plan for rheumatoid arthritis? *Int J Clin Rheumtol.* 2012;7:159-166.
48. Berger JR. Classifying PML risk with disease modifying therapies. *Mult Scler Relat Disord.* 2017;12:59-63.
49. Giovannoni G, Comi G, Cook S, et al. A placebo-controlled trial of oral cladribine for relapsing multiple sclerosis. *N Engl J Med.* 2010;362:416-426.
50. Cook S, Vermersch P, Comi G, et al. Safety and tolerability of cladribine tablets in multiple sclerosis: the CLARITY (CLAdRIbine Tablets treating multiple sclerosis orallY) study. *Mult Scler.* 2011;17:578-593.
51. Atkins HL, Bowman M, Allan D, et al. Immunoablation and autologous haemopoietic stem-cell transplantation for aggressive multiple sclerosis: a multicentre single-group phase 2 trial. *Lancet.* 2016;388:576-585.
52. Lublin FD, Baier M, Cutter G. Effect of relapses on development of residual deficit in multiple sclerosis. *Neurology.* 2003;61(11):1528-1532.

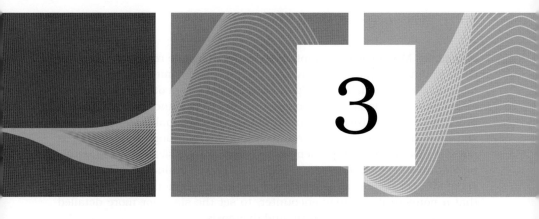

Evaluation and Diagnosis of the Multiple Sclerosis Patient

■ ■ ■ Hunter Vincent, Mary Ann Picone,
Constantine J. Pella, Annette F. Okai

Introduction

Evaluating a patient with intermittent neurologic symptoms can be a complex process with a myriad of differential diagnosis and diagnostic algorithms. Often times, the nonneurologist will overlook multiple sclerosis (MS) as a differential diagnosis, because traditionally MS has been viewed as a diagnosis of exclusion and other more common etiologies need to be ruled out. Although the diagnosis of MS is still uncommon, it is the most common neurologic disorder of young adults in the United States, affecting nearly 1 million people in the United States and 2.5 million globally, with the median prevalence estimated at nearly 33 per 100,000 globally as of 2013 and continuing to increase.[1] As the prevalence of MS increases, it is important for the nonneurologist to have a basic understanding of a neurologist's perspective on the evaluation and diagnosis of a patient with a high likelihood for MS. When considering MS as a diagnosis, there are telltale signs and symptoms that should stand out as more disease specific for MS, involving symptom timeline, magnetic resonance imaging (MRI) findings, physical examination findings, and common laboratory or diagnostic tests, which can help differentiate MS from other common disease mimics. Understanding some of the subtleties and atypical disease presentations can provide a nonneurologist with a valuable skillset to provide an earlier diagnosis and treatment options. Although this chapter is not intended to be a comprehensive reference for physicians, it will surely provide an efficient and effective framework for the evaluation and diagnosis of MS. Let us first start by demonstrating a common clinical scenario that a nonneurologist may encounter, to set the stage for more detailed discussion about further workup and diagnosis.

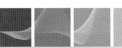

Case Study

A 29-year-old woman who was in her usual state of good health until 4 months ago began to notice some dragging of her right leg after walking 2 miles. This was especially noticed when she had been exercising and had increased body temperature. Resting and cooling down would quickly clear up her right leg weakness. She thought she might be out of shape and did not seek any medical attention. Other than some mild sense of fatigue, which she also attributed to increased stress at work, she had no other symptoms. Recently, she began to notice decreased sensation in the right buttocks that persisted over 24 hours and then she began to notice numbness in her right foot and leg, followed a few days later with numbness in the left leg. She went to an urgent care center where she was told she had a lower back problem, probably a "pinched nerve," and was given anti-inflammatory medication.

She began to notice hesitancy with urination, and it became more difficult for her to urinate. The numbness in her legs worsened, and she had increased weakness in her right leg. She then went to emergency department (ED), where she needed to be catheterized because of severe urinary retention. She had no cognitive deficits. On examination in the ED, cranial nerve testing was normal. Motor testing revealed 4+/5 weakness in the right lower extremity and T12 sensory level deficits. She also had a few beats of clonus at bilateral ankles.

MRI of the brain was performed in the ED and revealed greater than 10 scattered right and left periventricular ovoid gadolinium-enhanced lesions perpendicular to the ventricles and a demyelinating lesion in the T10-T12 levels of the spinal cord, extending more to the right side of the cord.

Disease Phenotypes and Time Course

One of the many difficulties with diagnosing MS lies in the fact that the disease presentation and neurologic symptoms are largely variable between each clinical case, depending on the location and severity of central nervous system (CNS) demyelinating lesions. To date, there are four different clinical phenotypes of MS, each presenting with a slightly different disease course: clinically isolated syndrome (CIS), relapsing remitting (RR), primary progressive (PP), and secondary progressive (SP). To complicate the clinical picture further, three of the phenotypes (RR, PP, SP) are technically classified as either "active" or "not active" and "worsening" or "not worsening"[2] (see Figure 3.1). Although proper disease classification is not essential for initial diagnostic purposes, it highlights the complexity of disease course and the burden that is bestowed upon the diagnosing physician.

Clinically Isolated Syndrome

CIS is characterized as the first episode of neurologic symptoms, lasting at least 24 hours, caused by an inflammatory or demyelinating lesion in the CNS, but not sufficient enough to satisfy the McDonald diagnostic criteria for MS. The neurologic symptoms can be monofocal, affecting only a single neurologic region such as the optic nerve in optic neuritis (seen in approximately 20% of initial symptoms), or multifocal, affecting multiple neurologic areas of the body.[3] The risk of CIS progressing to MS can vary depending on the presence of a CNS-occupying lesion.[3] When CIS is present with at least one demyelinating lesion in the CNS, the patient has a 60% to 80% risk of a second neurologic episode and being diagnosed with MS.[3] In patients with CIS without a CNS lesion, the risk decreases to approximately 20%.[3] Preliminary clinical trials show that early treatment of patients with CIS can decrease the risk of a second neurologic episode and the conversion to "clinically definite MS."[3]

Relapsing Remitting MS

RR MS is the most common disease course, encompassing approximately 85% of initial MS diagnosis. This MS disease classification is defined by exacerbations of disease symptoms, also known as relapses, followed by periods of remission where no apparent clinical worsening or progression of the disease occurs. However, changes can still be seen on MRI examination. Neurologic symptoms often include changes in vision, numbness, fatigue, spasticity, muscle spasms, bowel/bladder problems, and cognitive difficulty.[3] However, the presentation of RR MS is oftentimes extremely variable between patients and unique to each individual.

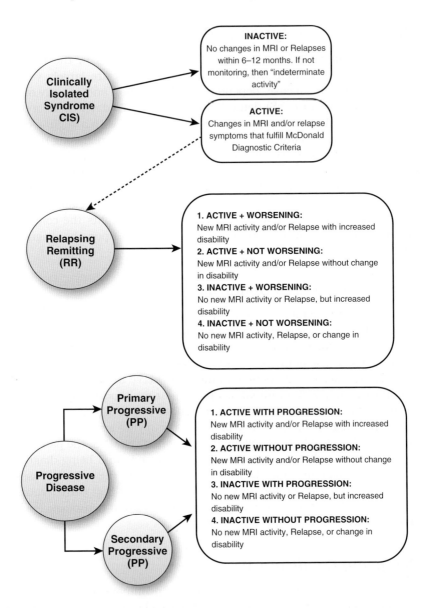

Figure 3.1. **Multiple sclerosis disease phenotypes.** Reprinted with permission from Picone MA, Vincent H, Blitz-Shabbir K, West CY, Akinsanya J. Lower Extremity Signs and Symptoms of Multiple Sclerosis. In: Positano RG, Borer JS, DiGiovanni CW, Trepal MJ, eds. *Systemic Disease Manifestation in the Foot, Ankle, and Lower Extremity.* Philadelphia, PA: Wolters Kluwer; 2017;284-300. Figure 25.1.

Patients may experience complete recovery of function and resolution of symptoms following a relapse or only partial recovery, leading to increased disability.

Primary Progressive MS

PP MS is a disease course characterized by worsening neurologic status from the onset of diagnosis, usually without relapses or remissions, affecting approximately 10% to 15% of patients with MS.[3] PP MS usually affects men and women equally and is often diagnosed later in life around the fourth or fifth decade.[3] In addition, PP MS tends to present with an increased number of spinal cord lesions with less inflammatory cells, versus RR MS, which usually presents with brain lesions ("plaques") containing a larger number of inflammatory cells.[3] It is common for patients with PP MS to experience difficulty with walking and mobility, which can potentially limit their ability to continue working.[3]

Secondary Progressive MS

Secondary progressive MS generally presents initially as a relapsing remitting disease course, in upward of 90% of cases,[3] but eventually transitions into a disease course defined by progressive disability that is independent of relapse activity. A majority of untreated patients with RR MS usually transition to secondary progressive MS approximately 10 years after diagnosis.[3] Although research is mixed, between 15% and upward of 50% of patients with relapsing remitting disease will advance to secondary progressive MS.[3] The onset of secondary progressive MS is of large clinical significance, because it has been shown to be the most important determining factor for long-term prognosis with MS, and its prevention is a crucial primary target for treatment.[3]

Diagnostic Criteria

Traditionally, MS has been defined as a diagnosis of exclusion. There is no single test or pathognomonic feature that is specific for MS, and although the advent of MRI has greatly improved ease of diagnosis, MS remains primarily a clinically diagnosed disease. However, in recent years, more concerted efforts have attempted to create more definitive diagnostic criteria for the disease. Since 2001, the McDonald criteria have been used as the gold standard for diagnostic criteria in MS. Over the past 2 decades they have been revised multiple times, most notably in 2010, with more minor clarifications made in 2017 (see Table 3.1) to add specificity to the 2010 criteria and improve diagnostic value.[4]

According to the 2017 criteria (see Table 3.1), for patients with a clinical course that begins with a neurologic attack, MS can be definitively diagnosed in two separate scenarios without the need of additional information. First, if a patient suffers at least two neurologic attacks with objective clinical evidence of at least two CNS lesions. Second, if a patient has at least two clinical attacks, with evidence of one CNS lesion and reasonable historical evidence of a prior attack involving a distinct anatomical region. However, there are other clinical presentations that do require other additional information to make the diagnosis of MS. Before we explain these clinical scenarios, there are specific terms that should first be explained.

Disseminated in Space (DIS): Although there is still some debate, DIS refers to the development of lesions in distinct anatomical locations within the CNS, indicating a multifocal CNS process. It can be demonstrated by one or more T2-hyperintense lesions that are characteristic of MS in two or more of four areas of the CNS: periventricular, cortical or juxtacortical, and infratentorial brain regions and the spinal cord.[4]

TABLE 3.1
2017 MCDONALD CRITERIA FOR DIAGNOSIS OF MULTIPLE SCLEROSIS

Number of Clinical Attacks	Number of Lesions With Objective Clinical Evidence	Additional Data Needed for a Diagnosis
≥2	≥2	None
≥2	1 (also containing definite historical evidence of a previous attack due to a lesion in a distinct anatomical location)	None
≥2	1	Attacks are **DIS** showing a different CNS site or by MRI scanning
1	≥2	Attacks are **DIT** with additional attacks, MRI scanning, or presence of CSF-specific oligoclonal bands
1	1	Attacks are **DIS** showing a different CNS site or by MRI scanning **And** Attacks are **DIT** with additional attacks, MRI scanning, or presence of CSF specific oligoclonal bands

Adapted from Thompson AJ, Banwell BL, Barkhof F, et al. Diagnosis of multiple sclerosis: 2017 revisions of the McDonald criteria. *Lancet Neurol.* 2018;17(2):162-173. Copyright © 2017 Elsevier. With permission.

CNS, central nervous system; CSF, cerebrospinal fluid; DIS, disseminated in space; DIT, disseminated in time; MRI, magnetic resonance imaging.

Disseminated in Time (DIT): The development or appearance of new CNS lesions over time. This can be demonstrated by the simultaneous presence of gadolinium-enhancing and nonenhancing lesions at any time or by a new T2-hyperintense or gadolinium-enhancing lesion on follow-up MRI, with reference to a baseline scan, irrespective of the timing of the baseline MRI.[4]

- *If a patient has at least two attacks + one CNS lesion, they will need the following:*
  - DIS demonstrated by additional clinical attack implicating a different CNS site or by MRI
- *If a patient has one clinical attack + at least two CNS lesions, they will need the following:*
  - DIT demonstrated by additional clinical attacks or by MRI
    Or
  - Cerebrospinal fluid (CSF)-specific oligoclonal bands
- *If a patient has one clinical attack + one CNS lesion, they will need the following:*
  - DIS demonstrated by additional clinical attack illustrating a different CNS site or by MRI
    And
  - DIT demonstrated by additional clinical attacks or by MRI
    Or
  - CSF-specific oligoclonal bands

In addition, the 2017 criteria provided further explanation for CIS, and understanding the nuances of this definition is important in the diagnostic algorithm of MS. CIS can be defined as a monophasic clinical episode reflecting a focal or multifocal inflammatory demyelinating CNS event, developing acutely/subacutely, lasting at least 24 hours, in the absence of fever or infection, in a patient not known to have MS. If the patient eventually satisfies the diagnostic criteria for MS, the Clinical Isolated Syndrome will be known as the patient's first attack/relapse.[4]

According to the 2013 revised classifications of MS phenotypes, the disease onset can be defined by MS with an attack onset or a progressive course onset.[2] Diagnosing patients with the PP subtype of MS, which is defined by its progressive disease course, also has its own unique diagnostic criteria (see Table 3.2).

- *Patient with 1 year of disability progression independent of clinical relapse, plus two of the following criteria:*
  - *One or more T2-hyperintense lesions characteristic of MS in one or more of the following brain regions: periventricular, cortical or juxtacortical, or infratentorial*
  - *Two or more T2-hyperintense lesions in the spinal cord*
  - *Presence of CSF-specific oligoclonal bands*

TABLE 3.2
2017 MCDONALD CRITERIA FOR THE DIAGNOSIS OF PRIMARY PROGRESSIVE MULTIPLE SCLEROSIS (MS)

Primary progressive MS can be diagnosed in patients with:
- 1 y of disability progression independent of clinical relapse

Plus two of any of the following:
- ≥1 T2-hyperintense lesion[a] that are characteristic of MS
- ≥1 of the following brain lesions
  - Periventricular
  - Cortical/juxtacortical
  - Infratentorial
- ≥2 T2-hypertense lesion[a] in the spinal cord
- Presence of CSF-specific oligoclonal bands

[a] For 2017 McDonald Criteria, there is no requirement for a distinction between symptomatic and asymptomatic MRI lesions.
Table adapted with permission from Carroll WM. 2017 McDonald MS diagnostic criteria: Evidence-based revisions. *Mult Scler.* 2018;24(2):92-95. Copyright © 2018 SAGE Publications.

Signs and Symptoms

Identifying signs and symptoms can often be difficult, as the disease process can be subtle and occur over a long time period, with large gaps between initial symptoms. Patients will often forget or downplay symptom significance, and it can be crucial for practitioners to ask detailed questions to elicit all necessary information. Furthermore, a detailed review of systems is often extremely valuable for collecting vital information. Often times, patients present to clinic for further evaluation after symptoms have already started to affect work performance, daily function, or quality of life. Identifying disease symptoms and establishing an accurate timeline of events is an essential step that will dictate further diagnostic workup and aid in quicker diagnosis and earlier treatment. Table 3.3 is a brief summary of common presenting symptoms for MS. This is by no means a comprehensive list but rather includes major neurologic red flags that a practitioner should identify. Furthermore, these symptoms can also be present in many other diseases and in a large severity spectrum, which will be discussed in the next section.

Physical Examination

A comprehensive neurologic examination is pivotal for identifying neurologic deficits and asymmetries that can lead to a proper diagnosis. This section will not delve into the comprehensive details of a neurologic physical examination but will rather highlight elements that are more characteristic of MS. As we have discussed, the clinical presentation of MS is quite variable and the physical examination findings may be similar to other neurologic diseases, in particular, diseases that affect upper motor

TABLE 3.3

COMMON PRESENTING SIGNS AND SYMPTOMS IN MULTIPLE SCLEROSIS (MS) (NOT A COMPREHENSIVE REVIEW OF SYSTEMS)

System	Common Presenting Signs or Symptoms
General	■ Fatigue ■ "Brain fog" ■ Reduced stamina: There are many metabolic and psychologic differentials for fatigue that need to be ruled out. But this can be a hallmark symptom in MS ■ Uhthoff phenomenon: worsening of MS symptoms when exposed to heat
HEENT	■ Decreased visual acuity ■ Blurred vision/unilaterally or bilaterally (like looking through a smudged window ■ Double vision ■ Decreased intensity of color ■ Eye pain with movement ■ Dysarthria ■ Dysphagia ■ Weakness with muscles of facial expression ■ Hearing loss ■ Dizziness/vertigo
GU	■ Urinary incontinence ■ Urinary retention ■ Increased urinary frequency ■ Increased frequency of UTIs (as a result of the above)
Endo	■ Intolerance to heat
Psych	■ Emotional lability ■ Pseudobulbar affect ■ Depression ■ Anxiety
Neuro	■ Paresthesias ■ Dysesthesias ■ Numbness ■ Focal motor weakness ■ Problems with balance ■ Problems with coordination (both upper and lower extremity) ■ Muscle spasticity ■ Cognitive issues such as word finding difficulty or memory problems

GU, genitourinary; HEENT, head, eyes, ears, nose, and throat.

neurons. As a nonneurologist, it is important to quickly and effectively collect the most significant data that can point to a diagnosis of MS. Here we will discuss specific areas of the neurologic examination that are the most pertinent for MS.

Mental Status

Patients often present to clinic reporting cognitive decline, including difficulty with word finding, memory, or slower processing speed at work or home. Although more extensive neurocognitive testing may be required to elicit more subtle cognitive deficits, the Montreal Cognitive Assessment (MoCA) is frequently used as a screening tool used at the point of care.[5] In addition, the Symbol Digits Modality Test (SDMT), in which the patient is asked to substitute a random list of symbols with digits based on a key, is used to assess information processing speed and has been shown to be a better measure of cognitive function over time in patients with MS.[6] Other neuropsychological tests have been studied in patients with MS, including the Brief International Cognitive Assessment for MS (BICAMS) and the Paced Auditory Serial Addition Test (PASAT), and will be covered more fully in the chapter titled *Cognitive Function in MS.*

Cranial Nerves

Complete cranial nerve examination is essential for any physical examination in a patient with concern for MS. Although isolated cranial neuropathies have been reported in the literature,[7] they are not commonly seen as presenting signs of MS and may be seen as a result of demyelinating lesions of the brainstem. Below is a brief summary of common findings with associated cranial nerves. Only the most common cranial nerve findings are listed, and this is merely a quick reference guide rather than a comprehensive reference.

CN II

Visual deficits are an extremely common presenting symptom with MS. Deficits can present as decreased visual acuity, blurred vision, diplopia, reduced color vision, or visual field deficits (Table 3.4).

The most common initial testing includes:

- Snellen eye examination
- Visual field test
- Funduscopic evaluation:
    - Assess for optic disc pallor, although disc may appear normal on funduscopic examination.
- Optical coherence tomography (OCT)[8]:
    - Provides high-resolution image of retinal nerve fiber layer. Although not a common first-line treatment, this technique has become more present as of late and can be a more advanced imaging technique to evaluate for neurodegeneration or progression of disease. Further discussion on OCT can be found in the ophthalmology chapter.

TABLE 3.4
HALLMARK MS FINDINGS—VISUAL SYSTEM[9]

Optic Neuritis
- Initial finding in 20% of patients with MS
- More often unilateral but can be bilateral
- Commonly seen with disc pallor on funduscopic examination
- *Caution:* common in NMO spectrum disease as recurrent optic neuritis can be a red flag for neuromyelits optica

Internuclear Ophthalmoplegia (INO)
- Inability of contralateral eye to medially deviate adduct with lateral gaze
- Secondary to lesions affecting the medial longitudinal fasciculus

Charcot Neurologie Triad
- Triad characterized by nystagmus, intention tremor, and scanning or staccato speech

CNs III, IV, VI[9]

A thorough examination of extraocular movement is essential, as dysfunction in the corresponding cranial nerves can precipitate diplopia, blurry vision, or visual field deficits.

- Important aspects to observe:
  - Symmetrical range of motion for ocular movement, assessing for unilateral CN dysfunction
  - Saccadic movements
  - Nystagmus
  - Coordinated eye movement, i.e., internuclear ophthalmoplegia

CN V

Facial numbness is a common presenting symptom with MS, as well as other conditions of upper motor neuron origin. Careful examination of the V1, V2, V3 branches of the facial dermatomes with light touch and pin prick is considered an important aspect for MS evaluation. In addition, absence of corneal reflex can indicate pathology involving any pathway of the reflex circuit.

CN VII

Proper assessment of the muscles of facial expression are crucial for identifying focal asymmetries or more global side-to-side differences in facial muscle tone. This can be important for evaluating other common differential diagnosis that need to be ruled out. Furthermore, in patients reporting changes in speech quality, facial motor strength is important to evaluate.

CN VIII

Although isolated hearing loss is not a common presenting feature of MS, it is still important to evaluate as part of an MS examination. Initial evaluation can be performed in office with standard high- and low-frequency tuning forks. It may be important to establish a baseline hearing level with more formalized audiological evaluation.

CN IX

Dysarthria and dysphagia can be common findings in early MS. Evaluating for midline symmetrical movement of the oropharynx and soft palate should not be overlooked. In some cases, formal swallow evaluation with a speech and language pathologist will be needed to conduct a barium swallow study particularly if a patient is complaining of choking on certain foods or any other swallowing complaints.

CN XI

Muscle testing should be performed on the sternocleidomastoid and trapezius muscles to assess for muscle tone symmetry.

CN XII

Midline tongue protrusion is important to evaluate for centrally mediated process involving the hypoglossal nerve.

Motor Testing

Outside the muscles of facial expression, complete motor testing should be performed involving C5-T1 and L1-S2 myotomes.

Sensory Testing

Complete sensory testing involving pin prick, light touch, vibration, and temperature are important for teasing out differential diagnosis. It is important to evaluate if the associated sensory deficits follow specific spinal root levels, stocking/glove distribution, or focal peripheral nerves. In addition, proprioceptive evaluation of the big toe/thumb, as well as Rhomberg test is important to evaluate. Furthermore, it is not uncommon for patients with MS to present with bandlike/bear hug dermatomal sensory distribution around the abdomen, often due to CNS lesions localized to thoracic spine. Identifying potential etiologies for isolated sensory symptoms could necessitate further evaluation with imaging or electrodiagnostic testing.

Reflex Testing

Reflexes are often normal or hyperreflexic in MS. Performing standard reflex testing at the biceps, brachioradialis, triceps, patella, and Achilles is considered standard for any neurologic examination.

- **High-yield tests for upper motor neuron involvement:**
  - *Babinski sign:*
    - Dorsiflexion of the great toe after irritation to plantar surface of the foot. Most common test for upper motor neuron damage
  - *Jaw jerk reflex:*
    - Stretch reflex for the masseter muscle, involving the trigeminal nerve CN V. Signifies a lesion above the foramen magnum
  - *Hoffman reflex:*
    - Test involves loosely holding the middle finger and flicking the fingernail downward. A positive response is seen when there is flexion and adduction of the thumb on the same hand
    - Positive result signifies upper motor neuron problem in the corticospinal tract
  - *Clonus:*
    - Involuntary, rhythmic, repetitive muscle contractions
    - Often seen with upper motor neuron damage and a sign of hyperexcitability
    - Most commonly elicited at the ankle, with abrupt dorsiflexion of a relaxed ankle joint
  - *Oppenheim sign:*
    - Dorsiflexion of the great toe after irritation of the medial tibia. Signifies upper motor neuron damage, similar to Babinski sign, involving corticospinal tract
  - *Chaddock sign:*
    - Dorsiflexion of the great toe with stroking of the lateral malleolus. Signifies upper motor neuron damage, similar to Babinski sign, involving corticospinal tract
  - *Lhermitte phenomenon:*
    - Electrical sensation that runs up and down the spine, often as a result of neck flexion. Typically represents damage in the upper cervical spine or lower brain stem.
    - Has been estimated to be present in 33% of patients with MS, and 16% reported this phenomenon in the first MS episode[10]
- **Other important considerations:**
  - *Spurling compression test*—Evaluate for potential cervical radiculopathy as cause for upper extremity paresthesias, pain, or focal weakness

- *Tinel test*—Perform at the wrist and elbow to assess for focal nerve entrapment involved with ulnar mononeuropathy at the elbow and carpal tunnel syndrome
- *Phalen/carpal compression*—These common physical examination maneuvers can also be used to further assess for carpal tunnel syndrome
- *Straight leg raise*—Evaluate for lumbar radiculopathy, which could be a cause for lower extremity paresthesia/dysesthesia

Spasticity

A hallmark sign of upper motor neuron damage is spasticity. This should be evaluated in both limbs of the upper and lower extremities. The modified Ashworth scale is the gold standard for spasticity evaluation (see Table 3.5).

Coordination

- Dysdiadochokinesia
  - Assess with rapid alternating movements, including finger pinching, hand tapping, or foot tapping
- Dysmetria
  - Finger-to-nose
  - Heel-to-shin test

TABLE 3.5
MODIFIED ASHWORTH SCALE

Grade	Description
0	No increased muscle tone
1	Slight increase in tone, spastic catch with release present or minimal resistance at end range of motion (ROM) during flexion and extension
1+	Slight increase in tone, spastic catch with minimal resistance throughout remainder of movement (less than half of ROM)
2	Further increased muscle tone throughout most ROM, but affected part easily moves
3	Considerable increase in muscle tone, passive movement difficult
4	Muscle rigid in flexion or extension

Reprinted with permission from Picone MA, Vincent H, Blitz-Shabbir K, West CY, Akinsanya J. Lower Extremity Signs and Symptoms of Multiple Sclerosis. In: Positano RG, Borer JS, DiGiovanni CW, Trepal MJ, eds. *Systemic Disease Manifestation in the Foot, Ankle, and Lower Extremity*. Philadelphia, PA: Wolters Kluwer; 2017:284-300. Table 25.3.

Gait

Gait analysis can be an important aspect of an initial evaluation in a patient with MS. It can reveal signs of ataxia illustrated through reduced balance and a wide-based gait pattern. In addition, it can reveal areas of focal muscle weakness, such as steppage gait seen with ankle dorsiflexor weakness, Trendelenburg gait seen with hip abductor weakness, or leg circumduction, which can be seen with hip flexor weakness. Spasticity can also affect gait patterns as illustrated by scissoring gait, which can result from adductor spasticity. However, depending on the area of spasticity, and presence of concomitant weakness, a wide variety of gait patterns and compensatory movements can be seen.

Although gait analysis at the initial visit is an important part of a comprehensive assessment, monitoring gait at subsequent follow-up appointments can often hold significant prognostic value and provide patients/physicians with evidence for disease worsening. Changes in ambulation/use of assistive device are directly correlated with disease severity, as illustrated by the Expanded Disability Status Scale (see Figure 3.2) and can be crucial for identifying disease course. Most

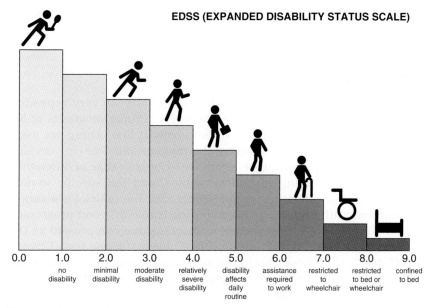

Figure 3.2. **Expanded Disability Status Scale (EDSS).** Reprinted with permission from Picone MA, Vincent H, Blitz-Shabbir K, West CY, Akinsanya J. Lower Extremity Signs and Symptoms of Multiple Sclerosis. In: Positano RG, Borer JS, DiGiovanni CW, Trepal MJ, eds. *Systemic Disease Manifestation in the Foot, Ankle, and Lower Extremity*. Philadelphia, PA: Wolters Kluwer; 2017:284-300. Figure 25.3. See eBook for color figure.

TABLE 3.6
HIGH-YIELD TESTS FOR GAIT ANALYSIS IN MULTIPLE
SCLEROSIS

Walking stamina	6′ or 2′ walk test
Walking speed	25-ft walk test
Assessing risk of falls	Tinetti Gait and Balance
Generalized balance/mobility	Timed Up and Go (TUG)

commonly, the timed 25-ft walk is used to assess ambulation speed, whereas the 6-minute walk has been validated to assess ambulatory stamina.[3] However, recently, the 2-minute walk test has been shown to have similar prognostic value to the 6-minute walking test in assessment of gait stamina.[11] In addition, the Tinetti gait and balance test can be used to assess risk for falls within the next year, whereas the Timed Up and Go test assesses dynamic balance and mobility (see Table 3.6). Decline in ambulation can be extremely important to identify, as it can lead to earlier use of assistive device, which can decrease fall risk and improve patient quality of life.

Major MS Mimics

As illustrated earlier, the clinical symptoms of MS can vary depending on the individual and the disease phenotype. Proper diagnosis of MS typically requires other diseases to be ruled out first. There are many diseases that can present with clinical symptoms and time courses similar to MS. It is important to be aware of the broad range of differential diagnosis, their defining clinical symptoms, and the specific workup that is needed to rule out that differential. See the tables for a variety of conditions with both relapsing-remitting (Table 3.7) and progressive disease courses (Table 3.8), as well as diseases that can present as DIS but not DIT (Table 3.9), DIT but not DIS (Table 3.10), and both DIS and DIT (Table 3.11). These charts are not comprehensive, but represent some of major differentials to be aware of and that should be considered with a comprehensive workup.

TABLE 3.7

DIFFERENTIAL DIAGNOSIS OF MULTIPLE SCLEROSIS WITH FOCUS ON SELECTED DISORDERS WITH A RELAPSING REMITTING COURSE

Disorder	Clinical Features	Other Data
Neuromyelitis optica spectrum disorder	Optic neuritis, especially bilateral or with poor visual recovery; transverse myelitis; intractable nausea and vomiting; paroxysmal tonic spasms	AQP4-IgG; MOG-IgG; sometimes OCT
Neurosarcoidosis	Optic neuropathy and myelopathy; facial palsy; early relapse after stopping steroids; with or without systemic involvement	Serum ACE concentration; chest radiograph, HRCT, lung function tests; CT/PET scan; slit-lamp examination; tissue biopsy
CNS vasculitis (primary or secondary)	Headache; acute CNS syndromes including hemiparesis and ataxia; early cognitive impairment; with or without systemic involvement	Serum ANCA (systemic vasculitis); tissue biopsy at systemic site or brain biopsy (if possible)
Susac syndrome	Encephalopathy, visual loss, deafness	Fluorescein angiogram looking for branch retinal artery occlusions; OCT; audiometry
CADASIL	Migraine, especially with complex or prolonged aura; recurrent acute hemiparesis and other vascular syndromes; neuropsychiatric disturbance; dementia	Testing for *NOTCH3* gene mutation; skin biopsy
Connective tissue disorders (SLE/ Sjögren syndrome, scleroderma, etc.)	Optic neuritis; longitudinally extensive transverse myelitis; systemic involvement; recurrent miscarriage, thrombosis (antiphospholipid syndrome)	Serological testing: ANA, ENA, antiphospholipid antibodies; AQP4-IgG
Behçet disease	Brainstem syndrome; myelopathy (rare); oral and genital ulceration; intraocular inflammation	Pathergy testing; HLA typing
CLIPPERS	Subacute ataxia, double vision, and slurred speech; early relapse after stopping steroids	Brain biopsy

(Continued)

TABLE 3.7

DIFFERENTIAL DIAGNOSIS OF MULTIPLE SCLEROSIS WITH FOCUS ON SELECTED DISORDERS WITH A RELAPSING REMITTING COURSE   (CONTINUED)

Disorder	Clinical Features	Other Data
Leber hereditary optic neuropathy	Bilateral sequential optic neuropathies with poor visual recovery; more common in men than in women	Genetic testing

Adapted from Brownlee WJ, Hardy TA, Fazekas F, et al. Diagnosis of multiple sclerosis: progress and challenges. *Lancet*. 2017;389(10076):1336-1346. Copyright © 2016 Elsevier. With permission.

ACE, angiotensin-converting enzyme; ANA, antinuclear antibodies; ANCA, antineutrophil cytoplasmic antibodies; AQP4, aquaporin 4; CADASIL, cerebral autosomal-dominant arteriopathy with subcortical infarcts and leukoencephalopathy; CLIPPERS, chronic lymphocytic inflammation with pontine perivascular enhancement responsive to steroids; CNS, central nervous system; ENA, extractable nuclear antigen; HRCT, high-resolution computed tomography; MOG, myelin oligodendrocyte glycoprotein; OCT, optical coherence tomography; SLE, systemic lupus erythematosus.

TABLE 3.8

DIFFERENTIAL DIAGNOSIS OF MULTIPLE SCLEROSIS WITH A FOCUS ON SELECTED DISORDERS WITH A PROGRESSIVE COURSE

Disorder	Clinical Features	Other Data
HTLV1-associated myelopathy	Progressive myelopathy; residence or travel to an endemic area (especially West Indies or Japan)	CSF HTLV1 antibody testing
Dural arteriovenous fistula	Subacute, progressive myelopathy	Spinal angiography
Nutritional myelopathy (vitamin B12 or copper deficiency)	Subacute progressive myelopathy or myeloneuropathy; optic atrophy (severe B12 deficiency); anemia or pancytopenia	Serum B12, methylmalonic acid; serum copper levels, ceruloplasmin
Primary lateral sclerosis	Spastic quadriparesis or hemiparesis; with or without bulbar involvement; with or without development of lower motor neuron signs	Electromyography looking for lower motor neuron involvement
Leukodystrophies: adrenomyeloneuropathy; Krabbe disease; Alexander disease; hereditary diffuse leukoencephalopathy with axonal spheroids	Progressive myelopathy (adrenomyeloneuropathy, Krabbe disease); bulbar symptoms, ataxia (Alexander disease); early cognitive impairment (hereditary diffuse leukoencephalopathy with axonal spheroids)	Very-long-chain fatty acids (adrenomyeloneuropathy); genetic testing available for some leukodystrophies

TABLE 3.8

DIFFERENTIAL DIAGNOSIS OF MULTIPLE SCLEROSIS WITH A FOCUS ON SELECTED DISORDERS WITH A PROGRESSIVE COURSE (CONTINUED)

Disorder	Clinical Features	Other Data
Hereditary spastic paraplegia (especially *SPG5*)	Slowly progressive myelopathy (spasticity greater than weakness) with or without other neurologic symptoms and family history	Genetic testing
Spinocerebellar ataxias	Progressive cerebellar ataxia, with or without other neurologic symptoms and family history	Genetic testing

Adapted from Brownlee WJ, Hardy TA, Fazekas F, et al. Diagnosis of multiple sclerosis: progress and challenges. *Lancet.* 2017;389(10076):1336-1346. Copyright © 2016 Elsevier. With permission.
CSF, cerebrospinal fluid.

TABLE 3.9

COMMON ETIOLOGIES THAT CAN BE DISSEMINATING IN SPACE (DIS) BUT NOT DISSEMINATING IN TIME (DIT)

DIS but _not_ DIT

1. Shower of the cerebral emboli
2. Thrombocytopenic purpura
3. CNS vasculitis
4. Mitochondrial encephalopathy
5. Drugs and toxins
6. Acute disseminated encephalomyelitis
7. Progressive multifocal leukoencephalopathy (PML)
8. Mycoplasma encephalopathy
9. Lyme disease
10. Vitamin B12 deficiency
11. Behçet disease
12. Sarcoidosis
13. Paraneoplastic syndromes
14. Periventricular leukomalacia
15. Psychiatric syndromes

CNS, central nervous system.
Adapted with permission from Rolak LA, Fleming JO. The Differential Diagnosis of Multiple Sclerosis. *Neurologist.* 2007;13(2):57-72.

TABLE 3.10

COMMON ETIOLOGIES THAT CAN BE DISSEMINATING IN TIME (DIT) BUT NOT DISSEMINATING IN SPACE (DIS)

DIT but _not_ DIS

1. Tumor (brain or spinal cord)
2. Arteriovenous malformation (brain or spinal cord)
3. Familial cavernous hemangiomata
4. Cervical spondylosis
5. Chiari malformation
6. Foramen magnum lesions
7. Peripheral neuropathy
8. Leber optic atrophy
9. Adult-onset leukodystrophies
10. Migraine
11. Sjögren disease
12. HTLV-1
13. Cerebellar degeneration
14. Syringomyelia

Adapted with permission from Rolak LA, Fleming JO. The Differential Diagnosis of Multiple Sclerosis. *Neurologist.* 2007;13(2):57-72.

TABLE 3.11

COMMON ETIOLOGIES THAT CAN BE DISSEMINATING IN BOTH TIME AND SPACE (DIT & DIS)

DIT & DIS

1. Cerebrovascular disease (including emboli)
2. Familial cavernous hemangiomata
3. CNS lymphoma
4. Subacute myelo-opticoneuropathy (SMON)
5. CNS vasculitis
6. Migratory sensory neuritis
7. Myasthenia gravis
8. Sjögren disease
9. HIV
10. Eale disease
11. Systemic lupus erythromatosus
12. Lyme disease
13. Porphyria

TABLE 3.11
**COMMON ETIOLOGIES THAT CAN BE DISSEMINATING IN BOTH
TIME AND SPACE (DIT & DIS)   (CONTINUED)**

DIT & DIS
14. Sarcoidosis
15. Anti-phospholipid antibody syndrome
16. Spinocerebellar degeneration
17. Cerebral autosomal-dominant arteriopathy with subcortical infarcts and lukoencephalopathy (CADASIL)
18. Psychiatric syndromes
19. NMO (aka Devic disease)

Adapted with permission from Rolak LA, Fleming JO. The Differential Diagnosis of Multiple Sclerosis. *Neurologist.* 2007;13(2):57-72.
CNS, central nervous system; HIV, human immunodeficiency virus.

Diagnostic Workup

If a patient presents with a clinical history and physical examination in which the list of differential diagnosis includes MS, it is important for the nonneurologist to have a basic framework for an effective MS diagnostic workup. Regardless of whether a referral is made to a neurologist or other medical specialist, preliminary data collection can be crucial for earlier diagnosis and targeted medical management. The following is a brief summary of the diagnostic tests that can be most effective for ruling out other etiologies and diagnosing MS.

Laboratory Tests

See Table 3.12 for a list of laboratory tests that should be sent to evaluate for the most important disease mimics of MS. Although a medical specialist or neurologist may elect for additional laboratory tests, such as specific genetic testing, the following list of tests are a good starting point for diagnostic workup.

Imaging

MRI continues to be the gold standard for supporting a diagnosis of MS, as well as searching for other possible radiological features to support another diagnosis. A standardized protocol for MRI in MS diagnosis has been created by MAGNIMS and the Consortium of Multiple Sclerosis Centers.[12] In short, the panel recommended that a brain MRI be obtained in all patients being considered for a diagnosis of MS. In addition, it was agreed upon that, although spinal MRI is not necessary in all cases, it is advised in the following cases: spinal cord localization, when there is a

TABLE 3.12
COMPREHENSIVE LABORATORY TESTS—MULTIPLE SCLEROSIS

HLA B27	SPEP
ANA	Rheumatoid factor
ACE	Anti SS-A/B
Anti-cardiolipin AB	FTA
Anti-DNA DS	Anti-thyroid peroxidase AB
Anti-ENA AB	Anti-thyroglobulin AB
CH 50	TSH
C3, C4 complement	T4
CBC	Urinalysis
CMP	Vitamin B6
Copper	Vitamin B12
Zinc	Vitamin D25
ESR	Hepatitis screen
Folate	JCV AB
Lipid panel	Varicella IgG/IgM
Lyme titer	Quantiferon TB
Lupus anticoagulant	Gad 65
EBV IgG/IgM	Celiac panel
SCL 70	NMO AB

AB, antibody; ACE, angiotensin-converting enzyme; ANA, antinuclear antibodies; CBC, complete blood count; CMP, comprehensive metabolic panel; DS, double strand; ESR, erythrocyte sedimentation rate; FTA, fluorescent treponema antigen; JCV, John Cunningham virus; NMO, neuromyelitis optica; SCL, scleroderma 70; SPEP, serum protein electrophoresis; TB, tuberculosis; TSH, thyroid stimulating hormone.

primary progressive course, when considering MS in less common populations (e.g., older individuals or nonwhite populations), or when additional data are needed to increase diagnostic confidence.[13] The specifics of MRI with MS will be discussed at length in the MRI chapter of this book.

CSF Analysis

A lumbar puncture with CSF analysis assessing for oligoclonal IgG bands has long been a mainstay in the diagnosis of MS. However, in recent years, less emphasis has been placed on using CSF findings for diagnostic purposes, and this analysis is no longer considered a mandatory clinical test in the setting of diagnostic MRI findings. That being said, CSF analysis does have a key prognostic value and role in clinical decision making.[14] Although the presence of oligoclonal bands in CSF can be a confirmatory test for MS, it is not specific for MS and can be found in a variety of other diseases of the CSF. In addition, the absence of CSF findings does not completely rule out an MS diagnosis, because CSF oligoclonal bands may be absent in individuals early in the disease process and in young children.[14] However, there continues to be diagnostic utility with the oligoclonal CSF test. The use of CSF testing for MS diagnosis is summarized in Table 3.1, in the revised 2017 McDonald criteria.

Electromyography

An electrodiagnostic evaluation can be an important part of the workup for MS. Although it is not highly specific for MS or essential to satisfy the diagnostic criteria, it can help to rule out other etiology that could explain the patient's symptoms. It can be helpful for diagnosing peripheral neuropathies, nerve entrapments such as carpal tunnel, or radiculopathies that could explain a patient's symptoms. One should consider referring a patient for electrodiagnostic evaluation if the clinical symptoms warrant such workup.

Evoked Potential

This diagnostic test measures electrical activity in the brain through stimulation of specific sensory nerve pathways. The test has been shown to detect decreased conduction velocity along the sensory pathways, which represents evidence of demyelination in the CNS pathways. In theory, any sensory pathway can be assessed, but typically visual EPs, short latency somatosensory EPs, and brainstem auditory EPs are tested most frequently. Evoked potential (EP) testing can detect changes in sensory pathway conduction for a variety of conditions besides MS, including optic neuropathies, myoclonus, and a variety of other CNS tumors and isolated brainstem lesions. It is often frequently used for intraoperative neurologic monitoring during spine surgery.[15] Previously, EP tests were used to establish dissemination in space by identifying different locations of CNS lesions in clinical cases with little or no changes clinically. However, recently, EP has been removed from the 2017 McDonald criteria, because of its lack of specificity compared with MRI imaging and CSF testing.[16]

Conclusion

Confirming a diagnosis of MS can be a difficult process because of the significant variability in disease presentation and the extensive workup needed to rule out other common neurologic conditions. Because of this, it is commonly overlooked by many general practitioners. However, MS continues to be the most common neurologic disorder affecting young adults, numbering nearly 1 million people in the United States, with prevalence continuing to rise. Often times, workup and diagnosis are performed by a neurologist after significant functional decline has already occurred. It is essential for nonneurologists to keep MS as a differential diagnosis when evaluating patients with intermittent neurologic symptoms, in an effort to facilitate earlier diagnosis and potentially earlier treatment. Understanding the different disease phenotypes, most common signs and symptoms, and effective preliminary workup is a crucial step for not only providing high-quality patient care but also identifying MS and minimizing functional decline.

References

1. National MS Society. MS Prevalence. https://www.nationalmssociety.org/About-the-Society/MS-Prevalence.
2. Lublin FD, Reingold SC, Cohen JA, et al. Defining the clinical course of multiple sclerosis. *Neurology.* 2014;83:1-9. doi:10.1212/WNL.0000000000000560.
3. Picone MA, Vincent H, Blitz-Shabbir K, West CY, Akinsanya J. Lower extremity signs and symptoms of multiple sclerosis. In: Positano RG, Borer J, DiGiovanni C, Trepal M, eds. *Systemic Disease Manifestation in the Foot, Ankle, and Lower Extremity.* Wolters Kluwer; 2017. vol. 3:284-300.
4. Thompson AJ, Banwell BL, Barkhof F, et al. Diagnosis of multiple sclerosis: 2017 revisions of the McDonald criteria. *Lancet Neurol.* 2018;17(2):162-173.
5. Parmenter BA, Weinstock-Guttman B, Garg N, Munschauer F, Benedict RHB. Screening for cognitive impairment in multiple sclerosis using the symbol digit modalities test. *Mult Scler J.* 2007;13(1):52-57. doi:10.1177/1352458506070750.
6. Smith A. *Symbol Digits Modalities Test: Manual.* Los Angeles: Western Psychological Services; 1973. https://www.communicate-ed.org.uk/assets/downloads/SDMT_Formula_Chart_Communicate-ed_2.pdf. Accessed on October 30, 2018.
7. Thömke F, Lensch E, Ringel K, Hopf HC. Isolated cranial nerve palsies in multiple sclerosis. *J Neurol Neurosurg Psychiatry.* 1997;63:682-685. https://www.ncbi.nlm.nih.gov/pmc/articles/PMC2169805/pdf/v063p00682.pdf.
8. Frohman EM, Fujimoto JG, Frohman TC, Calabresi PA, Cutter G, Balcer LJ. Optical coherence tomography: a window into the mechanisms of MS. *Nat Clin Pract Neurol.* 2008;4(12):664-675. doi:10.1038/ncpneuro0950.
9. Balcer LJ, Miller DH, Reingold SC, Cohen JA. Vision and vision-related outcome measures in multiple sclerosis. *Brain.* 2015;138(1):11-27. doi:10.1093/brain/awu335.
10. Khare S, Seth D. Lhermitte's sign: the current status. *Ann Indian Acad Neurol.* 2015;18(2):154-156. doi:10.4103/0972-2327.150622.
11. Gijbels D, Eijnde BO, Feys P. Comparison of the 2- and 6-minute walk test in multiple sclerosis. *Mult Scler.* 2011;17(10):1269-1272. doi:10.1177/1352458511408475.
12. Filippi M, Rocca MA, Ciccarelli O, et al. MRI criteria for the diagnosis of multiple sclerosis: MAGNIMS consensus guidelines. *Lancet Neurol.* 2016;15(3):292-303. doi:10.1016/S1474-4422(15)00393-2.
13. Traboulsee A, Simon JH, Stone L, et al. Revised recommendations of the consortium of MS centers task force for a standardized MRI protocol and clinical guidelines for the diagnosis and follow-up of multiple sclerosis. *AJNR Am J Neuroradiol.* 2016;37:394-401. doi:10.3174/ajnr.A4539.
14. Stangle M, Fredrikson SM, Meinl E, Petzold A, Stuve O, Tumani H. The utility of cerebrospinal fluid analysis in patients with multiple sclerosis. *Nat Rev Neurol.* 2013;9:267-276.
15. Walsh P, Kane N, Butler S. The clinical role of evoked potentials. *J Neurol Neurosurg Psychiatry.* 2005;76:16-22. doi:10.1136/jnnp.2005.068130.
16. National Multiple Sclerosis Center. Evoked Potentials. https://www.nationalmssociety.org/Symptoms-Diagnosis/Diagnosing-Tools/Evoked-Potentials. Accessed on November 4, 2018.

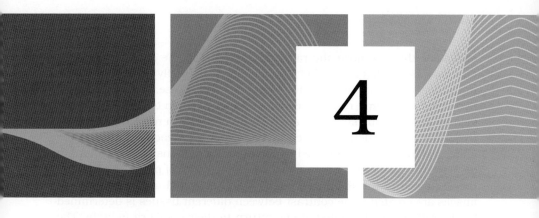

Magnetic Resonance Imaging in Multiple Sclerosis

■ ■ ■ Carlos A. Pérez, John A. Lincoln

Introduction

Since its clinical introduction in the 1980s, magnetic resonance imaging (MRI) has become an essential tool in supporting the diagnosis, longitudinal monitoring, and evaluation of therapeutic response in multiple sclerosis (MS).[1] Although the diagnosis of MS is mostly based on clinical findings, MRI has become an integral part of the overall diagnostic process because of its ability to sensitively and noninvasively demonstrate the spatial and temporal dissemination of demyelinating plaques in the brain and spinal cord.[2,3] In some cases, MRI can be useful for ruling out alternative neurological diseases.[4] In this chapter, we discuss the underlying principles and clinical utility of MRI with the aim of helping clinicians understand how to better apply this valuable tool in the assessment of MS and related conditions.

How MRI Works

MRI provides exquisite detail of the brain and the spinal cord in the axial, sagittal, and coronal planes.[5] Unlike computed tomography (CT) scans, it does not require the use of ionizing radiation. Instead, MRI uses a powerful magnetic field that aligns protons (hydrogen atoms) within water molecules that are normally randomly oriented in the same or opposite direction as the external field.[6] The alignment is briefly disrupted by the introduction of an external radiofrequency (RF) pulse, and the excited hydrogen atoms emit resonance signals as they return to their previously aligned (equilibrium) state that are then measured by a receiving coil.[3] The frequency information contained in the signal from each location in the imaged plane is then converted to corresponding intensity levels that are displayed as shades of gray in a matrix arrangement of pixels.[1] By varying the sequence of the RF pulses applied and collected, different types of images are created.[7] The contrast between different tissues is determined by the rate at which excited atoms return to their equilibrium state. The amount of time between successive RF pulses is referred to as repetition time, and the time between the delivery of the RF pulse and the receipt of the echo signal is referred to as the time to echo.[7]

T1-Weighted Sequencing

The longitudinal relaxation time, or T1, is the time constant that determines the rate at which the excited protons realign with the external magnetic field.[3] The more quickly the protons realign, the greater (and brighter) the signal. The rate at which this occurs is determined by the T1 properties of a tissue. Fat quickly realigns its longitudinal magnetization with the magnetic field, short T1, and it therefore appears bright (i.e., hyperintense) on a T1-weighted image.[8] Conversely, water has a much slower longitudinal magnetization realignment after an RF pulse, long T1, and therefore it appears dark (i.e., hypointense) on a T1-weighted image.[8] Therefore, tissues with high fat content (such as white matter) will be bright, and compartments filled with water (such as cerebrospinal fluid [CSF]) will be dark on T1-weighted scans. In this way, T1-weighted images are good for demonstrating anatomy (Figure 4.1).[8]

T1-weighted imaging can also be performed after the administration of gadolinium. Gadolinium is a paramagnetic contrast enhancement agent that facilitates the relaxation of hydrogen atoms (i.e., shortens T1).[1] It preferentially shortens T1 values in tissues where it accumulates, rendering them bright on T1-weighted images. Gadolinium-enhanced images are especially useful in looking at pathological tissues such as tumors, and areas of inflammation or infection, because these will demonstrate accumulation of contrast due to disruption of the blood-brain barrier (BBB), which will make them appear brighter than the surrounding tissue.[8]

T2-Weighted Sequencing

The transverse relaxation time, or T2, is the time constant that determines the rate at which the excited protons lose resonance perpendicular

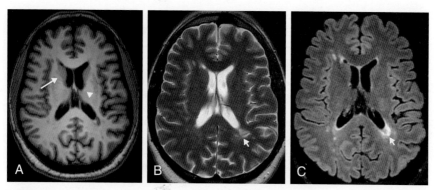

Figure 4.1. Appearance of tissue on T1, T2, and FLAIR (fluid attenuated inversion recovery) sequences. **(A)** T1 precontrast sequence showing the caudate nucleus (long arrow) and putamen (arrow head), **(B)** T2 sequence showing multiple sclerosis (MS) lesions (short arrow), **(C)** FLAIR sequence showing the same MS lesions (short arrow).

to the main field and become out of phase with each other after being excited by an RF pulse (i.e., dephasing).[6] Dephasing occurs because of random and time-dependent field variations induced by spins of neighboring atoms, because not all spins have exactly the same precession frequency.[6] The precession frequency of an atom refers to the rate of change in orientation of the rotational axis of protons due to an applied external magnetic field.[7] The addition of an external RF pulse results in augmentation of the angle of precession of the protons, and in doing so, it converts some of the magnetization that exists along the axis of the dominant magnetic field (longitudinal magnetization) into measurable magnetization along a perpendicular axis (transverse magnetization).[3,7] The rate at which this dephasing occurs is determined by the T2 properties of a tissue. The slower the dephasing, the greater (and brighter) the T2 signal.[3] On a T2-weighted scan, compartments filled with water (such as CSF) appear bright because of protons in phase with each other. To illustrate, as water molecules move around in all directions, their local magnetic fields fluctuate, averaging each other out. Without a significant net difference in internal magnetic fields, the protons stay in step with the applied external field for a longer period of time. Conversely, tissues with high fat content (such as white matter) appear dark. T2-weighted scans are good for demonstrating pathology because most, but not all, brain lesions tend to develop edema and are associated with an increase in water content, which will make them appear bright.[8] In general, T1- and T2-weighted images can be differentiated by looking at the CSF: CSF appears dark on T1-weighted imaging and bright on T2-weighted imaging[3] (Table 4.1).

TABLE 4.1
T1- AND T2-WEIGHTED MRI SIGNAL INTENSITIES

	T1	T2
Hyperintense (bright)	Fat, cholesterol, intravascular blood flow, protein-rich fluid, gadolinium, hemorrhage	Water, CSF, vasogenic edema, intravascular slow flow or thrombus, infarction, inflammation, infection
Hypointense (dark)	Water/CSF, air, bone, hemosiderin, edema, infection, gliosis, intravascular flow void	Bone, air, fat, protein-rich fluid, increased cellularity, intravascular flow void

Data from McMahon KL, Cowin G, Galloway G. Magnetic resonance imaging: The underlying principles. *J Orthop Sport Phys Ther.* 2011;41:806-819. doi:10.2519/jospt.2011.3576.
CSF, cerebrospinal fluid; MRI, magnetic resonance imaging.

FLAIR Sequencing

A third commonly used conventional sequence is the fluid attenuated inversion recovery (FLAIR). The FLAIR sequence is similar to a T2-weighted image, but the high signal of normal CSF fluid is attenuated and made dark.[5] The CSF signal is nullified by using a long inversion recovery sequence with a long inversion time (TI). A long inversion time suppresses the high CSF signal and improves the visualization of periventricular lesions.[9] As with the T2-weighted image, this sequence is very sensitive to pathology and makes the differentiation between CSF and brain parenchymal abnormalities much easier to distinguish.[9] FLAIR is particularly useful in the detection of subtle changes at the periphery of the hemispheres, near sulcal CSF, and in the periventricular region close to CSF (such as those typical of MS) (Figures 4.2A and 4.2B) where the high intensity of the CSF signal itself may attenuate visible contrast when compared with the high intensity of nearby lesions.[5,10]

Diagnostic Role of MRI in Multiple Sclerosis

Although there is no single diagnostic test for MS, MRI is routinely employed to evaluate a patient clinically suspected with MS. The diagnosis of MS is based on the principle of dissemination in time (DIT) and dissemination in space (DIS) of central nervous system (CNS) demyelination.[11-13] Conventional T1- and T2-weighted, as well as contrast-enhanced T1-weighted and FLAIR, images offer the most sensitive way of detecting lesions and are the current standard assessment methods to confirm the clinical diagnosis of MS.[9] The high conspicuity of MS-related abnormalities seen on MRI provide the best view of tissue injury, lesion activity, and disease accumulation compared with all other imaging modalities, including CT.[1]

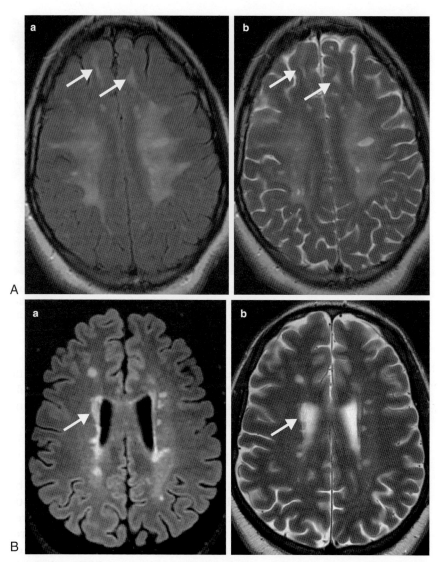

Figure 4.2. A. Juxtacortical multiple sclerosis (MS) lesions are more readily identified on FLAIR (fluid attenuated inversion recovery) (a) compared with T2 (b) sequences (long arrows). **B.** As with the prior figure, many periventricular MS lesions are more readily identified on FLAIR (a) compared with T2 (b) sequences (long arrows).

Although the diagnosis of MS can be straightforward in patients with a typical clinical history, when the symptoms are nonspecific or atypical of MS, MRI is the most commonly performed investigation that can support a clinical diagnosis.[14,15] For a considerable proportion of patients, MRI can replace some of the clinical criteria by revealing brain and spinal cord

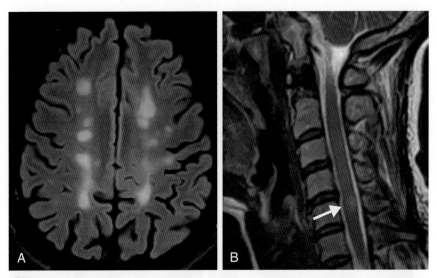

Figure 4.3. Characteristic multiple sclerosis (MS) lesions. **(A)** Axial FLAIR (fluid attenuated inversion recovery) sequence showing MS lesions that are perpendicular to the callosal plane with discrete lesion borders and most measuring more than 3 mm in diameter. **(B)** Sagittal T2 sequence showing discrete MS lesion at C5 (long arrow).

changes that are typical of MS[4] (Figure 4.3). The evolution of the diagnostic criteria for MS, from solely clinically based to the currently used McDonald criteria, reflects the increasing importance of MRI findings in establishing a timely and accurate diagnosis.[16]

Diagnostic Criteria for Multiple Sclerosis

The fundamental concept of DIT and DIS was first introduced by Schumacher et al. in 1965 as a first attempt to standardize diagnostic criteria for MS.[16] Initially, these criteria were based on clinical features alone, as well as the elimination of alternative diagnoses with similar presentations. In 1983, the Poser criteria were proposed, which incorporated paraclinical tests (evoked potentials, neuroimaging, and CSF analysis) to supplement clinical evidence for the diagnosis of MS in situations where clinical criteria were not met.[13]

With the advent of MRI, the need for early diagnosis and treatment prompted revision of the widely used Poser criteria.[17] In 2001, an international panel headed by Ian McDonald published new guidelines for the diagnosis of MS, commonly known as the 2001 McDonald criteria.[13,14,18] For the first time, these guidelines proposed the use of MRI findings as supporting evidence for lesion dissemination in time and space with the potential to enable an earlier diagnosis.[19] The concept of DIS was based

TABLE 4.2

BARKHOF CRITERIA FOR PREDICTION OF CIS CONVERSION TO CLINICALLY DEFINITE MS

- ≥1 Gadolinium-enhancing lesion or ≥9 T2-hyperintense lesions
- ≥1 Infratentorial lesion
- ≥1 Juxtacortical lesion
- ≥3 Periventricular lesions

CIS, clinically isolated syndrome; MS, multiple sclerosis.

on the Barkhof criteria[20] (Table 4.2), which were originally developed to predict conversion to clinically definite MS in patients presenting with an isolated first clinical symptom.[20] They require at least 3 of 4 of: (1) one gadolinium-enhancing lesion or nine T2-hyperintense lesions if gadolinium-enhancing lesions are not present; (2) at least one infratentorial lesion; (3) at least one juxtacortical lesion (i.e., involving the subcortical U-fibers); (4) at least three periventricular lesions. DIT was determined by a gadolinium-enhancing or a new T2 lesion detected on repeat MRI performed 3 months (90 d) or more after the baseline scan.[19]

When properly applied, the 2001 McDonald criteria showed high specificity (83%) and sensitivity (83%) for clinically definite MS at 3 years in patients presenting with a clinically isolated syndrome (CIS) suggestive of demyelinating disease.[13] In 2002, a retrospective analysis reported that, with MRI and the McDonald Criteria, 50% of patients with a first clinical attack would receive a diagnosis of definite MS within a year compared with only 20% when using the Poser criteria.[16] In the light of subsequent studies, the 2001 McDonald criteria were revised in 2005, 2010, and most recently in 2017,[11] further clarifying the role of MRI in the diagnosis of MS.

The first revision to the McDonald criteria was published in 2005.[18] One key difference from the prior iteration was that DIT could be established on the basis of a gadolinium-enhancing or a new T2 lesion in an MRI scan performed 30 days (rather than 90 d) or more after the baseline scan. In addition, for the first time, spinal cord lesions were incorporated in the total lesion count. These criteria maintained the high specificity of the original 2001 McDonald criteria[13] and achieved a sensitivity of 77% according to some studies.[13,21,22]

In 2010, new evidence and consensus using the Swanton/MAGNIMS (Magnetic Resonance Imaging in Multiple Sclerosis) criteria led to further revision of the McDonald criteria.[17,23,24] In the 2010 revision, the definition for DIS was simplified to include one or more T2 lesions in at least two of four key locations: juxtacortical, periventricular, infratentorial, and spinal cord.[14] Gadolinium-enhancing lesions were no longer required for the determination of DIS. The criteria for DIT were modified to include any new

T2 or gadolinium-enhancing lesions on follow-up scan at any time after the baseline scan or the simultaneous presence of asymptomatic enhancing and nonenhancing lesions on the same scan regardless of timing.[14] The sensitivity and specificity of the 2010 McDonald criteria reported by different studies range from 70% to 80% and 48% to 63%, respectively.[11,22,25]

The McDonald criteria were redefined in 2017 (Table 4.3). As with previous revisions, these newly revised criteria are expected to speed the diagnostic process with increased sensitivity while preserving specificity and to reduce the possibility of misdiagnosis, although this will need to be evaluated prospectively. The core requirement of the diagnosis of MS remains the objective demonstration of dissemination of CNS lesions in both space and time, based on either clinical findings alone or a combination of clinical and MRI findings.[12] DIS is demonstrated with MRI alone by one or more T2 lesions in at least two of the four MS-typical regions of the CNS: periventricular, juxtacortical (and now also cortical), infratentorial, and spinal cord, or by the development of a further clinical attack implicating a different CNS site.[26] Both symptomatic and asymptomatic lesions contribute to lesion count. DIT is demonstrated by the simultaneous presence of both symptomatic or asymptomatic gadolinium-enhancing and nonenhancing lesions at any point in time or a new T2 and/or gadolinium-enhancing lesion(s) on follow-up MRI irrespective of its timing with reference to a baseline MRI. Positive findings of oligoclonal bands in the spinal fluid can now substitute for demonstration of DIT in some settings.[12] Table 4.4 shows the definitions of DIS and DIT according to the newly revised 2017 McDonald criteria. The sensitivity and specificity of the complete set of the 2017 McDonald criteria have not been fully evaluated yet.

It should be noted that even with the wide utility of MRI, a diagnosis of MS should follow the exclusion of other possible etiologies that can mimic MS in clinical presentation and/or MRI findings.[13] MRI, like other clinical features or laboratory tests, is one piece of evidence that must be placed in the appropriate context to arrive at a correct diagnosis.

MRI in Multiple Sclerosis

Based on the chronologic changes to lesion morphology, MS lesion formation and activity can be divided into two phases: an acute phase characterized by contrast enhancement of lesions and a subacute phase characterized by changes in lesion signal intensity and size on unenhanced T1- and T2-weighted images.[2,27]

In the acute phase, lesions are typically isointense to the normal white matter on T1-weighted imaging and therefore cannot be seen on an unenhanced T1 scan.[1,2] However, the formation of new MS lesions is nearly always associated with a focal area of contrast enhancement on T1-weighted scans, which correlates with BBB disruption in the setting of acute perivascular

TABLE 4.3

2017 MCDONALD CRITERIA FOR DIAGNOSIS OF MULTIPLE SCLEROSIS (MS)

Clinical Presentation	Additional Data Needed for a Diagnosis of MS
≥2 Attacks and objective clinical evidence of ≥2 lesions ≥2 Attacks and objective clinical evidence of 1 lesion with historical evidence of prior attack involving a lesion in a different location	None. Dissemination in space (DIS) and dissemination in time (DIT) criteria have been met
≥2 Attacks and objective clinical evidence of 1 lesion	One of these criteria: ■ DIS: additional clinical attack implicating different CNS site ■ DIS: ≥1 symptomatic or asymptomatic MS-typical T2 lesions in ≥2 areas of the CNS: periventricular, cortical/juxtacortical, infratentorial, or spinal cord
1 Attack and objective clinical evidence of ≥2 lesions	One of these criteria: ■ DIT: additional clinical attack ■ DIT: simultaneous presence of both enhancing and nonenhancing symptomatic or asymptomatic MR-typical MRI lesions ■ DIT: new T2 or enhancing MRI lesion compared with baseline lesion scan (without regard to timing of baseline scan) ■ CSF-specific oligoclonal bands (not present in serum)
1 Attack and objective clinical evidence of 1 lesion	One of these criteria: ■ DIS: additional clinical attack implicating different CNS site ■ DIS: ≥1 symptomatic or asymptomatic MS-typical T2 lesions in ≥2 areas of the CNS: periventricular, cortical/juxtacortical, infratentorial, or spinal cord AND one of these criteria: ■ DIT: additional clinical attack ■ DIT: simultaneous presence of both enhancing and nonenhancing symptomatic or asymptomatic MR-typical MRI lesions ■ DIT: new T2 or enhancing MRI lesion compared with baseline lesion scan (without regard to timing of baseline scan)

CNS, central nervous system; CSF, cerebrospinal fluid.

TABLE 4.4
2017 McDONALD CRITERIA FOR DEMONSTRATION OF
DISSEMINATION IN SPACE AND TIME BY MRI

Dissemination in space

- ≥1 T2-hyperintense lesion(s) in two or more areas of the CNS: periventricular, cortical or juxtacortical, infratentorial, and spinal cord

Dissemination in time

- Simultaneous presence of gadolinium-enhancing and nonenhancing lesions at any time or by a new T2-hyperintense or gadolinium-enhancing lesion on follow-up MRI, irrespective of the timing of the baseline MRI

CNS, central nervous system; MRI, magnetic resonance imaging.

inflammation.[8,13] Gadolinium enhancement may last up to 2 months in acute lesions, although the average duration of enhancement is 3 weeks.[2] According to the pattern of contrast uptake, lesions can be classified as nodular or ringlike.[1] New contrast-enhanced lesions are usually associated with a hyperintense lesion in the same location on T2-weighted images but can also be detected before T2 abnormalities develop.[27] Clinical relapses often occur when a new lesion involves an eloquent area of the brain or cord. However, many new lesions occur in noneloquent or clinically silent brain regions. Because contrast-enhanced T1-weighted scans can detect disease activity 5 to 10 times more frequently than the clinical evaluation of relapses, it is generally believed that a significant number of these lesions can be clinically silent at any given time.[1,8,14,15,28]

The subacute phase of MS lesion morphology and activity can be subdivided into early and late periods.[3] In the early subacute period, observed within the initial 10 weeks, the T2-hyperintense lesion is a combination of an influx of inflammatory cells resulting in demyelination, axonal transection, and edema. During this time, there is also cessation of lesion contrast enhancement on postgadolinium T1-weighted imaging.[1] In the late subacute period, 3 to 5 months after initial inflammation, the T2-hyperintense lesion often decreases in size, because of not only decreased vasogenic edema but also a combination of degenerative and regenerative processes (gliosis and remyelination), respectively. Over the initial 6-month period, less than 40% of lesions become persistently hypointense on T1-weighted imaging, presumably secondary to permanent demyelination and severe axonal loss, and are referred to as "T1 black holes."[1] The accumulation of T1 black holes has been shown to correlate with disease progression and disability.[5,23] Although not uncommon in the brain, T1 black holes are rarely seen in the spinal cord, although, in part, this is because imaging of the spinal cord is more challenging because of the small cross-sectional size, motion artifacts, and low lesion contrast.[2]

Although MS lesions can occur anywhere in the CNS, above the tentorium cerebri, they have a predilection for periventricular white matter and tend to have an ovoid configuration with the major axes perpendicular to the ventricular surface (Dawson fingers)[1] (Figure 4.4). During their initial stage, the lesions are typically thin and appear to be linear, which is likely associated with the inflammatory changes around the long axis of the medullary vein that create the dilated perivenular space.[1,29] In addition to the periventricular regions, the corpus callosum, brainstem, U-fibers, optic nerves, and subcortical region are areas where MS lesions are frequently located.[30] In addition, lesions occur in the gray matter. Gray matter lesions are more easily detected on FLAIR imaging and other advanced sequencing techniques, including double inversion recovery (DIR)[31] and phase-sensitive inversion recovery (PSIR) (Figure 4.5).[32-34]

FLAIR and T2-weighted sequencing are the mainstays in the diagnostic workup of patients with MS (Figure 4.6).[35] The T2 and FLAIR lesion loads reflect the accumulation of gross tissue changes.[35] Although newly formed or enlarging T2 lesions might indicate new areas of MS-related tissue damage, T2 hyperintensities are nonspecific with respect to the actual pathological changes within the lesions and can represent areas of inflammation, edema, abnormal myelination, gliosis, or axonal loss.[4,15,36,37] Table 4.5 shows the MRI characteristics of brain lesions typical of MS.

The majority of conventional MRI scanners use different magnet strengths, typically 1.5 or 3.0 T. In general, an increase in magnet

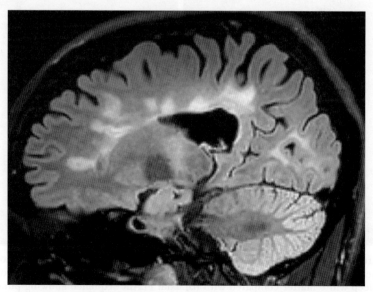

Figure 4.4. Dawson finger. Sagittal FLAIR (fluid attenuated inversion recovery) sequence showing "Dawson finger" appearance of multiple sclerosis (MS) lesions.

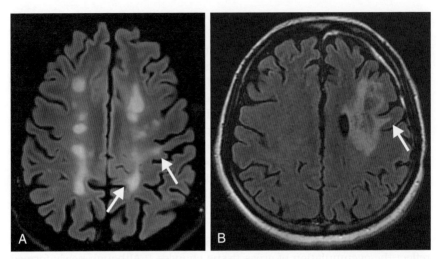

Figure 4.5. (A) Axial FLAIR (fluid attenuated inversion recovery) sequence showing "typical" multiple sclerosis (MS) lesions compared with **(B)** axial FLAIR sequence showing large amorphous tumefactive MS lesion. Demyelinating lesion often show early involvement of cortico-cortical fibers (U-fibers) as seen in this lesion (long arrows shown in both panels a and b).

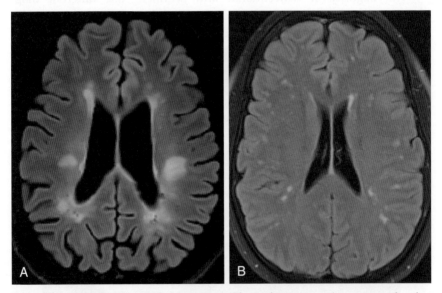

Figure 4.6. (A) Axial FLAIR (fluid attenuated inversion recovery) sequence showing "typical" multiple sclerosis (MS) lesions adjacent to the ventricles and involving the deep white matter compared with **(B)** axial FLAIR sequence showing punctate hyperintensities scattered throughout the subcortical and deep white matter.

> ▨ **TABLE 4.5**
> **MRI CHARACTERISTICS OF BRAIN LESIONS TYPICAL OF MS**
>
> ---
>
> ■ Lesion size: usually >5 mm
>
> ■ Asymmetric
>
> ■ Nonconfluent
>
> ■ Location: cortical/juxtacortical, periventricular (Dawson fingers), infratentorial, spinal cord, corpus callosum
>
> ■ Gadolinium-enhancing lesions (incomplete rim enhancement)
>
> ■ Central vein sign
>
> ■ New lesions on repeat imaging are common
>
> ---
>
> MRI, magnetic resonance imaging; MS, multiple sclerosis.

strength is expected to lead to an increase in the number of identifiable MS lesions.[38] Of note, open-configuration MRI scanners, which may be used when patients have difficulty tolerating a closed MRI machine, are usually less than 1.5 T, and the quality of images they provide is often suboptimal for detecting MS activity.[39] Additionally, there may be variability in scanning protocols and voxel size (resolution). Newer protocols use a "3D" image representing an isotropic voxel with dimensions of 1 × 1 × 1 mm cubed. By contrast, conventional "2D" images utilize a nonisotropic voxel with variable dimensions, commonly 2 × 2 × 5 mm. Because facilities may have different MRI scanners with different magnet strengths and imaging protocols, patients should be encouraged to use the same MRI facility for follow-up imaging. When possible, the same scanner should be used for a more accurate comparison of new and old MRI scans.

MRI of the Spinal Cord

The detection of spinal cord lesions or other intramedullary abnormalities is accomplished by MRI of the cervical and thoracic cord that includes sagittal and axial images with and without gadolinium.[40] Because of the higher density of eloquent axons in the cord, lesions in this region are more likely to be symptomatic. Clinically, spinal cord demyelination can manifest as motor weakness with accompanying ambulatory difficulties, sensory loss, neuropathic pain, paresthesias/dysesthesias, poor coordination, spasticity, and bladder/bowel dysfunction.[41] The length of the spinal cord lesion or lesions, the distribution of signal abnormality seen on axial plane imaging, and the pattern of gadolinium enhancement are all important clues that can help narrow the differential diagnosis.[42]

In MS, spinal cord lesions are typically one vertebral segment or less in craniocaudal length and rarely longitudinally extensive (i.e., three or more vertebral segments).[43] They are characteristically located peripherally along the cord within the dorsal or lateral columns and are mostly focal and asymmetric.[40] Detection of longitudinally extensive lesions in the craniocaudal plane or large central lesions involving >50% of the cord in the axial plane on MRI in patients with myelitis strongly suggests neuromyelitis optica spectrum disorder (NMOSD), with diagnostic specificity surpassed only by the presence of AQP4-IgG.[43] However, an initially longitudinally extensive spinal cord lesion can evolve over time and appear chronically as several small short-segment lesions.[29] Therefore, spinal cord MRI interpretation requires analysis in the clinical context and knowledge of the timing of the scan. It should also be noted that, although MS is rarely associated with an acute longitudinally extensive lesions in adults, the lesions may occur in up to 10% to 15% of patients with childhood-onset MS.[29] As with brain lesions, the detection of lesion enhancement after gadolinium administration implies BBB injury and the enhancement pattern can be informative.[44] Lesion enhancement is highly variable and can show a ringlike distribution of enhancement at the lesion periphery.[29] Table 4.6 shows the MRI characteristics of spinal cord lesions typical of MS.

Conventional MRI seems to lack sensitivity and specificity to MS-associated pathological changes in the spine.[43] Even though spinal cord lesions can be detected in up to 90% of patients with MS, only weak to moderate correlations have been observed between spinal cord abnormalities and clinical status.[45] This phenomenon has previously been described as the "clinicoradiological paradox."[41] A number of factors can contribute to the lower-than-expected correlation between spinal cord lesion load and clinical disability. Visible lesion contrast is decreased because the spinal cord represents a small fraction of the total imaged spinal volume that includes bone and CSF. In addition, the spine is a mobile structure

TABLE 4.6

MRI CHARACTERISTICS OF SPINAL CORD LESIONS TYPICAL OF MS

- Little to no cord swelling
- Size: at least 3 mm and less than two vertebral segments in length
- Focal (i.e., clearly delineated and circumscribed on T2-weighted sequences)
- Most commonly involve the cervical region compared with the rest of the spine
- On sagittal view, lesions rarely exceed two vertebral segments in length
- On cross-section, they typically occupy the lateral and posterior white matter columns and seldom occupy more than half of the cross-sectional area
- Enhancing spinal cord lesions are seen less frequently than in the brain but are commonly associated with new clinical symptoms when present

MRI, magnetic resonance imaging; MS, multiple sclerosis.

and artifacts related to breathing movements and intrinsic motion caused by cardiac and respiratory cycles can complicate image acquisition.[43] Sagittal views have been shown to underestimate the number of lesions in the spinal cord. Therefore, evaluation of both sagittal and axial images is recommended to improve the accuracy of identification of spinal cord lesions, as well as to reduce the risk of reporting equivocal abnormalities.[41] Lastly, spinal cord lesions, however small, can substantially contribute to disability.[27]

In addition to having diagnostic value, MRI evaluation of MS-associated spinal cord lesions can provide prognostic information. Reduced cross-sectional area of the upper cervical cord in patients with MS is thought to indicate disease-related atrophy.[43] Spinal cord atrophy in MS has shown a robust correlation with physical disability.[45] In a prospective study of patients with primary progressive MS, increased spinal cord atrophy over the first 2 years of the disease predicted worse outcomes at 5-year follow-up.[41] In this setting, spinal cord atrophy has been postulated as a potential outcome measure in clinical trials of putative neuroprotective therapies.

In a longitudinal study of patients with MS who presented with an inflammatory myelitis, a high number of cord lesions at baseline predicted worse clinical outcome and a higher number of relapses.[41] Although the relationship between spinal cord pathology and disease progression in MS is not completely understood, overall, extensive spinal cord abnormalities at presentation seem to confer an unfavorable prognosis.[41]

Cortical Lesions

Traditionally, MS has been considered a demyelinating white matter disease, but a number of pathologic studies have documented significant involvement of the gray matter in the deep nuclei and the cortex.[2,8] Although cortical lesions begin in the earliest stages of MS, they can be missed up to 95% of the time on conventional MRI.[46] DIR allows for better detection of cortical lesions by nulling the signal from the CSF and white matter.[46,47] PSIR is a T1-weighted sequence with higher signal to noise ratio, improved intensity, and gray-white matter contrast that has been shown to improve cortical lesion detection and classification.[33,34,48] With the use of advanced MRI techniques, such as DIR and PSIR, cortical lesions have been detected in up to 36% of patients with CIS and 97% of patients with MS.[33,34,38] In addition, in accordance to the newly revised 2017 McDonald criteria,[12] cortical lesions can now be used in fulfilling MRI criteria for DIS.

Histopathological and MRI studies show that gray matter damage becomes increasingly prominent with disease progression due to the accumulation of focal demyelinating cortical lesions, meningeal inflammation, neuronal injury, and Wallerian degeneration.[12] Over time, these degenerative changes will result in appreciable atrophy of gray matter.[49] Because cortical lesions can represent a substantial component of an individual's total disease burden, it has been hypothesized that cortical lesions contribute to disability not accounted for by T2-weighted lesion volume.[38,50] Moreover, in patients with CIS, the presence of cortical lesions correlates with a higher risk of conversion to clinically definite MS.[51]

Cross-sectional and longitudinal studies have shown correlations between the number and/or volume of cortical lesions and cognitive or physical impairment in MS.[51] A recent study of 42 patients with MS reported that patients with DIR-hyperintense cortical lesions showed significant global cortical thinning and episodic memory deficits.[51] Similarly, correlations were found between PSIR lesions and cortical volume and PSIR and symbol digit modalities test score (a cognitive component of the MS functional composite).[34] Although DIR and PSIR offers high sensitivity, specificity, and accuracy for the detection of gray matter lesions, these techniques have not been adopted as part of everyday clinical practice.

CNS Atrophy

Brain atrophy is evident on visual inspection of MRI scans of patients through all stages of MS, from CIS to relapsing-remitting, secondary progressive, and primary progressive (PP) disease, and is more pronounced in the latter groups.[52] Postmortem histopathological studies have shown that CNS atrophy predominantly results from axonal loss and neuronal shrinkage and is largely independent of demyelination.[53] Brain atrophy is the most accepted imaging biomarker of neurodegeneration and progression of disability in MS. When present early in the disease, brain atrophy can predict rapid disability progression.[54] Whole brain atrophy has been shown to correlate with cognitive dysfunction and mood disturbances, and measuring atrophy progression can provide clinically relevant information.[1,52,54,55] Patients with worsening disability have been shown to develop greater brain atrophy compared with those who are clinically stable.[56] In clinically stable and untreated patients with MS, brain volume loss occurs at a rate of about 0.5% to 1% per year, compared with 0.1% to 0.3% per year for healthy controls.[5,43,57] Patients with CIS who convert to clinically definite MS compared with those who do not typically have more pronounced brain atrophy.[21]

Gray matter atrophy is more pronounced in the deep gray matter nuclei than in the neocortical areas but can also occur in the thalamus, hippocampus, and cerebellum.[52] Within the brain, thalamic volume seems to be decreased even in patients with radiologically isolated syndrome (RIS). Thalamic atrophy has been shown to predict progression to clinically definite MS in patients who have had a single attack.[44] Corpus callosal atrophy is a key factor in cognitive impairment,[58] and hippocampal atrophy has been associated with impairment in memory encoding and retrieval.[57] The relationship between spinal cord atrophy and clinical disability is also strong.[41] In a prospective study of patients with PPMS, increased spinal cord atrophy over the first 2 years predicted worse outcome at 5-year follow-up.[41]

Quantification of brain volume on early scans provides prognostic measures of clinical status not only for long-term follow-up but also for short-term decline.[1] However, atrophy rates can be confounded by a number of influences, such as response to treatment, pseudoatrophy effects, genetics, and vascular risk factors.[38] There are currently several postprocessing and at-scanner methods to quantify whole-brain atrophy, although each may provide slightly different results.[59] Intertechnique variability is high,[53] and, thus far, large-scale trials have not been conducted to determine validity for a given measure.[45] At present, MRI atrophy metrics are not routinely used for diagnostic or prognostic purposes.[59] Efforts are currently underway to create a standardized protocol for image acquisition to allow for incorporation of brain atrophy quantification into clinical practice.

Central Vein Sign

Pathological studies have reported the presence of central vessels in MS lesions for many years.[44] CNS infiltration of mononuclear cells from peripheral blood develop around venules and cause white matter lesions in MS.[41] With the development of susceptibility-weighted imaging, which takes advantage of the T2-shortening effect of deoxyhemoglobin in venous blood (resulting in T2 hypointensity), the physical relationship between white mater lesions and venules can now be visualized.[45] The venocentric distribution of lesions, also termed the "central vein sign," has been observed across all MS clinical phenotypes.[60] Data from studies conducted with 3.0 and 7.0 T MRI scanners suggest that the high frequency of perivenular lesions is pathologically specific to MS, and therefore, the central vein sign is an important candidate for improving MRI diagnostic criteria and for reducing the rate of misdiagnosis.[60] One small prospective study of 22 patients with CIS who underwent a T2-weighted MRI scan found that all patients who eventually received a diagnosis of MS within a median follow-up period of 26 months had a central vein sign in >40% of brain lesions at baseline.[61] Those whose condition was not diagnosed as MS had a central vein sign in <40% of brain lesions at baseline. In this patient group, the central vein sign had a 100% positive and negative predictive value for a diagnosis of MS, However, given the small sample size, additional large prospective multicenter trials are needed to evaluate the clinical predictive value of the central vein sign in the diagnosis of MS.

MRI as a Measure of Cognitive Function

Cognitive impairment in MS has an estimated prevalence of 43% to 70% and can become evident in the earliest stages of the disease.[58] The most affected cognitive domains are information-processing speed, working memory, complex attention, executive functions, verbal fluency, and verbal and visuospatial learning and memory.[62] The accumulation of cognitive impairment is widely used as a predictor of conversion to clinically definite MS, disability progression, treatment compliance, depression, and low quality of life.[57] Cognitive dysfunction can, however, be subtle and require dedicated neuropsychological testing to be detected.[52] Recent efforts have highlighted the importance of evaluating the dynamics of cognition throughout the disease course.[8]

The most commonly used global MRI metrics for cognitive dysfunction in MS are volumes of the whole brain, gray matter, white matter, and white matter lesion burden.[52] Of these tissue fractions, cognitive impairment is most often associated with gray matter atrophy and lesion accumulation,[51] although correlations are weak. Two-dimensional MRI markers, such as third ventricle width, bicaudate ratio, and corpus callosal surface and index, have also been related to cognitive impairment in MS.[62] Other regions of interest include subcortical structures, such as the corpus callosum, thalamus, hippocampus, putamen, caudate nucleus, cerebellum, and cingulate gyrus, which have all been associated with cognitive function in MS.[52,53,63]

Available data suggest that focal white matter lesions play a role in cognition, but the overall effect of T2 lesions on MS-related cognitive impairment is limited.[45] The impact of white matter damage on cognition may be mediated by a disruption of crucial tracts or interference with specific functional nodes.[62] Therefore, the location of lesions in critical brain areas appears to be important and, in this context, the improved capability to detect cortical lesions is likely to provide additional pieces of information.[23] Correlations between various brain areas and cognition currently remain weak, and additional studies, possibly evaluating tract-specific changes, might be needed. Currently, normalized brain volume and lesion burden are mainly investigated in clinical trials as an important indirect predictor of cognitive outcome.[57]

Diagnostic Utility of Conventional MRI in Multiple Sclerosis

Despite the sensitivity of conventional MRI for the identification of focal white matter lesions in MS, there is a discrepancy between the white matter disease burden and clinical measures of physical disability and cognitive impairment.[23,45] This discrepancy is largely secondary to the intrinsic failure of conventional MRI to detect cortical lesions, as well other diffuse structural, metabolic, and functional abnormalities known to be present in the normal-appearing gray and white matter.[5,45] These limitations further decrease the specificity of MRI to the heterogeneous pathological substrates of the disease.

MRI scanners with high-field strengths (3.0 T and greater) may improve the early diagnosis of MS by increasing the sensitivity and specificity for the detection of enhancing and nonenhancing white matter lesions compared with 1.5-T scanners.[6,20,42,64] Total lesion counts can be up to 45% higher on high-field scanners compared with a 1.5 T scanner.[1] More recently, ultrahigh-field MRI strengths (7.0 T) have begun to help further elucidate our understanding of the underlying pathophysiologic mechanisms in MS.[65] However, because ultrahigh-field MRI is currently limited in widespread adoption owing to a lack of standardized protocols and large, well-controlled trials, 3.0-T MRI systems continue to be the most important paraclinical tool available in diagnosing and monitoring MS.

MRI in Clinically Isolated Syndrome

CIS is defined as the first clinical episode suggestive of demyelination or MS, which persists for at least 24 hours and occurs in the absence of fever, infection, or encephalopathy.[16,19,38] Symptoms usually develop over the course of hours to days and gradually remit over the ensuing weeks to months, although remission may not be complete in all cases.[13]

For patients presenting with CIS, the risk of conversion to MS is greater in those with abnormal T2-weighted imaging (>1 T2 lesion).[1] Patients with CIS will have abnormal T2 scans approximately 50% to 70% of the time.[63] Of those with an abnormal baseline MRI, 82% to 88% will convert to MS, compared with 19% to 21% of those with a normal baseline scan.[63] In various studies, the 10- to 20-year likelihood of developing MS for patients with CIS and MRI lesions characteristic of MS ranges from 60% to 80%.[66] In addition, recent studies have shown that asymptomatic spinal cord lesions in patients with CIS confer increased risk of conversion to clinically definite MS.[2,43]

All patients with CIS should have neuroimaging of the brain and spinal cord with a contrast-enhanced MRI to determine the risk of progression to clinically definite MS and potentially expedite treatment initiation with the goal of reducing future morbidity.

MRI in Radiologically Isolated Syndrome

The term radiologically isolated syndrome (RIS) refers to the incidental detection of radiological findings highly suggestive of MS in the absence of clinical signs and symptoms of CNS demyelination.[50] The MAGNIMS collaborative research network published new recommendations in 2016 to upgrade the imaging diagnostic criteria for MS in an effort to improve the previous 2010 McDonald criteria for MS.[67] These recommendations were partially incorporated into the revised 2017 McDonald criteria (Table 4.3), which should be applied for the establishment of DIT and DIS in patients with RIS.

Approximately one-third of individuals with RIS will be diagnosed with MS, and the remaining two-thirds will develop new lesions within 5 years of presentation.[12] According to a recent large, multicenter, retrospective study performed by the RIS Consortium, age (<37 y), sex (male), and the presence of demyelinating lesions in the spinal cord are the significant predictors for a first clinical event.[68] Specifically, around 58% of patients <37 years with spinal cord lesions are predicted to become symptomatic within 5 years and up to 90% if the male gender is added as an additional risk factor.[69] Other risk factors include high cerebral lesion load, gadolinium-enhancing lesions, CSF-specific oligoclonal bands, and abnormal visual evoked potentials.[12] Active monitoring of patients with clinical and radiological follow-up every 6 to 12 months is recommended.[70]

MRI Mimics in Multiple Sclerosis: Differential Diagnosis

More than 90% of patients with clinically definite MS have typical white matter lesions on MRI.[4] However, a key element in the diagnosis of MS is the exclusion of other possible disease entities. CNS lesions resulting from other disorders (e.g., ischemia, systemic lupus erythematosus, Behçet disease, other vasculitides, sarcoidosis) may appear similar to MS lesions on MRI[28,38] (Table 4.7). White matter changes related to normal aging can further complicate the diagnostic process.[2,59] In these cases, ancillary testing (blood work, CSF analysis, and evoked potentials) can help facilitate the diagnosis.[52] Careful assessment of MRI "red flags" can be helpful in suggesting a diagnosis other than MS.[8] These so-called red flags were described over a decade ago by the European Magnetic Resonance Network in MS (MAGNIMS) to help guide clinicians in the diagnosis of MS.[4] In addition, MAGNIMS also published a standardized MRI protocol for the diagnosis of MS to help increase diagnostic yield against possible MS mimics (Table 4.8).

Features have been described that distinguish MS from other demyelinating syndromes, including NMOSDs and acute demyelinating encephalomyelitis, as well as anti-myelin-oligodendrocyte glycoprotein antibody-related disease.[29] The location and shape of white matter lesions, as well as their signal characteristics on different MRI sequences, can be useful in differentiating MS from other white matter diseases[44] (Table 4.9). Specifically, lesions located in the juxtacortical/cortical regions, periphery of the brainstem, and the posterolateral cervical spinal cord are suggestive of MS.[4] In addition, elongated lesions along the subependymal veins that appear as Dawson fingers or the presence of a central vein sign is also characteristic of MS lesions.[40,65] Despite the intrinsic diagnostic challenges of MRI, most typical patients with MS receive a timely

TABLE 4.7
DIFFERENTIAL DIAGNOSIS OF WHITE MATTER LESIONS

- Hypoxic/ischemic
  - □ Atherosclerosis, stroke, hypertension, migraine, amyloid angiopathy, vasculopathy (CADASIL, Susac syndrome)
- Inflammatory
  - □ Multiple sclerosis, vasculitis (SLE, Sjögren syndrome, Behçet syndrome, primary CNS vasculitis), neurosarcoidosis
- Infectious
  - □ HIV, syphilis, Lyme disease, TB, PML
- Toxic/metabolic
- Traumatic
  - □ Posttraumatic, radiotherapy
- Metabolic
  - □ Leukodystrophies
- Neoplastic
  - □ Metastatic or primary disease
- Normal
  - □ Age-related or Virchow-Robin spaces

CADASIL, cerebral autosomal dominant arteriopathy with subcortical infarcts and leukoencephalopathy; CNS, central nervous system; HIV, human immunodeficiency virus; PML, progressive multifocal leukoencephalopathy; SLE, systemic lupus erythematosus; TB, tuberculosis.

TABLE 4.8
2015 MAGNIMS STANDARDIZED BRAIN AND SPINE MRI PROTOCOL

- Brain
  - □ Mandatory
    - Axial: proton-density and/or T2-FLAIR/T2-weigted
    - Sagittal: 2D or 3D T2-FLAIR
    - 2D or 3D contrast-enhanced T1-weighted
  - □ Optional
    - Unenhanced 2D or high-resolution isotropic 3D T1-weighted
    - 2D and/or 3D dual inversion recovery
    - Axial diffusion-weighted imaging
- Spinal cord
  - □ Mandatory
    - Dual-echo (proton-density and T2-weighted) conventional and/or fast spin-echo
    - STIR (as an alternative to proton-density-weighted)
    - Contrast-enhanced T1-weighted spin-echo (if T2 lesions present)
  - □ Optional
    - Phase-sensitive inversion recovery (as an alternative to STIR at the cervical segment)

FLAIR, fluid attenuated inversion recovery; MAGNIMS, Magnetic Resonance Imaging in Multiple Sclerosis; MRI, magnetic resonance imaging; STIR, short-TI inversion recovery.

owing to possible teratogenicity in the first trimester during organogenesis.[76] Gadolinium may cross the placenta in the second and third trimesters where it can be excreted into the amniotic fluid in small amounts (0.01% of the injected dose in animal models) and recirculated by the fetus.[77] This raises concern for gadolinium retention and associated NSF in the child. Although no cases of NSF in newborns have been reported to date, a large retrospective study evaluating the long-term safety of gadolinium exposure during pregnancy reported an increased fetal risk of rheumatologic, inflammatory, or infiltrative skin conditions in 123 children of women who were exposed to gadolinium during pregnancy versus 384,180 births (adjusted hazard ratio, 1.36; 95% confidence interval [CI], 1.09-1.69).[76] In addition, stillbirths and neonatal deaths also occurred more frequently among seven gadolinium MRI-exposed versus 9844 MRI-unexposed pregnancies (adjusted relative risk [RR], 3.70; 95% CI, 1.55-8.85), although there was no increased risk of harm to the fetus or in early childhood in children of women who were exposed to MRI without gadolinium.[76] A limitation of these conclusions is the use of a control group who did not undergo MRI (rather than patients who underwent MRI without gadolinium). Additional larger studies are needed to establish the risks of gadolinium administration to the developing fetus.

Although MRI is not contraindicated in pregnancy, until further studies are performed, current general consensus among the American College of Obstetricians and Gynecologists is that every effort should be made to avoid the administration of gadolinium to the pregnant woman and alternative imaging strategies such as ultrasound should be used whenever possible.[76]

Gadolinium Use During Lactation

The water solubility and minimal protein binding of gadolinium-based agents limit their excretion into breast milk.[74] Within 24 hours of gadolinium administration, less than 0.04% of the administered dose is excreted into breast milk and, of this amount, less than 1% will be absorbed by the infant's gastrointestinal tract.[72] Although theoretically any gadolinium excreted into breast milk could reach the infant, there are no reports of breastfeeding-related toxicity to date. However, the lack of knowledge about its long-term safety and the possible risks associated with immature renal function in the neonate are all causes for concern. Overall, the decision about whether to cease breastfeeding for a short period of time after gadolinium administration may be best made on a case-by-case basis, depending on the specific GBCA administered to the lactating mother. However, the current general consensus among the American College of Obstetricians and Gynecologists is that breastfeeding should not be interrupted after gadolinium administration.[76]

MRI Safety in Patients With Implanted Devices

Potential safety concerns exist regarding the safety of MRI evaluation in patients with implanted devices primarily because of factors that include electromagnetic field interactions, MRI-related heating, and the creation of image artifacts.[78] In the Unites States, the Food and Drug Administration (FDA) is responsible for reviewing the labeling provided by manufacturers regarding the safety of their devices and their compatibility for use in an MRI environment.[79] Clinicians should always include all medical devices (cardiac pacemakers, implantable infusion pumps, or other metal implants) in their assessment of a patient's suitability for MRI scanning. Strict adherence to basic screening and scanning protocols is also required.[79] Devices are classified as MR Safe, MR Conditional, or MR unsafe according to the FDA.[79] MR Safe devices have no known MRI contraindications, whereas MR Conditional devices should be used only within the MRI environment if all of the conditions for safe use provided by the manufacturer are followed.[80] Devices without information regarding MRI compatibility should be assumed to be unsafe. A complete list of FDA-approved implanted devices for use in MRI can be found at www.fda.gov. Additional recommendations regarding the various implantable devices are discussed in the following.

Cardiac Pacemakers

Although new implants are now required to be fully MRI compatible, not all implanted cardiac devices are considered safe for MRI.[81] The most commonly observed effect of MRI on a cardiac device is a change in the device parameters.[81,82] With the use of specific protocols of patients with pacemakers, reprogramming of the device before and after the MRI, or complete deactivation in some settings, MRI evaluations can be safely performed in most patients.[82]

Implantable Infusion Pumps

MRI scanning may affect the programming or function of implantable infusion pumps.[83] To prevent drug withdrawal or unintended medication overdose, some pump models may need to be reprogrammed before and/ or after the examination.[80] Therefore, it is important to be aware of the specific instructions and safety issues delivered by the manufacturer based on the specific model of the device. Depending on the medication being administered and the device model, some pumps may need to be emptied before an MRI in some situations.[80]

Vagus Nerve Stimulators

As with cardiac implantable devices or implantable infusion pumps, all vagus nerve stimulator devices should be interrogated and reprogrammed before and after an MRI by an appropriate health care professional.[84]

MRI-Compatible Metals

The strong magnetic field of an MRI scanner attracts ferrous, or iron-containing, metals and can cause serious injury to patients with certain implanted metallic devices.[3,78] Specific metals that have been cleared for use during MRI scans by safety experts include titanium, cobalt-chromium, copper, and stainless steel.[78] Nevertheless, careful patient screening before, during, and after an MRI scan is imperative in all patients with implantable devices.

Conclusion

MS and related CNS demyelinating disorders present unique diagnostic and management challenges in clinical practice. In the absence of definite diagnostic testing, MRI serves as an important diagnostic tool and a reliable and sensitive surrogate biomarker of disease activity and progression that is also commonly employed as a key outcome measure in pharmaceutical clinical trials. Rapidly advancing neuroimaging techniques will continue to improve our understanding of the underlying pathophysiology of this disease.

References

1. Ge Y. Multiple sclerosis: the role of MR imaging. *AJNR Am J Neuroradiol.* 2006;27:1165-1176.
2. Hemond CC, Bakshi R. Magnetic resonance imaging in multiple sclerosis. *Cold Spring Harb Perspect Med.* 2018:a028969. doi:10.1101/cshperspect.a028969.
3. McMahon KL, Cowin G, Galloway G. Magnetic resonance imaging: the underlying principles. *J Orthop Sport Phys Ther.* 2011;41:806-819. doi:10.2519/jospt.2011.3576.
4. Geraldes R, Ciccarelli O, Barkhof F, et al. The current role of MRI in differentiating multiple sclerosis from its imaging mimics. *Nat Rev Neurol.* 2018;14. doi:10.1038/nrneurol.2018.14.
5. Klawiter EC. Current and new directions in MRI in multiple sclerosis. *Continuum (Minneap Minn).* 2013;19:1058-1073.
6. Ropele S, De Graaf W, Khalil M, et al. MRI assessment of iron deposition in multiple sclerosis. *J Magn Reson Imaging.* 2011;34:13-21. doi:10.1002/jmri.22590.
7. Sands MJ, Levitin A. Basics of magnetic resonance imaging. *Semin Vasc Surg.* 2004;17:66-82. doi:10.1053/j.semvascsurg.2004.03.011.
8. Sicotte NL. Magnetic resonance imaging in multiple sclerosis: the role of conventional imaging. *Neurol Clin.* 2011;29:343-356. doi:10.1016/j.ncl.2011.01.005.
9. Sahraian MA, Eshaghi A. Role of MRI in diagnosis and treatment of multiple sclerosis. *Clin Neurol Neurosurg.* 2010;112:609-615. doi:10.1016/j.clineuro.2010.03.022.
10. Pretorius PM, Quaghebeur G. The role of MRI in the diagnosis of MS. *Clin Radiol.* 2003;58:434-448. doi:10.1016/S0009-9260(03)00089-8.

11. Filippi M, Preziosa P, Meani A, et al. Prediction of a multiple sclerosis diagnosis in patients with clinically isolated syndrome using the 2016 MAGNIMS and 2010 McDonald criteria: a retrospective study. *Lancet Neurol.* 2018;17:133-142. doi:10.1016/S1474-4422(17)30469-6.

12. Thompson AJ, Banwell BL, Barkhof F, et al. Diagnosis of multiple sclerosis: 2017 revisions of the McDonald criteria. *Lancet Neurol.* 2018;17:162-173. doi:10.1016/S1474-4422(17)30470-2.

13. Milo R, Miller A. Revised diagnostic criteria of multiple sclerosis. *Autoimmun Rev.* 2014;13:518-524. doi:10.1016/j.autrev.2014.01.012.

14. Polman CH, Reingold SC, Banwell B, et al. Diagnostic criteria for multiple sclerosis: 2010 Revisions to the McDonald criteria. *Ann Neurol.* 2011;69:292-302. doi:10.1002/ana.22366.

15. Neema M, Stankiewicz J, Arora A, Guss Z, Bakshi R. MRI in multiple sclerosis: what's inside the toolbox? *Neurotherapeutics.* 2007;4:602-617. doi:10.1016/j.nurt.2007.08.001.

16. Gafson A, Giovannoni G, Hawkes CH. The diagnostic criteria for multiple sclerosis: from Charcot to McDonald. *Mult Scler Relat Disord.* 2012;1:9-14. doi:10.1016/j.msard.2011.08.002.

17. Nielsen JM, Uitdehaag BMJ, Korteweg T, Barkhof F, Polman CH. Performance of the Swanton multiple sclerosis criteria for dissemination in space. *Mult Scler.* 2010;16:985-987. doi:10.1177/1352458510369244.

18. Polman CH, Reingold SC, Edan G, et al. Diagnostic criteria for multiple sclerosis: 2005 revisions to the McDonald criteria. *Ann Neurol.* 2005;58:840-846. doi:10.1002/ana.206703.

19. McDonald WI, Compston A, Edan G, et al. Recommended diagnostic criteria for multiple sclerosis: guidelines from the International Panel on the diagnosis of multiple sclerosis. *Ann Neurol.* 2001;50:121-127. doi:10.1002/ana.1032.

20. Barkhof F, Filippi M, Miller DH, et al. Comparison of MRI criteria at first presentation to predict conversion to clinically definite multiple sclerosis. *Brain.* 1997;120:2059-2069.

21. Filippi M, Absinta M, Rocca MA. Journal of the neurological sciences sleep disturbances in multiple sclerosis. *J Neurol Sci.* 2013;331:14-18. doi:10.1016/j.jns.2011.07.015.

22. Sefidbakht S, Babaeinejad M, Jali R, et al. The McDonald criteria for dissemination in space in the differential diagnosis of multiple sclerosis and neuro-Behçet's disease. *Neurol Asia.* 2014;19:47-52.

23. Filippi M, Agosta F. Imaging biomarkers in multiple sclerosis. *J Magn Reson Imaging.* 2010;31:770-788. doi:10.1002/jmri.22102.

24. Schäffler N, Köpke S, Winkler L, et al. Accuracy of diagnostic tests in multiple sclerosis – a systematic review. *Acta Neurol Scand.* 2011;124:151-164. doi:10.1111/j.1600-0404.2010.01454.x.

25. Hyun J-W, Huh S-Y, Kim W, et al. Evaluation of 2016 MAGNIMS MRI criteria for dissemination in space in patients with a clinically isolated syndrome. *Mult Scler.* 2017;18:1-9. doi:10.1177/1352458517706744.

26. Carroll WM. 2017 McDonald MS diagnostic criteria: evidence-based revisions. *Mult Scler.* 2018;24:92-95. doi:10.1177/1352458517751861.

27. Rovira A, Auger C, Alonso J. Magnetic resonance monitoring of lesion evolution in multiple sclerosis. *Ther Adv Neurol Disord.* 2013;6:298-310. doi:10.1177/1756285613484079.

28. Olek MJ. Differential diagnosis, clinical features, and prognosis of multiple sclerosis. *Curr Clin Neurol Mult Scler.* 2005:15-53.

29. Wingerchuk DM. Immune-mediated myelopathies. *Continuum (Minneap Minn)*. 2018;24:497-522. doi:10.1212/CON.0000000000000582.

30. Ge Y, Law M, Herbert J, Grossman RI. Prominent perivenular spaces in multiple sclerosis as a sign of perivascular inflammation in primary demyelination. *AJNR Am J Neuroradiol*. 2005;26:2316-2319.

31. Bedell BJ, Narayana PA. Implementation and evaluation of a new pulse sequence for rapid acquisition of double inversion recovery images for simultaneous suppression of white matter and CSF. *J Magn Reson Imaging*. 1998;8:544-547. doi:10.1002/jmri.1880080305.

32. van Munster CEP, Jonkman LE, Weinstein HC, Uitdehaag BMJ, Geurts JJG. Gray matter damage in multiple sclerosis: impact on clinical symptoms. *Neuroscience*. 2015;303:446-461. doi:10.1016/j.neuroscience.2015.07.006.

33. Nelson F, Poonawalla AH, Hou P, Huang F, Wolinsky JS, Narayana PA. Improved identification of intracortical lesions in multiple sclerosis with phase-sensitive inversion recovery in combination with fast double inversion recovery MR imaging. *AJNR Am J Neuroradiol*. 2007;28:1645-1649. doi:10.3174/ajnr.A0645.

34. Harel A, Ceccarelli A, Farrell C, et al. Phase-sensitive inversion-recovery MRI improves longitudinal cortical lesion detection in progressive MS. *PLoS One*. 2016;11:1-11. doi:10.1371/journal.pone.0152180.

35. Filippi M. Magnetic resonance techniques in multiple sclerosis. *Arch Neurol*. 2011;68:1514. doi:10.1001/archneurol.2011.914.

36. Okuda DT. Incidental lesions suggesting multiple sclerosis. *Continuum (Minneap Minn)*. 2016;22:730-743. doi:10.1212/CON.0000000000000339.

37. Neema M, Stankiewicz J, Arora A, et al. T1- and T2-based MRI measures of diffuse gray matter and white matter damage in patients with multiple sclerosis. *J Neuroimaging*. 2007;17:16-21. doi:10.1111/j.1552-6569.2007.00131.x.

38. Balashov K. Imaging of central nervous system demyelinating disorders. *Continuum (Minneap Minn)*. 2016;22:1613-1635. doi:10.1212/CON.0000000000000373.

39. Hong C, Lee DH, Han BS. Characteristics of geometric distortion correction with increasing field-of-view in open-configuration MRI. *Magn Reson Imaging*. 2014;32:786-790. doi:10.1016/j.mri.2014.02.007.

40. Chen JJ, Carletti F, Young V, Mckean D, Quaghebeur G. MRI differential diagnosis of suspected multiple sclerosis. *Clin Radiol*. 2016;71:815-827. doi:10.1016/j.crad.2016.05.010.

41. Kearney H, Miller DH, Ciccarelli O. Spinal cord MRI in multiple sclerosis-diagnostic, prognostic and clinical value. *Nat Rev Neurol*. 2015;11:327-338. doi:10.1038/nrneurol.2015.80.

42. Stankiewicz JM, Neema M, Alsop DC, et al. Spinal cord lesions and clinical status in MS: 1.5T and 3T MRI study. *J Neurol Sci*. 2009;279:99-105. doi:10.1016/j.jns.2008.11.009.Spinal.

43. Rovira A, Auger C. Spinal cord in multiple Sclerosis: magnetic diagnosis. *Semin Ultrasound CT MRI*. 2016;37:396-410. doi:10.1053/j.sult.2016.05.005.

44. Wattjes MP, Steenwijk MD, Stangel M. MRI in the diagnosis and monitoring of multiple sclerosis: an update. *Clin Neuroradiol*. 2015;25:157-165. doi:10.1007/s00062-015-0430-y.

45. Miller TR, Mohan S, Choudhri AF, Gandhi D, Jindal G. Advances in multiple sclerosis and its variants: conventional and newer imaging techniques. *Radiol Clin N Am*. 2014;52:321-336.

46. Geurts JJG, Vrenken H. Toward understanding cortical lesions in multiple sclerosis. *Neurology*. 2010;75:1224-1225.

47. Kolber P, Montag S, Fleischer V, et al. Identification of cortical lesions using DIR and FLAIR in early stages of multiple sclerosis. *J Neurol*. 2015;262:1473-1482. doi:10.1007/s00415-015-7724-5.

48. Sethi V, Yousry TA, Muhlert N, et al. Improved detection of cortical MS lesions with phase-sensitive inversion recovery MRI. *J Neurol Neurosurg Psychiatry.* 2012;83:877-882. doi:10.1136/jnnp-2012-303023.

49. Radue EW, Bendfeldt K, Mueller-Lenke N, Magon S, Sprenger T. Brain atrophy: an in-vivo measure of disease activity in multiple sclerosis. *Swiss Med Wkly.* 2013;143:1-11. doi:10.4414/smw.2013.13887.

50. Granberg T, Martola J, Kristoffersen-Wiberg M, Aspelin P, Fredrikson S. Radiologically isolated syndrome – incidental magnetic resonance imaging findings suggestive of multiple sclerosis, a systematic review. *Mult Scler.* 2013;19:271-280. doi:10.1177/1352458512451943.

51. Geisseler O, Pflugshaupt T, Bezzola L, et al. The relevance of cortical lesions in patients with multiple sclerosis. *BMC Neurol.* 2016;16:1-8. doi:10.1186/s12883-016-0718-9.

52. Rocca MA, Battaglini M, Benedict RHB, et al. Brain MRI atrophy quantification in MS. *Neurology.* 2017;88:403-413. doi:10.1212/WNL.0000000000003542.

53. Jacobsen CO, Farbu E. MRI evaluation of grey matter atrophy and disease course in multiple sclerosis: an overview of current knowledge. *Acta Neurol Scand Suppl.* 2014;129:32-36. doi:10.1111/ane.12234.

54. Calabrese M, Favaretto A, Martini V, Gallo P. Grey matter lesions in MS from histology to clinical implications. *Prion.* 2013;7:20-27. doi:10.4161/pri.22580.

55. Calabrese M, Agosta F, Rinaldi F, et al. Cortical lesions and atrophy associated with cognitive impairment in relapsing-remitting multiple sclerosis. *Arch Neurol.* 2009;66:1144-1150.

56. Information A. Cortical lesions in multiple sclerosis clinical: relevance for a hidden disease burden. *JAMA Neurol.* 2015;72:979-980. doi:10.1002/mus.24642.profile.

57. Artemiadis A, Anagnostouli M, Zalonis I, Chairopoulos K, Triantafyllou N. Structural MRI correlates of cognitive function in multiple sclerosis. *Mult Scler Relat Disord.* 2018;21:1-8. doi:10.1016/j.msard.2018.02.003.

58. Ouellette R, Bergendal Å, Shams S, et al. Lesion accumulation is predictive of long-term cognitive decline in multiple sclerosis. *Mult Scler Relat Disord.* 2018;21:110-116. doi:10.1016/j.msard.2018.03.002.

59. Inglese M, Petracca M. MRI in multiple sclerosis: clinical and research update. *Curr Opin Neurol.* 2018;31:1-7. doi:10.1212/01.CON.0000389933.77036.14.

60. Sati P, Oh J, Todd Constable R, et al. The central vein sign and its clinical evaluation for the diagnosis of multiple sclerosis: a consensus statement from the North American Imaging in Multiple Sclerosis Cooperative. *Nat Rev Neurol.* 2016;12:714-722. doi:10.1038/nrneurol.2016.166.

61. Cortese R, Magnollay L, Tur C, et al. Value of the central vein sign at 3T to differentiate MS from seropositive NMOSD. *Neurology.* 2018;90:e1183-e1190. doi:10.1212/WNL.0000000000005256.

62. Filippi M, Rocca MA, Benedict RH, et al. The contribution of MRI in assessing cognitive impairment in multiple sclerosis. *Neurology.* 2010;75:2121-2128. doi:10.1212/WNL.0b013e318200d768.

63. Odenthal C, Coulthard A. The prognostic utility of MRI in clinically isolated syndrome: a literature review. *Am J Neuroradiol.* 2015;36:425-431. doi:10.3174/ajnr.A3954.

64. Bakshi R, Thompson AJ, Rocca MA, et al. MRI in multiple sclerosis: current status and future prospects. *Lancet Neurol.* 2008;7:615-625. doi:10.1016/S1474-4422(08)70137-6.

65. Sparacia G, Agnello F, Gambino A, Sciortino M, Midiri M. Multiple sclerosis: high prevalence of the 'central vein' sign in white matter lesions on susceptibility-weighted images. *Neuroradiol J.* 2018;31(4):356-361. doi:10.1177/1971400918763577.

66. Rocca MA, Messina R, Filippi M. Multiple sclerosis imaging: recent advances. *J Neurol.* 2013;260:929-935. doi:10.1007/s00415-012-6788-8.

67. Filippi M, Rocca MA, Ciccarelli O, et al. MRI criteria for the diagnosis of multiple sclerosis: MAGNIMS consensus guidelines. *Lancet Neurol.* 2016;15:292-303. doi:10.1016/S1474-4422(15)00393-2.

68. Lebrun C. Radiologically isolated syndrome should be treated with disease-modifying therapy – commentary. *Mult Scler.* 2017;23:1821-1823. doi:10.1177/1352458517727149.

69. Yamout B, Al Khawajah M. Radiologically isolated syndrome and multiple sclerosis. *Mult Scler Relat Disord.* 2017;17:234-237. doi:10.1016/j.msard.2017.08.016.

70. De Stefano N, Giorgio A, Tintoré M, et al. Radiologically isolated syndrome or subclinical multiple sclerosis: MAGNIMS consensus recommendations. *Mult Scler.* 2018;23:214-221. doi:10.1177/1352458517717808.

71. Ramalho J, Ramalho M. Gadolinium deposition and chronic toxicity. *Magn Reson Imaging Clin N Am.* 2017;25:765-778.

72. Webb JAW, Thomsen HS. Gadolinium contrast media during pregnancy and lactation. *Acta Radiol.* 2013;54:599-600. doi:10.1177/0284185113484894.

73. Ramalho J, Ramalho M, Jay M, Burke LM, Semelka RC. Gadolinium toxicity and treatment. *Magn Reson Imaging.* 2016;34:1394-1398. doi:10.1016/j.mri.2016.09.005.

74. Puac P, Rodríguez A, Vallejo C, Zamora CA, Castillo M. Safety of contrast material use during pregnancy and lactation. *Magn Reson Imaging Clin N Am.* 2017;25:787-797.

75. FDA. *FDA Drug Safety Communication: FDA Warns that Gadolinium-based Contrast Agents (GBCAs) Are Retained in the Body; Requires New Class Warnings.* 2017. Available at https://www.fda.gov/Drugs/DrugSafety/ucm559007.htm.

76. Ray JG, Vermeulen MJ, Bharatha A, Montanera WJ, Park AL. Association between MRI exposure during pregnancy and fetal and childhood outcomes. *JAMA.* 2016;316:952-961. doi:10.1001/jama.2016.12126.

77. Prola-Netto J, Woods M, Roberts VHJ, et al. Gadolinium chelate safety in pregnancy. *Radiology.* 2017;286:122-128. doi:10.1148/radiol.2017162534.

78. Dill T. Contraindications to magnetic resonance imaging. *Heart.* 2008;94:943-948. doi:10.1136/hrt.2007.125039.

79. Shellock FG, Woods TO, Crues JV III. MR labeling information for implants and devices: explanation of terminology. *Radiology.* 2009;253:26-30. doi:10.1148/radiol.2531091030.

80. Sunder R. *Magnetic Resonance Imaging (MRI) Safety.* 2018. https://www.fda.gov/MedicalDevices/ScienceandResearch/ResearchPrograms/ucm477387.htm.

81. Nazarian S, Hansford R, Rahsepar A, Weltin V, MvVeigh D. Safety of magnetic resonance imaging in patients with cardiac devices. *N Engl J Med.* 2017;377:2555-2564. doi:10.1016/j.cogdev.2010.08.003.

82. Shulman RM, Hunt B. Cardiac implanted electronic devices and MRI safety in 2018 — the state of play. *Eur Radiol.* 2018;28(10):4062-4065. doi:10.1007/s00330-018-5396-0.

83. De Andres J, Villanueva V, Palmisani S, et al. The safety of magnetic resonance imaging in patients with programmable implanted intrathecal drug delivery systems: a 3-year prospective study. *Anesth Analg.* 2011;112:1124-1129. doi:10.1213/ANE.0b013e318210d017.

84. De Jonge JC, Melis GI, Gebbink TA, De Kort GAP, Leijten FSS. Safety of a dedicated brain MRI protocol in patients with a vagus nerve stimulator. *Epilepsia.* 2014;55:e112-e115. doi:10.1111/epi.12774.

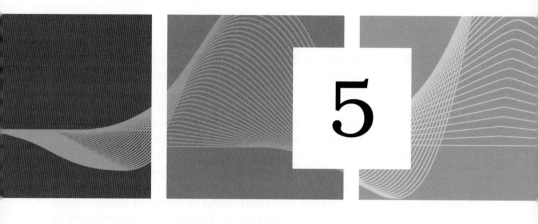

Internal Medicine I

■ ■ ■ Mary Ann Picone

Introduction

The primary care provider is a vital member of the multiple sclerosis (MS) multidisciplinary team who often has the role of coordinator of care and who is often called upon to refer patients to neurologists or other specialists. Considering the increased number of disease-modifying therapies (DMTs) for patients with MS, this also leads to an increase in monitoring and safety recommendations. It is of paramount importance for internists to optimize and prevent comorbid medical conditions. How to recognize a relapse, what vaccinations are safe to use, what monitoring needs to be done with the various DMTs are several of the topics that will be discussed below. In this era of more efficacious therapies, it is increasingly important that primary care practitioners work in partnership with neurologists to help educate and maintain patients in the best overall medical health possible to improve care.

Relapse Assessment

One facet of MS that internists should be prepared to check for is an acute exacerbation of symptoms or a relapse. A relapse is considered development of any new symptom lasting at least 24 hours in the absence of fever or infection or recurrence of a previous symptom such as optic neuritis separated by a period of at least 30 days of stability.[1] For example, if a patient had left optic neuritis that improved and was stable for at least 30 days and then began to note blurred vision again in the left eye for more than 24 hours, this would be considered a new relapse. Increase in body temperature by overheating can also cause transient worsening of symptoms but should improve once a patient cools down. Patients should be asked whether they have any new or worsening MS symptoms and, if so, how long they have been going on.

MS relapse tends to evolve over the course of 24 hours to a few days. Vascular events, on the other hand, tend to be very abrupt in onset. Inquiring whether the patient has been under a period of undue stress or has not been sleeping well can also be helpful. An exacerbation of symptoms during a period of infection, often urinary tract infection, is considered a pseudorelapse. Urinary tract or other infections can worsen previous symptoms such as optic neuritis. Infections, even if a patient is afebrile, can cause worsening of underlying disease activity. Patients may have increase in symptoms such as spasticity and present to a physician's office, and this could be due to infection.

Many patients may not present with typical symptoms of dysuria, so urinalysis is recommended during suspected relapse. Discerning the presence of a urinary tract or any underlying infection is vital since initiating steroid treatments when there is an underlying infection is unnecessary and risks worsening the underlying condition. However, if symptoms persist even when the infection clears, especially if symptoms are interfering with daily activities, then this would be true relapse that would require acute treatment, usually with steroids.[1] A typical steroid course for treatment is Solu-Medrol 1 g administered intravenously over 1 to 2 hours daily for 3 to 5 days. If no underlying infection is present and there is worsening of neurologic symptoms, referral to neurologist should be made. See Figure 5.1 for algorithm for MS relapse management. Although there is no guarantee that treatment with steroids will bring about complete recovery from a relapse, they do tend to expedite recovery. Occasionally, a second course of steroids may be needed. Steroid taper is usually not needed. The effects of a relapse can last days, weeks, or even months before improvement is seen. Magnetic resonance imaging (MRI) of the brain with gadolinium contrast at the time of relapse will often show areas of acute inflammation.

Malignancies in MS

In recent years, patients with MS are getting diagnosed earlier and initiating treatment with DMTs. These treatments are not without their drawbacks; in addition to the close monitoring required with the DMTs, concerns arise about an increased risk of malignancy with immunosuppressive therapies. This is especially a concern in MS patients that have been diagnosed with

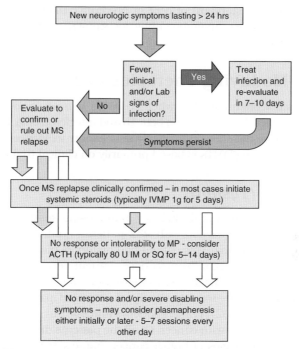

Figure 5.1. Flow chart showing the algorithm for multiple sclerosis (MS) relapse management. Adapted by permission from Springer: Berkovich R. Treatment of acute relapses in multiple sclerosis. *Neurotherapeutics.* 2013;10(1):97-105. Copyright © 2012 The American Society for Experimental NeuroTherapeutics, Inc.

cancer: Does the diagnosis mean they need to stop their DMT's?[2] Are there any DMT's that patients may need to avoid if they have history of cancer? And finally, is there a higher incidence of cancer in MS patients?

A review was done by Marrie et al,[3] utilizing PUBMED, SCOPUS, Web of Knowledge, and EMBASE databases to investigate incidence and prevalence of cancer in persons with MS. Although the findings were inconsistent, the review demonstrated that risk of any cancer was most often reported to be lower in MS than in the general population. If anything, the incidence of meningioma and urinary system cancer appeared to be slightly higher than expected; however, this finding could be a result of the increased number of brain MRIs done as part of MS disease monitoring and findings from referrals to urologists because of urinary tract issues common to MS.[3]

Oftentimes, once patients are diagnosed with MS, they have been known to neglect their general medical care and assume that many symptoms may be related to MS. MS patients are typically not immune deficient, and there has not been increased cancer risk seen in the disease itself.[2] As patients age, however, there can be increased malignancy risk, so it is important to follow established standard of care of preventive maintenance, such as screening colonoscopies, mammography for women, and prostate-specific antigen testing for men.

Disease-Modifying Therapies and Malignancies

Another question often asked is whether DMTs increase cancer risk. The interferon therapies, both interferon beta 1b and interferon beta 1a, and glatiramer acetate have not shown any increase in cancer incidence. Information regarding the following DMTs is based primarily on clinical trial information:

Natalizumab (Tysabri)

In the NAtalizumab Safety and EFFIcacy in Relapsing Remitting MS clinical trial of Tysabri versus placebo with 932 patients studied, 1 patient died from malignant melanoma. This patient had history of melanoma and noted a skin lesion after first natalizumab dose. Patient received a total of five doses before melanoma diagnosis. Six cases of cancer were noted in the AFFIRM trial. Five cases were in the Tysabri-treated patients and one in placebo. Five out of the 627 Tyasbri patients and one out of the 315 placebo patients were diagnosed with cancer. Of all the patients diagnosed with cancer, there were three cases of breast cancer, one cervical cancer, and one new malignant melanoma. There has not been any increased cancer signal seen in postmarketing surveillance, and no increased screening requirements are required for patients on natalizumab.[4,5]

Fingolimod (Gilenya)

In the clinical trial of fingolimod versus placebo with 281 patients studied, 189 received treatment for the full 24 months. During the core study, one basal cell and one squamous cell carcinoma were reported in the fingolimod group.[6] The patient with basal cell carcinoma had a history of multiple skin lesions. During the extension phase of the trial, one case of basal cell carcinoma was reported in the placebo-fingolimod group. Among all reported clinical trials, basal cell carcinoma was reported in 2% of patients receiving fingolimod.[7] A potential increased risk of basal cell carcinoma has been added to the fingolimod prescribing label. A skin examination before initiation of treatment is recommended and should be repeated yearly.

Ocrelizumab (Ocrevus)

In ocrelizumab clinical trials, six cases of breast cancer were reported. None were seen in the placebo-treated patients. There has not been any increased postmarketing signal noted since the drug became approved in 2017. No additional screening is recommended.[8]

Alemtuzumab (Lemtrada)

Alemtuzumab may increase the risk of **thyroid cancer**. In clinical trials, three of 919 (0.3%) Lemtrada-treated patients developed thyroid cancer. This may have been related to increased vigilance and screening during clinical trial protocol. Two additional instances of thyroid cancer were noted in uncontrolled studies. Patients and clinicians are encouraged to monitor for any lumps or swellings in the neck, persistent hoarseness, voice changes, trouble swallowing, and any persistent cough not related to underlying upper respiratory tract infection. Greater concern with alemtuzumab is secondary thyroid autoimmunity, which can occur in approximately 34% of alemtuzumab-treated patients.[9] Patients on alemtuzumab are also recommended to have baseline and yearly general skin checks to monitor for skin cancer. In uncontrolled studies, four of 1486 (0.3%) alemtuzumab-treated patients developed **melanoma** or melanoma in situ.

Cases of lymphoma and lymphoproliferative disorders have occurred in alemtuzumab-treated patients. Careful consideration has to be given regarding initiating therapy with alemtuzumab with anyone who has any preexisting or existing cancer.[9] Yearly dermatologic screening for all patients on DMT is generally recommended as good medical practice.

Comorbidities

Comorbidity is the occurrence of one or more other diseases in individuals with an index disease, in this case, MS.[10] MS is a chronic illness often associated with escalating disability over time that impacts an individual's quality of life and ability to function independently.[11] Many medical conditions can often be present concurrently with MS and can impact disease activity. Recognizing comorbidities and treating them appropriately can improve outcomes of patients with MS. As we will discuss, there are worsened disease outcomes when MS is complicated by comorbid conditions. As new treatment options become available, MS patients are able to live longer with the disease. This presents a challenge to internists treating MS because they must discern whether MS, part of the normal aging process, or an underlying comorbidity causes symptoms.

Although there is a need for further investigation into the incidence of comorbidities in MS, a review of existing studies found that the comorbidities with the highest incidence noted were cancer, hypertension, and stroke, and those with the highest prevalence were depression, anxiety, hypertension, hyperlipidemia, and chronic lung disease.[12] As this study was based on information from mostly North America and Western Europe, there is a need for data regarding comorbidity in MS populations of Africa and Central or South America. The potential role of underlying comorbidities remains a challenge for physicians and researchers alike, owing to the heterogeneous outcomes of patients with MS. Other factors contributing to the difficulty of discerning MS symptoms from other comorbidities are the frequency of relapse rate, age at onset, and initial presenting neurological symptoms. Comorbidities can lead to diagnostic delays, can increase disability, and have an impact on quality of life, mortality, and cognition.[13,14] Given the complexity of comorbidities in MS, collaboration between physicians from relevant specialties is essential to improving patient outcomes.

Impact of Medical Comorbidities on Multiple Sclerosis Activity

Management of medical comorbidities is important not only for overall good medical health and quality of life, but also can prevent the rate at which a patient relapses. Kowalec et al showed that high comorbidity burden (three or more conditions) such as hypertension, depression, and hyperlipidemia can increase relapse rate activity in MS patients.[15] Migraine was also associated with an increase in relapse rate. As conditions like hypertension and diabetes are seen more frequently in the aging MS population, close monitoring is required to optimize medical treatment, with the goal of minimizing, or preventing, hospitalizations. The internist should assure that the patient is being effectively counseled and managed to try to achieve healthy weight, optimal diet, and exercise regimen.

A retrospective electronic medical review study looking at influence of hypertension, diabetes, obstructive lung disease, and hyperlipidemia showed that patients with three comorbidities had slower walking abilities and self-reported worse outcomes compared with those who did not have these coexisting conditions.[16] Analysis of patients from the North American Research Committee on MS (NARCOMS) registry showed that the presence of 1 vascular comorbidity at the time of MS diagnosis was associated with a 51% increased risk of early gait disability, and the presence of 2 comorbidities was associated with a 228% increased risk of ambulatory disability.[16]

Existence of Comorbidities Can Impact Treatment Initiation

Studies have shown the greater the number of comorbidities a patient has, the less likely they are to initiate a DMT.[14] Considering what we know about the importance of initiating therapy early to slow the progression of disability, this delay can be significant. Presence of comorbidities can also impact adherence to therapy once initiated, for example, there is strong evidence demonstrating that MS patients with underlying migraines could experience migraine worsening if the patient is treated with interferon beta.[17] This often necessitates a shift in DMT to another therapy that would help reduce migraines but be less effective in combating MS progression. Comorbidities can also worsen underlying MS symptoms.[18] In particular, pain and fatigue can be exacerbated by a comorbid condition. Rheumatoid arthritis, inflammatory bowel disease, migraine, chronic obstructive pulmonary disease, hypertension, autoimmune thyroid disease, and depression have been associated with increased pain complaints.[19]

When evaluating patients with preexisting comorbidities who present with new symptoms of potential neurologic origin, the nonneurologist must investigate whether the new symptom is due to the preexisting disease or new diagnosis. Consider a patient with diabetes who presents with sensory symptoms; these may be related to diabetic neuropathy or MS disease progression, and determining the origin of these symptoms is critical for treatment.

Communication between neurologists and other medical specialties may help to avoid drug-drug interactions and adverse events such as hospitalization. As essential as it is to make an accurate MS diagnosis and begin an appropriate DMT, preventing and managing comorbidities can be equally important in slowing the progression of disability. The greater the number of comorbidities a patient has, the more likely they are to switch from their first DMT therapy and less likely they are to remain on DMT that may be most effective at preventing MS progression.[20]

Comorbidities Can Increase Mortality

Compared with the general population, mortality in MS is increased, with a life expectancy on average 10 years shorter.[21] It stands to reason that the addition of comorbidities has the potential to further decrease life expectancy.[21] One Canadian study found ischemic heart disease, depression, diabetes, and lung comorbidities to increase mortality in MS.[22] Managing underlying comorbidities, treating depression and anxiety are challenges often faced by internists caring for MS patients.[13] Counseling on smoking cessation is also often a challenge, but very important as smoking has been shown to contribute to disability progression.

Comorbidities Can Affect Disability

Several cross sectional studies have suggested that an increase in comorbidities correlates to an increase in disability. For example, one study examining cardiovascular risk scores in MS found a direct relationship between the Framingham General Cardiovascular Disease Risk Score and MS severity scale.[23] The NARCOMS had suggested that increased vascular comorbidities such as heart disease and diabetes increased risk of walking difficulties.[16]

Lifestyle Choices Affect Disease Progression

Neurologists, MS specialists, and other nonneurological specialists must coordinate to formulate a treatment approach, the ultimate objective being overall wellness. Diet has proven to play an important role in symptom severity and disability. Diet and exercise have been associated with decreased disability and also decrease in symptoms such as fatigue, depression, and pain.[19] Maintaining a healthy diet can contribute to the slowing of disease progression. A recent study found an increase in lesions on MRI imaging in MS patients with hyperlipidemia.[24,25] It is essential to encourage and educate patients about the benefits of optimal health behaviors, such as smoking cessation, maintaining a healthy weight and physical activity benefits. Some of the health measures important in MS management include smoking cessation, normalizing vitamin D levels, maintaining healthy body weight (with BMI < 25), encouraging a diet high in fruits and vegetables and whole grains and low in sugar and red meat, exercise, and social stimulation.[24,26] Smoking is particularly injurious, given the effects it can have not only on MS disability but many common comorbid vascular conditions such as hypertension and heart disease. Identification of comorbidities, increasing patient awareness of the severity and need for treatment of these diseases, and coordinating with the primary care doctor can have a positive impact on health-related outcomes.[27] An example of a patient case study where interdisciplinary coordination improved overall level of functioning is the following.

A 44-year-old woman, with a history of relapsing MS, who although had been relapse free while being treated with Tysabri, became John Cunningham virus antibody positive, and decision was made to switch to rituximab. She was experiencing severe frequent migraines, occurring at least 15 times monthly. She also had history of chronic low-back pain which had led her to become dependent on narcotic medications. Depression was also present in part due to chronic pain and decreased ability to function. Sleep was impaired and this was contributing to increase in day time fatigue. She was unable to work. To best manage this patient, a multi-pronged approach was necessary. She was switched to rituximab for her DMT and has responded well. She has no new MRI lesions or relapses. For her lower back pain, physical therapy was recommended and she was also referred to pain specialist who did try epidural injections to decrease pain but what did eventually provide patient with significant overall pain relief was the use of medicinal marijuana. She was able to eliminate use of narcotics and other anticonvulsant medications she had taken for pain relief such as gabapentin. Magnesium supplement helped with nighttime cramping that she experienced. She was referred to psychiatry who treated her with low-dose venlafaxine for depression. Botox injections have been used for chronic migraine, and these are significantly improved. She has resumed part time work and is also doing yoga, which has been beneficial for her back pain. Regarding vaccinations, she received Shingrix first dose 4 weeks before rituximab infusion.

In the next chapter, we will have greater discussion of vaccination use in MS patients and the various DMTs and their monitoring requirements.

References

1. Olek MJ, Howard J. *Treatment of Acute Exacerbations of Multiple Sclerosis in Adults.* In: Dashe JF, ed. Wolters Kluwer; 2018 (19). https://www.uptodate.com/contents/treatment-of-acute-exacerbations-of-multiple-sclerosis-in-adults?-search=multiple%20sclerosis%20relapse&source=search_result&selectedTitle=1~99&usage_type=default&display_rank=1. Accesed November 10, 2018.
2. Nielsen NM, Rostgaard K, Rasmussen S, et al. Cancer risk among patients with multiple sclerosis: a population based register study. *Int J Cancer.* 2006;118:979-984.
3. Marrie RA, Reider N, Cohen J, et al. Systematic review of the incidence and prevalence of cancer in multiple sclerosis. *Mult Scler J.* 2014;21(3):294-304.
4. Tysabri (Natalizumab). Biogen. 2018. https://www.tysabri.com/?cid=PPC-GGL-TY.DTC.Tysabri_DTC_Branded_Phrase.Phrase-NA-19104&gclid=EAIaIQobC hMI5qr74aLV3gIVxFqGCh0oFAH4EAAYASAAEgI1PPD_BwE&gclsrc=aw.ds. Accessed November 14, 2018.
5. Polman CH, O'Connor PW, Havrdova E, et al. A randomized, placebo-controlled trial of natalizumab for relapsing multiple sclerosis. *NEJM.* 2006;354(9):899-910.
6. Oconnor P, Comi G, Montalban X, et al. Oral fingolimod (FTY720) in multiple sclerosis: two-year results of a phase II extension study. *Neurology.* 2009;72(1):73-79. doi:10.1212/01.wnl.0000338569.32367.3d.
7. Olek MJ. *Disease-Modifying Treatment of Relapsing-Remitting Multiple Sclerosis in Adults.* In: Dashe JF, ed. Wolters Kluwer; 2018 (84). https://www.uptodate.com/contents/disease-modifying-treatment-of-relapsing-remitting-multiple-sclerosis-in-adults?search=copaxone&source=search_result&selectedTitle=2~15&usage_type=default&display_rank=1. Accessed November 10, 2018.
8. Ocrevus (Ocrelizumab). Genentech. 2018. https://www.ocrevus.com/hcp.html?cid=ocr_PS_MNOVMSH0396_14&c=MNOVMSH0396&gclid=EAIaIQobChMIzKuqa TV3gIVCVqGCh3jzgR0EAAYASAAEgLEdfD_BwE&gclsrc=aw.ds. Accessed November 14, 2018.
9. Lemtrada (Alemtuzumab). Genzyme. 2018. https://www.lemtradahcp.com/?s_mcid=ps-LP-google-BRinfo-BRsafety-BROfficialSite. Accessed November 14, 2018.
10. Gijsen R, Hoeymans N, Schellevis FG, Ruwaard D, Satariano WA, van Den Bos GAM. Causes and consequences of comorbidity: a review. *J Clin Epidemiol.* 2001:54:661-674.
11. Marrie RA, Horvitz R, Cutter G, Tyry T, Campagnolo D, Vollmer T. Comorbidity, socioeconomic status and multiple sclerosis. *Mult Scler.* 2008;14:1091-1098.
12. Marrie RA, Reider N, Cohen J, et al. A systematic review of the incidence and prevalence of sleep disorders and seizure disorders in multiple sclerosis. *Mult Scler.* 2015;21:342-349.
13. Marrie RA. Comorbidity in multiple sclerosis: implications for patient care. *Nat Rev Neurol.* 2017;13:375-382.

14. Zhang T, Tremlett H, Leung S, et al. Examining the effects of comorbidities on disease modifying therapies in multiple sclerosis. *Neurology.* 2016;86:1287-1295.
15. Kowalec K, McKay K, Patten S, et al. Comorbidity increases the risk of relapse in multiple sclerosis. *Neurology.* 2017;89:2455-2461.
16. Marrie RA, Rudick R, Horwitz R, et al. Vascular comorbidity is associated with more rapid disability progression in multiple sclerosis: overview. *Mult Scler.* 2015;21(3):263-281.
17. Villani V, Prosperini L, De Giglio L, Pozzilli C, Salvetti M, Sette G. The impact of interferon beta and natalizumab on comorbid migraine in multiple sclerosis. *Headache.* 2012;52(7):1130-1135. doi: 10.1111/j.1526-4610.2012.02146.x. PubMed PMID: 22486199.
18. Laroni A, Signori A, Maniscalco G, et al. Assessing association of comorbidities with treatment choice, and persistence in MS. *Neurology.* 2017;89:2222-2229.
19. Feist KM, Fisk JD, Patten SB, et al. Comorbidity is associated with pain related activity limitations in multiple sclerosis. *Mult Scler Relat Disord.* 2015;4:470-476.
20. Fitzgerald KC, Tyry T, Salter A, et al. Diet quality is associated with disability and symptom severity in multiple sclerosis. *Neurology.* 2017;90(1):e1-e11.
21. Thorman A, Sorenson P, Koch-Hendriksen N, Laursen B, Magyar M. Comorbidity in MS is associated with diagnostic delays and increased mortality. *Neurology.* 2017;89:1668-1675.
22. Marrie RA, Elliott L, Marriott J, et al. Effect of comorbidity on mortality in multiple sclerosis. *Neurology.* 2015;85:240-247.
23. Moccia M, Lanzillo R, Palladino R, et al. The Framingham cardiovascular risk score in multiple sclerosis. *Eur J Neurol.* 2015;22(8):1176-1183. doi: 10.1111/ene.12720. PubMed PMID: 25912468.
24. Conway DS, Thompson NR, Cohen JA. Influence of hypertension, diabetes, hyperlipedmia, and obstructive lung disease on multiple sclerosis disease course. *Mult Scler.* 2017;23:277-285.
25. Weinstock-Guttman B, Ziavadinov R, Mahfooz N, et al. Serum lipid profiles are associated with disability and MRI outcomes in multiple sclerosis. *J Neuroinflammation.* 2011:8:127.
26. Fitzgerald KC, Tyry T, Salter A, et al. Diet quality is associated with disability and symptom severity in multiple sclerosis. *Neurology.* 2018;90(1):e1-e11.
27. Moss BP, Rensel MR, Hersh CM. Wellness and the role of comorbidities in multiple sclerosis. *Neurotherapeutics.* 2017;14:999-1017.

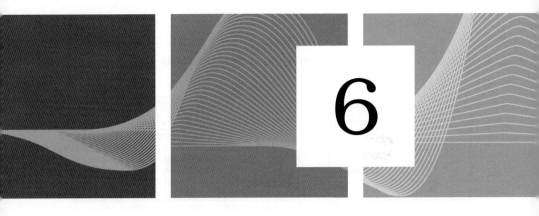

Internal Medicine II: Disease-Modifying Therapies and Adverse Effects

■ ▓ ▒ Mary Ann Picone, Constantine J. Pella

Introduction

Disease-modifying therapies (DMTs) are at the forefront of treatment for the progression of multiple sclerosis (MS). It is important for the internist and nonneurologist to understand the administration of DMTs and the adverse effects and infection risks associated with some of the newer DMTs. For more information on the mechanism of action of DMTs, please refer to the Immunology chapter.

As you can see from Figure 6.1, there are multiple DMTs available now with different mechanisms of actions. Table 6.1 shows the stratification of the different therapies organized by efficacy. These are approved for relapsing forms of MS, and ocrelizumab is approved also for primary progressive MS. The challenge in choosing treatment is trying to do the best to individualize treatment for a heterogeneous disease. Choosing the optimal individualized treatment regimen involves evaluating patient lifestyle, comorbidities, support system, benefits and risks of treatment, timing of pregnancy, and prognostic disease profile and encouraging the patient to

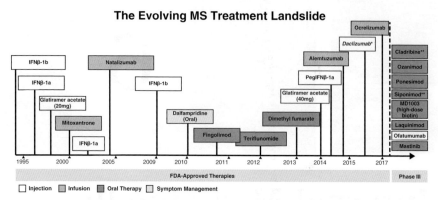

Figure 6.1. Time plot showing the evolution of different disease-modifying therapies for the treatment of MS. *Voluntary withdrawal from market announced March 2018. Republished with permission of Intellisphere, LLC from Owens GM. Managed care aspects of managing multiple sclerosis. *Am J Manag Care.* 2013;19 (16 Suppl):s307-s312; permission conveyed through Copyright Clearance Center, Inc. See eBook for color figure. **Recently received FDA approval March 2019.

have realistic expectations of what the therapies can do. Although none of the treatments are cures, the goal is to achieve as close to what is referred to as NEDA, no evidence of disease activity. This refers to no new activity noted on magnetic resonance imaging (MRI), no relapses, and no clinical disease progression. Considering the higher-efficacy agents available today, there is a lower threshold to keep a patient on a therapy that may be suboptimal. It is important that patients are followed closely, particularly early on in the disease course and when new therapies are initiated to monitor for efficacy and adverse events. We have no biomarkers at present to predict which patients will respond to a certain therapy; however, neurofilament light protein is a proposed biomarker for MS disease activity and treatment response. This is a structural component of neurons and axons. Neurofilaments are released into the cerebrospinal fluid (CSF) after axonal injury. Levels increase during relapse, and initial CSF levels may help to predict disease course. These are still investigational at this point.

Injections

Copaxone (Glatiramer Acetate)

This is an immunomodulator used for patients with relapsing-remitting MS. It consists of the acetate salts of synthetic polypeptides, containing four naturally occurring amino acids: L-glutamic acid, L-alanine, L-tyrosine, and L-lysine. Designed to mimic a protein in myelin, Copaxone binds to major histocompatibility complex molecules and competes with myelin antigens for T cells, which induces specific suppressor cells of

TABLE 6.1
VARIOUS DISEASE-MODIFYING TREATMENTS (DMTS)
STRATIFIED BY EFFICACY

DMT	Route of Administration	Dosage	Monitoring	Adverse Effects
Low Efficacy				
Interferon-ß (Betaseron, Extavia, Rebif, Avonex, Plegridy)	SC/IM	Depends on type of interferon therapy	Every 6 mo: CBC, LFTs Every 12 mo: TSH	Injection site reaction, flulike symptoms, headache, lymphopenia, hepatotoxicity, depression, spasticity
Glatiramer acetate (Copaxone)	SC	20 mg/mL daily or 40 mg/ mL twice a week (~48 h apart)	–	Immediate postinjection reaction, uncommon idiosyncratic reaction, lipoatrophy
Teriflunomide (Aubagio)	PO	7.0 and 14.0 mg daily	Once per month for 1st 6 months LFTs Every 6 mo: CBC, LFTs	Diarrhea, nausea, alopecia, bone marrow suppression, hepatotoxicity, peripheral neuropathy, teratogenicity
Medium Efficacy				
Dimethyl fumarate (Tecfidera)	PO	Titrated up from 120 mg twice a day to 240 mg twice a day	Every 6 mo: CBC, LFTs	Dyspepsia, nausea, vomiting, abdominal pain, diarrhea, flushing, PML
Fingolimod (Gilenya)	PO	0.5 mg daily	In 3 mo: repeat CBC with diff, LFTs, Macula Eval. Every 6 mo: LFTs, CBC with diff	Headache, hypertension, transaminitis, lymphopenia, HSV, macular edema, bradycardia, PML, dermatological cancers

(Continued)

TABLE 6.1

VARIOUS DISEASE-MODIFYING TREATMENTS (DMTS) STRATIFIED BY EFFICACY   (CONTINUED)

DMT	Route of Administration	Dosage	Monitoring	Adverse Effects
High Efficacy				
Natalizumab (Tysabri)	IV	300 mg every 4 wk	Every 3 months, CBC with diff, LFTS. Every 6 mo: JCV Ab, MRI. After 6 mo: natalizumab neutralizing antibodies	Infusion reactions, hepatotoxicity, PML, HSV, encephalitis, headache
Alemtuzumab (Lemtrada)	IV	12 mg/d 5 consecutive days followed by 12 mg/d for 3 consecutive days 1 y later	Every 3 mo: TSH. Yearly skin examination, GYN, MRI	Secondary autoimmunity, infusion reactions, malignancies, infections, pneumonitis
Ocrelizumab (Ocrevus)	IV	600 mg every 6 mo[a]	Hepatitis B screen before use, yearly MRI	Infusion reactions, reactivation of hepatitis B and tuberculosis, possible malignancy, PML, upper respiratory infections

Adapted with permission from Mahajan KR, Rae-Grant A. New American Academy of Neurology Disease-Modifying Treatment Guidelines: Impact on Clinical Practice. In: Practical Neurology. Bryn Mawr Communications III, LLC; 2018;17(6):22-27.

Patients are premedicated with IV solumedrol or an equivalent corticosteroid and an antihistamine before the infusion.

APC, antigen presenting cells; BUN, blood urea nitrogen; CBC, complete blood count; CNS, central nervous system; Cr, creatinine; ECG, electrocardiography; GYN, gynecological screening for HPV; HSV, herpes simplex virus; IM, intramuscular; IV, intravenous; JCV, John Cunningham virus; LFT, liver function test; MRI, magnetic resonance imaging; OCT, optical coherence tomography; PML, progressive multifocal leukoencephalopathy; PO, orally, dihydro-orotate dehydrogenase; SC, subcutaneous; TSH, thyroid stimulating hormone; UA, urine analysis.

the T helper 2 (Th2) type that migrate to the brain where they express the anti-inflammatory cytokines interleukin 10 and transforming growth factor beta, in addition to brain-derived neurotrophic factor.[1] Recent evidence suggests that Copaxone directly inhibits dendritic cells and monocytes, both of which are circulating antigen-presenting cells.[7] There is no required blood work monitoring with Copaxone.

Interferon

Interferons as a class need to have complete blood count (CBC) with differential and liver function profile monitored generally every 6 months. Depression has been reported with interferons, although in clinical trials versus noninterferon therapy, no increased risk of depression was noted in patients treated with interferon. Flulike symptoms are the most common side effects, but dose titration can help to mitigate flulike symptoms. Injection-site reactions can also be seen, particularly with subcutaneous injections. Seizures have also been reported in patients given interferon therapy. Dosing with interferons (for adults) varies based on the brand:

1. **Interferon beta-1b (Betaseron, Extavia)**: Initial: 0.0625 mg every other day, increase dose by 0.0625 mg every 2 weeks to target dose of 0.25 mg every other day.[2]
2. **Interferon beta-1a**
   a. **Avonex:** 30 µg administered intramuscularly once weekly or 7.5 µg once weekly to reduce flulike side effects, increasing dose in increments of 7.5 µg once weekly till target dose of 30 µg a week is reached.
   b. **Rebif:** Target dose either 22 or 44 µg administered subcutaneously three times weekly.[3]
   c. **Plegridy:** A pegylated version of Avonex that allows for longer-lasting binding to interferon receptor sites; thus, this only needs to be administered subcutaneously twice monthly. Initial dose 63 µg on day 1, 94 µg on day 15. Maintenance 125 µg every 14 days beginning on day 29.[4]

Oral Therapies

Aubagio (Teriflunomide)

As the active metabolite of leflunomide, it acts as an immunomodulatory agent by inhibiting pyrimidine synthesis and disrupts T cells from interacting with antigen-presenting cells.[5] It is approved for the treatment of relapsing forms of MS in adults and is available in 7- and 14-mg doses. No titration is needed. Side effects include hair thinning, abdominal pain, diarrhea, and often soft stools. Liver enzymes have to be monitored monthly for the first 6 months and then periodically thereafter. Aubagio can cause increased blood pressure, and although this is not considered a contraindication for use of the drug, patients with a history of high blood pressure should be monitored closely.[5] If a patient needs to stop the drug abruptly because of tolerability issues or pregnancy considerations, an elimination procedure can be undertaken with the use of cholestyramine or activated charcoal to quickly decrease serum levels of Aubagio.[5] Pediatric use is being evaluated in clinical trials.

Gilenya (Fingolimod)

This is a sphingosine 1-phosphate receptor modulator indicated and approved for the treatment of relapsing forms of MS.[6] It binds to sphingosine receptors to block the egress of lymphocytes (B cells, central memory and naïve T cells) from lymphoid tissue, reducing the number of lymphocytes in peripheral blood. Gilenya does not destroy lymphocytes but does sequester them in lymphoid tissue; thus, CBC testing will demonstrate lymphopenia, often with absolute lymphocyte counts below $0.2 \times 10^9/L$.[7] This is an expected finding. Within 8 weeks of discontinuation of fingolimod, lymphocyte counts usually return to the normal range, but CD4 and CD8 central memory cells decrease and remain decreased over time. It was recently approved for pediatric use.

There are some concerns relating to fingolimod adverse reactions that should be noted by the internist. Bradycardia and atrioventricular (AV) block can occur. Six-hour first-dose electrocardiogram (EKG) monitoring is required for Gilenya for monitoring of bradycardia and risk of first-degree AV block at the initiation of dosing and at the 6-hour mark, along with hourly blood pressure and heart rate monitoring.[6] Ophthalmological evaluation before the first dose, 3 to 4 months after therapy initiation, and yearly thereafter for macular edema is also required.

There is an increased risk of macular edema if the patient has underlying diabetes or uveitis. If noted, macular edema is reversed once Gileny is discontinued.[7] Gilenya can elevate liver enzymes; thus, patients need to have liver enzymes monitored periodically. Progressive multifocal leukoencephalopathy (PML) cases have been reported with Gilenya, not thought to be related to lymphopenia.[8] The age of the patient may play a role in increased PML risk. Other opportunistic infections also have occurred; these include pulmonary tuberculosis (TB), asymptomatic pulmonary cryptococcus, and cutaneous cryptococcus, and also a case of disseminated cryptococcus, ocular and cerebral toxoplasmosis, visceral leishmaniasis, Kaposi sarcoma, and Merkel cell carcinoma.

Respiratory and herpetic infections also can occur. If patients have frequent herpetic infections, they may not be ideal candidates for Gilenya use; however, there can be consideration of maintaining the patient on low-dose acyclovir or famvir while on Gilenya. Drug-drug interactions between Gilenya and other medications that have the potential to prolong QT interval have to be considered. The following is not an exhaustive list but includes some of the more frequently used classes of drugs that can prolong QT interval and should be avoided with Gilenya use[6]:

- **Antimicrobials:** Levofloxacin, ciprofloxacin, erythromycin, keto-conazole, azithromycin, chloroquine, clarithromycin, fluconazole, moxi-floxacine, pentamidine
- **Antidepressants:** Amitriptyline, desipramine, imipramine, fluoxetine, sertraline, venlafaxine, escitalopram, citalopram
- **Antipsychotics:** Haloperidol, quetiapine, chlorpromazine, thioridazine
- **Others:** Sumatriptan, zolmitriptan, methadone, ondansetron, propofol, donepezil, droperidol
- **Antiarrhythmics:** Amiodarone, quinidine, procainamide

Tecfidera (Dimethyl Fumarate)

Tecfidera is indicated for relapsing forms of MS. It is a twice-daily oral medication, recommended usually to be taken with breakfast and dinner. In the 2-year DEFINE trial, comparing Tecfidera with placebo, there was a 49% relative risk reduction of relapses compared with placebo.[9] Taking Tecfidera with food decreases flushing and abdominal pain. Flushing and abdominal pain seen with Tecfidera are most common within the first month of use and then significantly decrease thereafter. Non-enteric-coated aspirin before dosing also decreases flushing. CBC with differential and liver function tests (LFTs) should be drawn before Tecfidera use and repeated at least every 6 months. If someone has a serious infection, then it is important to hold treatment with Tecfidera until infection is resolved.

In the clinical trials, mean lymphocyte counts decreased about 30% during the first year of treatment. If lymphocyte count is less than 500 and persists greater than 6 months, then the drug should be discontinued. Repeat lymphocyte testing should be performed until counts return to normal. Tecfidera should not be used during pregnancy or breastfeeding. If anyone does become pregnant while taking Tecfidera, she should discontinue treatment and enroll in Tecfiderapregnancyregistry.com. Increased LFTs have been observed with Tecfidera, and because of this it is important to check LFTs periodically, on average every 6 months. Tecfidera may cause liver injury. PML cases have been seen with Tecfidera and seem to be associated with lower lymphocyte counts. Infections other than PML appear to be rare with Tecfidera.

Monoclonal Antibodies (Infusion Therapies)

Lemtrada (Alemtuzumab)

This is a monoclonal antibody given in two treatment cycles. Year 1 it is administered 5 days in a row and then year 2, 3 days in a row. Lemtrada targets the CD52 molecule expressed on T and B leukocytes. Because intravenous administration of Lemtrada causes lysis of these cells, infusion reactions can occur as a result of these cells being depleted, causing cytokine release syndrome. Pretreatment with steroids and antihistamines helps to decrease these reactions. Once the immune system starts to reconstitute, secondary autoimmunity can occur. Monthly CBC with differential to monitor for autoimmune thrombocytopenia, and urinalysis and serum creatinine to monitor for Goodpasture syndrome, is required monthly up to 4 years after the last infusion. The urine protein to creatinine ratio needs to be obtained before starting the drug and at periodic intervals up to 48 months after last infusion. Thyroid function testing is required every 3 months. Human immunodeficiency virus testing before starting the drug is also required by the US Food and Drug Administration (FDA). Hepatitis B and hepatitis C carriers who receive Lemtrada may be at risk of irreversible liver damage relative to potential virus reactivation. Yearly skin examination is also required because of increased risk of melanoma. Annual HPV screening is recommended for women. Before starting Lemtrada the following tests are recommended:

- TB screen
- Varicella zoster titer
- CBC with differential
- Urinalysis
- Thyroid function profile
- Serum creatinine
- Urine protein to creatinine ratio

If a woman is of childbearing potential, it is important to make sure that she is not pregnant before initiating treatment. Contraceptive therapy is recommended, and patients should not try to get pregnant for at least 6 months after Lemtrada infusion. Anyone who has any active infection should not proceed with the infusion but should wait until the infection is cleared before treating. Tattoos also should be avoided for at least 8 weeks after infusion to help prevent infection. Acyclovir must be given at the start of treatment and continued for at least 2 months. If the CD4 count is still below 200 at that time, acyclovir needs to be continued until the count is 200 or above. Regarding lymphopenia, even though repopulation of cells occurs, 20% of patients had below normal lymphocyte counts after 12 months. The following are certain infections and other safety precautions with Lemtrada that should be recognized:

- **Acute acalculous cholecystitis** was seen in eight patients who received Lemtrada for relapsing MS. Seven developed acute acalculous cystitis during or shortly after receiving Lemtrada, and one person developed it 6 to 7 weeks after infusion. Frequency of this risk is estimated at 0.2%[10]

- **Acute coronary syndrome** is possible. A young otherwise healthy woman developed cardiac ischemia midway through a Lemtrada infusion. The mechanism may have been related to increased endothelial and myocyte membrane permeability and vasodilation via cytokine release syndrome and could lead to an increased demand and ischemia of the myocardium. This underscores the need for monitoring of vital signs during infusion and vigilance for potential cardiac events. EKG monitoring at this point is not required but may be up to the discretion of the treating neurologist[11]

- **Listeria** was first reported with Lemtrada use in 2008.Dietary precautions are important to emphasize to patients, particularly avoiding uncooked meats and fish, unpasteurized soft cheeses, dairy products, and juices for at least 4 months after infusion. The risk of *Listeria* meningitis is the highest in the first month after each Lemtrada cycle. However, owing to the concern that patients may not follow dietary precautions, preventive treatment with sulfamethoxazole-trimethoprim is now recommended in the United Kingdom. If it is unlikely that the patient will be compliant with diet, co-trimoxazole 960 mg three times weekly for 1 month is recommended. If patients are adherent to following a *Listeria*-free diet, another treatment option is 8 days of amoxicillin 1 g three times daily or co-trimoxazole 960 mg twice daily, which would eliminate *Listeria* colonization before treatment

- **Hemophagocytic lymphohistiocytosis** occurred in two patients treated with Lemtrada for leukemia, but this was not seen in MS

- **Pulmonary nocardia beijingensis infection**

- **Pneumonitis**

- **Ischemic and hemorrhagic stroke and cervicocephalic arterial dissection** is a rare but serious complication that can occur shortly after Lemtrada use. Health care providers need to advise patients at every Lemtrada infusion to seek emergency medical attention if they have symptoms of numbness, or weakness, visual symptoms, sudden difficulty with walking or balance, or sudden severe headache or neck pain[12]

Ocrevus (Ocrelizumab)

Ocrevus is a B cell–directed humanized monoclonal antibody, targeting the CD20 antigen expressed on mature B cells. It is the first FDA-approved therapy for primary progressive MS and FDA approved for relapsing forms of MS. It targets pro-B cells in the bone marrow but spares CD20-negative plasma cells that produce antibodies. The main effect of the anti-CD 20 therapy seems to maintain adequate antibody levels but reduces antigen presenting and cytokine secreting functions of B cells. Compared with rituximab, Ocrevus has a higher capacity for direct, antibody-dependent cell toxicity.

In the OPERA study comparing ocrelizumab with interferon beta-1a, the infection rate was 58.4% in the Ocrevus-treated group and 52.4% in the interferon beta-1a group. Main infections noted were upper respiratory tract infections and nasopharyngitis. Most infections were considered mild to moderate. There were no deaths related to infection in OPERA, which analyzed relapsing patients, and in the ORATORIO study, which analyzed progressive patients and compared ocrelizumab with placebo, there were two deaths, due to pneumonia, one of which was aspiration pneumonia, not thought to be related to ocrelizumab. Since ocrelizumab has been FDA approved there have been six cases of PML reported all in patients who had transitioned to Ocrevus from Tysabri who were John Cunningham virus (JCV) antibody positive. Ocrevus can cause reactivation of hepatitis B infection, and hepatitis panel is required before its use.

Tysabri (Natalizumab)

Tysabri is the first monoclonal antibody approved to treat relapsing MS. The mechanism of action includes blocking alpha4 integrin on lymphocytes, decreasing trafficking of lymphocytes into the central nervous system. There are risks of infection when using Tysabri that should be noted. Patients who are taking Tysabri and have positive JCV antibodies have a higher risk of developing PML. The risk is higher for patients who are JCV antibody positive who have been taking Tysabri for longer than 2 years and have been on prior immunosuppressive therapy. Besides being able to detect if a patient is JCV antibody positive, the clinician can use the JCV index to know the exact titer level. For those taking Tysabri for 25 to 36 months without prior immunosuppressive use, the PML risk is 0.2/1000 in those with index of 0.9 or less, 0.3/1000 with index of 0.9 to 1.5, and 3/1000 in those with index greater than 1.5.

Herpes infections have also been reported with natalizumab.[13] An important point to keep in mind is that PML can be mistaken for relapse activity or worsening of underlying MS symptoms and may not be recognized. Sometimes the only change that is noticed is cognitive change or altered mental status, and MRI may be the only way that early changes of PML may be noted, so consistent monitoring and being alert to any change in behavior or function are important. Clinical trials studying extended interval dosing of natalizumab from every 28 days to every 6 weeks to possibly maintain efficacy and decrease risk of PML are ongoing.

Rituxan (Rituximab)

Rituximab is a chimeric monoclonal antibody directed against the CD 20 antigen on B cells (the epitope is different from that of Ocrevus). It is not FDA approved for MS but has been used particularly for patients who have failed other MS therapies and is the standard of care for the treatment of neuromyelitis optica.[14] It is used for the treatment of B cell lymphoma, lymphoproliferative disorders, rheumatoid arthritis, and systemic lupus erythematosus refractory to other treatments. Many of the infections seen with rituximab have occurred in the setting of its use in the treatment of patients with rheumatoid arthritis where it was used in combination with other immunosuppressive therapies, for example, cyclophosphamide or methotrexate. It varies also from ocrelizumab in that rituximab has a greater effect on complement-dependent cytotoxicity than ocrelizumab.

Dalfampridine (Ampyra)

Dalfampridine is not a DMT but is a treatment that is often used as an adjunct for patients who are experiencing walking difficulties. It is a potassium channel blocker that helps to improve conduction along demyelinated nerve fibers. Approximately 33% to 40% of patients are positive responders to the drug, measured in clinical trials by improvement in 25-foot timed walking speed. On average, patients who were positive responders had an approximately 25% improvement in walking speed. This correlated with clinically meaningful quality-of-life measures. The main concern with Ampyra is that patients need to have a creatinine clearance rate above 50. The standard dose is 10 mg twice daily, taken 12 hours apart. Seizures can be a side effect of the medication. A decrease in the creatinine clearance or taking the drug too close together could increase levels of dalfampridine within the blood stream.

So What Will the Future Hold?

Progress is still being made to develop new DMT for the patient with MS. Many potential DMT that are in clinical trials show great potential for future treatment. The following are several of the agents currently in clinical trials:

- Ofatumumab (subcutaneous anti-CD20-directed monoclonal antibody) for relapsing forms of MS
- Ublituximab (intravenous anti-CD20 monoclonal antibody)
- Cladribine, FDA approved March 2019, oral agent, purine antimetabolite, considered cytotoxic. It is administered in two oral yearly treatment courses, causing prolonged lymphopenia. It will generally be recommended for patients who have either tolerability or efficacy failure with prior DMT. It is also contraindicated in patients with chronic infections, HIV, current malignancy and TB. It should not be used during pregnancy or breastfeeding.[40]
- Ozanimod, siponimod (these are both more selective S1P1 receptor agonists). Siponimod recently received FDA approval for use in relapsing and active secondary progressive patients
- Biotin (vitamin B7) is a water-soluble vitamin, currently in phase 3 trial; high-dose biotin 100 mg three times daily for progressive MS. Early studies have shown improvement in slowing disability progression
- Ibudilast—oral phosphodiesterase-4 and 10 inhibitor showed slowing of whole brain atrophy and may be a future treatment for progressive disease
- Therapeutic approaches using autologous hematopoietic stem cells and mesenchymal stem cells are being investigated in clinical trials as MS treatments. To date, the best success has been seen in younger patients with highly active disease. Helpful websites for patients to get information on stem cell research are http://www.iscr.org and http://www.celltherapysociety.org[15]
- Diets to help modulate the gut microbiome and vaccine targeting EBV are also being studied

Vaccinations

Vaccinations play an important role in public health by prevention of communicable illnesses.[16] Benefits of long-term preventive immunity often outweigh risks associated with the vaccine. Infections can often worsen MS symptoms, so vaccinations that help in the prevention of febrile illnesses can decrease infections and minimize relapse risk.[17] Generally, inactivated vaccines that have killed viral components have a low risk versus benefit.[16] Even with these considerations, patients with MS are still often discouraged to get vaccinations.

Two main concerns regarding immunizations are whether they may trigger relapse activity or whether the patient is able to mount a sufficient immune response to the vaccine. Use of the hepatitis B vaccine in France had raised concern of increased risk of MS relapse after this vaccination. The Vaccines in MS Study (VACCIMUS) conducted by Confavareux et al. utilizing the European Database for MS for vaccination history studied tetanus, influenza, and hepatitis B and concluded that vaccinations did not increase the short-term risk of relapse in MS.[18] Mailand and Fredericksen in 2016 conducted a PubMed literature review analyzing the risk of developing MS following vaccinations. The study did not find any change in the development of MS with vaccination against hepatitis B, human papillomavirus (HPV), seasonal influenza, variola, tetanus, measles mumps rubella, polio, diphtheria, or Bacillus Calmette–Guérin (BCG).[19] A case control study conducted by DeStefano et al examining cases of MS or optic neuritis among adults aged 18 to 49 years did not reveal any increased risk of MS exacerbation or optic neuritis following vaccination against hepatitis B, influenza, tetanus, measles, or rubella.[20]

Live Attenuated Vaccines

Live attenuated vaccines are obtained from the virus or bacteria and are weakened in the laboratory. A small dose of the pathogen grows in the immunized host, and antibodies are developed. These are generally not recommended in MS because the vaccine's ability to cause disease has been decreased but the vaccine is not entirely inactivated.[21] Exposure to a family member or child who has had live virus injection and subsequent risk is not certain. The following are examples of live attenuated vaccines.

Measles Mumps Rubella

Adult patients may need to have antibody titers checked. If the titer is low, a booster dose should be given. This vaccine is generally safe when given to patients taking interferon therapies and glatiramer acetate. However, because measles mumps rubella is a live attenuated virus, it is not recommended to be used during treatment with cell-depleting therapies alemtuzumab, ocrelizumab, rituximab, and also fingolimod, dimethyl fumarate, cladribine, and terifluonimide.

Varicella Vaccine

Varicella immunization appears to be safe for patients with MS. Before treatment with fingolimod, if there is no evidence of varicella antibodies, patients are required to have the vaccine, wait 4 weeks, and then start taking fingolimod. All nonimmune adults are recommended to have two doses of the vaccine 4 to 8 weeks apart. Varicella vaccine in general is recommended by the Centers for Disease Control and Prevention (CDC) to be given to people of any age who are seronegative for varicella. If patients have untreated or active TB, they cannot get the vaccine but need to wait until the TB is treated. It is also recommended before alemtuzumab use if patient is IgG antibody negative. Live attenuated vaccine should be given at least 4 weeks before ocrelizumab infusion.

Yellow Fever

Encephalitis and meningitis may occur following the vaccine. Studies have shown an increased risk of relapses following the yellow fever vaccine. Individuals taking immunosuppressant medications should generally not use this vaccine.[19] However, this risk of increased relapses does need to be weighed against the risk of contracting yellow fever, which is potentially fatal.

Generally, it is best to avoid this vaccine unless risk when traveling to an endemic country (South America, Africa) is great.

Bacillus Calmette–Guérin

One small pilot trial had suggested that the BCG vaccine could reduce exacerbation in MS. However, in the United States, the CDC, because of the low risk of *Mycobacterium tuberculosis* infection, does not generally recommend this.

Smallpox Vaccine

This is a live vaccine and is generally not recommended for anyone with MS; however, if there is exposure, then the risk of developing smallpox outweighs the risk of its use.

Other Live Attenuated Vaccines

■ Oral polio
■ Intranasal influenza
■ Oral typhoid-directed against bacteria

Inactivated Vaccines (Killed Microbes)

Inactivated vaccines, or "killed microbes," in general are safer to use than live attenuated vaccines, regardless of what DMT the patient is taking.[21] Oftentimes, repeated doses are given because the immune response generated is weaker. Generally, inactivated vaccines are considered safe to use in patients taking interferon therapies, Aubagio, Copaxone, mitoxantrone, Gilenya, Lemtrada, Tysabri, Tecfidera, Ocrevus, and Rituxan.

The following vaccines are inactivated whole virus vaccines that are accepted for use in patients with MS:

■ **Polio (injection)**
■ **Rabies**
■ **Hepatitis A**
■ **Varicella**

Subunit and Conjugate Vaccines

Subunit vaccines involve microbial antigens that stimulate the immune system. Conjugate vaccines are polysaccharides attached to an antigen to boost efficacy and include conjugate polysaccharide vaccines (*Haemophilus influenza* type B, pneumococcal, meningococcal) and meningococcal quadrivalent conjugate and meningococcal polysaccharide vaccines.

Influenza Vaccination (Seasonal Flu)

Two types of influenza vaccines are commonly used. The first is the inactivated vaccine, which is typically used by most facilities. The second is the live attenuated vaccine (nasal spray). This should be avoided. The National MS Society has stated in its guidelines that the seasonal flu vaccine is considered safe and generally recommended in all patients with MS, regardless of the DMT they are taking. Not only can influenza infection worsen MS disease symptoms but also it is associated with significant morbidity on its own.[22]

The influenza vaccine is particularly recommended for patients with MS who are nonambulatory, wheelchair or bed-bound, use motorized scooters, and have impaired respiratory function[23] and is given on an annual basis. For patients who are taking the cell-depleting therapies Lemtrada and rituximab, the influenza vaccine should be given 6 weeks before the infusion cycle. For Ocrevus, it should be administered at least 2 weeks before infusion. Note that it is only the inactivated flu vaccine (standard dose) that is recommended. More data are needed to make recommendations regarding the high-dose inactivated flu vaccine (Fluzone High-Dose).

The immune response in patients receiving interferon beta-1b/1a and glatiramer acetate was shown to be similar to that of controls in the study done by Olberg.[24] Regarding influenza efficacy with natalizumab use, there have been conflicting studies. One study done by Vagberg et al showed that a humoral immune response to the influenza vaccination was maintained in natalizumab-treated patients, and the study done by Kaufman et al[25] also showed no decrease in immune response in relapsing patients treated with natalizumab. However, a Norwegian study done by Olberg et al evaluated 90 patients who received fingolimod, glatiramer acetate, interferon beta-1a/1b, natalizumab, or no therapy and compared them with 62 healthy controls. Serum samples were collected before vaccination and 3, 6, and 12 months after vaccination. The results showed reduced protection rates with patients treated with natalizumab or fingolimod but not interferon beta-1a/1b or glatiramer, suggesting that patients receiving fingolimod or natalizumab should be considered for a second dose of the flu vaccine.[26]

A vaccine study (study to investigate the immune response to influenza vaccine in patients with multiple sclerosis on teriflunomide) analyzing humoral response rates following teriflunomide use showed effective response, although it slightly decreased with the 14-mg dose. Immune response was also maintained in patients taking Tecfidera. The influenza vaccine is contraindicated in patients who are allergic to eggs. Patients who have an acute febrile illness or active infection should wait until they are infection free before getting the vaccine. If a patient does contract the flu, use of Tamiflu or antivirals such as amantadine may be helpful in decreasing symptoms.

Hepatitis B Vaccine

For the hepatitis B vaccine, there are two to three vaccinations recommended. This is considered safe in MS. The VACCIMUS study group did not find any association between hepatitis B vaccination and increased risk of relapse. The Institute of Medicine study also found no association with the onset of MS disease activity. According to the CDC guidelines, the hepatitis B vaccine is recommended for all children, teenagers, and adults who are at risk of contracting this disease, that is:

- Anyone working in a job that involves contact with human blood
- Anyone with diabetes and under age 60 years
- Anyone living in a house or having sex with someone who has hepatitis B infection
- Anyone having sex with more than one partner
- People who live or travel outside the United States for more than 6 months out of the year
- A 2002 report by the Institute of Medicine did not find any causal relationship between the hepatitis B vaccine and development of MS

Human Papillomavirus Vaccine (Gardasil) Inactivated

This is recommended for males and females for the prevention of genital warts and anal and cervical cancer. There is a three-dose series to the vaccine, the second and third doses given 2 and 6 months from the first dose. In a cohort study utilizing nationwide registries in two Scandinavian countries conducted by Scheller et al,[27] HPV vaccinations were not associated with the development of MS or other demyelinating illness. This study included 3,983,824 females, aged 10 to 44 years, during the years 2006 to 2013, among whom 789,082 received a total of 1,927,581 HPV vaccine doses. This study added to the body of data supporting a favorable overall safety profile of the HPV vaccine. There was one case report,[28] however, of acute disseminated encephalomyelitis following the second immunization with Gardasil. A recent large-scale study utilizing patient registries in Denmark and Sweden among nearly 800,000 patients who received the vaccine found no increased risk of developing MS.

Zoster (Shingrix) Recombinant Vaccine Subunit

The CDC recommendation for zoster vaccination is administration of two doses of recombinant zoster vaccine (RZV-Shingrix) 2 to 6 months apart to adults 50 years or older regardless of prior history of herpes zoster or having received the live zoster vaccine (Zostavax, ZVL). Recombinant Shingrix vaccine is preferred in MS because of both its increased safety and efficacy. The efficacy of Shingrix in preventing zoster is 97.2% compared with Zostavax, a 51% decrease in preventing zoster. No studies have been done of Shingrix in MS; however, no increase in autoimmune disease was noted in two clinical studies with Shingrix.

The Zostavax vaccine is not recommended if a patient is taking Aubagio. Zostavax in general is not recommended because Shingrix has become available owing to improved efficacy and decreased risk. Also, for Lemtrada use, the patient would need to wait 6 weeks after receiving the vaccine before getting Lemtrada.

Pneumococcal (Conjugate Polysaccharide Vaccine)

Pneumovax 23 and Prevnar 13 are inactivated and considered safe.

Generally, CDC guidelines for the general population are also recommended for patients with MS, particularly for patients who are wheelchair dependent who have impaired pulmonary function. The humoral response after Lemtrada use was similar to that of controls.

Other Subunit/Conjugated Vaccines

- Typhoid
- Tick-borne encephalitis

Toxoid Vaccine

Toxoid vaccines are derived from a toxin treated to destroy its toxic properties but that can elicit an immune response to the original toxin. Toxoid vaccines are present for diphtheria, tetanus, and botulism.

Diphtheria, Tetanus Toxoids, and Pertussis

The CDC recommends that all adults be vaccinated for diphtheria/tetanus. Tetanus vaccination appears to be safe for patients with MS. Tetanus booster should be given every 10 years (Table 6.2).

TABLE 6.2

MOST COMMONLY USED VACCINATIONS ORGANIZED BY TYPE OF VACCINE AND RANKED LOW RISK (CONSIDERED SAFE) TO HIGH RISK (NOT RECOMMENDED)

Vaccine	Type	Use in People With Multiple Sclerosis
Injectable seasonal flu vaccine	Inactivated	Considered safe
Hepatitis B vaccine	Inactivated	Considered safe
Pneumovax 23 and Prevnar 13 pneumococcal vaccines	Inactivated	Considered safe
Tetanus vaccine	Inactivated	Considered safe; may reduce relapses
Gardasil human papillomavirus vaccine (HPV)	Inactivated	Probably safe
Polio	Inactivated (in most countries)	Probably safe
Rabies	Inactivated	Probably safe; benefit likely outweighs any risks
Measles-mumps-rubella vaccine	Live attenuated	Probably safe in individuals not on immunosuppressant medications
Varivax varicella vaccines	Live attenuated	Probably safe. Required before treatment with fingolimod and alemtuzumab in patients without previous exposure
Yellow fever vaccine	Live attenuated	May not be safe; should not be used by individuals on immunosuppressant medications
Shingrix vaccine	Recombinant	Considered safe

During Relapses

According to the Immunization Panel of the MS Council for Clinical Practice Guidelines:

During relapses vaccination should be delayed until patients have stabilized or have shown signs of improvement, usually 4 to 6 weeks after the start of the relapse. The exception being if a patient required immediate tetanus vaccination.

Corticosteroid Use and Vaccinations

Corticosteroid use could decrease the efficacy of a vaccination, so it is advisable to wait usually 4 to 6 weeks before administering the vaccine.[27] This is because corticosteroids are usually administered during the time of relapse. Short-term use of glucocorticoids is usually not a contraindication to receiving the vaccine or if doses <40 mg are used.[23]

Lemtrada (Alemtuzumab)

The recommendation is to vaccinate before treatment, 6 weeks before infusion. The live virus vaccine should not be administered following a course of Lemtrada. There is no specific recommendation regarding the administration of inactivated vaccines following infusion.

A study showed that adequate antibody levels were produced to seasonal flu vaccine and pneumococcal and meningococcal vaccines.

Ocrevus

The Veloce study was done in the United States and Canada evaluating the humoral response of Ocrevus to selected vaccines. Vaccines studied were tetanus toxoid, pneumococcal polysaccharide vaccine, seasonal influenza, 20-valent pneumococcal conjugate vaccine, and keyhole limpet hemocyanin. Ocrelizumab does deplete CD20$^+$ B cells but preserves the ability for B cells to reconstitute and preserves preexisting humoral immunity. Humoral responses were decreased at all time points in patients following ocrelizumab use because of B cell depletion compared with controls. Patients were, however, able to mount humoral responses to the vaccines and neoantigen studied. Cellular immune responses were not studied.

Live attenuated vaccines or live vaccines are not recommended to be taken during treatment but can be given up to 4 weeks before infusion. Findings from the Veloce study confirm that all inactivated vaccines should be given at least 2 weeks before the infusion. Flu vaccine is recommended because a potentially protective humoral response is generated, even if attenuated.[29] No live attenuated or live virus should be given during treatment or following treatment until B cells have returned to normal levels.

Tecfidera

Live vaccines are not recommended. Immune response to vaccines is maintained after Tecfidera exposure.[60] Three vaccine types were evaluated: tetanus/diphtheria toxoid to test T cell–dependent recall response, pneumococcal vaccine polyvalent to test T cell–independent humoral response, and meningococcal oligosaccharide conjugate to test T cell–dependent neoantigen response.

Gilenya (Fingolimod)

Humoral responses are decreased to influenza, pneumococcal vaccine, and tetanus toxoid. That being said, administration of flu vaccine is still recommended for patients. Avoid live vaccines during treatment and for 2 months after treatment discontinuation.

Tysabri (Natalizumab)

In the Natalizumab Safety and Efficacy in Relapsing Remitting MS phase 3 clinical trial of Tysabri monotherapy in relapsing MS, Tysabri 300 mg was administered versus placebo and administered every 28 days for up to 116 weeks. During this trial, 20% of patients received vaccinations. These vaccinations included influenza, either polyvalent or monovalent; hepatitis A; hepatitis B; typhoid; inactivated polio; pneumococcal; tick-borne encephalitis; yellow fever; diphtheria (Tysabri group only); diphtheria and tetanus; tetanus antitoxin; tetanus toxoid; diphtheria, tetanus toxoids, and pertussis (DTP); measles, mumps, rubella (Tysabri group only); and live rubella vaccines (placebo group only). No vaccine-related adverse events were reported in this trial other than one patient having an allergy to the influenza vaccine in the Tysabri group.

A phase 4 open-label randomized study was done to evaluate the effects of Tysabri treatment on the immune response to vaccination in patients with relapsing MS. This study measured memory antibody responses to neoantigen (keyhole limpet hemocyanin) and analyzed the effects of Tysabri on circulating lymphocyte subsets at 3 and 6 months of treatment. No significant differences were noted between Tysabri-treated and vaccines-only groups in the proportion of responders to recall immunization with Td or primary immunization with KLH, and all subjects had protective levels of Td antibodies.

Sleep Disorders in MS

Another common presenting complaint from a patient with MS is problem with sleep, either due to difficulty falling asleep or staying asleep. Poor sleep patterns can aggravate daytime fatigue, which is often a common symptom for up to 90% of patients with MS at some point during their disease course.[30] It can also aggravate problems with poor cognition. Insomnia, obstructive sleep apnea, and restless leg syndrome need to be investigated because treatment can not only improve restful sleep and decrease fatigue but also improve overall quality of life.

Up to 40% of patients with MS may have insomnia.[30] Many symptoms such as spasticity, anxiety, depression, pain, and overactive bladder can contribute to difficulty falling asleep. Identification of these issues and treatment can help in decreasing insomnia. Discussion with patient should be had about improving sleep hygiene, maintaining a cool bedroom temperature, and exercise except not close to bedtime. Patients who are taking CNS stimulants, such as modafinil or methylphenidate, have to be counseled not to take these close to bedtime but should restrict use to the morning or early afternoon at the latest. Use of antihistamines should be avoided because of risk of psychomotor impairment and daytime grogginess. Benzodiazepines or benzodiazepine agonists are preferred. Behavioral modification strategies, meditation, and yoga can also be helpful.

Sleep apnea is often overlooked, but especially if a patient or spouse is noting that snoring is present, frequent nighttime awakenings occur, or daytime sleepiness is present, this should be investigated. Overnight sleep study and referral to a sleep specialist can help to diagnose this. Patients who have brainstem dysfunction could be at an increased risk for this. If this condition is diagnosed, positive airway pressure is usually the preferred treatment. Restless leg syndrome, defined as uncomfortable sensation or restlessness of the lower extremities, usually present in the evening, helped with movement, and worsened by rest can be seen in patients with MS. Studies have shown that restless leg movements are three times more common in patients with MS than in the general population. Treatment should be individualized based on the frequency and severity of symptoms.

Lymphedema

Lymphedema is the abnormal accumulation of interstitial fluid resulting from injury, infection, or congenital deformities of the lymphatic system. It is classified as primary lymphedema, which is the presence of lymphedema without any inducing factor, often a result of a congenital condition of the lymphatic vessels, or secondary lymphedema, which occurs as the result of a separate underlying condition or treatment. Common causes of secondary lymphedema are cancer and cancer treatment, infection, obesity, venous insufficiency, and inflammatory disorders. The main cause of lymphedema in conditions such as MS is reduction in the muscle movements that usually enable the lymphatic fluid to flow properly. Often there is greater lymphedema in the weaker extremity. Unlike most other causes of lymphedema, in MS it is not caused by venous insufficiency, or cardiac failure, but in patients who are less ambulatory there should be a high index of suspicion for deep vein thrombosis and cellulitis.[31] Treating with diuretics is usually not recommended. For mild cases of lymphedema, compression socks and keeping legs elevated help. For more severe cases, lymphatic therapy and the use of compression pumps are recommended.

Wellness and Coordination of Care

An important goal of MS treatment is to best maintain and enhance the central nervous system reserve. What may seem to be a common sense approach can make significant difference. Cessation of tobacco use, increasing vitamin D levels, optimizing body weight, regular exercise, healthy diet, controlling comorbidities, and improving intellectual and social stimulation and emotional well-being are measures that need to be reinforced to patients and have them understand their importance. A healthier lifestyle can help the CNS age well and preserve the CNS reserve.

Because there has been an increased focus on alternative and complementary therapies in MS, there is greater discussion presently regarding integrative medicine. This refers to integration of approved DMTs, complementary therapies, and lifestyle medicine that emphasize overall wellness mindset, with diet and exercise incorporated into what we consider conventional medicine. Behavioral change often is necessary for patients to adopt a healthier lifestyle. Of increased importance is understanding the lifestyle of patients, what their specific treatment goals are, and what might interfere with adherence to treatment plan.

As discussed earlier in this chapter, the presence of comorbidities decreased patients' quality of life and affected treatment adherence. Time spent in educating patients on the importance of exercise and diet and their role in improving overall MS disease management can produce long-term positive ripple effects. Complementary therapies can include acupuncture, yoga, tai chi, mindfulness, therapeutic massage, reflexology, art and music therapy, magnetic therapy,[32] and hippotherapy.[33] One study even showed benefits of cha cha dancing in MS![34] Small positive steps should be encouraged and reinforced. Discussion of being active versus inactive should be stressed.

As to diet, this is discussed in greater detail in another chapter. In general, there is not one specific best diet for MS; however, much research is ongoing studying the Mediterranean diet, which emphasizes fruits, vegetables, whole grains, legumes, and fish.[35] Cannabis use in MS can play a role particularly for pain and spasms.[36] Certain states have legalized marijuana for medicinal use; however, because it is not approved on the federal level, patients may be at risk for federal offenses when traveling from state to state. Bee venom was thought to be possibly helpful for the treatment of MS; however, studies show that there is no significant effect.[37] Opiate antagonist medications have also been in the discussion for the treatment of MS, particularly naltrexone. Low-dose naltrexone has not shown benefit in long-term disease progression; however, some studies have shown benefit in decreasing fatigue.[38]

In general, patients should be counseled to check with their health care provider regarding any supplements because some can be immune stimulating, such as echinacea, and are not generally recommended. The most important supplement to monitor is vitamin D, because not only can low vitamin D levels can play a role in disease development but also increased vitamin D levels can play a role in decreasing CNS inflammatory activity in patients who already have MS. Studies have shown benefit in achieving blood vitamin D levels in the 60- to 80-ng/mL range.[36,39]

Awareness of increased infection risks with certain DMTs, possible drug-drug interactions, emphasis on wellness and good health practices, and attention to treatment of comorbidities can potentially lead to not only improved overall health but also improvement in MS disease activity. Collaboration between internists, family practitioners, nurse practitioners, and physicians assistants with neurologists is key to improved patient outcomes.

References

1. Copaxone (glatiramer acetate injection). Teva Neuroscience Inc. Available at https://www.copaxonehcp.com/. Accessed November 17, 2018.
2. *Interferon Beta-1b: Drug Information.* Lexicomp; 2018. Available at https://www.uptodate.com/contents/interferon-beta-1b-drug-information?-search=betaseron&source=panel_search_result&selectedTitle=1~11&usage_type=panel&kp_tab=drug_general&display_rank=1. Accessed November 10, 2018.
3. *Interferon Beta-1a: Drug Information.* Lexicomp; 2018. Available at https://www.uptodate.com/contents/interferon-beta-1a-drug-information?-search=rebif&source=panel_search_result&selectedTitle=1~23&usage_type=panel&kp_tab=drug_general&display_rank=1. Accessed November 10, 2018.
4. *Pegylated Interferon (Peginterferon) Beta-1a: Drug Information.* Lexicomp; 2018. Available at https://www.uptodate.com/contents/pegylated-interferon-peginterferon-beta-1a-drug-information?search=plegridy&source=panel_search_result&selectedTitle=1~4&usage_type=panel&kp_tab=drug_general&display_rank=1. Accessed November 10, 2018.
5. *Teriflunomide: Drug Information.* Lexicomp; 2018. Available at https://www.uptodate.com/contents/teriflunomide-drug-information?source=see_link. Accessed November 10, 2018.
6. *Fingolimod: Drug Information.* Lexicomp; 2018. Available at https://www.uptodate.com/contents/fingolimod-drug-information?search=gilenya&-source=panel_search_result&selectedTitle=1~12&usage_type=panel&kp_tab=drug_general&display_rank=1. Accessed November 10, 2018.
7. Warnke C, Dehmel T, Ramanujam R, et al. Initial lymphocyte count and low BMI may affect fingolimod-induced lymphopenia. *Neurology.* 2014;83(23): 2153-2157.

8. Berger JR, Cree BA, Greenberg B, et al. Progressive multifocal leukoenceph-alopathy after fingolimod treatment. *Neurology*. 2018;90(20):e1815-e1821. doi:10.1212/WNL.0000000000005529.

9. *Tecfidera (Dimethyl Fumarate) [Prescribing Information]*. Cambridge, MA: Biogen Idec Inc; December 2017. Available at https://www.uptodate.com/contents/dimethyl-fumarate-drug-information?search=tecfidera&source=panel_search_result&selectedTitle=1~9&usage_type=panel&kp_tab=drug_general&display_rank=1. Accessed November 10, 2018.

10. Croteau D, Flowers C, Kulick C, Brinker A, Kortepeter C. Acute acalculous cholecystitis. A new safety risk for patients with MS treated with alemtuzumab. *Neurology*. 2018;90:e1548-e1552. doi:10.1212/WNL.0000000000005422.

11. Ferraro D, Camera V, Vitetta F, et al. Acute coronary syndrome associated with alemtuzumab infusion in multiple sclerosis. *Neurology*. 2018;90:852-854.

12. *FDA Warns About Rare but Serious Risks of Stroke and Blood Vessel Wall Tears With Multiple Sclerosis Drug Lemtrada (Alemtuzumab)*. U.S Food and Drug Administration; 2018. Available at http://app.info.fda.gov/e/er?utm_campaign=FDA%20MedWatch%20-%20Lemtrada%20%28alemtu-zumab%29%3A%20Drug%20Safety%20Communication&utm_medium=e-mail&utm_source=Eloqua&s=2027422842&lid=5793&elqTrackId=1503e36ae3524f5494e6245f2c93585f&elq=21cc624b86584094afd347b4ba3637b1&elqa-id=6087&elqat=1. Accessed November 29, 2018.

13. Rae Grant A, Day G, Marrie R, et al. Practice guideline recommendations sum-mary: disease modifying therapies for adults with multiple sclerosis. *Neurology*. 2018;90;777-788. doi:10.1212/WNL.0000000000005347.

14. Rituxan (Rituximab). Genentech. Available at http://www.rituxan.com/. Accessed November 17, 2018.

15. Freedman M. The promise of stem cell therapy for MS. *IOMSNews*. 2018;2(3): 17-19.

16. Williamson EML, Chahin S, Berger JR. Vaccines in multiple sclerosis. *Curr Neurol Neurosci Rep*. 2016;16:36.

17. Loebermann M, Winkelmann A, Hartung H,Hengel H, Reisinger E, Zetti U. Vaccination against infection in patients with multiple sclerosis. *Nat Rev Neurol*. 2012;8:143-151.

18. Confavreux C,Suissa S, Saddier P, Bourdes V, Vukusic S. Vaccinations and the risk of relapse in multiple sclerosis. *N Engl J Med*. 2001;344:319-326.

19. Mailand MT, Frederiksen JL. Vaccines and multiple sclerosis: a systematic review. *J Neurol*. 2017;264(6):1035-1050. doi:10.1007/s00415-016-8263-4.

20. DeStefano F, Verstraeten T, Jackson LA, et al. Vaccinations and risk of central nervous system demyelinating diseases in adults. *Arch Neurol*. 2003;60(4):504-509.

21. Living Well with MS. National Multiple Sclerosis Society. Available at https://www.nationalmssociety.org/Living-Well-With-MS. Accessed November 15, 2018.

22. Living Well with MS: Vaccinations. National Multiple Sclerosis Society. Available at http://www.nationalmssociety.org/Living-Well-With-MS/Health-Wellness/Vaccination. Accessed November 15, 2018.

23. Russell AF, Parrino J, Fisher CL, et al. Safety, tolerability, and immunogenicity of zoster vaccine in subjects on chronic/maintenance corticosteroids. *Vaccine.* 2015;33(27):3129-3134. doi:10.1016/j.vaccine.2015.04.090.

24. Olberg H, Cox R, Nostbakken J, Aarseth J, Vedeler C, Myhr KM. Immunotherapies influence the influenza vaccination response in multiple sclerosis patients: an explorative study. *Mult Scler.* 2014;20(8):1074-1080.

25. Kaufman M, Pardo G, Rossman H, Sweetser M, Forrestal F, Duda P. Natalizumab treatment shows no clinically meaningful effects on immunization responses in patients with relapsing-remitting multiple sclerosis. *J Neurol Sci.* 2014;341:22-27.

26. Olberg HK, Eide GE, Cox J, et al. Antibody response to seasonal influenza vaccination in patients with multiple sclerosis receiving immunomodulatory therapy. *Eur J Neurol.* 2018;25(3):527-534.

27. Scheller NM, Svanstrom H, Pasternak B, et al. Quadrivalent HPV vaccination and risk of multiple sclerosis and other demyelinating diseases of the central nervous system. *JAMA.* 2015;313(1):54-61.

28. Stokmaier D, Winthrop K, Chognot C, Evershed J, Manfrini M, McNamara J, Bar-Or A. Effect of Ocrelizumab on Vaccine Responses in Patients With Multiple Sclerosis. Presented at the 70th American Academy of Neurology (AAN) Annual Meeting; April 21-27, 2018. Los Angeles, CA, USA. Platform presentation number S36.002.

29. Hehn V, Howard J, Liu S, et al. Immune response to vaccines is maintained in patients treated with dimethyl fumarate. *Neurol Neuroimmunol Neuroinflamm.* 2018;5(1):409.

30. Braley TJ. Sleep disorders in patients with multiple sclerosis. *Pract Neurol.* Bryn Mawr Communications. 2018;17(6):47-55.

31. Mehrara B, Eidt JF, Mills JL, et al. *Clinical Features and Diagnosis of Peripheral Lymphedema.* UpToDate; 2018. Available at https://www.uptodate.com/contents/clinical-features-and-diagnosis-of-peripheral-lymphedema. Accessed November 28, 2018.

32. *New Results Show That Magnetic Stimulation of Brain May Improve Working Memory and Brain Connectivity in People with MS.* National Multiple Sclerosis Society; 2017. Available at https://www.nationalmssociety.org/About-the-Society/News/New-Results-Show-that-Magnetic-Stimulation-of-Brai. Accessed November 28, 2018.

33. Bowling A. *Optimal Health With Multiple Sclerosis.* Demos Health; 2014: 3-17.

34. Baron JR. Dance as integrative medicine. *Altern Complement Ther.* Marry Anne Liebert Inc. 2016;22(3). doi:10.1089/act.2016.29053.jrb.

35. Sand IK, Digga E, Benn E, et al. *A Modified Mediterranean Dietary Intervention for Multiple Sclerosis: Results of A Pilot Study and Lessons Learned for Future Dietary Research in MS;* 2018. Available at https://onlinelibrary.ectrims-congress.eu/ectrims/2018/ectrims 2018/228487/ilana.katz.sand.a.modified.mediterranean.dietary.intervention.for.multiple.html. Accessed November 26, 2018.

36. Claflin SB, van der Mei IAF, Taylor BV. Complementary and alternative treatments of multiple sclerosis: a review of the evidence from 2001 to 2016. *J Neurol Neurosurg Psychiatry.* 2018;89;34-41.

37. Wesselius T, Heersema DJ, Mostert JP, et al. A randomized crossover study of bee sting therapy for multiple sclerosis. *Neurology.* 2005;65(11): 1764-1768.

38. Low-Dose Naltrexone. National Multiple Sclerosis Society. Available at https://www.nationalmssociety.org/Treating-MS/Complementary-Alternative-Medicines/Low-Dose-Naltrexone. Accessed November 28, 2018.

39. Munger KL, Levin LI, Hollis BW, Howard NS, Ascherio A. Serum 25-hydroxyvitamin D levels and risk of multiple sclerosis. *JAMA*. 2006;296(23):2832-2838.

40. Mavenclad (cladribine): Drug Information. EMD Serono; 2019. Available at https://www.emdserono.com/us-en/expertise/neurology-and-immunology.html. Accessed April 2, 2019.

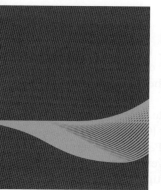
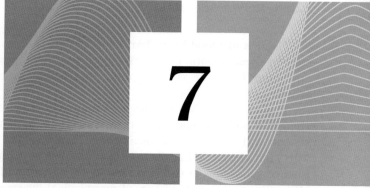

7

Multiple Sclerosis in Emergency Medicine

■ ▓ ▓ Richard I. Lappin

Introduction

Multiple sclerosis is an immune-mediated inflammatory demyelinating disease of the central nervous system whose cause and pathogenesis are still unclear. Both genetic and environmental factors seem to influence susceptibility to the disease. With an incidence of 2 to 10 cases per 100,000 persons per year (in the United States, Canada, and Europe), MS is a relatively uncommon disease, but because it usually begins early in life it is a major cause of disability in young adults.[1]

The classic lesion of MS is the plaque, seen in the white matter of the brain or spinal cord. In the acute phase, plaques show a combination of inflammatory cell infiltration, extensive demyelination, and some degree of axonal damage. White matter lesions are typically found in the periventricular region, corpus callosum, centrum semiovale, deep white matter, and basal ganglia.[2] More recently, histopathology and imaging have shown that gray matter lesions are common even in early MS and may be critical to the progression of disease. Gray matter lesions can be found in the cerebral cortex, deep structures such as the thalamus, the cerebellum, and the gray matter of the spinal cord. They are difficult to detect without specialized magnetic resonance imaging (MRI) sequences such as double inversion recovery. Although they do show demyelination, gray matter lesions are not marked by massive inflammatory infiltration or evidence of blood-brain barrier (BBB) breakdown; the inflammatory cells in these lesions may derive from the meninges or choroid plexus and enter from the cerebrospinal fluid (CSF) via the pial surface or ventricles.[3]

It is clear that MS lesions are often asymptomatic. Autopsy studies show that some persons have central nervous system (CNS) lesions consistent with MS and no clinical evidence of disease. Patients presenting with what appears clinically to be a first attack of demyelination (clinically isolated syndrome, or CIS) are often found to have multiple old plaques on MRI without any prior history of neurological disease. Repeat imaging of patients in the relapsing phase of MS shows that new lesions appear at a rate 5- to 10-fold greater than in clinical relapses.

Advanced MS is also associated with diffuse atrophy of the brain and spinal cord, which is closely correlated with disability. The connection between the acute lesions of MS and later atrophy is unclear.

Natural History of Multiple Sclerosis

The median age of onset of multiple sclerosis is approximately 30 years, although the disease can begin anywhere from early childhood to the seventh decade of life. For approximately 85% of patients with MS, the disease will begin with a relapsing-remitting pattern. The hallmark of relapsing-remitting MS (RRMS) is the relapse (also called attack or exacerbation), defined as an episode of neurological dysfunction lasting at least 24 hours and not associated with fever or infection. Attacks develop over a period of hours to days and resolve over weeks to months. They are currently believed to be episodes of acute demyelination. On average, patients with RRMS will have a clinically apparent relapse every 2 years; more frequent assessment of patients tends to yield higher estimates of relapse rate. Relapses tend to be more frequent early in the disease and wane over time. Each relapse may have complete clinical resolution, or there may be permanent sequelae. In the relapsing-remitting phase, there is relatively little disease progression between acute relapses.[4-6]

Some clinical features at the very beginning of the disease, for example, residual deficit after the first relapse and number of relapses during the first 2 years, correlate with a shorter time to reach disability milestones during the relapsing-remitting phase. By contrast, relapses over the remainder of the relapsing-remitting phase appear to have little effect on the speed at which disability accumulates.

Most patients with RRMS will, after 10 to 20 years, gradually transition to a secondary progressive phase, dominated by steadily worsening disability with few or no relapses. By 9 years after disease onset, only half of patients will still have relapses. The frequency of relapses and rate of accumulation of disability during the relapsing-remitting phase vary tremendously from patient to patient. However, once relapsing patients reach an Extended Disability Status Scale (EDSS) score of 3 or begin a progressive phase, they enter a period of steady decline, which is similar from patient to patient and only weakly influenced by the speed of the relapsing-remitting phase.[7]

About 15% of patients will present with primary-progressive MS (PPMS), characterized by slowly worsening disability from the onset of the disease. The distinction between RRMS and PPMS is made exclusively by history; there are no examination or imaging findings that distinguish the two variants. The most common presentation of PPMS is a gradually worsening spinal cord syndrome with spastic paraparesis and no clear sensory level.

Pseudorelapses

MS symptoms can be worsened in the presence of infection or other physiologic stress, a situation referred to as a pseudorelapse.[3,4] Worsening of symptoms via increased body temperature (Uthoff phenomenon) may underlie some of these episodes. Classical pseudorelapses are exacerbations of previous symptoms and typically include worsened generalized fatigue and spasticity. In the emergency department (ED), any patient with MS with worsened symptoms should be screened for infection, especially of the respiratory and urinary tract. The presence of a plausible infectious process, along with an MRI showing no acute lesion, is generally taken to diagnose a pseudorelapse. Occasionally, patients with known MS will also present with psychologically based symptoms in the setting of depression or severe life stresses.[8]

However, some caution is justified in making the diagnosis of pseudorelapse. There is evidence that new MS lesions can be triggered by infection, so the presence of a urinary tract infection (UTI) or viral respiratory illness does not in itself exclude a true relapse. Furthermore, current MR technology does not detect all acute lesions; gray matter lesions, for example, are not well seen without specialized sequences. Given that MRI lesions accumulate at a rate at least 5 to 10 times greater than clinical relapses, it seems likely that some true attacks are misdiagnosed as pseudorelapses.

Initial Presentation of MS

A single focal attack of demyelination does not in itself constitute MS. The diagnosis of MS requires the demonstration of CNS lesions disseminated in both space and time, based on either clinical findings alone or a combination of clinical findings and MRI or CSF-specific oligoclonal bands

(OCBs).[9] The initial presentation of MS may be a CIS, that is, an attack compatible with MS but not yet fulfilling diagnostic criteria. For patients with a CIS and an otherwise normal MRI, the long-term likelihood (>10 y) of developing MS is approximately 20%.

Just as there are no clinical presentations that are unique to MS, any of the manifestations of MS can be an initial presentation. Common presenting syndromes include optic neuritis, spinal cord sensory or motor symptoms, transverse myelitis, and brainstem and cerebellar syndromes.

Optic Neuritis

Optic neuritis typically begins with eye pain, worse with eye movement, followed by blurred or dimmed central vision. **Complete unilateral loss of vision is rare.** On examination, there is usually an afferent pupillary defect. Retinal examination may reveal mild optic disc swelling (papillitis), although if the lesion is located some distance from the fundus (retrobulbar neuritis), the retinal examination may be normal. The presence of retinal hemorrhages or exudates should suggest a diagnosis other than acute demyelination.[10]

Spinal Cord Syndromes

Spinal cord lesions can cause a variety of sensory and motor symptoms or mixtures of the two. Persistent tingling and numbness are common and may be bilateral, leading them to be mistaken for the intermittent tingling of hyperventilation. Strange sensations that the legs are swollen, cold, tightly wrapped, or swaddled in soft gauze or severe pains that radiate upward from the feet are characteristic of spinal cord lesions and are easily dismissed as anxious or delusional. Motor symptoms include leg weakness or clumsiness, often with enhanced reflexes and extensor plantar responses. Transverse myelitis is the most fulminant spinal cord syndrome, with profound bilateral weakness, sensory loss, and bowel and bladder dysfunction. Partial and incomplete spinal syndromes with asymmetric signs are much more common.[11]

Brainstem and Cerebellar Lesions

Brainstem and cerebellar lesions can cause various combinations of vertigo, diplopia, dysarthria, limb incoordination, and tremor. An internuclear ophthalmoplegia is common and if bilateral is almost pathognomonic of MS. MS can cause an attack of acute vertigo, but there are generally other brainstem symptoms and signs such as diplopia, dysarthria, facial numbness, limb weakness, or clumsiness to indicate that this is not simply a peripheral vestibular syndrome.

New Paroxysmal Symptoms

New **paroxysmal symptoms** lasting seconds to minutes at a time can indicate an acute attack if they recur over a period of weeks or more. An example of this is Lhermitte symptom, an electric shocklike sensation, typically induced by neck flexion, which radiates down the back into the legs and often indicates a lesion within the cervical spinal cord affecting the spinothalamic tracts. Other paroxysmal symptoms include tonic contractions of the face or limbs and fleeting episodes of dysarthria or sensory disturbance. Trigeminal neuralgia associated with atypical features such as onset before age 50 years, bilateral presentation, or facial numbness should raise suspicion for MS. Painful paroxysmal symptoms associated with MS are best treated with agents such as carbamazepine and gabapentin, rather than opioids.

Imaging

Although computed tomography can sometimes demonstrate MS lesions, MRI is currently the imaging modality of choice. In many cases, MRI can establish a diagnosis of MS at the time of the first attack by demonstrating not only the acute lesion but also additional lesions disseminated in both time and space. On MRI, brain lesions appear ovoid in shape and are typically aligned at right angles to the corpus callosum, forming a pattern on sagittal imaging referred to as "Dawson fingers." The most valuable sequences are T2/T2-fluid attenuation inversion recovery, used to identify old (chronic) lesions, and contrast-enhanced T1, which detects breakdown of the BBB associated with acute white matter lesions. Enhancement typically resolves within a month, usually leaving a T2-hyperintense lesion that persists indefinitely. T2 lesions that are hypointense on T1 ("black holes") are thought to represent areas of severe white matter destruction and axonal loss. Diffuse brain and spinal cord atrophy are also commonly seen in advanced MS and correlate more strongly with clinical disability than does total lesion burden. Spinal cord lesions are common in patients with MS, although isolated spinal involvement is uncommon.[12,13]

All patients with suspected MS should have MRI of the brain with and without contrast. Neurology consultation can help choose appropriate imaging to maximize diagnostic yield.

Oligoclonal Bands

Activation of an IgG (humoral) immune response leads to the appearance on electrophoresis of multiple distinct bands of IgG corresponding to the activation of multiple B cell clones. This response can be seen in a variety of systemic infectious, inflammatory, and neoplastic diseases. OCBs found in the CSF and not in the serum indicate an immune response originating within the CNS. This is seen not only in MS but also in meningitis, neurosyphilis, progressive multifocal leukoencephalopathy (PML), tumors, and many other CNS disorders. CSF-specific OCBs are found in up to 95% of patients with clinically definite MS.[14]

Before the advent of MRI, OCBs were a vital factor in establishing dissemination in time for the diagnosis of MS. One meta-analysis found that the presence of OCBs in a patient with a CIS was associated with an odds ratio of approximately 10 for the development of MS. In the MRI era, OCBs are often unnecessary for diagnosis. The neurology consultant should decide whether lumbar puncture for OCBs is needed, and because the results will not be immediately available to influence management, the test is most appropriately performed when the patient is admitted.

Differential Diagnosis

The differential diagnosis for a young adult who presents with a classic history of two or more acute episodes of neurological dysfunction with at least partial resolution is limited. For patients with a single attack of CNS disturbance, the differential is broad and includes many infectious, inflammatory, ischemic, neoplastic and genetic disorders.[15] Given the complexities of the differential and the profound consequences of a diagnosis of multiple sclerosis, emergency medicine (EM) clinicians would be prudent to ask for neurology consultation to help with the evaluation of these patients.

A number of clinical "red flags" suggest that a diagnosis other than MS should be considered. Hyperacute onset of symptoms (over seconds to minutes) or very short duration (minutes to hours) suggests an ischemic or hemorrhagic lesion, seizure, or syncope. Diffuse encephalopathy with confusion or depressed level of awareness points toward a systemic process (toxic or metabolic) or a multifocal CNS disorder such as encephalitis, vasculitis, or posterior reversible encephalopathy syndrome.

A significant number of patients eventually receive an incorrect diagnosis of MS, especially when difficult-to-localize symptoms of dizziness, fatigue, and cognitive difficulties are combined with nonspecific white matter T2-hyperintense lesions.[16] Studies suggest that the most common diagnoses for these patients are psychiatric disorders, migraine, and chronic pain disorders such as fibromyalgia.

Complications of Established MS

Lower Urinary Tract Dysfunction

Lower urinary tract dysfunction is almost universal in MS, appearing on average 6 years after onset. Normal bladder function requires the bladder to fill at low pressure, preventing damage to the kidneys, and then contract efficiently under conscious control, avoiding urine stasis and infection. MS can interfere at multiple levels—conscious control in the frontal lobe, the reflex control center in the pons, and reflex arcs in the spinal cord. Dysfunction can be broadly divided into abnormal urinary storage (overactive bladder caused by detrusor muscle overactivity) and abnormal emptying caused by detrusor underactivity or detrusor-sphincter dyssynergia. Overactive bladder symptoms classically include urgency, frequency, and urge incontinence, whereas voiding dysfunction causes hesitancy, weak stream, and sensation of incomplete emptying. In patients with MS, however, urinary symptoms correlate poorly with the underlying urodynamics. Patients with chronic urinary symptoms may benefit from urological referral.[17,18]

UTIs are exceedingly common in patients with MS and are responsible for up to half of all hospital admissions in these patients. The likelihood of a UTI increases with longer duration of disease and increasing disability; additional risk factors include female gender, elevated postvoid residual volume, and the presence of an indwelling urinary catheter. Intermittent self-catheterization may be useful in decreasing the risk in patients who develop recurrent UTIs. Asymptomatic bacteriuria should not be treated, except perhaps in patients about to begin high-dose steroid for an acute relapse. Local symptoms and signs of possible UTI include suprapubic or flank pain, worsening of chronic urinary urgency or frequency, catheter blockage, and cloudy or malodorous urine; general symptoms and signs include fever, lethargy, and worsening of previous deficits. Patients with significant sensory deficits may not perceive symptoms such as dysuria but may have other complaints such as increased fatigue and spasticity secondary to their infection.

Spasticity

Spasticity (increased tone and stiffness in limbs) as well as spontaneous or movement-induced muscle **spasms** are common in MS, especially with spinal cord involvement. Spasms can be quite painful and interfere with activities of daily living. Spasms may be triggered by touching a limb or by lower-body conditions that the patient may not perceive, such as bladder infection, fecal impaction, and decubitus ulcers. Painful spasm may respond to oral magnesium; spasticity may be treated with gamma-aminobutyric acid agonists such as baclofen and tizanidine.[19]

Constipation

Constipation is present in more than 30% of patients, whereas fecal urgency or incontinence is much less common. Severe, chronic constipation can lead to complications such as impaction, sigmoid volvulus, large-bowel obstruction, and perforation.

Generalized Fatigue

Generalized fatigue, although poorly understood, is almost universal in MS and an important cause of work-related disability. Sleep disorders (sometimes from bladder dysfunction), pain, depression, and anxiety can contribute to fatigue in these patients. Pharmacologic agents such as amantadine, modafinil, and methylphenidate are sometimes prescribed.

Cognitive Dysfunction

Cognitive dysfunction affects a large proportion of patients with MS and may be underrecognized in routine clinical assessment. Most often, there are impairments of episodic memory and information processing speed.[20]

Pain

Pain is a common and underrecognized complication of MS. Spinal lesions can cause both localized back pain and painful dysesthesias felt in the limbs. Other causes of pain include painful tonic spasms and paroxysmal conditions such as Lhermitte sign and trigeminal neuralgia. Antidepressants, such as the tricyclic antidepressants and serotonin-norepinephrine reuptake inhibitors, or antiepileptics, such as gabapentin, are currently recommended for chronic pain. Opioids are not recommended as first-line agents because of their limited efficacy and potential for causing tolerance and addiction.

Emergency Department Issues in Multiple Sclerosis

Although the neurologist must attend to the nuances of diagnosis and choice of long-term treatment, the emergency physician has a different set of questions. For a previously healthy patient with new neurological symptoms, the primary questions are: Could this patient have multiple sclerosis? What evaluation and testing should be done in the ED setting? Should the patient be admitted?

For a patient with an established diagnosis of MS and new or worsened neurological symptoms, the questions include: What evaluation should be performed to decide whether they are having a relapse? What testing might help? How important is this determination? Should this patient be admitted?

Emergency Department Identification of Patients With a Potential First Attack

Because the median age of onset for MS is approximately 30 years, MS should be considered in the differential diagnosis of young patients presenting with new neurological symptoms. Unfortunately, several cognitive biases can prevent MS from being considered. The possibility of serious disease is more easily set aside in young healthy persons. Clinicians may be tempted to attribute unusual symptoms to anxiety, emotional stress, or even a somatiform disorder.

A 2013 retrospective study at Mount Sinai Medical Center in New York analyzed ED visits before an initial diagnosis of MS. Over a 5-year period, there were 49 MS diagnoses and 98 ED visits before the diagnosis, 50% of which were for neurological symptoms. Of those, 88% were retrospectively felt by the study reviewers to have been a first presentation of MS and included in the study.[21]

The initial ED impression was MS for only 10% of patients, whereas 57% received no specific initial diagnosis and 16% received an incorrect diagnosis, such as stroke, neuropathy, tumor, or muscle spasm. However, 78% of the ED presentations resulted in a neurology consult and 76% were admitted to the hospital, 82% of those to the neurology service. Ultimately, 61% received a diagnosis of MS during their admission, and 74% were diagnosed within a week. Of the remainder, an additional 4% were diagnosed within a month, 8% within 6 months, and another 6% within the year. Demographic factors of age, sex, and insurance status did not predict diagnostic delay, but admitted patients were diagnosed sooner. The authors concluded that ED presentation for acute neurological symptoms represents an opportunity for rapid diagnosis and treatment of early MS and that neurology consultation and admission expedites the process.

Emergency Department Evaluation of Patients With Known MS

Surprisingly little study has been devoted to the evaluation of established patients with MS in the ED setting.

A 2014 observational study from Mount Sinai Medical Center in New York examined ED utilization by patients with established MS over a 3-year period in a population that included a significant number of poor and uninsured patients.[22] Almost 75% of visits were for nonneurological symptoms, such as musculoskeletal pain, fever, and gastrointestinal complaints. More than half of the patients had severe disability, defined as an EDSS of 6 or greater (needing an assistive device such as a cane or crutch to walk 100 m). Presentations directly related to MS, such as exacerbations, were diagnosed in only 20% of patients with mild to moderate disease (EDSS < 6) and 13.2% of visits overall. For patients with mild to moderate disease (EDSS < 6), most visits were for medical issues unrelated to MS; for those with severe disease, most visits were for medical issues that were related to MS but indirectly, such as UTI or pneumonia, decubitus ulcers, or falls. Only half of the patients with RRMS were receiving disease-modifying treatment.

A 2016 observational study from Johns Hopkins examined the value of ED MRI in the evaluation of patients with MS who present with a possible exacerbation. Over a 2-year period, 115 encounters resulted in MRI; 37% had active MRI findings, 42% were diagnosed with a true exacerbation, and 18% were diagnosed with a pseudoexacerbation. When spine imaging was performed, 20% showed acute activity, although only 10% showed activity only in the spine. MRI only occasionally (8%) revealed an alternative diagnosis, such as radiculopathy, compressive myelopathy, and stroke. Of those diagnosed with an exacerbation, 92% were admitted and almost all received steroids.[23]

The study demonstrated clinicians' reliance on MRI to decide disposition and treatment in large centers with ready access to this resource. Indeed, the authors point out that "no (nonpregnant) patient with MS presenting to the ED was admitted for treatment of an MS exacerbation without either ED MRI imaging or inpatient MR imaging, despite the current definition of MS exacerbations as a clinical diagnosis."

A 2017 observational study from the Cleveland Clinic divided ED visits into three categories: category 1 comprised new neurological symptoms, category 2 comprised worsening of preexisting symptoms, and category 3 comprised nonneurological complications of MS. Over a calendar year, there were 97 MS-related ED visits, divided almost equally among the three categories. In category 1, 64% of patients had an MRI performed, of which 52% showed acute activity. Although 33% of patients in this category therefore had a positive MRI, almost twice that number (61%) were diagnosed with a true exacerbation. In category 2, 48% of patients had an MRI, and 29% of studies were positive. Although only 14% of patients in this category had a positive study, almost twice that number (24%) were diagnosed with a true exacerbation. The authors do not specify what proportion of the patients diagnosed with an exacerbation in the absence of a positive MRI had no MRI done (i.e., judged not to need one for diagnosis) and what proportion had a negative MRI but nevertheless received the diagnosis on clinical grounds.[24] The authors state that ED mistriage results in a large number of unnecessary MRIs and admissions to the neurology service, but they do not present data regarding who (EM or Neurology) decided to perform an MRI and who decided on admission.

The study refutes some common assumptions regarding the diagnosis of true and pseudorelapses. Patients with clinical or laboratory findings suggestive of infection, especially UTI, are often assumed to have a pseudorelapse. In this study, however, patients diagnosed with true relapse had an overall rate of suspected infection (30%) only slightly lower than those with nonrelapse (53%) and had a rate of UTI (23%) similar to those with nonrelapse (34%).

Treatment of Acute Attacks

Most acute attacks (relapses) are treated with glucocorticoids. Steroid treatment appears to accelerate the recovery from an attack, improving outcome assessed at 4 to 5 weeks. However, steroid treatment does not appear to alter the long-term outcome of the attack or reduce the long-term risk of further attacks.[25-27] A typical course of steroid consists of 3 to 7 days of either intravenous (IV) (500-1000 mg of methylprednisolone daily) or oral steroid (626-1250 mg of oral prednisone). There does not appear to be any significant benefit for IV over oral route of administration. The potential side effects of short courses of high-dose steroids are familiar to emergency practitioners and include psychiatric disturbances, gastrointestinal symptoms, increased susceptibility to infection, and hyperglycemia in diabetics.

Adrenocorticotropic hormone (ACTH), which stimulates adrenal production of glucocorticoids, is occasionally used for patients who cannot tolerate or do not respond to direct administration of corticosteroids. Some investigators have suggested that there may be additional anti-inflammatory and immunomodulatory effect of ACTH mediated through melanocortin pathways.

Several very small trials have suggested that **plasmapheresis** might improve the short-term resolution of acute attacks. The American Academy of Neurology recommends consideration of plasmapheresis as a second-line therapy for patients whose relapse does not respond to steroid.

Disease-Modifying Agents

Several immunomodulatory agents have been demonstrated to slow the rate of clinical relapse and the rate of accumulation of MRI brain lesions in patients with RRMS. Most of these therapies are started as soon as a patient receives a diagnosis of MS and are continued indefinitely unless side effects become intolerable. Many are unique to MS treatment and relatively unfamiliar to ED clinicians. Progression of clinical or radiographic disease may cause clinicians to change to a different agent.[28,29]

Treatment of the progressive forms of MS (primary and secondary) has proved more challenging. Ocrelizumab has been shown to slow disability progression in PPMS, and siponimod may be beneficial in the secondary-progressive phase.

Injectable Therapies

Interferon Beta-1b (Betaseron)

Interferon beta-1b (Betaseron) is a cytokine that modulates immune responsiveness by a variety of mechanisms and was the first disease modifying therapy approved for treatment of MS. It is administered by self-injection every other day. A pegylated form of interferon beta-1a (Plegridy) is now available that can be given every other week. Side effects of interferons include injection-site reactions, infections and necrosis, and flu-like symptoms. There is a high prevalence of asymptomatic liver function test (LFT) elevations and possibly an association with leukopenia.

Glatiramer Acetate (Copaxone)

Glatiramer acetate (Copaxone) is a mixture of random polymers of four amino acids, designed to be antigenically similar to myelin basic protein; it appears to compete with myelin antigens for presentation to T cells and induce T helper and T suppressor cells to modulate immune response. Glatiramer acetate is given by subcutaneous injection three times per week. Side effects include injection-site reactions, transient flushing, as well as occasional chest pain, dyspnea, and palpitations.

Infusion Therapies

Natalizumab (Tysabri)

Natalizumab (Tysabri) is a recombinant monoclonal antibody against alpha4 integrin. The integrins are a family of cell-adhesion molecules; alpha4 integrin, which is expressed on the surface of inflammatory lymphocytes and monocytes, modulates adhesion to endothelium and migration of leukocytes into the brain. It is usually given as an infusion every 4 weeks. The most important side effect of natalizumab is development of PML, a potentially fatal neurological disease caused by reactivation of the JC virus. Risk factors for natalizumab-induced PML include previous immunosuppression, presence of anti-JC virus antibody, and duration of treatment. Any patient given natalizumab presenting with new neurological symptoms, especially confusion, change in behavior, aphasia, or hemiparesis should have an evaluation by the neurology service that includes MRI and possibly lumbar puncture to assess JC virus DNA titer.[30]

Alemtuzumab (Campath, Lemtrada)

Alemtuzumab (Campath, Lemtrada) is a humanized monoclonal antibody (also used to treat chronic lymphocytic leukemia and T cell lymphoma) against the cell-surface molecule CD52, which causes the depletion of CD52-positive immune cells such as T lymphocytes, natural killer cells, and monocytes. Treatment is given as a course of infusions on five consecutive days, followed a year later by a course of three daily infusions. Immediate infusion reactions include headache, nausea, rash, and fever. Longer-term complications include susceptibility to viral infections such as herpes simplex and zoster and autoimmune disorders such as thyroid dysfunction and immune thrombocytopenia.[31]

Ocrelizumab (Ocrevus)

Ocrelizumab (Ocrevus) is a recombinant human monoclonal antibody against CD20, a cell-surface marker found on B lymphocytes. Adverse reactions include immediate infusion reactions; its use is contraindicated in patients with active hepatitis B infection because of virus reactivation seen in patients treated with other CD20 antibodies such as rituximab.[32]

Oral Therapies

Dimethyl Fumarate (Tecfidera)

Dimethyl fumarate (Tecfidera) is an organic compound recently found to have efficacy in MS. It has anti-inflammatory and immunomodulatory properties. Common adverse effects include flushing and gastrointestinal complaints, as well as decreased lymphocyte counts.

Teriflunomide (Aubagio)

Teriflunomide (Aubagio) is an inhibitor of pyrimidine synthesis that has immunomodulatory effects via reduced proliferation of activated T and B lymphocytes. Adverse effects include gastrointestinal complaints, hair thinning, and elevation of LFTs. Leflunomide, a compound metabolized to teriflunomide, is associated with embryo lethality and teratogenesis in animal testing; although there is no evidence of fetal harm in babies born to mothers taking teriflunomide, it is considered contraindicated in patients who are pregnant or trying to conceive.

Fingolimod (Gilenya)

Fingolimod (Gilenya) is a sphingosine-1-phosphate receptor modulator, which causes lymphocytes to be sequestered in lymph nodes. Common adverse effects include headache, cough, diarrhea, back pain, leukopenia, and elevated liver enzymes. There have also been reports of dose-dependent bradyarrhythmias, atrioventricular block, and QT prolongation associated with its use. This is commonly seen with first-dose administration. Use of fingolimod with other drugs that can cause QT interval prolongation such as escitalopram should be avoided.

Goals of Emergency Department Evaluation

For patients with a possible first attack of MS, a thorough ED evaluation, including MRI, is important. Neurology consultation and hospital admission appear to markedly increase the rate of early diagnosis for these patients. An accurate diagnosis will allow them to begin disease-modifying treatment early, perhaps delaying or preventing later disability.

For patients with established MS and new symptoms, the goal of ED evaluation is more ambiguous. As the Mount Sinai study showed, ED evaluation of these patients often focuses on distinguishing true from pseudorelapse, usually with MRI as the deciding factor. Most patients with presumed relapse are then admitted.

Both components of this approach are flawed. The determination of a true relapse effectively means a decision to consider steroids, which are the only commonly used treatment for relapses. However, steroids do not alter the eventual outcome of a relapse; they only speed up the eventual resolution of symptoms. This means that the diagnosis of a relapse is not critical for the patient's long-term well-being and the use of advanced MRI must be weighed against the costs in time, money, and use of a limited resource.

There is good reason to question the need to admit all patients with relapses. Evidence suggests that high-dose oral steroid is as effective as IV steroid.[27] If a patient's acute symptoms are not severe or disabling, a basic medical evaluation shows no serious infection, and the patient has good outpatient neurological follow-up, there is no reason that the patient with relapse needs to be admitted. Even when IV steroid is selected, patients may be able to receive the treatment as an outpatient.

The Cleveland Clinic authors proposed an evaluation algorithm for MS in which most patients avoid the ED entirely. Patients should be instructed to contact their neurologist before presenting to the hospital. Those who appear medically stable and are able to care for themselves should be managed outside of the hospital, with a prompt outpatient visit to screen for infection and oral or outpatient IV steroid for suspected relapse. Patients with new neurological symptoms should receive imaging only if their symptoms are severe.[21]

Although this protocol is reasonable, it assumes the existence of resources that might not be present in most hospitals, such as easy telephone access to a neurologist, prompt outpatient follow-up, and an MS team able to provide outpatient IV steroids. In the absence of such resources, many symptomatic patients will come to the ED and many patients will be admitted for IV steroids.

Conclusion

Multiple sclerosis is a complex neurological disorder whose diagnosis and management present many challenges for EM clinicians. A better understanding of the natural history and complications of MS, as well as the many therapies used for the disease, can help clinicians provide the best care for these patients.

Key Points

The role that acute relapses play in the long-term accumulation of disability in patients with MS remains unclear.

Steroids given for acute attacks speed up resolution of symptoms but do not affect long-term disability. Oral steroids appear to be as effective as IV ones.

In a patient with known MS and new or worsened symptoms, the most important goals are excluding significant infection or other acute medical condition, assessing the functional severity of the symptoms, and assuring that the patient has good outpatient neurological follow-up.

Patients with mild symptoms, no evidence of severe infection, and good follow-up can generally be treated as outpatients.

The decision to start steroids for a suspected relapse should ideally be made in collaboration with the patient's neurologist or the neurology consultant. For patients with mild symptoms, the potential side effects may outweigh the symptomatic benefit.

Patients with severe acute symptoms, significant acute medical illness, poor follow-up, or limited ability to care for themselves because of advanced disease may require admission.

References

1. Compston A, Coles A. Multiple sclerosis. *Lancet.* 2008;372(9648):1502-1517.
2. Herndon RM, The pathology of multiple sclerosis and its variants. In: Herndon RM ed. *Multiple Sclerosis: Immunology, Pathology and Pathophysiology.* New York, NY: Demos; 2002:185-197.
3. Prins M, Schul E, Geurts J, et al. Pathological differences between white and grey matter multiple sclerosis lesions. *Ann NY Acad Sci.* 2015;1351:99-113.
4. Galea I, Ward-Abel N, Heesen C. Relapse in multiple sclerosis. *BMJ.* 2015;350:h1765.
5. Vollmer T. The natural history of relapses in multiple sclerosis. *J Neurol Sci.* 2007;256:S5-S13.
6. Confavreux C, Vukisic S. Natural history of multiple sclerosis: a unifying concept. *Brain.* 2006;129:606-616.
7. Leray E, Yaouanq J, Le Page E, et al. Evidence for a two-stage disability progression in multiple sclerosis. *Brain.* 2010;133(7):1900-1913.
8. Merwick A, Sweeney BJ. Functional symptoms in clinically definite MS – pseudo-relapse syndrome. *Int MS J.* 2008;15(2):47-51.
9. Thompson AJ, Banwell BL, Barkhof F, et al. Diagnosis of multiple sclerosis: 2017 revisions of the McDonald criteria. *Lancet Neurol.* 2018;17(2):162-173.
10. Wilhelm H, Schnabet M. The diagnosis and treatment of optic neuritis. *Dtsch Arztbel Int.* 2015;112:616-626.
11. Patten JP. The anatomy, physiology and clinical features of spinal cord disease. In: *Neurological Differential Diagnosis.* London: Springer-Verlag; 1996:213-225.

12. Filippi M, Rocca MA, De Stefano N, et al. Magnetic resonance techniques in multiple sclerosis. *Ach Neurol.* 2011;68(12):1540-1520.

13. Kaunzner UW, Gauthier SA. MRI in the assessment and monitoring of multiple sclerosis: an update on best practice. *Ther Adv Neurol Disord.* 2017;10(6):247-261.

14. Arrambide G, Tintore M, Espejo C, et al. The value of oligoclonal bands in the multiple sclerosis diagnostic criteria. *Brain.* 2018;141(4):1075-1084.

15. Toledano M, Weinshenker BG, Solomon AJ. A clinical approach to the differential diagnosis of multiple sclerosis. *Curr Neurol Neurosci Rep.* 2015;15(8):57.

16. Liu S, Kullnat J, Bourdette D, et al. Prevalence of brain magnetic resonance imaging meeting Barkhof and McDonald criteria for dissemination in space among headache patients. *Mult Scler J.* 2013;19(8):1101-1105.

17. Sadiq A, Brucker BM. Management of neurogenic lower urinary tract dysfunction in multiple sclerosis patients. *Curr Urol Rep.* 2015;16(7):44.

18. Panicker JN, Fowler CJ. Lower urinary tract dysfunction in patients with multiple sclerosis. *Handb Clin Neurol.* 2015;130:371-381.

19. Crabtree-Hartmann E. Advanced symptom management in multiple sclerosis. *Neurol Clin.* 2018;36:197-218.

20. Rocca MA, Amato MP, De Stefano N, et al. Clinical and imaging assessment of cognitive dysfunction in multiple sclerosis. *Lancet Neurol.* 2015;14(3):302-317.

21. Farber R, Hannigan C, Alcauskas M, et al. Emergency department visits before the diagnosis of MS. *Mult Scler Relat Disord.* 2014;3(3):350-354.

22. Oynhausen S, Alcauskas M, Hannigan C, et al. Emergency medical care of multiple sclerosis patients: primary data from the Mount Sinai resource utilization in multiple sclerosis project. *J Clin Neurol.* 2014;10(3):216-221.

23. Pakpoor J, Saylor D, Izbudak I, et al. Emergency department MRI scanning of patients with multiple sclerosis: worthwhile or wasteful? *AJNR Am J Neuroradiol.* 2017;38(1):12-17.

24. Abboud H, Mente K, Seay M, et al. Triaging patients with multiple sclerosis in the emergency department: room for improvement. *Int J MS Care.* 2017;19(6):290-296.

25. Filippini G, Brusaferri F, Sibley WA, et al. Corticosteroids or ACTH for acute exacerbations in multiple sclerosis. *Cochrane Database Syst Rev.* 2000;4:CD001331.

26. Brusaferri F, Candelise L. Steroids for multiple sclerosis and optic neuritis: a meta-analysis of randomized controlled trials. *J Neurol.* 2000;247(6):435-442.

27. Burton JM, O'Connor PW, Hohol M, et al. Oral versus intravenous steroids for treatment of relapses in multiple sclerosis. *Cochrane Database Sust Rev.* 2012;12:CD006921.

28. Tramacere I, Del Giovane C, Salanti G, et al. Immunomodulators and immunosuppressants for relapsing-remitting multiple sclerosis: a network meta-analysis. *Cochrane Database Syst Rev.* 2015;9:CD011381.

29. Rae-Grant A, Day GS, Marrie RA, et al. Practice guideline recommendations summary: disease-modifying therapies for adults with multiple sclerosis: Report of the Guideline Development, Dissemination, and Implementation Subcommittee of the American Academy of Neurology. *Neurology.* 2018;90(17):777-788.

30. Pucci E, Giuliani G, Solari A, et al. Natalizumab for relapsing remitting multiple sclerosis. *Cochrane Database Syst Rev.* 2011;10:CD007621.

31. Ruck T, Bittner S, Wiendi H, et al. Alemtuzumab in multiple sclerosis: mechanism of action and beyond. *Int J Mol Sci.* 2015;16(7):16414-16439.

32. Hauser SL, Bar-Or A, Comi G, et al. Ocrelizumab versus interferon beta-1a in relapsing multiple sclerosis. *N Engl J Med.* 2017;376(3):221-234.

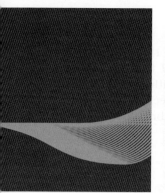
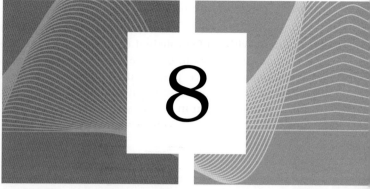

8

Visual Dysfunction in Multiple Sclerosis

■ ▨ ▧ Doria M. Gold, Janet C. Rucker, Steven Galetta

Introduction

Multiple sclerosis (MS) is the most common and familiar disease in a class of inflammatory demyelinating disorders that cause myelin inflammation and destruction and neuronal and axonal loss.[1] Visual symptoms occur in 50% to 80% of patients with MS at some point in the disease course and are a significant source of disability.[2] Visual loss is frequently the initial disease manifestation, with 20% of patients presenting with idiopathic demyelinating optic neuritis.[1,3] Effects on the visual system can be divided into disorders of the *afferent* visual system, including the optic nerves and intracranial visual pathways, and the *efferent* visual system of eye movement control.

Afferent Visual Disturbances

Optic Neuritis

Idiopathic demyelinating optic neuritis is the most common optic neuropathy under the age of 40 years. It may occur as an initial clinically isolated demyelinating event in the absence of a diagnosis of MS or in a patient with an established diagnosis of MS (Case 1). Typical presentation is vision loss in one eye that progresses over 1 to 2 weeks and is accompanied by eye pain that is typically worse with eye movement.[4] Bilateral simultaneous optic neuritis can occur, especially in children,[5] but it is uncommon in adults and should generate a broader differential diagnosis.[6]

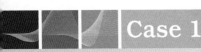

Case 1

Idiopathic demyelinating optic neuritis with no prior established MS diagnosis

A 36-year-old man presented with a "white spot" in the vision of his left eye, and left eye pain increased with movement. Upon further questioning, he reported numbness over his left cheek that occurred when he was out in the heat.

Examination revealed visual acuity of 20/20 in the right eye and 20/15 in the left eye and normal color vision in each eye on Ishihara color plate testing. The left pupil was sluggishly reactive to light, and a left afferent pupillary defect was present. Optic discs appeared normal without swelling or obvious pallor; however, optical coherence tomography (OCT) revealed elevation of the retinal nerve fiber layer in the left eye (Figure 8.1A), suggesting subclinical disc edema and strongly suggesting acute optic neuritis. No objective sensory deficit was noted. Automated visual field testing revealed a very subtle temporal visual field defect in the left eye.

Magnetic resonance imaging (MRI) of the orbits and brain with gadolinium demonstrated left optic nerve T2 hyperintensity and enhancement (Figure 8.2A and B), thus confirming acute demyelinating optic neuritis. There were periventricular, deep white matter, juxtacortical, and left pontine T2-hyperintense lesions compatible with demyelination (Figure 8.2C). He was diagnosed with optic neuritis and MS. Corticosteroids were discussed for immediate treatment of optic neuritis, and a decision was made between the doctor and the patient not to administer corticosteroid treatment. He was given peginterferon beta-1a. At follow-up, his vision improved in the absence of steroid treatment and retinal nerve fiber layer thinning had developed in the left eye (Figure 8.1B).

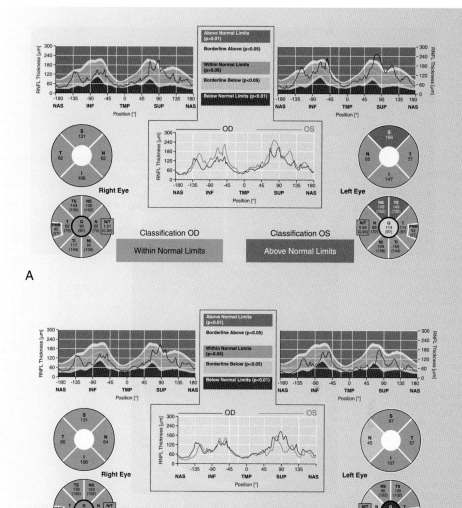

Figure 8.1. Retinal nerve fiber layer (RNFL) optical coherence tomography. A. Average RNFL thickness of 90 is normal in the right eye and elevated to 114 μm in the left eye in Case 1 at initial presentation with acute vision loss in the left eye, suggesting mild optic nerve swelling in the left eye. B. Average RNFL thickness remains 90 and normal in the right eye and has declined to 76, now thin, in the left eye, as expected several months after acute optic neuritis. See eBook for color figure.

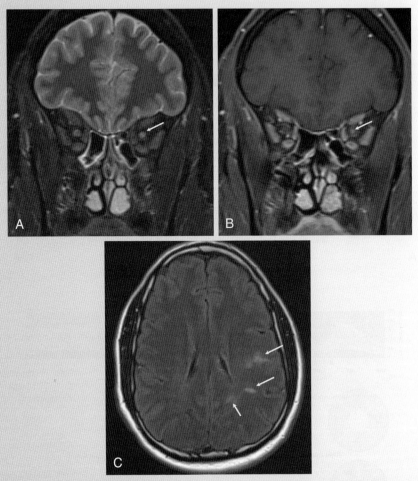

Figure 8.2. MRI orbits and brain with gadolinium. A. Coronal T2-weighted image through the orbits shows increased T2 signal in the left optic nerve (arrow). B. Coronal T1-weighted image with gadolinium through the orbits shows left optic nerve enhancement (arrow). C. Axial T2-weighted FLAIR image shows multiple demyelinating lesions (arrows).

Commentary Our patient had visual symptoms suggestive of optic neuritis; however, his visual acuity, color vision, and low contrast vision were normal. Nonetheless, an afferent pupillary defect and mild visual field defect are two of the most characteristic features of an optic neuropathy. OCT confirmed mild subclinical disc swelling supporting the diagnosis of an acute optic neuropathy. The visual symptoms, presence of subclinical optic nerve swelling in the left eye, and the orbital MRI findings established the diagnosis of acute optic neuritis in our patient. The transient numbness of his face likely reflected a prior demyelinating event exacerbated by a small rise in body temperature.

TABLE 8.1
FEATURES SUGGESTING ATYPICAL OPTIC NEURITIS

No pain

No light perception vision

Retinal hemorrhages

Macula exudates

Severe optic nerve swelling

Bilateral visual loss

No visual recovery

Visual loss progresses beyond 2 wk

Visual acuity, color vision, low contrast vision, pupils, visual fields, and funduscopic examination are the key elements of the examination to perform in the patient with suspected optic neuritis. Optic neuritis is a clinical diagnosis, and it is important to keep in mind a list of red flags (Table 8.1) that would be atypical for idiopathic demyelinating optic neuritis and may suggest an alternative cause of optic neuropathy. The degree of vision loss is highly variable in optic neuritis and can range from mild to severe, with initial visual acuity typically between 20/25 and 20/200.[4] However, the presence of no light perception vision is a red flag and should suggest other potential causes of an acute optic neuropathy, including ischemic and systemic causes. The patient's best visual acuity should always be assessed using corrective lenses or pinhole correction. Color vision is typically formally tested with Ishihara or Hardy Rand Rittler (HRR) color plates that display differentially colored numbers or geometric shapes. The advantage of the HRR plates is that they contain blue and purple shapes, which can sometimes be more affected than the red-green plates contained in the Ishihara series. A simple beside assessment of color vision can be performed by comparing the brightness of a red object between the affected and unaffected eyes, seeking "red desaturation" in the affected eye. Other color tops can also be tried. Detection of an afferent pupillary defect is critical in determining that the vision loss is attributable to an optic nerve process. The afferent pupillary defect may be detected by moving a light back and forth rhythmically between the two pupils. With an optic neuropathy, there will be an asymmetric response and the affected pupil will often paradoxically dilate to the light stimulus.[7] Central visual field loss, called a central scotoma, can often be found on confrontation or automated visual field examination. On ophthalmoscopy, most adults with optic neuritis will have a normal-appearing fundus, suggesting that most of the swelling is retrobulbar or behind the optic nerve head.[4] However, OCT may reveal subclinical optic disc swelling in some of these patients (Case 1). The optic disc will demonstrate mild swelling on ophthalmoscopy in about one-third of patients. Terms to describe this optic nerve head swelling include anterior optic neuritis or papillitis. Children are more likely than adults to have anterior optic neuritis.[8] The presence of severe optic disc swelling in an adult with vision loss in one eye is unlikely to be idiopathic demyelinating optic neuritis, and other etiologies should be considered. Bilateral optic neuropathy is also unusual for typical optic neuritis, and other causes, such as sarcoid, syphilis, vasculitis, and viral processes, should be sought. It should be remembered that papilledema, which is the term used to describe optic nerve head swelling from raised intracranial pressure, usually does not affect the visual acuity like a case of optic neuritis.

Visual improvement in optic neuritis typically occurs over several weeks independent of whether or not corticosteroid treatment is administered, with 90% of patients recovering visual acuity to 20/40 or better.[9] Nonetheless, patients with good high contrast acuity recovery often report reduced visual quality of life and have residual visual dysfunction, particularly for low contrast vision.[10] In the ensuing weeks to months after a bout of optic neuritis, retinal nerve fiber layer thinning can be documented by OCT (Case 1) and optic atrophy occurs. Uhthoff phenomenon, or transient blurring of vision when overheated from exercise or a hot shower, is a common complaint following optic neuritis.

Ancillary testing in the clinic includes formal automated visual field testing and OCT, which is a retinal and optic nerve imaging tool that uses light waves to take cross-sectional images and has wide application in interrogation of optic nerve health in optic neuritis and MS.[11]

Initiated over 20 years ago, the Optic Neuritis Treatment Trial (ONTT) is a landmark clinical trial in which patients were followed for 15 years following an initial clinically isolated idiopathic demyelinating optic neuritis. Participants were randomized to three acute treatment arms: intravenous corticosteroids for 3 days followed by an oral corticosteroid tapered for 11 days, oral corticosteroids in 1 mg/kg/d dosing tapered over 14 days, or oral placebo. At 6 months, the intravenously treated cohort experienced faster recovery of vision[12]; however, there was no difference in final visual outcome at 1 year among the groups.[9] The oral corticosteroid cohort had an increased risk of recurrent optic neuritis, resulting in a recommendation not to treat patients with optic neuritis solely with oral corticosteroids in standard 1 mg/kg/d dosing.

Given that optic neuritis can be the harbinger of a diagnosis of MS, much attention has been given to assessment of factors that may shed light on prognosis. It is clear that the presence of brain lesions on MRI at the time of the initial demyelinating event has the highest predictive value.[13,14] Fifteen years after the bout of optic neuritis diagnosis, the risk of MS was 25% in the patients with no MRI brain lesions, whereas 72% of patients with one or more brain lesions had developed MS in the ONTT study.[13]

Other Afferent Disorders in MS

Many patients with MS have reduced visual quality or visual symptoms in the absence of acute optic neuritis, and referral of any patient with MS for visual and OCT assessment can be helpful in establishing a baseline and to follow the disease course. Subclinical visual system involvement may also occur and deficits of low contrast vision and structural optic nerve injury with retinal nerve fiber layer thinning on OCT are well documented in the absence of acute optic neuritis (Case 2).[15-17]

Case 2

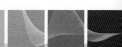

Subclinical optic neuropathy

A 58-year-old man with past medical history of hypertension, asthma, and recently diagnosed MS presented with pressure and discomfort of his right eye for several weeks. He described the discomfort as a feeling that something was in his eye. There was no change with eye movements and no vision change in his right eye. He had no history of vision loss.

On examination, vision was 20/15 in the right eye and 20/20 in the left eye. He perceived all Ishihara color plates correctly with each eye. Formal automated visual fields were normal. Low contrast vision was slightly reduced in each eye. Pupils were equal and briskly reactive to light without an afferent pupillary defect. Eye movements were normal. Optic discs were normal without swelling or pallor. Retinal nerve fiber layer OCT was thin in the right eye and slightly thin in the left eye (Figure 8.3). Slit lamp examination showed an impaired right eye tear film.

Commentary Although this patient had a diagnosis of MS and a symptom of eye pain, his eye pain was more suggestive of an irritative process affecting the cornea rather than an optic neuritis. Although asymptomatic of any visual deficit, he was found to have slightly reduced low contrast vision in each eye and retinal nerve fiber layer thinning on OCT, findings likely suggesting subclinical demyelinating optic neuropathy. The presence of a thin retinal nerve fiber layer is not consistent with acute optic neuritis, as it often takes weeks to months for retinal thinning to occur after a bout of acute visual loss.

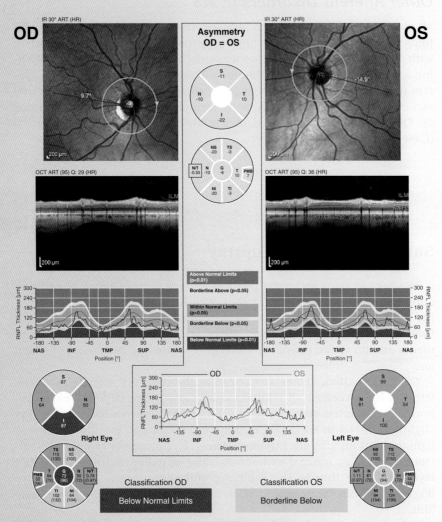

Figure 8.3. Retinal nerve fiber layer (RNFL) optical coherence tomography for Case 2, showing thinning in the right eye and a borderline low average thickness in the left eye. See eBook for color figure.

Not all vision loss in MS is due to optic nerve involvement. Other conditions to be aware of that may require ophthalmology consultation include steroid-induced cataracts and serous retinopathy from repetitive steroid treatment of demyelinating exaccerbations[18] and macular edema (Figure 8.4). The latter may occur as the result of the MS medication fingolimod.[19]

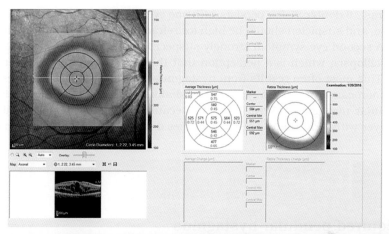

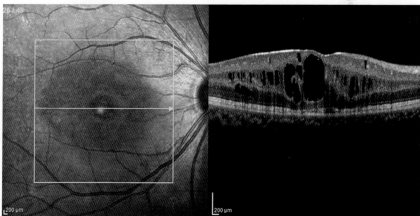

Figure 8.4. Optical coherence tomography through the macula showing fingolimod-induced macular edema. *Courtesy of Ari Green, MD.* See eBook for color figure.

Efferent Visual Disturbances

Visual symptoms attributable to abnormalities of eye movements, such as unstable fixation, impaired range of eye movements, or misalignment of the eyes are common in MS[20-23] and often reflect acute or chronic demyelinating lesions in the brainstem or cerebellum. Symptoms can be quite debilitating and are associated with worse functional and quality of life outcomes in patients with MS.[23,24]

With regard to symptoms, diplopia that is only present with both eyes open and resolves with closure of either eye, so-called binocular diplopia, is due to a misalignment of the two eyes due to demyelination of an ocular motor cranial nerve or connecting pathways that govern ocular motility. In contrast, if double vision persists with one eye covered, MS is not likely the cause, and suspicion should be high for refractive error or ocular problem.

A second eye symptom strongly suspect for abnormal eye movements is oscillopsia, which is a perception that the world is jumping or bouncing. This most often results from nystagmus, or oscillations of the eyes. A common cause in MS is a type of slow shaking of the eyes called acquired pendular nystagmus (APN) (Case 3). Because of persistent movement of the eyes with APN, there is also sometimes decreased central visual acuity.

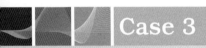

Case 3

Acquired pendular nystagmus

A 34-year-old woman with a 10-year history of MS with substantial gait impairment and chronically poor vision was evaluated for oscillopsia, as she reported constant visual motion. On examination, visual acuity was 20/40 in the right eye and 20/80 in the left eye, color vision was reduced in each eye, and both optic nerves appeared pale. When asked to hold her eyes steady and look straight ahead, small horizontal oscillations of the eyes were seen (Video 8.1 in eBook) consistent with APN. She walked with a walker. MRI brain revealed several chronic demyelinating lesions in the brain, including in the brainstem. She was started on gabapentin to treat her nystagmus and resultant oscillopsia. The dose was gradually increased over several months from a starting dose of 300 mg once a day to 900 mg three times a day, at which point, her oscillopsia was substantially reduced and the nystagmus was less visible on examination.

Commentary   This patient with long-standing MS was quite disabled with chronic bilateral optic nerve demyelination and gait dysfunction requiring a walker. Although some component of her reduced visual acuity and visual impairment was from optic nerve disease, her nystagmus directly caused oscillopsia and also likely contributed to her poor visual acuity and visual function. She was symptomatically helped and her nystagmus was reduced by moderately high doses of gabapentin to treat APN.

Examination of eye movements in patients with MS should include observation for any abnormal movement of the eyes as the patient looks straight ahead, side to side, and up and down; assessment of whether each eye moves completely up, down, and to each side; evaluation of the smoothness of eye motion as the eyes follow a slowly moving target (e.g., smooth pursuit); evaluation of the accuracy and speed of fast eye movements called saccades; and determination of whether or not the eyes are aligned and making coordinated movements.

Abnormal smooth pursuit is common in MS; however, it is typically not a cause of visual symptoms. A more typical cause of visual symptoms is internuclear ophthalmoplegia, abbreviated INO, which is caused by demyelination in a structure called the medial longitudinal fasciculus (MLF) that coordinates horizontal eye movements. INO leads to impaired adduction (motion of an eye toward the nose) in one eye on the same side as the demyelinating lesion in the brainstem and abducting nystagmus in the opposite eye (to and fro spontaneous motion of the opposite eye when it is placed in a lateral or outward position toward the ear). For example, when looking left, the right eye will incompletely, or more slowly, turn in toward the nose because of a lesion in the right MLF. In this scenario, the left (abducting) eye will try to maintain paired gaze and as a result will manifest with nystagmus when looking left, which can result in diplopia, blurry vision or "just not seeing right." INO can be the presenting feature of MS or can occur acutely or be chronically present in established MS. On occasion, INO can be simultaneously present on both sides at the same time, in which case each eye has difficulty moving toward the nose on horizontal gaze in the opposite direction.

MRI is indicated when a patient develops new diplopia or oscillopsia, although sometimes the examination is more sensitive than the MRI in detecting an abnormality. For example, the MLF is a very tiny structure, and although examination may definitely prove the presence of an INO, a lesion may not be detectable in the MLF on MRI. Several specific treatment options are available for patients with chronic diplopia or oscillopsia. Patching of one eye or prisms in glasses can be used to eliminate diplopia. Prisms redirect the angle of entry of a visual stimulus to realign the images so that the two eyes again become "yoked." For chronic diplopia with stable ocular misalignment, for example, with chronic bilateral INO, eye muscle surgery to mechanically realign the eyes and better approximate the visual stimulus on the two retinas can be considered.

In the case of APN, medications can be quite effective in minimizing oscillopsia and maximizing visual acuity. Gabapentin and memantine are the first choices for APN in MS and have been shown to be effective in small randomized controlled studies.[25]

Conclusions

Systematic assessment of optic nerve function and eye movements are required to detect the myriad visual manifestations of MS. Steroids are the mainstay of acute therapy but can have consequences, both ophthalmological and systemic. It is important to realize that steroids may help accelerate recovery from an MS attack but do not affect the long-term natural history of MS. Fortunately, there are now many options for the long-term treatment of MS. A low threshold should be maintained for obtaining neuro-ophthalmologic consultation in patients with MS, as MS is a condition that affects all parts of the central nervous system, with frequent and significant impact on vision.

References

1. Balcer LJ. Multiple sclerosis and related demyelinating diseases. In: Miller NR, Newman NJ, eds. *Walsh & Hoyt's Clinical Neuro-ophthalmology.* 6th ed. Philadelphia: Lippincott Williams & Wilkins; 2005:3430-3525.
2. Mowry EM, Loguidice MJ, Daniels AB, et al. Vision related quality of life in multiple sclerosis: correlation with new measures of low and high contrast letter acuity. *J Neurol Neurosurg Psychiatry.* 2009;80:767-772.
3. Miller D, Barkhof F, Montalban X, Thompson A, Filippi M. Clinically isolated syndromes suggestive of multiple sclerosis, part I: natural history, pathogenesis, diagnosis, and prognosis. *Lancet Neurol.* 2005;4:281-288.
4. The Clinical Profile of Optic Neuritis. Experience of the optic neuritis treatment trial. Optic neuritis study group. *Arch Ophthalmol.* 1991;109:1673-1678.
5. Wilejto M, Shroff M, Buncic JR, Kennedy J, Goia C, Banwell B. The clinical features, MRI findings, and outcome of optic neuritis in children. *Neurology.* 2006;67:258-262.
6. de la Cruz J, Kupersmith MJ. Clinical profile of simultaneous bilateral optic neuritis in adults. *Br J Ophthalmol.* 2006;90:551-554.
7. Cox TA, Thompson HS, Corbett JJ. Relative afferent pupillary defects in optic neuritis. *Am J Ophthalmol.* 1981;92:685-690.
8. Morales DS, Siatkowski RM, Howard CW, Warman R. Optic neuritis in children. *J Pediatr Ophthalmol Strabismus.* 2000;37:254-259.
9. Beck RW, Cleary PA. Optic neuritis treatment trial. One-year follow-up results. *Arch Ophthalmol.* 1993;111:773-775.
10. Sabadia SB, Nolan RC, Galetta KM, et al. 20/40 Or better visual acuity after optic neuritis: not as good as we once thought? *J Neuroophthalmol.* 2016;36:369-376.
11. Frohman EM, Fujimoto JG, Frohman TC, Calabresi PA, Cutter G, Balcer LJ. Optical coherence tomography: a window into the mechanisms of multiple sclerosis. *Nat Clin Pract Neurol.* 2008;4:664-675.
12. Beck RW, Cleary PA, Anderson MM Jr, et al. A randomized, controlled trial of corticosteroids in the treatment of acute optic neuritis. The Optic Neuritis Study Group. *N Engl J Med.* 1992;326:581-588.
13. Optic Neuritis Study G. Multiple sclerosis risk after optic neuritis: final optic neuritis treatment trial follow-up. *Arch Neurol.* 2008;65:727-732.
14. Optic Neuritis Study G. The 5-year risk of MS after optic neuritis. Experience of the optic neuritis treatment trial. *Neurology.* 1997;49:1404-1413.
15. Walter SD, Ishikawa H, Galetta KM, et al. Ganglion cell loss in relation to visual disability in multiple sclerosis. *Ophthalmology.* 2012;119:1250-1257.
16. Balcer LJ, Baier ML, Pelak VS, et al. New low-contrast vision charts: reliability and test characteristics in patients with multiple sclerosis. *Mult Scler.* 2000;6:163-171.
17. Saidha S, Syc SB, Ibrahim MA, et al. Primary retinal pathology in multiple sclerosis as detected by optical coherence tomography. *Brain.* 2011;134:518-533.

18. Dinning WJ. Steroids and the eye–indications and complications. *Postgrad Med J.* 1976;52:634-638.

19. Jain N, Bhatti MT. Fingolimod-associated macular edema: incidence, detection, and management. *Neurology.* 2012;78:672-680.

20. de Seze J, Vukusic S, Viallet-Marcel M, et al. Unusual ocular motor findings in multiple sclerosis. *J Neurol Sci.* 2006;243:91-95.

21. Nerrant E, Tilikete C. Ocular motor manifestations of multiple sclerosis. *J Neuroophthalmol.* 2017;37:332-340.

22. Prasad S, Galetta SL. Eye movement abnormalities in multiple sclerosis. *Neurol Clin.* 2010;28:641-655.

23. Derwenskus J, Rucker JC, Serra A, et al. Abnormal eye movements predict disability in MS: two-year follow-up. *Ann NY Acad Sci.* 2005;1039:521-523.

24. Serra A, Derwenskus J, Downey DL, Leigh RJ. Role of eye movement examination and subjective visual vertical in clinical evaluation of multiple sclerosis. *J Neurol.* 2003;250:569-575.

25. Thurtell MJ, Joshi AC, Leone AC, et al. Crossover trial of gabapentin and memantine as treatment for acquired nystagmus. *Ann Neurol.* 2010;67:676-680.

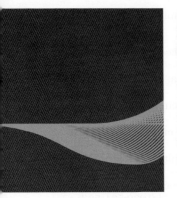
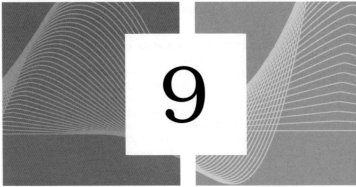

9

Cutaneous Disorders Associated With Multiple Sclerosis

■■■ Anna-Marie Hosking, Joseph L. Jorizzo

Introduction

Patients with multiple sclerosis (MS) suffer from a variety of characteristic cutaneous disorders. Patients with MS often experience paroxysmal itching and dysesthesias and are at an increased risk for injection site reactions or cutaneous neoplasms with certain medications. In this chapter, we review the cutaneous signs and symptoms seen in patients with MS, the cutaneous side effects of disease-modifying therapies, and the medication contraindications physicians should be aware of when managing patients with MS and concomitant skin disease.

Signs and Symptoms—Paroxysmal Dysesthesias and Pruritus

MS is characterized by paroxysmal symptoms, including dysesthesias, pruritus, and phantom sensations. Paresthesias, frank dysesthesias, or pruritus may be the first presenting symptom in a patient with MS. In 1979, Yabuki and Hayabara reported seven cases of segmental burning dysesthesias of the upper extremities in patients with MS.[1] Dysesthesias

154

include pins and needles sensations as well as burning, stabbing, or tearing pain. Most commonly, chronic pain syndromes present with dysesthetic discomfort in the legs but may also involve the trunk and upper extremities.[2]

Itching is a rare sensory symptom in neurological diseases, including MS.[3] Paroxysmal itching as a manifestation of MS was first recognized by Osterman and Westerberg in 1975.[4] Pruritus with MS is transient, comes on with intensity, and is triggered by heat, movement, or sensory stimulation.[2] It has been described on the upper and lower limbs as well as the face and trunk. In a study of 377 patients, 17 presented with paroxysmal itching, with one patient presenting with itching as the only initial MS symptom.[3] Often, the itching is intense, leading to vigorous scratching with subsequent skin excoriation. Many patients also experience persistent dysesthesias or sensory changes in the same location in between paroxysmal episodes. Itching has been associated with other paroxysmal symptoms, including tonic seizures or trigeminal neuralgia.[3] Yamamoto et al reported three Japanese women with MS with paroxysmal itching attacks with abrupt onset and resolution, ranging from seconds to minutes, occurring five to six times daily, often during sleep. These itching attacks presented as the first and only MS symptom or as a predictive symptom of MS exacerbation.[5] The mechanism of itching in MS is unknown. It is thought to be related to transversely spreading ephaptic activation of axons in a partially demyelinated fiber tract in the central nervous system, rendering the nerve fiber hypersensitive to minor irritation.[4,6]

Cutaneous Side Effects of Disease-Modifying Therapy

Injectable Therapies

Interferon-beta (IFN-β) and glatiramer acetate are both effective disease-modifying therapies for MS. IFN-β is available in four preparations: IFN-β 1b (Betaseron® or Extavia®, Bayer Schering Pharma, Berlin, Germany) subcutaneous injection every other day; IFN-β 1a (Rebif®, Merck Serono, Darmstadt, Germany) subcutaneous injection three times weekly; IFN-β 1a (Avonex®, Biogen, Cambridge, Massachusetts, USA) intramuscular injection once weekly; and pegylated IFN-β 1a (Plegridy®, Biogen) subcutaneous injection every 2 weeks.[7] Glatiramer acetate (Copaxone®, Teva Sanofi Aventis, Paris, France) is an amino acid polymer analog of myelin basic protein administered via subcutaneous injection either daily (20 mg/mL) or three times a week (40 mg/mL). These medications have excellent safety profiles; however, injection site reactions are an important limitation in the use of subcutaneous IFN-β and glatiramer acetate.[8,9] In a prospective study of 412 patients with MS treated with disease-modifying therapy for 2 years, none of the patients given intramuscular IFN-β 1a reported missing a dose because of injection site reactions, whereas 5.7% of patients given subcutaneous IFN-β 1b, 7.1% of patients given subcutaneous IFN-β 1a, and 4.3% of patients given subcutaneous glatiramer acetate reported missing doses because of injection site reactions. This is concerning, as missed doses were associated with twice the likelihood of treatment discontinuation.[10] Nonadherence to disease-modifying therapy is associated with poor clinical outcomes and increased risk of MS relapse.[11,12] Management of injection site reactions requires an ongoing dialogue between the neurologist and dermatologist to manage adverse cutaneous side effects and to tailor the appropriate dose and type of disease-modifying therapy.

Injection Site Reactions

Injectable disease-modifying therapies can cause a wide range of injection site reactions, from transient erythema and eczemalike reactions to severe ulcers and necrosis, which may require treatment cessation and surgical intervention. The most common injection site reactions include erythema, bruising, induration, immune-mediated inflammatory reactions, lipoatrophy, cutaneous necrosis, and ulceration.[9] Rare cutaneous reactions have been reported, including psoriasis exacerbation,[13] granulomatous dermatitis with focal sarcoidal features,[14] Raynaud phenomenon,[15] panniculitis,[16,17] vasculitis,[18] subacute cutaneous lupus erythematosus,[19] morphea,[20] localized pigmentation disorders,[21] cutaneous mucinoses,[22] and fixed drug eruptions.[23] Injection site reactions most commonly occur during the first month of treatment but have been reported up to 29 months after initiating therapy.[24] Some reports suggest a decrease in the incidence with increasing treatment duration.[25] Injection-site reactions are observed more frequently in injection sites with reduced subcutaneous fat (i.e., thighs and arms) than in areas with increased subcutaneous fat (i.e., buttocks and abdomen).[26] There is a higher predominance in females than in males, ranging from 2:1 to 8:1, although this may be an artifact of the higher overall incidence of MS in women.[24,27]

Interferon-beta

Along with flulike symptoms, injection site reactions are the most common side effect observed in patients using injectable IFN-β, occurring in up to 90% of patients using subcutaneous formulations and up to 33% of those using intramuscular formulations.[9,28] In three controlled clinical trials investigating the use of IFN-β 1b (Betaseron®), injection site reactions occurred in 86% of patients compared with 37% with placebo. Injection site necrosis occurred in 5% of patients compared with none in the placebo cohort. Other reactions, including inflammation (53%), pain (18%), hypersensitivity (3%), and edema (3%) were significantly associated with IFN-β 1b treatment. Approximately 76% of patients who developed injection site reactions did so in the first 3 months of treatment.[29] In addition, a placebo-controlled randomized trial of IFN-β 1b for secondary progressive MS reported injection site reactions in 43.6% of patients versus 10.3% with placebo. Necrosis occurred in 4.7% compared with zero in the placebo group and inflammation in 50% compared with 4.2% in the placebo group.[30] A 30-month postlicensure study reviewed the adverse event reports for IFN-β 1b following Food and Drug Administration (FDA) approval in 1993. Adverse events included erythema (51%), pain (30%), and necrosis (13%), with 6% of patients with injection site reactions subsequently discontinuing therapy and 21% of patients with injection site necrosis requiring surgical intervention.[24]

In two multicenter studies evaluating the safety and efficacy of IFN-β 1a (Rebif®) in patients with relapsing remitting MS, injection site reactions occurred in 89% and 92% of patients taking 22 μg and 44 μg three times weekly, respectively, compared with 39% with placebo. Injection site necrosis occurred in six patients (3%) taking 44 μg three times weekly and two patients (1%) taking 22 μg three times weekly over the course of 2 years.[31]

Intramuscular administration (Avonex®) is associated with fewer skin reactions when compared with subcutaneous administration of IFN-β. In pooled placebo-controlled clinical studies, injection site pain, inflammation, and injection site reactions occurred in 8%, 6%, and 3% of patients, respectively, compared with 6%, 2%, and 1% with placebo. To date, there have been no reports of necrosis with the use of Avonex®. However, lipoatrophy can occur when improperly injecting intramuscular formulations subcutaneously, due to an incorrect injection angle.[9,28]

Panniculitis and Lipoatrophy

Panniculitis, the inflammation of subcutaneous adipose tissue, has been described in patients treated with IFN-β therapy, with subsequent lipoatrophy seen in up to 46% of patients.[9,32] Localized lipoatrophy is characterized by loss of subcutaneous adipose tissue in the area of the injection site, resulting in well-circumscribed areas of skin depression, seen most commonly on the anterolateral surface of thighs or upper arms. Histopathology shows atrophic and diminutive fat lobules in the subcutaneous fat (Figure 9.1). Proposed mechanisms include a direct toxic effect on adipocytes, inciting an inflammatory response followed by a hypersensitivity reaction and residual loss of subcutaneous fat.[33] Patients generally present with pain, erythema, and induration at injection sites of the arms or thighs (abdomen and buttocks are less common). A minority of reactions

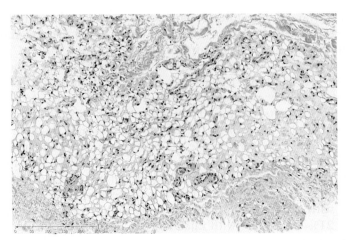

Figure 9.1. Lipoatrophy. Atrophic and diminutive fat lobules in the subcutaneous fat with minimal surrounding inflammation (hematoxylin and eosin, 14×). See eBook for color figure.

are severe enough to cause difficulty with ambulation or require surgical debridement.[34] Reports of both septal and lobular panniculitis have been described with or without accompanying vascular thrombosis.[13,16,17,32,35-40] Lipoatrophy is a concerning side effect, as it may be irreversible, resulting in disfiguring contours of the thighs and arms. It is more commonly observed with glatiramer acetate injection than with IFN-β. There are multiple potential explanations for the occurrence of lipoatrophy with IFN-β, including incorrect injection into the dermis, secondary reaction from the high immunogenicity of IFN-β, and administration of nonprewarmed medication.[10,22]

Morphea

A rare and more recently reported cutaneous side effect of IFN-β therapy is localized scleroderma, or morphea. Morphea is a cutaneous fibrosing connective tissue disorder characterized by excessive collagen deposition leading to thickening of the dermis, subcutaneous tissue, or both (Figure 9.2). Cases of morphea have been reported with both IFN-β 1a and IFN-β 1b.[20,41,42] In one case, woody induration consistent with morphea appeared on the anterior thighs 6 months after injection of IFN-β 1a.[20] Another case reported a morpheaform reaction to IFN-β 1b injection on the thighs and abdomen after 10 years of IFNβ-1b therapy.[42] Histopathologically, these cases were consistent with morphea, with thickened collagen bundles extending into the subcutaneous fat, paucity of adnexal structures, and a deep reticular lymphocytic infiltrate (Figure 9.3).[41] The authors proposed a possible dysregulation of inflammatory cytokines, trauma, or a combination of both as the underlying cause.

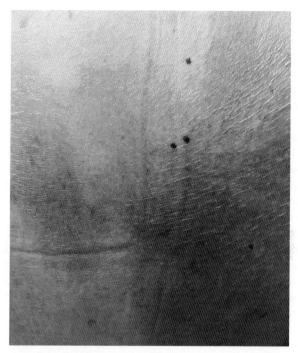

Figure 9.2. Clinical presentation of morphea showing multiple hyperpigmented atrophic plaques with an erythematous border. Also pictured are a few scattered cherry angiomas and seborrheic keratoses. See eBook for color figure.

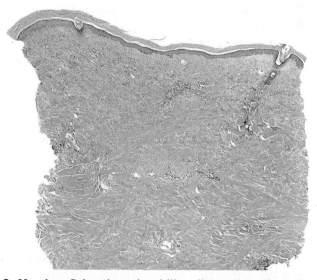

Figure 9.3. Morphea. Sclerotic eosinophilic collagen throughout the dermis with a dense perivascular and periadnexal infiltrate composed of lymphocytes and plasma cells and trapping of adnexal structures (hematoxylin and eosin, 3×). See eBook for color figure.

Cutaneous Ulceration and Necrosis

Injection site ulceration and necrosis typically occur within the first 4 months of therapy but have been reported greater than 1 year after initiating therapy. Necrosis is generally limited to an area 3 cm or less in diameter with extension into the subcutaneous fat, although larger lesions with involvement of the fascia overlying muscle have been reported.[29] Healing is usually associated with scarring. In rare cases, debridement with subsequent skin grafting may be required. Histologically, perivascular and interstitial lymphohistiocytic infiltrates, panniculitis, and thrombosis of deeper vessels have been reported.[13,29,43-50] Proposed mechanisms include thrombosis and necrosis of dermal vessels secondary to abnormal aggregation of platelets as well as a hypersensitivity reaction within blood vessels.[43,51-53] Incorrect injection technique and improper depth of injection have been identified as risk factors.[54] The decision of whether to continue treatment depends on the extent of necrosis. Some patients have experienced healing of necrotic skin lesions while continuing therapy. Patients should be advised not to administer therapy into the affected area.[23] If multiple lesions are present, the general consensus is that therapy should be discontinued.[29]

Pathogenesis

The pathogenesis of injection site reactions with IFN-β therapy is not fully understood. Direct toxic and proinflammatory mechanisms, as well as IgE-mediated and delayed hypersensitivity reactions have been proposed as potential causes. Furthermore, immune-mediated necrotizing vasculitis and platelet-dependent thrombosis may play a role. Patients with MS have clotting abnormalities at baseline secondary to abnormal platelet activation, which may be further exacerbated by the immunomodulatory treatments used in MS.[37,51,55] IFN-β administered subcutaneously can induce inflammatory skin reactions due to local chemokine induction with immune cell extravasation. More specifically, studies have demonstrated an upregulation of chemokines (CCL2 and CXCL10), with recruitment of circulating T cells to evolving skin lesions.[56] Histologically, reports have demonstrated a lupuslike reaction with superficial and deep perivascular and periadnexal lymphocytic infiltrate with focal interface damage and interstitial mucin.[23,57,58] In severe cases, thrombosis of deeper vessels may be seen.[13,29,43-49]

Systemic Reactions

Rare systemic reactions have been reported with the use of IFN-β therapy in patients with MS, although a direct correlation between disease onset and the use of IFN therapy could not be proven in all cases. Twelve cases of sclerosing skin disorders, including both limited and diffuse cutaneous sclerosis, have been reported in patients with MS.[59] In five of these patients, IFN-β had been administered between 1 and 8 years before the onset of sclerosis, which the authors suggested may have been the trigger.[59] One case of cutaneous vasculitis with renal impairment was reported in a patient injecting IFN-β for 10 weeks who developed purpura, proteinuria, and hematuria after an injection.[18] In another case, a middle-aged female developed disseminated cutaneous lesions after her third IFN-β injection, which reappeared after a subsequent injection and resolved upon discontinuation of therapy.[60] A diffuse maculopapular rash was reported in one patient after her second IFN-β injection, which resolved with antihistamines and corticosteroids but reappeared after the third injection.[61] In addition, there was one report of severe, new-onset dermatomyositis in a male patient after 5 years of IFN-β therapy. There was a temporal association between exacerbation of symptoms and repeated injections, with in vitro studies revealing enhanced type I IFN signaling in lymphoid cells in response to IFN-β.[62] Furthermore, IFN-induced sarcoidosis is a rare reaction but has been reported in seven patients with MS, as well as one with multiple myeloma and one patient with renal cell carcinoma.[14,63-70] In one case, a patient developed noncaseating granulomas in her skin and in pulmonary lymph nodes after 3 years of therapy. The authors proposed that the development of sarcoidosis was due to a dysregulation in the modulatory role of IFN-β (and more generally type I interferon) expression in chronic inflammation.[64] In addition, multiple reports of new-onset psoriasis, psoriatic arthritis, and psoriasis exacerbations have been reported with the use of IFN therapy, with some lesions lasting as long as 6 years after the cessation of IFN-β.[13,71-74] The mechanism is thought to be due to IFN-β's proinflammatory effect in psoriasis, with upregulation of the interleukin (IL)-23/ T helper cell (Th)17 pathway.[72,75]

Glatiramer Acetate

Injection site reactions have been reported in 20% to 80% of patients taking glatiramer acetate, including erythema (66%), inflammation (49%), pain (73%), and pruritus (40%).[76-78] These injection site reactions are generally mild or moderate in severity and disappear spontaneously in hours to days. Similar rates of injection site reactions are seen with the 20- and 40-mg dosing regimens.[76] Aviv et al recently proposed three distinct histologic responses to glatiramer acetate injections: (1) erythematous plaques and nodules with superficial and sometimes deep inflammatory infiltrates seen in an acute response, (2) morpheaform plaques with perivascular and interstitial dermatitis and thick collagen bundles seen in chronic cases, and (3) lipoatrophy initially present as deep infiltrates of lymphocytes, neutrophils, eosinophils, and plasma cells, leading to a more chronic infiltration, loss of subcutaneous adipose tissue, and delicate fibrosis.[79] Average onset of injection site reactions after glatiramer acetate therapy is 1.75 years, but reactions may occur as early as the first injection.[79] Possible causes of injection site reactions include the high immunogenicity of glatiramer acetate, repeated trauma to the fat inciting an inflammatory reaction, as well as an allergic reaction to glatiramer acetate components.[80,81]

Panniculitis and Lipoatrophy

Glatiramer acetate is characteristically associated with frank panniculitis and subsequent lipoatrophy.[33,82-86] Of all the injectable disease-modifying therapies for MS, glatiramer acetate is associated with the highest prevalence of lipoatrophy. This occurrence was originally reported to be rare, occurring in 2% of patients in clinical studies, but in a recent study involving full skin examinations in patients taking glatiramer acetate, prevalence was as high as 45%.[84,87] Trauma alone can cause lipoatrophy, such as the lipoatrophy seen with acupuncture. It is thought that this type of lipoatrophy is caused by the activation of macrophages and release of cytokines such as tumor necrosis factor (TNF) and IL-1.[82] Histologically, acupuncture-induced lipoatrophy is characterized by an involutional pattern with thin and elongated fat lobules, with only a few surrounding macrophages. However, on histopathologic examination of glatiramer acetate–associated lipoatrophy, a lobar panniculitis predominates with histiocytes engulfing lipids from necrotic adipocytes and T lymphocytes in the fat lobules. Thickened septa with scattered lymphoid follicles composed of B lymphocytes may also be seen.[33] This type of adverse event appears to be independent of injection technique.[84] Glatiramer acetate panniculitis is thought to be secondary to the drug's high immunogenicity, as a robust immune response is required for glatiramer acetate to be therapeutic in MS treatment.[33,80,85] In mild cases, cutaneous lesions may resolve with treatment discontinuation but can reappear if injections are restarted. However, two recent reports suggested that glatiramer acetate–associated lipoatrophy can persist and even progress despite discontinuing treatment.[80,88]

Nicolau syndrome (embolia cutis medicamentosa) is a rare complication of the injection of several drugs, leading to cutaneous, subcutaneous, or muscular aseptic necrosis. There are multiple cases of Nicolau syndrome reported in the literature secondary to glatiramer acetate injections.[53,89,90] One patient who had been given 20 mg glatiramer acetate for 7 years experienced severe, lancinating pain with injection into her lower abdomen after recently increasing the dosage and decreasing the frequency of her injections.[90] Histological examination of the excised specimen revealed predominately lobar panniculitis with lymphocytes and plasma cells surrounding necrotic adipocytes as well as diffuse subcutaneous sclerosis. The authors proposed that this morphealike sclerosis is likely an underreported aspect of glatiramer acetate injection site reactions.[90]

Management

Prompt treatment of injection site reactions is important, as it may contribute to continued patient compliance. For the management of injection site reactions, ibuprofen and topical corticosteroids or calcineurin inhibitors have been shown to be beneficial in decreasing inflammation.

Adherence to proper injection protocol can help reduce the risk, including prewarming the injection solution, sterile technique, proper needle length, subcutaneous injection (vs. intradermal injection), and regularly changing injection sites.[91] Therefore, the injection technique should be regularly reviewed with patients to ensure competence and reduce the incidence of secondary complications.

Injection site care is another important aspect in preventing complications. Warm compress application before injection has been shown to be effective in decreasing injection site reactions.[87] The use of firm pressure and ice packs after injections can also help minimize swelling and bruising. If swelling persists for longer than a day, warm compresses can be applied to the site. If swelling continues to persist, the patient should be instructed to consult a physician to rule out possible infection.[91]

In the case of mild to moderate injection site reactions, disease-modifying therapy should not be discontinued. For injection site necrosis, temporary dose reduction or discontinuation may be indicated depending on the severity.[26,29] Local treatment may include topical antibacterials, but it is important to avoid topical corticosteroids in the case of necrosis, as they can prolong wound healing and increase the risk of infection.[91] Surgical excision and grafting may be indicated in more severe cases. It is important to note that some injection site reactions (i.e., postinflammatory hyperpigmentation, scars, and disfiguring lipoatrophy) may persist.

Infusion Therapies (Alemtuzumab, Natalizumab, Ocrelizumab, Rituximab)

Cutaneous Infusion-Associated Reactions

Alemtuzumab. Alemtuzumab (Lemtrada, Campath-1H®, Genzyme Corporation, Cambridge, MA, USA) is a humanized monoclonal antibody directed against cluster of differentiation (CD)52, which is present on the surface of B and T cells. In two phase 3 trials of alemtuzumab in relapsing remitting MS (12 mg on 5 consecutive days and 3 consecutive days 12 mo later), cutaneous infusion-associated reactions occurred in 66% of patients, including rash (47%), urticaria (13%), pruritus (11%), and erythema (4%).[92] Two subsequent studies including a retrospective chart review and a prospective cohort study reported lower rates of cutaneous side effects in 34.2% and 33.3% of patients, respectively.[93,94] This difference was attributed to a higher dose of corticosteroids and suggests that pretreatment with corticosteroids and antihistamines may help ameliorate the cutaneous side effects of alemtuzumab infusion.[93]

The histopathologic spectrum of hypersensitivity reactions associated with alemtuzumab was recently described.[95] Biopsies of five patients with cutaneous T cell lymphoma or chronic lymphocytic leukemia who were treated with alemtuzumab and developed pruritic, erythematous papules, and plaques were reviewed. Histopathologic examination revealed subacute spongiotic dermatitis with multifocal parakeratosis, endothelial activation, and perivascular lymphocytic infiltrate, without prominent eosinophils. The authors hypothesize that the cutaneous reaction may be due to an immunologic response secondary to resident memory T cells in the skin.[95]

One case report demonstrated severe generalized bullous drug eruption occurring 10 days after infusion of alemtuzumab. The rash resolved with high-dose oral corticosteroids. A subsequent infusion was given 1 year later with concomitant intravenous and postinfusion corticosteroids. Following the second infusion, the patient developed a more limited, asymptomatic macular dermatitis.[96] Alopecia is another reported adverse effect of alemtuzumab, with two cases of alopecia universalis and three cases of alopecia areata in the literature.[97-99] Immune thrombocytopenic purpura was initially reported in six patients in a 2008 study, including a fatal case in a patient receiving alemtuzumab 24 mg.[100-103] Across all clinical trials, immune thrombocytopenic purpura incidence was 2% in patients receiving alemtuzumab 12 or 24 mg. Therefore, patients should be advised to monitor for the development of petechiae, increased bleeding, or easy bruising.

In uncontrolled studies of alemtuzumab for MS, melanoma occurred in 4 of 1486 (0.3%) of alemtuzumab-treated patients. One patient had evidence of locally advanced disease.[104] Postmarketing reports of melanoma include a 34-year-old woman who developed superficial spreading melanoma in a long-standing nevus after 6 months of treatment with alemtuzumab. The authors hypothesized that alemtuzumab led to impairment of immunosurveillance predisposing to tumorigenesis.[105] Two additional cases of melanoma with alemtuzumab therapy have been reported in a retrospective study of Austrian patients with B cell chronic lymphocytic leukemia.[106] These findings have led the FDA to recommend routine skin examination at the start of treatment and annually thereafter to monitor for melanoma.[107]

Natalizumab. Natalizumab (Tysabri®, Biogen Idec, Cambridge, MA, USA and Elan Pharmaceuticals, Dublin, Ireland) is an adhesion-molecule inhibitor, specifically a humanized monoclonal antibody targeting α4 integrins on the surface of lymphocytes. As a result, natalizumab blocks leukocyte trafficking across the blood-brain barrier.[108] Cutaneous side effects associated with natalizumab infusions include urticaria, allergic dermatitis, and hypersensitivity reactions, including serum sickness reactions.[109-111] Less common reactions have been reported in the literature. One patient reportedly developed acquired perforating dermatosis after 6 infusions (300 mg per month).[112] Skin lesions were temporally associated with infusions, appearing 3 to 5 days after each infusion, resolving 15 days later. In another case, a patient with a 12-year history of MS developed a generalized erythematous drug eruption, edema, and nausea after 1 month of natalizumab.[113]

Natalizumab may also induce or aggravate psoriasis in patients with MS. One patient with a family history of psoriasis developed plaque psoriasis 6 years after the initiation of natalizumab. Her disease was well controlled with topical therapies.[114] Another patient in her 30s with a history of mild psoriasis in adolescence developed a severe disseminated psoriasis eruption that was resistant to topical treatment and phototherapy after six natalizumab infusions. The authors hypothesized a paradoxical immune reaction due to upregulation of other pathways after blocking the migration of lymphocytes across the blood-brain barrier.[115] A middle-aged man without any history of psoriasis developed severe psoriasis on his extremities after two doses of natalizumab. Treatment was discontinued after six doses because of persistent psoriasis and new-onset foot pain that made walking difficult.[116] Finally, another patient without any prior history of psoriasis developed biopsy-proven psoriasis on the scalp, trunk, and extremities with associated arthralgias after 19 natalizumab infusions.[117] Treatment was switched to dimethyl fumarate, and the plaques cleared within 3 months.

The role of natalizumab in the development of melanoma is unclear. A meta-analysis of safety data from clinical trials on natalizumab reported a similar incidence of melanoma among patients who received natalizumab (3/4250; 0.07%) compared with placebo (2/2059; 0.10%).[118] Multiple case reports of melanoma have been reported with natalizumab therapy, including a case of ocular melanoma as well as urethral melanoma.[119-125] On review of the FDA's Adverse Event Reporting System database up until 2014, 137 cases of natalizumab-associated melanoma were identified. The median onset was 4 months after starting therapy, and there were two mucosal melanomas, five ocular melanomas, and nine melanoma-related deaths.[119] In normal melanocytes, $\alpha 4$ integrin is not expressed; however, it is expressed on melanoma cells. Downregulation of $\alpha 4$ integrin has been shown to be involved with melanoma invasion. Thus, one proposed mechanism of natalizumab-potentiated melanoma involves binding $\alpha 4$ integrin to directly promote melanoma cell replication, invasion, and migration.[119] Conversely, the role of natalizumab in inducing melanoma was challenged by the results of a 4-year dermoscopic study following 74 patients with MS with 775 monitored melanocytic skin lesions. This investigation yielded substantial dermoscopic changes in only 1.54% of cases.[126] All excised lesions were benign, and immunohistological studies and proliferation and invasion assays revealed a lack of detectable levels of melanoma progression markers (secreted protein acidic and rich in cysteine [SPARC] and β_3 integrin) in nevi. This study concluded that natalizumab therapy does not increase the risk for nevus transformation.[126] Nevertheless, further data are needed to clarify if an association exists. Patients taking natalizumab should be warned regarding the potential risk of melanoma, and physicians should remain vigilant in screening for melanoma, especially in patients with a history of atypical moles.

Ocrelizumab. Ocrelizumab (Ocrevus®, Genentech, Inc, San Francisco, CA, USA) is a humanized monoclonal antibody targeting CD20 antigen on B cells that is FDA approved for the treatment of relapsing and primary progressive MS.[127,128] There has been one report of biopsy-proven psoriasiform dermatitis in an elderly woman 3.5 months after starting ocrelizumab. This was determined to be a "probable" drug reaction by the authors.[129]

Rituximab. Rituximab (Rituxan®, Biogen-IDEC/Genentech, San Francisco, CA, USA) is a chimeric mouse/human anti-CD20 antibody that results in selective reduction of mature B lymphocytes and has been shown to be effective in MS treatment.[130] In a nonrandomized, single-arm study of rituximab for the treatment of primary cutaneous B cell lymphoma, 356 patients (37%) developed infusion-associated reactions, including itching, rash, and urticaria.[131] Mucocutaneous reactions, including fatal cases of Stevens-Johnson syndrome or toxic epidermal necrolysis, are less commonly reported complications after treatment with rituximab. Other reactions include paraneoplastic pemphigus, lichenoid dermatitis, and vesiculobullous dermatitis.[131] The onset of these reactions varies but can be seen as soon as the first infusion. In one case, toxic epidermal necrolysis developed 12 hours post rituximab infusion and demonstrated a successful response to etanercept.[132] In another case, a 36-year-old man developed mucositis and fevers after the first two infusions and maculopapular rash with severe urogenital ulceration after the third.[133] However, this case was later reported to be more likely due to a paraneoplastic pemphigus and not consistent with Stevens-Johnson syndrome given the chronic nature of the disease.[134] Another report described a fatal case of Stevens-Johnson syndrome/toxic epidermal necrolysis overlap in a patient receiving his first cycle of allopurinol, rituximab, and bendamustine treatment for non-Hodgkin B cell lymphoma.[135] The combination of rituximab and bendamustine in contributing to fatal toxic epidermal necrolysis has been previously reported.[136] In addition, seven cases of iatrogenic Kaposi sarcoma in human immunodeficiency virus–negative patients have been reported with the use of rituximab.[137-140] The authors suggest screening for human herpesvirus-8 in high-risk patients before initiating rituximab. Similarly, a few cases of cutaneous vasculitis as well as serum sickness reactions have been reported.[141-144]

Oral Therapies

Teriflunomide

Teriflunomide (Aubagio®, Genzyme Corporation) is a once-daily oral immunomodulator for the treatment of relapsing remitting MS. Teriflunomide inhibits dihydro-orotate dehydrogenase, a key enzyme in de novo pyrimidine synthesis required for lymphocyte proliferation.[145] Teriflunomide is the active metabolite of leflunomide, which was approved for the treatment of rheumatoid arthritis in 1998.[146] The primary dermatologic side effect associated with teriflunomide is hair thinning. Pooled safety and tolerability data from four placebo-controlled studies and extension studies with treatment duration exceeding 12 years and a cumulative exposure to teriflunomide exceeding 6800 patient-years reported dose-dependent hair thinning.[147] Hair thinning, defined as decreased hair density or hair loss, occurred more frequently in the 14-mg cohort (13.9%) compared with the 7-mg (10.0%) and placebo (5.1%) groups. Sixteen patients discontinued treatment because of hair thinning. Onset was during the first 6 months, and most cases improved during treatment continuation.[147]

Fingolimod

Fingolimod (Gilenya, Novartis Pharma AG, Basel, Switzerland) is an immunomodulatory medication approved by the FDA in 2010 for the treatment of MS.[148] Fingolimod is a sphingosine-1-phosphate receptor modulator that causes internalization of the receptor. As a result, immune cells are unable to receive signals to leave the lymphoid tissue and enter the central nervous system.[149,150]

Clinical trials support an increased incidence of cutaneous malignancy in patients taking fingolimod compared with placebo.[151,152] A phase 3 clinical trial of fingolimod reported an increased risk of basal cell carcinoma in 14 (4%) patients compared with 9 (2%) patients in the placebo cohort. Squamous cell carcinoma occurred in 6 (2%) compared with 1 (<1%) in the placebo group, whereas melanoma occurred in 1 (<1%) versus 0 in the placebo group.[151] Another phase 3 clinical trial reported basal cell carcinoma in 6 (2%) patients in the 1.25-mg cohort and 10 (3%) in the 0.5-mg cohort compared with 2 (1%) in the placebo group.[152] In addition, there have been multiple reports of Merkel cell carcinoma, a rare neuroendocrine skin cancer, with fingolimod therapy.[153-156]

Melanoma was reported in some of the safety and efficacy trials for fingolimod, with the majority of cases determined to be melanoma in situ.[157-159] In a phase 3 trial, three cases of melanoma in situ occurred in 429 patients treated with 0.5 mg daily, whereas none occurred in 420 patients treated with 1.25 mg daily.[157] It has since been postulated that the increased incidence of melanoma in situ is possibly due to the increased monitoring for adverse events during study periods.[160] In another 24-month placebo-controlled clinical trial, one melanoma occurred in 429 patients treated with 1.25 mg daily, no melanomas in 425 patients treated with 0.5 mg daily, and 1 melanoma in 418 patients in the placebo cohort.[158] Furthermore, a 3-year phase 2 study showed no difference in melanoma incidence between the fingolimod and placebo cohorts.[159]

A recent case series reported five cases of superficial spreading melanoma (Breslow depth 0.5-2.3 mm) in 1000 patients taking fingolimod after 12 to 32 months of treatment in the Netherlands.[160] The authors hypothesized that the decreased number of circulating lymphocytes leads to a decrease in immune surveillance of melanoma. Additional reports include melanoma arising in a preexisting nevus in a middle-aged Caucasian woman (Breslow depth 0.9 mm) 57 months after starting fingolimod 1.25 mg daily as well as another middle-aged Caucasian woman (Breslow depth 1.125 mm) after taking fingolimod 0.5 mg for 61 months.[161,162] Another case of melanoma arising in a long-standing nevus was reported after 2 months of fingolimod 0.5 mg daily. Histopathology confirmed superficial spreading melanoma (Breslow depth 1.5 mm).[163]

In contrast, there are in vitro studies suggesting a protective role for fingolimod in the development of melanoma.[164,165] In general, patients should be informed regarding a potentially higher risk for skin cancers with fingolimod. Patients should have routine full-body skin examinations with a dermatologist to monitor for skin cancers, especially if the duration of therapy is greater than 6 months.[162]

Drug Interactions and Contraindications in Patients With MS: What to Know When Treating Skin Conditions

Psoriasis

A Canadian population-based study in 2008 reported a 54% higher risk of incident psoriasis in the population with MS.[166] More recent Danish and United States–based studies also support a significant association between psoriasis and MS.[167,168] Although the exact mechanism has not been elucidated, there appears to be similar pathophysiology as well as overlapping genetic risk variants between MS and psoriasis.[167] This argument is challenged by other studies that do not support such an association.[169-172]

In managing patients with MS and concomitant psoriasis, it is important to be aware of specific drug interactions and contraindications. It is well known that IFN-β can exacerbate or induce de novo psoriasis.[13,71,74,173,174] As discussed previously, worsening of psoriasis has also been reported in patients taking natalizumab.[114-116] In addition, there are reports of patients developing psoriatic arthritis while on IFN-β therapy.[73,117] TNF-α inhibitors can worsen demyelination and are therefore contraindicated in demyelinating disorders, including MS and Guillain-Barré syndrome. Demyelinating disorders such as optic neuritis and MS have been reported with the use of etanercept, infliximab, adalimumab, and golimumab, with an incidence of 0.02% to 0.2%.[175-182] For any patient taking a TNF-α inhibitor, regular neurological examinations are recommended.[183]

Traditional agents used to treat psoriasis, including methotrexate and cyclosporine, have shown benefit in MS.[184-188] Newer biologic agents have been evaluated for the treatment of MS. In a phase 2 clinical trial of ustekinumab, a neutralizing monoclonal antibody against the IL-12/23 p40 chains, there was no demonstrated benefit or harm in the treatment of relapsing remitting MS.[189] Although there is no clear benefit for MS, ustekinumab has been safely used to treat psoriasis in patients with MS.[190] Secukinumab, a monoclonal antibody that inhibits IL-17A, has been shown to significantly reduce the cumulative number of new enhancing T1 magnetic resonance imaging lesions compared with placebo. Secukinumab was well tolerated in patients with MS with no reports of worsening disease.[191] Data are limited for apremilast and IL-23 inhibitors; however, there are no reports of MS worsening with these drugs.[183]

Skin Cancer

Screening for skin cancer in patients with MS requires an evolving partnership between neurologists and dermatologists. Before the era of disease-modifying therapies, patients with MS had a lower risk of developing both melanoma and nonmelanoma skin cancer.[192,193] However, with the use of immunosuppressive medications, the risk of cutaneous malignancy has been shown to be increased.[193] More specifically, alemtuzumab and fingolimod require a routine skin examination by a dermatologist at the start of treatment and yearly thereafter to monitor for skin cancer.[107,156] Although the association between melanoma and natalizumab is controversial, yearly skin cancer screening is recommended.

Cosmetic Procedures

Although there are no specific MS-associated medical contraindications to most cosmetic procedures, caution should be exercised and individual medical history should be reviewed for each patient. For example, when injecting dermal fillers in patients with MS, physicians should ensure that patients have normal vascular supply to ensure appropriate wound healing in the area of desired treatment.[194] In patients with MS taking immunosuppressive medications, infection awareness and prevention is important for cosmetic procedures, as well as manicures, pedicures, and tattoos. Furthermore, patients with MS may require screening for loss of sensation to the affected areas before undergoing laser treatments.[195]

References

1. Yabuki S, Hayabara T. Paroxysmal dysesthesia in multiple sclerosis. *Folia Psychiatr Neurol Jpn.* 1979;33(1):97-104.
2. Taylor R. *Multiple sclerosis potpourri. Paroxysmal symptoms, seizures, fatigure, pregnanacy, and more.* In: *Multiple Sclerosis: A Rehabilitative Approach.* Vol 9. 3rd ed. Royal Oak, Michigan; 1998.
3. McAlpine D. Symptoms and signs. In: Multiple Sclerosis. A Reappraisal. 2nd ed. Baltimore, Maryland: Williams and Wilkins; 1972:132.
4. Ostermann PO, Westerberg CE. Paroxysmal attacks in multiple sclerosis. *Brain.* 1975;98(2):189-202.
5. Yamamoto M, Yabuki S, Hayabara T, Otsuki S. Paroxysmal itching in multiple sclerosis: a report of three cases. *J Neurol Neurosurg Psychiatry.* 1981;44(1):19-22. doi:10.1136/jnnp.44.1.19.
6. Lee SS, Lee HS, Baek SH. Paroxysmal pruritus as the first relapsing symptom of neuromyelitis optica. *Neurology Asia.* 2010;15(2):185-187.
7. Bayas A, Rieckmann P. Managing the adverse effects of interferon-β therapy in multiple sclerosis. *Drug Saf.* 2000;22(2):149-159. doi:10.2165/00002018-200022020-00006.
8. Balak DM, Hengstman GJ, Hajdarbegovic E, van den Brule RJ, Hupperts RM, Thio HB. Prevalence of cutaneous adverse events associated with long-term disease-modifying therapy and their impact on health-related quality of life in patients with multiple sclerosis: a cross-sectional study. *BMC Neurol.* 2013;13:146. doi:10.1186/1471-2377-13-146.
9. Balak DM, Hengstman GJ, Çakmak A, Thio HB. Cutaneous adverse events associated with disease-modifying treatment in multiple sclerosis: a systematic review. *Mult Scler.* 2012;18(12):1705-1717. doi:10.1177/1352458512438239.
10. Beer K, Müller M, Hew-Winzeler AM, et al. The prevalence of injection-site reactions with disease-modifying therapies and their effect on adherence in patients with multiple sclerosis: an observational study. *BMC Neurol.* 2011;11:144. doi:10.1186/1471-2377-11-144.
11. Tan H, Cai Q, Agarwal S, Stephenson JJ, Kamat S. Impact of adherence to disease-modifying therapies on clinical and economic outcomes among patients with multiple sclerosis. *Adv Ther.* 2011;28(1):51-61. doi:10.1007/s12325-010-0093-7.
12. Al-Sabbagh A, Bennet R, Kozma C. Medication gaps in disease modifying therapy for multiple sclerosis are associated with an increased risk of relapse: findings from a national managed care database. *J Neurol.* 2008;255(S79).
13. Webster GF, Knobler RL, Lublin FD, Kramer EM, Hochman LR. Cutaneous ulcerations and pustular psoriasis flare caused by recombinant interferon beta injections in patients with multiple sclerosis. *J Am Acad Dermatol.* 1996;34(2, Part 2):365-367. doi:10.1016/S0190-9622(07)80010-7.

14. Mehta CL, Tyler RJ, Cripps DJ. Granulomatous dermatitis with focal sarcoidal features associated with recombinant interferon β-1b injections. *J Am Acad Dermatol.* 1998;39(6):1024-1028. doi:10.1016/S0190-9622(98)70285-3.
15. Linden D. Severe Raynaud's phenomenon associated with interferon-β treatment for multiple sclerosis. *Lancet.* 1998;352(9131):878-879. doi:10.1016/S0140-6736(05)60005-0.
16. Cuesta L, Moragon M, Perez-Crespo M, Onrubia J, Garcia M. Mixed panniculitis secondary to interferon beta-1a therapy in a woman with multiple sclerosis. *Actas Dermo-Sifiliográficas.* 2013;104(3):175-266.
17. Heinzerling L, Dummer R, Burg G, Schmid-Grendelmeier P. Panniculitis after subcutaneous injection of interferon beta in a multiple sclerosis patient. *Eur J Dermatol.* 2002;12(2):194-197.
18. Debat Zoguereh D, Boucraut J, Beau-Salinas F, Bodiguel E. Cutaneous vasculitis with renal impairment complicating interferon-beta 1a therapy for multiple sclerosis. *Rev Neurol.* 2004;160(11):1081-1084.
19. Nousari HC, Kimyai-Asadi A, Tausk FA. Subacute cutaneous lupus erythematosus associated with interferon beta-1a. *Lancet.* 1998;352(9143):1825-1826. doi:10.1016/S0140-6736(05)79887-1.
20. Bezalel SA, Strober BE, Ferenczi K. Interferon beta-1a–induced morphea. *JAAD Case Rep.* 2015;1(1):15-17. doi:10.1016/j.jdcr.2014.10.002.
21. Coghe G, Atzori L, Frau J, et al. Localized pigmentation disorder after subcutaneous pegylated interferon beta-1a injection. *Mult Scler.* 2018;24(2):231-233. doi:10.1177/1352458517708465.
22. Benito-León J, Borbujo J, Cortés L. Cutaneous mucinoses complicating interferon beta-1b therapy. *Eur Neurol.* 2002;47(2):123-124. doi:10.1159/000047965.
23. Tai YJ, Tam M. Fixed drug eruption with interferon-β-1b. *Australas J Dermatol.* 2005;46(3):154-157. doi:10.1111/j.1440-0960.2005.00168.x.
24. Gaines AR, Varricchio F. Interferon beta-1b injection site reactions and necroses. *Mult Scler.* 1998;4(2):70-73. doi:10.1177/135245859800400205.
25. Interferon beta-1b in the treatment of multiple sclerosis: final outcome of the randomized controlled trial. The IFNB Multiple Sclerosis Study Group and the University of British Columbia MS/MRI Analysis Group. *Neurology.* 1995;45(7):1277-1285.
26. Walther EU, Dietrich E, Hohlfeld R. Therapy of multiple sclerosis with interferon-beta-1b. Educating the patient and managing side-effects. *Nervenarzt.* 1996;67(6):452-456.
27. The IFNB Multiple Sclerosis Study Group. Interferon beta-1b is effective in relapsing-remitting multiple sclerosis. I. Clinical results of a multicenter, randomized, double-blind, placebo-controlled trial. *Neurology.* 1993;43(4):655-661.
28. Weise G, Hupp M, Kerstan A, Buttmann M. Lobular panniculitis and lipoatrophy of the thighs with interferon-β1a for intramuscular injection in a patient with multiple sclerosis. *J Clin Neurosci.* 2012;19(9):1312-1313. doi:10.1016/j.jocn.2011.11.026.
29. Berlex Laboratories. Richmond, CA: Betaseron® (Interferon Beta-1b) Product Monograph; 1993.
30. Placebo-controlled multicentre randomised trial of interferon beta-1b in treatment of secondary progressive multiple sclerosis. European Study Group on interferon beta-1b in secondary progressive MS. *Lancet.* 1998;352(9139):1491-1497.

31. Ebers G. Randomised double-blind placebo-controlled study of interferon beta-1a in relapsing/remitting multiple sclerosis. PRISMS (Prevention of Relapses and Disability by Interferon beta-1a Subcutaneously in Multiple Sclerosis) Study Group. *Lancet.* 1998;352(9139):1498-1504.

32. Ball N, Cowan B, Hashimoto S. Lobular panniculitis at the site of subcutaneous interferon beta injections for the treatment of multiple sclerosis can histologically mimic pancreatic panniculitis. A study of 12 cases. *J Cutan Pathol.* 2009;36:331-337.

33. Soares Almeida LM, Requena L, Kutzner H, Angulo J, de Sa J, Pignatelli J. Localized panniculitis secondary to subcutaneous glatiramer acetate injections for the treatment of multiple sclerosis: a clinicopathologic and immunohistochemical study. *J Am Acad Dermatol.* 2006;55(6):968-974. doi:10.1016/j.jaad.2006.04.069.

34. Beiske AG, Myhr KM. Lipoatrophy: a non-reversible complication of subcutaneous interferon-beta 1a treatment of multiple sclerosis. *J Neurol.* 2006;253(3):377-378. doi:10.1007/s00415-006-0898-0.

35. O'Sullivan SS, Cronin EM, Sweeney BJ, Bourke JF, Fitzgibbon J. Panniculitis and lipoatrophy after subcutaneous injection of interferon β-1b in a patient with multiple sclerosis. *J Neurol Neurosurg Psychiatry.* 2006;77(12):1382-1383. doi:10.1136/jnnp.2006.094813.

36. Nakamura Y, Kawachi Y, Furuta J, Otsuka F. Severe local skin reactions to interferon beta-1b in multiple sclerosis-improvement by deep subcutaneous injection. *Eur J Dermatol.* 2008;18(5):579-582.

37. Poulin F, Rico P, Côté J, Bégin LR. Interferon beta-induced panniculitis mimicking acute appendicitis. *Arch Dermatol.* 2009;145(8):916-917. doi:10.1001/archdermatol.2009.106.

38. Ziegler V, Kranke B, Soyer P, Aberer W. Extensive cutaneous-subcutaneous infiltration as a side-effect of interferon-beta injection. *Hautarzt.* 1998;49(4):310-312.

39. Soria A, Maubec E, Henry-Feugeas M, et al. Panniculitis induced by interferon beta-1a vascular toxicity. *Ann Dermatol Venereol.* 2007;134(4 Pt 1):374-377. Available at https://www.ncbi.nlm.nih.gov/pubmed/17483759. Accessed September 26, 2018.

40. Mazzon E, Guarneri C, Giacoppo S, et al. Severe septal panniculitis in a multiple sclerosis patient treated with interferon-beta. *Int J Immunopathol Pharmacol.* 2014;27(4):669-674. Available at http://journals.sagepub.com/doi/abs/10.1177/039463201402700425?url_ver=Z39.88-2003&rfr_id=ori:rid:crossref.org&rfr_dat=cr_pub%3dpubmed. Accessed September 26, 2018.

41. Lee EY, Glassman SJ. Deep morphea induced by interferon-β1b injection. *JAAD Case Rep.* 2016;2(3):236-238. doi:10.1016/j.jdcr.2016.04.003.

42. McCall M, Owen C. Morpheaform reaction caused by interferon-beta 1b. *J Am Acad Dermatol.* 2013;68(4):AB71. doi:10.1016/j.jaad.2012.12.296.

43. Feldmann R, Löw-Weiser H, Duschet P, Gschnait F. Necrotizing cutaneous lesions caused by interferon beta injections in a patient with multiple sclerosis. *Dermatology (Basel).* 1997;195(1):52-53. doi:10.1159/000245687.

44. Radziwill AJ, Courvoisier S. Severe necrotising cutaneous lesions complicating treatment with interferon beta-1a. *J Neurol Neurosurg Psychiatry.* 1999;67(1):115. doi:10.1136/jnnp.67.1.115

45. Sheremata WA, Taylor JR, Elgart GW. Severe necrotizing cutaneous lesions complicating treatment with interferon beta-1b. 2009;5(27):1-6. doi:10.1056/NEJM199506083322316.

46. Casoni F, Merelli E, Bedin R, Martella A, Cesinaro A, Bertolotto A. Necrotizing skin lesions and NABs development in a multiple sclerosis patient treated with IFNβ 1b. *Mult Scler.* 2003;9(4):420-423. doi:10.1191/1352458503ms933sr.

47. Ohata U, Hara H, Yoshitake M, Terui T. Cutaneous reactions following subcutaneous β-interferon-1b injection. *J Dermatol.* 2010;37(2):179-181. doi:10.1111/j.1346-8138.2009.00783.x.
48. Koontz D, Alshekhlee A. Letter to the editor: embolia cutis medicamentosa following interferon beta injection. *Int J Dermatol.* 2006;45:1326-1328.
49. Wells J, Kossard S, McGrath M. Abdominal wall ulceration and mucinosis secondary to recombinant human interferon-β-1b. *Australas J Dermatol.* 2005;46(3):202-204.
50. Faghihi G, Basiri A, Pourazizi M, Abtahi-Naeini B, Saffaei A. Multiple cutaneous necrotic lesions associated with Interferon beta-1b injection for multiple sclerosis treatment: a case report and literature review. *J Res Pharm Pract.* 2015;4(2):99-103. doi:10.4103/2279-042X.155762.
51. Elgart GW, Sheremata W, Ahn YS. Cutaneous reactions to recombinant human interferon beta-1b: the clinical and histologic spectrum. *J Am Acad Dermatol.* 1997;37(4):553-558. doi:10.1016/S0190-9622(97)70170-1.
52. Weinberg JM. Cutaneous necrosis associated with recombinant interferon injection. *J Am Acad Dermatol.* 1998;39(5):807. doi:10.1016/S0190-9622(98)70061-1.
53. Feldmann R, Schierl M, Rauschka H, Sator PG, Breier F, Steiner A. Necrotizing skin lesions with involvement of muscle tissue after subcutaneous injection of glatiramer acetate. *Eur J Dermatol.* 2009;19(4):385. doi:10.1684/ejd.2009.0675.
54. Inafuku H, Kasem Khan M, Nagata T, Nonaka S. Cutaneous ulcerations following subcutaneous interferon beta injection to a patient with multiple sclerosis. *J Dermatol.* 2004;31(8):671-677.
55. Sheremata WA, Jy W, Horstman LL, Ahn YS, Alexander JS, Minagar A. Evidence of platelet activation in multiple sclerosis. *J Neuroinflammation.* 2008;5:27. doi:10.1186/1742-2094-5-27.
56. Buttmann M, Goebeler M, Toksoy A, et al. Subcutaneous interferon-beta injections in patients with multiple sclerosis initiate inflammatory skin reactions by local chemokine induction. *J Neuroimmunol.* 2005;168(1–2):175-182. doi:10.1016/j.jneuroim.2005.07.011.
57. Conroy M, Sewell L, Miller OF, Ferringer T. Interferon-beta injection site reaction: review of the histology and report of a lupus-like pattern. *J Am Acad Dermatol.* 2008;59(suppl 2):S48-S49. doi:10.1016/j.jaad.2007.12.013.
58. Arrue I, Saiz A, Ortiz-Romero PL, Rodríguez-Peralto JL. Lupus-like reaction to interferon at the injection site: report of five cases. *J Cutan Pathol.* 2007;34(suppl 1):18-21. doi:10.1111/j.1600-0560.2007.00715.x.
59. Hugle T, Gratzl S, Daikeler T, Frey D, Tyndall A, Walker UA. Sclerosing skin disorders in association with multiple sclerosis. Coincidence, underlying autoimmune pathology or interferon induced? *Ann Rheum Dis.* 2008;68(1):47-50. doi:10.1136/ard.2007.083246.
60. Szilasiova J, Gdovinova Z, Jautova J. Cutaneous vasculitis associated with interferon β-1b treatment for multiple sclerosis. *Clin Neuropharmacol.* 2009;32(5):301-303.
61. Serarslan G, Okuyucu E, Melek I, Hakverdi S, Duman T. Widespread maculopapular rash due to intramuscular interferon beta-1a during the treatment of multiple sclerosis. *Mult Scler.* 2008;14(2):259-261. doi:10.1177/1352458507079945.
62. Somani AK, Swick AR, Cooper KD, McCormick TS. Severe dermatomyositis triggered by interferon beta-1a therapy and associated with enhanced type I interferon signaling. *Arch Dermatol.* 2008;144(10):1341-1349. doi:10.1001/archderm.144.10.1341.

63. O'Reilly S, White A, Florian A. Mediastinal sarcoidosis in a patient receiving interferon-beta for multiple sclerosis. *Chest.* 2005;128(4):450S. doi:10.1378/chest.128.4_MeetingAbstracts.450S-a

64. Chakravarty SD, Harris ME, Schreiner AM, Crow MK. Sarcoidosis triggered by interferon-beta treatment of multiple sclerosis: a case report and focused literature review. *Semin Arthritis Rheum.* 2012;42(2):206-212. doi:10.1016/j.semarthrit.2012.03.008.

65. Sahraian MA, Moghadasi AN, Owji M, et al. Cutaneous and pulmonary sarcoidosis following treatment of multiple sclerosis with interferon-β-1b: a case report. *J Med Case Rep.* 2013;7:270. doi:10.1186/1752-1947-7-270.

66. Petousi N, Thomas EC. Interferon-β-induced pulmonary sarcoidosis in a 30-year-old woman treated for multiple sclerosis: a case report. *J Med Case Rep.* 2012;6(1):344. doi:10.1186/1752-1947-6-344.

67. Carbonelli C, Montepietra S, Caruso A, et al. Sarcoidosis and multiple sclerosis: systemic toxicity associated with the use of interferon-beta therapy. *Monaldi Arch Chest Dis.* 2012;77(1):29-31. doi:10.4081/monaldi.2012.165.

68. Viana de Andrade AC, Brito ÉA, Harris OM, Viana de Andrade AP, Leite MF, Pithon MM. Development of systemic sarcoidosis and xanthoma planum during multiple sclerosis treatment with interferon-beta 1a: case Report. *Int J Dermatol.* 2015;54(5):e140-145. doi:10.1111/ijd.12676.

69. Bobbio-Pallavicini E, Valsecchi C, Tacconi F, Moroni M, Porta C. Sarcoidosis following beta-interferon therapy for multiple myeloma. *Sarcoidosis.* 1995;12(2):140-142.

70. Abdi EA, Nguyen GK, Ludwig RN, Dickout WJ. Pulmonary sarcoidosis following interferon therapy for advanced renal cell carcinoma. *Cancer.* 1987;59(5):896-900.

71. Navne JE, Hedegaard U, Bygum A. Activation of psoriasis in patients undergoing treatment with interferon-beta. *Ugeskr Laeger.* 2005;167(32):2903-2904.

72. Kolb-Mäurer A, Goebeler M, Mäurer M. Cutaneous adverse events associated with interferon-β treatment of multiple sclerosis. *Int J Mol Sci.* 2015;16(7):14951-14960. doi:10.3390/ijms160714951.

73. La Mantia L, Capsoni F. Psoriasis during interferon beta treatment for multiple sclerosis. *Neurol Sci.* 2010;31(3):337-339. doi:10.1007/s10072-009-0184-x.

74. López-Lerma I, Iranzo P, Herrero C. New-onset psoriasis in a patient treated with interferon beta-1a. *Br J Dermatol.* 2009;160(3):716-717. doi:10.1111/j.1365-2133.2008.09005.x.

75. Axtell R, Raman C, Steinman L. Interferon-β exacerbates Th17 inflammatory diseases. *Trends Immunol.* 2011;32(6):272-277. doi:10.1016/j.it.2011.03.008.

76. Khan O, Rieckmann P, Boyko A, Selmaj K, Zivadinov R. Three times weekly glatiramer acetate in relapsing–remitting multiple sclerosis. *Ann Neurol.* 2013;73(6):705-713. doi:10.1002/ana.23938.

77. Boster A, Bartoszek MP, O'Connell C, Pitt D, Racke M. Efficacy, safety, and cost-effectiveness of glatiramer acetate in the treatment of relapsing–remitting multiple sclerosis. *Ther Adv Neurol Disord.* 2011;4(5):319-332. doi:10.1177/1756285611422108.

78. Teva Neuroscience. *Copaxone [Package Insert].* Kansas City, MO: Teva Neuroscience; 2009.

79. Aviv B, Yaron Z, Anat A, Sharon B. Patterns of local site reactions to subcutaneous glatiramer acetate treatment of multiple sclerosis: a clinicopathological study. *Int J Clin Exp Pathol.* 2018;11(6):3126-3133.

80. Ball NJ, Cowan BJ, Moore GRW, Hashimoto SA. Lobular panniculitis at the site of glatiramer acetate injections for the treatment of relapsing-remitting multiple sclerosis. A report of two cases. *J Cutan Pathol.* 2008;35(4):407-410. doi:10.1111/j.1600-0560.2007.00819.x.

81. Sánchez-López J, Rodríguez del Rio P, Cases-Ortega B, Martínez-Cócera C, Fernández-Rivas M. Allergy workup in immediate-type local reactions to glatiramer acetate. *J Investig Allergol Clin Immunol.* 2010;20(6):521-523.

82. Drago F, Rongioletti F, Battifoglio ML, Rebora A. Localised lipoatrophy after acupuncture. *Lancet.* 1996;347(9013):1484. doi:10.5555/uri:pii:S0140673696917195.

83. Mancardi GL, Murialdo A, Drago F, et al. Localized lipoatrophy after prolonged treatment with copolymer 1. *J Neurol.* 2000;247(3):220-221. doi:10.1007/s004150050568.

84. Edgar CM, Brunet DG, Fenton P, McBride EV, Green P. Lipoatrophy in patients with multiple sclerosis on glatiramer acetate. *Can J Neurol Sci.* 2004;31(1):58-63.

85. Soós N, Shakery K, Mrowietz U. Localized panniculitis and subsequent lipoatrophy with subcutaneous glatiramer acetate (Copaxone) injection for the treatment of multiple sclerosis. *Am J Clin Dermatol.* 2004;5(5):357-359.

86. Hwang L, Orengo I. Lipoatrophy associated with glatiramer acetate injections for the treatment of multiple sclerosis. *Cutis.* 2001;68(4):287-288.

87. Jolly H, Simpson K, Bishop B, et al. Impact of warm compresses on local injection-site reactions with self-administered glatiramer acetate. *J Neurosci Nurs.* 2008;40(4):232-239.

88. Hashimoto S, Ball N, Tremlett H. Progressive lipoatrophy after cessation of glatiramer acetate injections: a case report. *Mult Scler.* 2009;15(4):521-522. doi:10.1177/1352458508100504.

89. Harde V, Schwarz T. Embolia cutis medicamentosa following subcutaneous injection of glatiramer acetate. *J Dtsch Dermatol Ges.* 2007;5(12):1122-1123. doi:10.1111/j.1610-0387.2007.06391.x.

90. Mott SE, Peña ZG, Spain RI, White KP, Ehst BD. Nicolau syndrome and localized panniculitis: a report of dual diagnoses with an emphasis on morphea profunda-like changes following injection with glatiramer acetate. *J Cutan Pathol.* 2016;43(11):1056-1061. doi:10.1111/cup.12791.

91. McEwan L, Brown J, Poirier J, et al. Best practices in skin care for the multiple sclerosis patient receiving injectable therapies. *Int J MS Care.* 2010;12(4):177-189. doi:10.7224/1537-2073-12.4.177.

92. Caon C, Namey M, Meyer C, et al. Prevention and management of infusion-associated reactions in the comparison of alemtuzumab and Rebif® efficacy in multiple sclerosis (CARE-MS) program. *Int J MS Care.* 2015;17(4):191-198. doi:10.7224/1537-2073.2014-030.

93. Šega-Jazbec S, Barun B, Horvat Ledinek A, Fabekovac V, Krbot Skorić M, Habek M. Management of infusion related reactions associated with alemtuzumab in patients with multiple sclerosis. *Mult Scler Relat Disord.* 2017;17:151-153. doi:10.1016/j.msard.2017.07.019.

94. Thomas K, Eisele J, Rodriguez-Leal FA, Hainke U, Ziemssen T. Acute effects of alemtuzumab infusion in patients with active relapsing-remitting MS. *Neurol Neuroimmunol Neuroinflamm.* 2016;3(3):e228. doi:10.1212/NXI.0000000000000228.

95. Clark SL, Tse JY, Fisher DC, et al. Histopathologic spectrum of hypersensitivity reactions associated with anti-CD52 therapy (alemtuzumab). *J Cutan Pathol.* 2016;43(11):989-993. doi:10.1111/cup.12800.

96. Ngu S, Shaffrali F. A case of severe drug reaction secondary to alemtuzumab with successful re-exposure. *Clin Exp Dermatol.* 2017;42(8):925-926. doi:10.1111/ced.13230.

97. Willis MD, Harding KE, Pickersgill TP, et al. Alemtuzumab for multiple sclerosis: long term follow-up in a multi-centre cohort. *Mult Scler.* 2016;22(9):1215-1223. doi:10.1177/1352458515614092.

98. Ghodasara R, Smith S, Mosley M. Serious adverse events (SAE), autoimmunity (AI), and infections following alemtuzumab (ALE) therapy in a large, high disability, treatment-refractory MS clinic cohort. *ECTRIMS Online Libr.* 2016. Available at https://onlinelibrary.ectrims-congress.eu/ectrims/2016/32nd/145865/samuel.f.hunter.serious.adverse.events.28sae29.autoimmunity.28ai29.and.infections.html. Accessed October 8, 2018.

99. Zimmermann J, Buhl T, Müller M. Alopecia universalis following alemtuzumab treatment in multiple sclerosis: a barely recognized manifestation of secondary autoimmunity—report of a case and review of the literature. *Front Neurol.* 2017;8. doi:10.3389/fneur.2017.00569.

100. CAMMS223 Trial Investigators, Coles AJ, Compston DA, Selmaj KW, et al. Alemtuzumab versus interferon beta-1a in early multiple sclerosis. *N Engl J Med.* 2008;359(17):1786-1801. doi:10.1056/NEJMoa0802670.

101. Lambert C, Dubois B, Dive D, et al. Management of immune thrombocytopenia in multiple sclerosis patients treated with alemtuzumab: a Belgian consensus. *Acta Neurol Belg.* 2018;118(1):7-11. doi:10.1007/s13760-018-0882-3.

102. Cuker A, Coles AJ, Sullivan H, et al. A distinctive form of immune thrombocytopenia in a phase 2 study of alemtuzumab for the treatment of relapsing-remitting multiple sclerosis. *Blood.* 2011;118(24):6299-6305. doi:10.1182/blood-2011-08-371138.

103. Cuker A, Stasi R, Palmer J, Oyuela P, Margolin D, Bass A. Successful detection and management of immune thrombocytopenia in alemtuzumab-treated patients with active relapsing-remitting multiple sclerosis (P2.198). *Neurology.* 2014;82(suppl 10). Available at http://n.neurology.org/content/82/10_Supplement/P2.198.abstract.

104. *Lemtrada FDA Prescribing Information*; 2014. Avaialble at https://www.accessdata.fda.gov/drugsatfda_docs/label/2014/103948s5139lbl.pdf.

105. Pace AA, Zajicek JP. Melanoma following treatment with alemtuzumab for multiple sclerosis. *Eur J Neurol.* 2009;16(4):e70-e71. doi:10.1111/j.1468-1331.2009.02552.x.

106. Fiegl M, Gastl G, Hopfinger G, et al. Alemtuzumab in chronic lymphocytic leukaemia, other lymphoproliferative disease and autoimmune disorders. *Memo.* 2008;1(4):211-222. doi:10.1007/s12254-008-0064-8.

107. FDA Approves Lemtrada™ (alemtuzumab) for Relapsing MS – UPDATE. National Multiple Sclerosis Society. http://www.nationalmssociety.org/About-the-Society/News/FDA-Approves-LemtradaTM-(alemtuzumab)-for-Relapsing. Accessed November 12, 2018.

108. Davenport RJ, Munday JR. Alpha4-integrin antagonism–an effective approach for the treatment of inflammatory diseases? *Drug Discov Today.* 2007;12(13-14):569-576. doi:10.1016/j.drudis.2007.05.001.

109. Phillips JT, O'Connor PW, Havrdova E, et al. Infusion-related hypersensitivity reactions during natalizumab treatment. *Neurology.* 2006;67(9):1717-1718. doi:10.1212/01.wnl.0000242629.66372.33.

110. Krumbholz M, Pellkofer H, Gold R, Hoffmann LA, Hohlfeld R, Kümpfel T. Delayed allergic reaction to natalizumab associated with early formation of neutralizing antibodies. *Arch Neurol.* 2007;64(9):1331-1333. doi:10.1001/archneur.64.9.1331.

111. Lapucci C, Gualandi F, Mikulska M, et al. Serum sickness (Like Reaction) in a patient treated with alemtuzumab for multiple sclerosis: a case report. *Mult Scler Relat Disord*. 2018;26:52-54. doi:10.1016/j.msard.2018.09.006.

112. Piqué-Duran E, Eguía P, García-Vázquez O. Acquired perforating dermatosis associated with natalizumab. *J Am Acad Dermatol*. 2013;68(6):e185-e187. doi:10.1016/j.jaad.2012.11.004.

113. André MC, Pacheco D, Antunes J, Silva R, Filipe P, Soares de Almeida LM. Generalized skin drug eruption to natalizumab in a patient with multiple sclerosis. *Dermatol Online J*. 2010;16(6). Available at https://escholarship. org/uc/item/2w71s2mx. Accessed October 31, 2018.

114. Lambrianides S, Kinnis E, Leonidou E, Pantzaris M. Does natalizumab induce or aggravate psoriasis? A case study and review of the literature. *CRN*. 2018;10(3):286-291. doi:10.1159/000492891.

115. Millán-Pascual J, Turpín-Fenoll L, Del Saz-Saucedo P, Rueda-Medina I, Navarro-Muñoz S. Psoriasis during natalizumab treatment for multiple sclerosis. *J Neurol*. 2012;259(12):2758-2760. doi:10.1007/s00415-012-6713-1.

116. Clark SJ, Wang Q, Mao-Draayer Y. Switching from natalizumab to fingolimod: case report and review of literature. *J Immunol Clin Res*. 2016;3(1):1030.

117. Vacchiano V, Foschi M, Sabattini L, Scandellari C, Lugaresi A. Arthritic psoriasis during natalizumab treatment: a case report and review of the literature. *Neurol Sci*. 2018;39(1):181-183. doi:10.1007/s10072-017-3112-5.

118. Panzara MA, Bozic C, Sandrock AW. More on melanoma with transdifferentiation. *N Engl J Med*. 2008;359(1):99; author reply 99-100. doi:10.1056/ NEJMc086089.

119. Sabol RA, Noxon V, Sartor O, et al. Melanoma complicating treatment with natalizumab for multiple sclerosis: a report from the Southern Network on Adverse Reactions (SONAR). *Cancer Med*. 2017;6(7):1541-1551. doi:10.1002/ cam4.1098.

120. Selewski DT, Shah GV, Segal BM, Rajdev PA, Mukherji SK. Natalizumab (tysabri). *Am J Neuroradiol*. 2010;31(9):1588-1590. doi:10.3174/ajnr.A2226.

121. Bergamaschi R, Montomoli C. Melanoma in multiple sclerosis treated with natalizumab: causal association or coincidence? *Mult Scler*. 2009;15(12):1532-1533. doi:10.1177/1352458509347154.

122. Ismail A, Kemp J, Sharrack B. Melanoma complicating treatment with natalizumab (Tysabri) for multiple sclerosis. *J Neurol*. 2009;256(10):1771-1772. doi:10.1007/s00415-009-5200-9.

123. Laroni A, Bedognetti M, Uccelli A, Capello E, Mancardi GL. Association of melanoma and natalizumab therapy in the Italian MS population: a second case report. *Neurol Sci*. 2011;32(1):181-182. doi:10.1007/s10072-010-0427-x.

124. Mullen JT, Vartanian TK, Atkins MB. Melanoma complicating treatment with natalizumab for multiple sclerosis. *N Engl J Med*. 2008;358(6):647-648. doi:10.1056/NEJMc0706103.

125. Vavricka BMP, Baumberger P, Russmann S, Kullak-Ublick GA. Diagnosis of melanoma under concomitant natalizumab therapy. *Mult Scler*. 2011;17(2):255-256. doi:10.1177/1352458510389629.

126. Pharaon M, Tichet M, Lebrun-Frénay C, Tartare-Deckert S, Passeron T. Risk for nevus transformation and melanoma proliferation and invasion during natalizumab treatment: four years of dermoscopic follow-up with immunohistological studies and proliferation and invasion assays. *JAMA Dermatol*. 2014;150(8):901-903. doi:10.1001/jamadermatol.2013.9411.

127. Kausar F, Mustafa K, Sweis G, et al. Ocrelizumab: a step forward in the evolution of B-cell therapy. *Expert Opin Biol Ther*. 2009;9(7):889-895. doi:10.1517/14712590903018837.

128. Press Announcements – FDA Approves New Drug to Treat Multiple Sclerosis. https://www.fda.gov/NewsEvents/Newsroom/PressAnnouncements/ ucm549325.htm.

129. Darwin E, Romanelli P, Lev-Tov H. Ocrelizumab-induced psoriasiform dermatitis in a patient with multiple sclerosis. *Dermatol Online J.* 2018;24(7), pii:13030/qt220859qb.

130. Granqvist M, Boremalm M, Poorghobad A, et al. Comparative effectiveness of rituximab and other initial treatment choices for multiple sclerosis. *JAMA Neurol.* 2018;75(3):320-327. doi:10.1001/jamaneurol.2017.4011.

131. FDA. *RITUXAN (Rituximab)*. Genentech Package Insert; 2010. Available at https:// www.accessdata.fda.gov/drugsatfda_docs/label/2010/103705s5311lbl.pdf.

132. Didona D, Paolino G, Garcovich S, Caro RDC, Didona B. Successful use of etanercept in a case of toxic epidermal necrolysis induced by rituximab. *J Eur Acad Dermatol Venereol.* 2016;30(10):e83-e84. doi:10.1111/jdv.13330.

133. Lowndes S, Darby A, Mead G, Lister A. Stevens–Johnson syndrome after treatment with rituximab. *Ann Oncol.* 2002;13(12):1948-1950. doi:10.1093/ annonc/mdf350.

134. Henning JS, Firoz BF. Rituxan is not associated with Stevens Johnson syndrome. *Ann Oncol.* 2011;22(6):1463-1464. doi:10.1093/annonc/mdr254.

135. Fallon MJ, Heck JN. Fatal Stevens–Johnson syndrome/toxic epidermal necrolysis induced by allopurinol–rituximab–bendamustine therapy. *J Oncol Pharm Pract.* 2015;21(5):388-392. doi:10.1177/1078155214533368.

136. Robinson KS, Williams ME, van der Jagt RH, et al. Phase II multicenter study of bendamustine plus rituximab in patients with relapsed indolent B-cell and mantle cell non-Hodgkin's lymphoma. *J Clin Oncol.* 2008;26(27):4473-4479. doi:10.1200/JCO.2008.17.0001.

137. Ureshino H, Ando T, Kojima K, et al. Rituximab-containing chemotherapy (R-CHOP)-induced kaposi's sarcoma in an HIV-negative patient with diffuse large B cell lymphoma. *Intern Med.* 2015;54(24):3205-3208. doi:10.2169/ internalmedicine.54.5103.

138. Jerdan K, Brownell J, Singh M, Braniecki M, Chan L. A case report of iatrogenic cutaneous Kaposi sarcoma due to rituximab therapy for thrombotic thrombocytopenic purpura. *Acta Oncol.* 2017;56(1):111-113. doi:10.1080/02 84186X.2016.1253867.

139. Périer A, Savey L, Marcelin AG, Serve P, Saadoun D, Barete S. Brief report: de novo human herpesvirus 8 tumors induced by rituximab in autoimmune or inflammatory systemic diseases. *Arthritis Rheumatol.* 2017;69(11):2241-2246. doi:10.1002/art.40217.

140. Billon E, Stoppa AM, Mescam L, et al. Reversible rituximab-induced rectal Kaposi's sarcoma misdiagnosed as ulcerative colitis in a patient with HIV-negative follicular lymphoma. *Clin Sarcoma Res.* 2018;8(1):11. doi:10.1186/ s13569-018-0097-7.

141. Kandula P, Kouides PA. Rituximab-induced leukocytoclastic vasculitis: a case report. *Arch Dermatol.* 2006;142(2):246-247. doi:10.1001/ archderm.142.2.246.

142. Dereure O, Navarro R, Rossi JF, Guilhou JJ. Rituximab-induced vasculitis. *Dermatology (Basel).* 2001;203(1):83-84. doi:10.1159/000051713.

143. D'Arcy CA, Mannik M. Serum sickness secondary to treatment with the murine–human chimeric antibody IDEC-C2B8 (rituximab). *Arthritis Rheum.* 2001;44(7):1717-1718. doi:10.1002/1529-0131(200107)44:7<1717::AID-ART299>3.0.CO;2-C.

144. Herishanu Y. Rituximab-induced serum sickness. *Am J Hematol.* 2002;70(4):329. doi:10.1002/ajh.10127.

145. Bar-Or A, Pachner A, Menguy-Vacheron F, Kaplan J, Wiendl H. Teriflunomide and its mechanism of action in multiple sclerosis. *Drugs*. 2014;74(6):659-674. doi:10.1007/s40265-014-0212-x.

146. *Drug Approval Package: Arava (Leflunomide Tablet) NDA# 20905*. U.S. Food and Drug Administration; 1998. Available at https://www.accessdata.fda. gov/drugsatfda_docs/nda/98/20905_arava.cfm.

147. Comi G, Freedman MS, Kappos L, et al. Pooled safety and tolerability data from four placebo-controlled teriflunomide studies and extensions. *Mult Scler Relat Disord*. 2016;5:97-104. doi:10.1016/j.msard.2015.11.006.

148. *FDA Approves First Oral Drug to Reduce MS Relapses*; 2010. Available at https://www.prnewswire.comfda-approves-first-oral-drug-to-reduce-ms-re-lapses-103518384.

149. Groves A, Kihara Y, Chun J. Fingolimod: direct CNS effects of sphingosine 1-phosphate (S1P) receptor modulation and implications in multiple sclerosis therapy. *J Neurol Sci*. 2013;328(1):9-18. doi:10.1016/j.jns.2013.02.011.

150. Matloubian M, Lo CG, Cinamon G, et al. Lymphocyte egress from thymus and peripheral lymphoid organs is dependent on S1P receptor 1. *Nature*. 2004;427(6972):355-360. doi:10.1038/nature02284.

151. Lublin F, Miller DH, Freedman MS, et al. Oral fingolimod in primary progressive multiple sclerosis (INFORMS): a phase 3, randomised, double-blind, placebo-controlled trial. *Lancet*. 2016;387(10023):1075-1084. doi:10.1016/S0140-6736(15)01314-8.

152. Calabresi PA, Radue EW, Goodin D, et al. Safety and efficacy of fingolimod in patients with relapsing-remitting multiple sclerosis (FREEDOMS II): a double-blind, randomised, placebo-controlled, phase 3 trial. *Lancet Neurol*. 2014;13(6):545-556. doi:10.1016/S1474-4422(14)70049-3.

153. Mahajan KR, Ko JS, Tetzlaff MT, Hudgens CW, Billings SD, Cohen JA. Merkel cell carcinoma with fingolimod treatment for multiple sclerosis: a case report. *Mult Scler Relat Disord*. 2017;17:12-14. doi:10.1016/j.msard.2017.06.004.

154. Calvi A, Riz MD, Lecchi E, et al. Merkel cell carcinoma in a patient with relapsing-remitting multiple sclerosis treated with fingolimod. *J Neurol Sci*. 2017;381:296-297. doi:10.1016/j.jns.2017.09.003.

155. Beadnall HN, Gill AJ, Riminton S, Barnett MH. Virus-related Merkel cell carcinoma complicating fingolimod treatment for multiple sclerosis. *Neurology*. 2016;87(24):2595-2597. doi:10.1212/WNL.0000000000003434.

156. FDA. *Gilenya (Fingolimod) Prescribing Information*; 2018. Available at https://www.accessdata.fda.gov/drugsatfda_docs/label/2018/022527s024lbl.pdf.

157. Cohen JA, Barkhof F, Comi G, et al. Oral fingolimod or intramuscular interferon for relapsing multiple sclerosis. *N Engl J Med*. 2010;362(5):402-415. doi:10.1056/NEJMoa0907839.

158. Kappos L, Radue E-W, O'Connor P, et al. A placebo-controlled trial of oral fingolimod in relapsing multiple sclerosis. *N Engl J Med*. 2010;362(5):387-401. doi:10.1056/NEJMoa0909494.

159. Comi G, O'Connor P, Montalban X, et al. Phase II study of oral fingolimod (FTY720) in multiple sclerosis: 3-year results. *Mult Scler*. 2010;16(2):197-207. doi:10.1177/1352458509357065.

160. Killestein J, Leurs CE, Hoogervorst ELJ, et al. Five cases of malignant melanoma during fingolimod treatment in Dutch patients with MS. *Neurology*. 2017;89(9):970-972. doi:10.1212/WNL.0000000000004293.

161. Conzett KB, Kolm I, Jelcic I, et al. Melanoma occurring during treatment with fingolimod for multiple sclerosis: a case report. *Arch Dermatol*. 2011;147(8):991-992. doi:10.1001/archdermatol.2011.212.

162. Robinson CL, Guo M. Fingolimod (gilenya) and melanoma. *BMJ Case Rep.* 2016;2016. doi:10.1136/bcr-2016-217885. pii:bcr2016217885.

163. Haebich G, Mughal A, Tofazzal N. Superficial spreading malignant melanoma in a patient on fingolimod therapy for multiple sclerosis. *Clin Exp Dermatol.* 2016;41(4):433-434. doi:10.1111/ced.12770.

164. Tay KH, Liu X, Chi M, et al. Involvement of vacuolar H(+)-ATPase in killing of human melanoma cells by the sphingosine kinase analogue FTY720. *Pigment Cell Melanoma Res.* 2015;28(2):171-183. doi:10.1111/pcmr.12326.

165. Ishitsuka A, Fujine E, Mizutani Y, et al. FTY720 and cisplatin synergistically induce the death of cisplatin-resistant melanoma cells through the down-regulation of the PI3K pathway and the decrease in epidermal growth factor receptor expression. *Int J Mol Med.* 2014;34(4):1169-1174. doi:10.3892/ijmm.2014.1882.

166. Marrie RA, Patten SB, Tremlett H, Wolfson C, Leung S, Fisk JD. Increased incidence and prevalence of psoriasis in multiple sclerosis. *Mult Scler Relat Disord.* 2017;13:81-86. doi:10.1016/j.msard.2017.02.012.

167. Egeberg A, Mallbris L, Gislason GH, Skov L, Hansen PR. Risk of multiple sclerosis in patients with psoriasis: a Danish nationwide cohort study. *J Invest Dermatol.* 2016;136(1):93-98. doi:10.1038/JID.2015.350.

168. Guido N, Cices A, Ibler E, et al. Multiple sclerosis association with psoriasis: a large U.S. population, single centre, retrospective cross-sectional study. *J Eur Acad Dermatol Venereol.* 2017;31(9):e397-e398. doi:10.1111/jdv.14205.

169. Langer-Gould A, Albers K, Van Den Eeden S, Nelson L. Autoimmune diseases prior to the diagnosis of multiple sclerosis: a population-based case-control study. *Mult Scler.* 2010;16(7):855-861. doi:10.1177/1352458510369146.

170. Edwards LJ, Constantinescu CS. A prospective study of conditions associated with multiple sclerosis in a cohort of 658 consecutive outpatients attending a multiple sclerosis clinic. *Mult Scler.* 2004;10(5):575-581. doi:10.1191/1352458504ms1087oa.

171. Ramagopalan SV, Dyment DA, Valdar W, et al. Autoimmune disease in families with multiple sclerosis: a population-based study. *Lancet Neurol.* 2007;6(7):604-610. doi:10.1016/S1474-4422(07)70132-1.

172. Kwok T, Loo WJ, Guenther L. Psoriasis and multiple sclerosis: is there a link? *J Cutan Med Surg.* 2010;14(4):151-155. doi:10.2310/7750.2010.09063.

173. Munschauer FE, Kinkel RP. Managing side effects of interferon-beta in patients with relapsing-remitting multiple sclerosis. *Clin Ther.* 1997;19(5):883-893. doi:10.1016/S0149-2918(97)80042-2.

174. Hong J, Bernstein D. A review of drugs that induce or exacerbate psoriasis. *Psoriasis Forum.* 2012;18a(1):2-11. doi:10.1177/247553031218a00101.

175. Lozeron P, Denier C, Lacroix C, Adams D. Long-term course of demyelinating neuropathies occurring during tumor necrosis factor-α–blocker therapy. *Arch Neurol.* 2009;66(4):490-497. doi:10.1001/archneurol.2009.11.

176. Tristano AG. Neurological adverse events associated with anti-tumor necrosis factor alpha treatment. *J Neurol.* 2010;257(9):1421-1431. doi:10.1007/s00415-010-5591-7.

177. Mohan N, Edwards ET, Cupps TR, et al. Demyelination occurring during anti-tumor necrosis factor alpha therapy for inflammatory arthritides. *Arthritis Rheum.* 2001;44(12):2862-2869.

178. Gomez-Gallego M, Meca-Lallana J, Fernandez-Barreiro A. Multiple sclerosis onset during etanercept treatment. *Eur Neurol.* 2008;59(1–2):91-93. doi:10.1159/000109576.

179. Cruz Fernández-Espartero M, Pérez-Zafrilla B, Naranjo A, et al. Demyelinating disease in patients treated with TNF antagonists in rheumatology: data from BIOBADASER, a pharmacovigilance database, and a systematic review. *Semin Arthritis Rheum.* 2011;41(3):524-533. doi:10.1016/j.semarthrit.2011.05.003.

180. Kemanetzoglou E, Andreadou E. CNS demyelination with TNF-α blockers. *Curr Neurol Neurosci Rep.* 2017;17(4):36. doi:10.1007/s11910-017-0742-1.

181. Kay J, Fleischmann R, Keystone E, et al. Golimumab 3-year safety update: an analysis of pooled data from the long-term extensions of randomised, double-blind, placebo-controlled trials conducted in patients with rheumatoid arthritis, psoriatic arthritis or ankylosing spondylitis. *Ann Rheum Dis.* 2015;74(3):538-546. doi:10.1136/annrheumdis-2013-204195.

182. Caminero A, Comabella M, Montalban X. Tumor necrosis factor alpha (TNF-α), anti-TNF-α and demyelination revisited: an ongoing story. *J Neuroimmunol.* 2011;234(1):1-6. doi:10.1016/j.jneuroim.2011.03.004.

183. Kaushik SB, Lebwohl MG. CME part I psoriasis: which therapy for which patient psoriasis comorbidities and preferred systemic agents. *J Am Acad Dermatol.* 2019;80(1):27-40. doi:10.1016/j.jaad.2018.06.057.

184. Neumann JW, Ziegler DK. Therapeutic trial of immunosuppressive agents in multiple sclerosis. *Neurology.* 1972;22(12):1268-1271.

185. Currier RD, Haerer AF, Meydrech EF. Low dose oral methotrexate treatment of multiple sclerosis: a pilot study. *J Neurol Neurosurg Psychiatry.* 1993;56(11):1217-1218. doi:10.1136/jnnp.56.11.1217.

186. Ashtari F, Savoj MR. Effects of low dose methotrexate on relapsing-remitting multiple sclerosis in comparison to Interferon β-1α: a randomized controlled trial. *J Res Med Sci.* 2011;16(4):457-462.

187. Goodkin DE, Rudick RA, VanderBrug Medendorp S, et al. Low-dose (7.5 mg) oral methotrexate reduces the rate of progression in chronic progressive multiple sclerosis. *Ann Neurol.* 1995;37(1):30-40. doi:10.1002/ana.410370108.

188. Zhao GJ, Li DKB, Wolinsky JS, et al. Clinical and magnetic resonance imaging changes correlate in a clinical trial monitoring cyclosporine therapy for multiple sclerosis. *J Neuroimaging.* 1997;7(1):1-7. doi:10.1111/jon1997711.

189. Segal BM, Constantinescu CS, Raychaudhuri A, Kim L, Fidelus-Gort R, Kasper LH. Repeated subcutaneous injections of IL12/23 p40 neutralising antibody, ustekinumab, in patients with relapsing-remitting multiple sclerosis: a phase II, double-blind, placebo-controlled, randomised, dose-ranging study. *Lancet Neurol.* 2008;7(9):796-804. doi:10.1016/S1474-4422(08)70173-X.

190. Chang S, Chambers CJ, Liu FT, Armstrong AW. Successful treatment of psoriasis with ustekinumab in patients with multiple sclerosis. *Dermatol Online J.* 2015;21(7). Available at https://escholarship.org/uc/item/3bs971cr. Accessed November 8, 2018.

191. Havrdová E, Belova A, Goloborodko A, et al. Activity of secukinumab, an anti-IL-17A antibody, on brain lesions in RRMS: results from a randomized, proof-of-concept study. *J Neurol.* 2016;263(7):1287-1295. doi:10.1007/s00415-016-8128-x.

192. Goldacre MJ, Seagroatt V, Yeates D, Acheson ED. Skin cancer in people with multiple sclerosis: a record linkage study. *J Epidemiol Community Health.* 2004;58(2):142-144. doi:10.1136/jech.58.2.142.

193. Lebrun C, Vermersch P, Brassat D, et al. Cancer and multiple sclerosis in the era of disease-modifying treatments. *J Neurol.* 2011;258(7):1304-1311. doi:10.1007/s00415-011-5929-9.

194. Lafaille P, Benedetto A. Fillers: contraindications, side effects and precautions. *J Cutan Aesthet Surg.* 2010;3(1):16-19. doi:10.4103/0974-2077.63222.
195. Laser Hair Removal. Herron Dermatology & Laser. Available at https://www.herrondermatology.com/cosmetic/laser-hair-removal/. Accessed November 12, 2018.

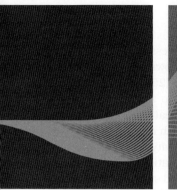
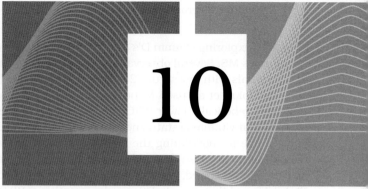

Endocrine Disorders in Multiple Sclerosis

■ ▓▓ ▓ Tiffany Yeh, Michele Yeung, Dorothy A. Fink

Introduction

Multiple sclerosis (MS) is largely thought to be an inflammatory autoimmune disease; however, there is significant cross talk between the endocrine and immune systems leading to observations of certain endocrine abnormalities, such as vitamin D deficiency potentially modulating MS risk and relapse rates. Additionally, many key treatments of MS, such as alemtuzumab, glucocorticoids (GC), and biotin, have a number of effects on the endocrine system, such as thyroid dysfunction, osteoporosis, hypothalamic-pituitary-adrenal (HPA) axis suppression, iatrogenic Cushing syndrome, and diabetes/metabolic syndrome. Here we provide an overview of these topics and encourage all clinicians treating patients with MS in their practice to be well versed in identifying and treating endocrine comorbidities in patients with MS.

Metabolic Bone Health

The Role of Vitamin D Supplementation in MS

Expression of both vitamin D receptors and the rate-limiting enzyme for vitamin D synthesis, 1-alpha-hydroxylase, has been reported in most immune cells.[1] The suggestion that vitamin D potentially can have immunomodulatory effects in the body has prompted dedicated research in the last

2 decades exploring vitamin D's role in the disease process that leads to and perpetuates MS. Several observational studies have shown a higher MS risk in individuals with low serum 25-dihydroxyvitamin D [25(OH)D].[2,3] Others, such as Mokry et al, used Mendelian randomization to show that individuals with genetically lower 25(OH)D had a twofold greater odds of MS.[4] It appears that vitamin D status not only is associated with risk of MS but also plays a role in modulating the degree of disease activity.[5-7] Other studies have demonstrated an effect of vitamin D supplementation on MS disease activity. A randomized, double-blind, placebo-controlled study conducted in Finland found that vitamin D3 supplementation at 20,000 IU weekly had no adverse effects, but the vitamin D3 (add-on treatment to interferon [IFN]-b) group had a significantly lower number of gadolinium-enhancing lesions on brain magnetic resonance imaging (MRI).[8] The double-blind, multicenter, 48-week SOLAR (double blind placebo controlled study of high dose cholecalciferol oil add on treatment to subcutaneous interferon beta 1a) study is the largest study to date.[9] The authors found no statistical significant differences in disease-free activity between the placebo group and the vitamin D group. However, there was a nonsignificant trend toward lower relapse rates in the vitamin D-treated group as well as a statistically significant reduction in new lesions at 48 weeks. Several other randomized controlled studies are currently underway to further elucidate the role of vitamin D in MS.

It is recommended that all patients with MS or MS risk factors be screened for vitamin D deficiency. 25(OH)D should be the assay used to evaluate vitamin D status. Vitamin D deficiency is defined as a 25(OH)D below 20 ng/mL, and vitamin D insufficiency as a 25(OH)D of 21 to 29 ng/mL.[10] Vitamin D comes in multiple forms. Vitamin D2 (ergocalciferol) is the plant form of vitamin D and is primarily manufactured. Vitamin D3 (cholecalciferol) is found in animal-based foods and synthesized in humans in the skin by a photolytic process.[11]

Foods rich in vitamin D include fatty fish (e.g., salmon, mackerel), cod liver oil, egg yolk, and shiitake mushrooms. Cholecalciferol and ergocalciferol are also available from fortified foods (e.g., milk, cereal, orange juice, and cheeses). In general, diet by itself is often a poor source of vitamin D, providing only 40 to 400 IU per food serving. It is also important to note that sunlight (ultraviolet B) exposure and vitamin D production in the skin is highly variable. Factors such skin pigmentation, age, use of sunscreen, and environmental factors such as winter season, high latitude, pollution, cloud cover, and ozone levels will alter an individual's vitamin D production through the skin.[12]

Vitamin D supplementation through food and production through sunlight will often be inadequate and unpredictable. Therefore, in the setting of vitamin D deficiency or insufficiency, it is not recommended for individuals to use food or sunlight as their main source of repletion. Vitamin D supplementation can be administered daily, weekly, or monthly. Vitamin D3 (cholecalciferol) is widely preferred over vitamin D2 (ergocalciferol), as it has been proved to be the more potent form of vitamin D in humans.[13] The Endocrine Society recommends a daily supplement dose of 600 to 800 IU to satisfy the requirements for optimal bone health, but a higher intake (1500-2000 IU) may be needed to achieve and maintain 25(OH)D levels at 30 ng/mL.[10] Considering current evidence, many clinicians who treat patients with MS may choose to empirically supplement to a higher vitamin D level goal, such as 40 to 60 ng/mL, until more conclusive data are found. To obtain such levels, patients may need to take between 2000 and 5000 IU/d of vitamin D.[11]

Vitamin D toxicity is a rare event caused by inadvertent or intentional ingestion of excessively high amounts of vitamin D.[10] The Endocrine Practice Guidelines Committee expressed concerns in individuals with 25(OH)D levels of 150 ng/mL or higher, when daily doses of vitamin D exceed 10,000 IU or when high intake of vitamin D is combined with high intake of calcium (>1200 mg daily).[10] Although the study was of limited duration, Kimball et al showed that large doses of vitamin D supplementation ranging from 28,000 to 280,000 IU/wk was well tolerated and had no significant adverse effects such as hypercalcemia or hypercalciuria.[14] Other studies performed in pregnant patients demonstrate safety with giving doses of 50,000 IU weekly for up to 12 weeks or a dose as high as two doses of 300,000 IU intramuscularly.[15] Additionally, there have been several studies conducted specifically in patients with MS that showed safety using doses of vitamin D above 10,000 IU/d.[14,16,17] Follow-up in these studies ranged from 12 weeks to 1 year. To date, there is a paucity of evidence supporting the use of higher doses of vitamin D over a prolonged time; therefore, regardless of the dose of supplementation initiated, we recommend that 25(OH)D levels are checked 3 months after initiating supplementation and trended over time to ensure levels are within goal and to adjust vitamin D dose. Caution should be taken in patients with impairment of renal function or other disease states such as sarcoidosis or lymphoma that could compound the effects of vitamin D supplementation and lead to hypercalcemia. Additionally, there is some evidence to suggest that higher doses of vitamin D is associated with an increased risk of falls in the elderly.[18]

Case Study

Case: A 55-year-old woman with history of MS is referred to you for a low 25(OH)D level. Three months ago, she was found to have a 25(OH)D of 15. She was administered vitamin D3 400 IU twice a day by her primary care physician. Repeat laboratory tests today show a 25(OH)D of 16. What should you recommend to treat this patient's vitamin D deficiency?

She should be given ergocalciferol (D2) 50,000 IU weekly for 8 weeks. Following that, she should be maintained on vitamin D3 2000 to 5000 IU daily. 25(OH)D levels should be determined again in 3 months for further dose adjustments for a goal 25(OH)D level of 40 to 60 ng/mL.

Management of Glucocorticoid-Induced Osteoporosis

GCs have a particularly large impact on bone loss and fractures.[19] The highest rate of bone loss occurs within the first 3 to 6 months of GC treatment followed by a slower decline with continued GC use.[20] Both high daily and high cumulative GC doses increase the risk of fracture, particularly vertebral fracture, because of the greater effects of GCs on trabecular bone than on cortical bone. However, this effect is largely reversible. Once GC treatment is terminated, bone mineral density increases and fracture risk declines.[20]

Physicians should take a thorough history evaluating the details of GC use (dose, duration, pattern of use) and assess for risk factors for osteoporosis and fractures (falls, history of fractures, frailty, low body weight, hypogonadism, secondary hyperparathyroidism, thyroid disease, family history of hip fracture, history of alcohol use or smoking). In patients older than 40 years, it is recommended that the FRAX calculator (https://www.sheffield.ac.uk/FRAX/) be used to assess fracture risk if the patient does not have osteoporosis. When GC use is included as a risk factor in FRAX, the risk generated is associated with a prednisone dose of ≤7.5 mg/d; therefore, fracture risk should be increased if patients are on a dose above 7.5 mg/d (15% for major osteoporotic fracture and 20% for hip fracture risk).[21] Patients treated with long-term or high-dose GC who have concomitant osteoporosis risk factors are the individuals at the highest risk of GC-induced osteoporosis. These patients should undergo bone mineral density testing within 6 months of beginning GC treatment.[22]

In addition to causing bone loss and fractures, steroid use puts individuals at risk for avascular bone necrosis (AVN). Steroids are now the second most common cause of AVN after trauma, and the prevalence of AVN varies between 3% and 38%.[23] The pathogenesis of GC-induced AVN is not fully understood, but it has been hypothesized to involve progressive destruction of bone vasculature and death of osteocytes, ultimately leading to alteration of bone architecture.[23] The duration of steroid treatment, the total cumulative dose, and the highest daily dose of steroids have been implicated as important factors in the development of avascular necrosis. AVN is typically characterized by pain that is gradual in onset, worsens with activity, relieved by rest, and radiates from the joint down the affected limb. It is important for clinicians to be mindful of these symptoms in their patients taking steroids, as early diagnosis is crucial to prognosis. Conventional radiography is generally the first-line test, with MRI being the most sensitive modality in diagnosing AVN.[23]

The American College of Rheumatology 2017 Guidelines recommend that all patients taking prednisone ≥2.5 mg/d for ≥3 months should have a calcium intake of 1000 to 1200 mg/d and 600 to 800 IU/d of vitamin D in addition to lifestyle modifications of smoking cessation, limiting alcohol intake, and incorporating resistance exercises into daily routine.[22] Those with moderate to high risk of fracture should be treated with oral bisphosphonates (BPs) such as alendronate 70 mg weekly, ibandronate 150 mg monthly, or risedronate 35 mg once weekly. Oral BPs are preferred for safety, cost, as well as the lack of evidence of superior antifracture benefits from other osteoporosis medications. An advantage of oral BPs is that they can be stopped if GCs are discontinued; however, because they are poorly absorbed in the gastrointestinal tract, they should be used with caution in patients with upper gastrointestinal disease because of the potential for worsening of gastrointestinal symptoms. For those who do not tolerate oral BPs because of gastrointestinal side effects, intravenous BPs (zoledronic acid 5 mg intravenously per year) can be used. All BPs are contraindicated in patients with hypocalcemia and renal impairment (creatinine clearance below 30 mL/min) and in those who are pregnant or lactating. Rare but recognized side effects of long-term BP use include osteonecrosis of the jaw and atypical subtrochanteric or diaphyseal femoral fractures. Given these concerns, patients on BPS should discuss the medications with their dentist/oral health care provider. Additionally, the need to continue treatment should be reviewed at regular intervals. After 5 years of oral alendronate, risedronate, or ibandronate or after 3 years of intravenous zoledronic acid, fracture risk should be reassessed and a drug holiday should be strongly considered. Lastly, if oral or intravenous BPs are contraindicated, other options include recombinant parathyroid hormone (teriparatide 20 µg subcutaneous daily) and monoclonal antibody RANK ligand inhibitors (denosumab 60 mg subcutaneous every 6 mo).

Adrenal Gland

Evaluation and Management of Adrenal Insufficiency

Another major complication that comes with GC use for longer durations is the suppression of the HPA axis.[24] With exogenous steroid use, the adrenocorticotropic hormone (ACTH)-secreting cells of the pituitary atrophy so that when steroids are withdrawn, the pituitary fails to respond appropriately and low ACTH with subsequently low cortisol levels are observed. The longer an individual takes exogenous steroids, the more likely the adrenal gland itself also atrophies leading to an impairment of the adrenals to respond to ACTH. Depending on the duration and dose of GC use, the degree of HPA axis suppression can vary. In general, patients who are more likely to develop HPA axis suppression are those who receive high doses (>20-30 mg prednisone or equivalent) of systemic GCs for long periods (>3 wk) and those who appear to have Cushingoid features.[25] Individuals with adrenal insufficiency typically exhibit nonspecific symptoms such as fatigue, decreased appetite, and abdominal discomfort; however, when they are exposed to any stressor, these same individuals can become critically ill with nausea, vomiting, orthostatic hypotension, and even hemodynamic instability. The full recovery of the HPA axis varies from 1 week to several months after discontinuation of GCs.[26]

Before starting any course of GC, clinicians should educate their patients about the risk and symptoms of adrenal insufficiency. It is important for clinicians treating patients with MS to have a high suspicion for adrenal insufficiency particularly in patients after discontinuation of high-dose or long-term treatment of GC or patients with nonspecific symptoms after discontinuing steroids of any dose or duration.

To identify patients with suppressed endogenous cortisol production, the standard high-dose cosyntropin stimulation test should be performed. This test consists of measuring serum cortisol immediately before and 30 and 60 minutes after administration of 250 µg of cosyntropin, a synthetic derivative of ACTH. Normal adrenal function is indicated by a serum cortisol concentration ≥18. Those patients with cortisol concentration ≤18 need to be considered for GC replacement therapy under the guidance of an endocrinologist. The stimulation test should be performed once the patient has stopped taking steroids or is given a physiologic dose of steroids (hydrocortisone 10 mg in the morning and 5 mg in the evening or prednisone 5 mg daily). If a patient continues to take steroids at physiologic dosing, then he or she must not take the steroid on the morning of the stimulation test and instead must wait until completing the stimulation test.

Management of Iatrogenic Cushing Syndrome

Development of iatrogenic Cushing syndrome (CS) is another potential complication seen in patients receiving long-term high-dose steroids. Although patients taking steroids of higher doses and longer durations are at higher risk of developing CS, it is difficult to predict exact doses and the time course at which CS will develop owing to factors such as varying GC potency, formulations, and administration method, in addition to other medications that the patient may be taking that can influence steroid metabolism.[27] Exogenous CS presents with the same signs and symptoms as spontaneous CS. The CS stigmata includes central obesity, dorsocervical and supraclavicular fat pads, moon facies, thin skin, straie, and proximal muscle weakness.

The diagnosis of iatrogenic CS requires clinical suspicion. These individuals will have surprisingly very low morning serum cortisol particular for their degree of Cushingoid features.[28] ACTH levels will also be low because of suppressed pituitary production. The treatment for iatrogenic CS is dose reduction or discontinuation of steroid therapy. However, this often poses a clinical challenge because of concern of HPA-axis suppression (as discussed earlier) or exacerbation of underlying MS symptoms for which steroids were initiated. For this reason, clinicians should always initiate GC therapy judiciously; using the minimum dose for the shortest duration possible along with frequent follow-up to reassess for MS-related symptoms.

Glycemic Control and Metabolic Syndrome

Type 1 Diabetes Mellitus and Multiple Sclerosis

Type 1 diabetes mellitus (T1D) is caused by autoimmune destruction of pancreatic islet cells, resulting in irreversible insulin deficiency. Similarly in MS, there is an autoimmune destruction of myelin in the central nervous system. Both diseases have been noted to occur at a higher rate in patients with one of the diagnoses. The similarity in epidemiology, clinical, and immunologic features suggest a possible common mechanism of development or genetic predisposition.[29-31]

In a cohort study done in Sardinia, the prevalence of T1D in patients with MS was five times greater than that of the general population sample. The prevalence was three times greater when compared with healthy siblings. Healthy patients with a first- or second-degree relative with MS also had an increased risk of developing T1D.[29] Other studies analyzing the reverse (development of MS in patients with T1D) have resulted in similar rates of concurrence.[30,31] The etiology of the association is unclear. There may be a shared HLA-DR,DQ genetic locus, although the haplotype is unclear. In a genome-wide linkage scan, there were two specific regions at 10q21.1 and 20p12.3 that coincided.[32] Currently, the precise genetic or environmental link between the two conditions is yet to be fully understood.

Microvascular and Macrovascular Complications of Diabetes Mellitus and Multiple Sclerosis

In addition to the diagnosis of diabetes itself, microvascular and macrovascular complications of T1D affect the overall health of patients with MS. Diabetic neuropathy damages the peripheral nervous system, resulting in paresthesias, sensory loss, neuropathic pain, and autonomic dysfunction. Uncontrolled hyperglycemia can result in increased risk of cerebrovascular accidents. Recurrent severe hypoglycemia can result in cerebral ischemia, cognitive dysfunction, or impairment of coordination and executive function.[31] Macular edema is a prominent adverse event in patients treated with fingolimod (a sphingosine-1-phosphate receptor modulator) for relapsing forms of MS. Diabetes itself is a risk factor for macular edema, by weakening the retinal vasculature, and approximately 10% of patients with diabetes develop macular edema. Therefore, patients with diabetes being treated with fingolimod may have a higher predisposition to developing fingolimod-associated macular edema (FAME) and should be screened at baseline as well as 3 to 4 months into treatment. It is not an absolute contraindication to therapy. FAME does appear to be dose dependent and typically resolves with cessation of therapy.[33] Therefore, appropriate diagnosis and timely treatment of patients with T1D is essential.

Metabolic Syndrome and Multiple Sclerosis

Patients with MS often have reduced exercise capacity, increased immobility, and a sedentary lifestyle, which may lead to metabolic syndrome and cardiovascular disease. In a study of 130 patients with MS, 30% had metabolic syndrome, 56% had central obesity, 28% had hypertension, and 10% had type 2 diabetes mellitus (T2D).[34] Other studies have shown greater body fat mass and fat percentage, higher blood pressure, resting heart rates, triglyceride levels, and impaired glucose tolerance.[35] The likelihood for cardiovascular mortality is significantly greater than in the general population (up to 2.4-fold increased rate).[34,36] Metformin is often used as a first-line therapy to decrease insulin resistance in patients with metabolic syndrome, especially if patients are taking steroids. Therefore, it is important for patients to maintain regular follow-up with their primary care doctor to prevent and manage metabolic syndrome. Of note, the body mass index is not an accurate measurement for patients with MS, as the lower ratio of muscle to fat leads to an underestimation of the amount of adipose tissue.[34]

Treatment-Associated Glucose Intolerance

In addition to having increased risk of metabolic syndrome, patients are frequently on courses of GC therapy. Approximately 44% of patients with MS have at least one acute exacerbation a year, the primary treatment of which is high-dose corticosteroids. Repeated exposure to steroids has been known to result in steroid-induced hyperglycemia, and even T2D. Some patients respond well to lifestyle changes, including limited processed carbohydrates and increase activity. Patients with preexisting diabetes require adjustments to their antihyperglycemic regimens. Insulin resistance associated with steroids profoundly affects postprandial hyperglycemia. Insulin may be needed depending on when patients are taking or have stopped taking steroid therapy. It is essential to work with an endocrinologist to determine the best regimen to counter the hyperglycemia associated with steroids. Fluctuations in glycemic control may lead to complications. Therefore, checking and maintaining steady glucose control during an MS exacerbation is important.[37]

H.P. Acthar Gel (ACTH hormone) is a cosyntropin injection that is occasionally used in lieu of high-dose steroids for MS relapses. ACTH acts by stimulating the adrenal cortex to produce endogenous corticosteroids rather than using solumedrol, an exogenous synthetic steroid. There have been reports of hyperglycemia after Acthar Gel administration. Therefore, it should be used with caution in patients with known diabetes or prior hyperglycemia, and these patients should undergo serial glucose monitoring during treatment.[37] If indicated, consider treatment with metformin to help decrease overall insulin resistance and insulin therapy in conjunction with steroid or Acthar Gel doses.

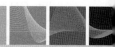

Case Study

Case: A 40-year-old man with a history of MS presents to you for new-onset hyperglycemia. He has no prior history of diabetes mellitus. Three days ago, administration of methylprednisone 500 mg daily was started for symptoms of an acute MS. He takes methylprednisone every morning and is to complete 4 days of steroids for a total of 7 days. He reports symptoms of polyuria and polydipsia that started yesterday. You do a fingerstick glucose test, and the result is 389. He weighs 95 kg. What is the best way to manage this patient's hyperglycemia?

This patient has no prior history of diabetes but now has steroid-induced hyperglycemia. NPH insulin can often be used safely in patients with steroid-induced hyperglycemia, as its duration of action matches steroids with an intermediate half-life (methylprednisone, prednisone). The total daily insulin dose can be calculated by multiplying 0.2 U/kg. Half of this would be the patient's basal requirement. NPH insulin has a duration of action of 12 hours; thus, taking half of the basal requirement would be an appropriate starting NPH dose. Therefore, this patient should be given NPH 10 U daily to be administered with the steroid dose. Also, metformin can be used with the insulin to optimize glucose control. Although insulin promotes weight gain, metformin may help attenuate weight changes and often helps with weight loss.[38]

Thyroid Disorders

Autoimmune Thyroid Disorder

In the general population, autoimmune thyroid disorder (AITD) has an estimated prevalence of 5% and is higher in females as well as patients with other autoimmune disorders. In one meta-analysis, a summary estimate of prevalence of AITD in patients with MS was 6.44%.[39] AITD presents as three clinical phenotypes: autoimmune hypothyroidism (Hashimoto), autoimmune hyperthyroidism (Graves disease [GD]), and silent thyroiditis.

Autoimmune hypothyroidism, characterized by elevated thyroid peroxidase (TPO) antibodies, is the most common. It is a painless, chronic lymphocytic thyroiditis that develops over years, eventually resulting in hypothyroidism. Treatment involves thyroid replacement hormone and is routinely managed in primary care. Autoimmune hyperthyroidism is the second most common phenotype, caused by uncontrolled stimulation of the TSH or thyrotropin receptor by thyroid receptor antibodies (TRAbs), resulting in thyroid hormone overproduction. Clinically, patients present like GD and can even develop orbitopathy. Treatment is a bit more complicated, involving months of antithyroid medications (i.e., methimazole) or definitive treatment with radioactive iodine or thyroidectomy. Symptomatic treatment with a beta-blocker (i.e., propranolol) is often used. Finally, AITD can be exhibited as silent thyroiditis, a painless, self-limited subacute lymphocytic thyroiditis. There are often positive TPO antibodies, similar to hypothyroidism, but the clinical course is different. It starts with hyperthyroid symptoms due to inflammation and leakage of thyroid hormone and then leads to transient hypothyroidism, with gradual return of normal thyroid function over weeks to months. Ultrasound uptake and scan of the thyroid during the hyperthyroid state often shows decreased uptake (as opposed to increased uptake in Graves). Treatment is primarily supportive care and close monitoring.

Screening for AITD would entail evaluating clinical symptoms for hypothyroidism or hyperthyroidism and checking serum TSH and free T4. Diagnosis of AITD is made via clinical symptoms and laboratory studies: serum TSH, free T4, and antibodies (TPO antibodies for hypothyroidism, TRAbs for hyperthyroidism). Treatment depends on diagnosis, and close follow-up with endocrinology is recommended.[40,41]

Thyroid Nodules

Thyroid nodules are often found incidentally, either on clinical examination or on imaging done for another purpose. They are very common, occurring in up to 50% of the general population by age 60 years. They are most often benign (over 90%), but all nodules should be further evaluated for hyperactivity or malignancy. A formal thyroid ultrasound scan should be ordered, as well as serum TSH and free T4 to assess if the nodule is producing any excessive thyroid hormone. Most thyroid nodules are nonfunctioning and do not cause any symptoms. Rarely, if a nodule is large enough, it can cause compressive symptoms, such as dysphagia or hoarseness. If on ultrasound scan the nodule has suspicious features, such as size >2 cm, calcifications, irregular margins, taller than wide, or evidence of extrathyroidal extension, patients should be referred to endocrinology for a fine-needle biopsy and further evaluation.[42]

Alemtuzumab (Lemtrada)-Related Thyroid Dysfunction

Alemtuzumab is a monoclonal anti-CD52 used to treat relapsing forms of MS. The precise mechanism is not fully understood, but it appears to be depletion then repopulation of T and B lymphocytes in an attempt to shift the immunologic balance. This immune reconstitution phase may result in the formation of autoantibodies, including those targeting the thyroid.[40,43] Autoimmune thyroid disease (AITD) is the most common autoimmune disorder after treatment, followed by immune thrombocytopenia and glomerular nephropathies. In phase 3 clinical trials, there was a 40.7% chance of thyroid-related adverse events within 5 years, with a peak at 3 years post treatment (16% in the CARE-MS trials [phase 3 comparison of alemtuzumab vs interferon beta 1a in relapsing remitting MS]).[40,43,44] Hyperthyroidism was four times more prevalent than hypothyroidism and more common than subacute thyroiditis.[41,43] Thyroid dysfunction was typically mild to moderate, its incidence peaked at year 3, and it either self-resolved (one in three cases of hyperthyroidism) or was treatable along current guidelines. In the 10-year phase 2 CAMMS223 (phase 2 study of alemtuzumab vs interferon beta 1 a in early relapsing remitting MS) study as well as the phase 3 CARE-MS (phase 3 comparison of alemtuzumab and interferon beta 1a efficacy in RRMS) study, no deaths occurred as a result of thyroid events.[40,43,44]

A 2016 Belgian task force proposed a clinical management algorithm to address alemtuzumab treatment-related thyroid adverse events (Figure 10.1).[40] The clinical management algorithm and recommendations are similar to those proposed by Devonshire et al, in the *Journal of Neurology*, 2018.[44] Before starting alemtuzumab, patients should be evaluated for risk factors for thyroid disease (family history, prior head/ neck irradiation, or smoking), current or prior treatment for thyroid disease, and baseline thyroid function tests, including TPO antibodies. It is also important to ask female patients about contraception or pregnancy plans, as thyroid dysfunction and its treatment can lead to pregnancy-related complications. After starting alemtuzumab, patients should have routine clinical screening for symptoms of hyperthyroidism or hypothyroidism, along with biochemical monitoring. Thyroid function tests (TSH and free T4) should be checked every 3 months during therapy, until up

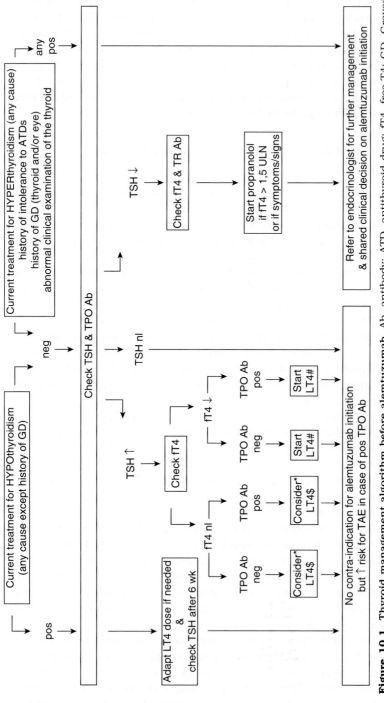

Figure 10.1. Thyroid management algorithm before alemtuzumab. Ab, antibody; ATD, antithyroid drug; fT4, free T4; GD, Graves disease; LT4, levothyroxine; neg, negative; nl, normal; pos, positive; TAE, thyroid adverse event; TPO, thyroperoxidase; TR, thyrotropin receptor; TSH, thyroid stimulating hormone; ULN, upper limit of normal. *Symptoms/signs of hypothyroidism or TSH > 10 mU/L favor initiation of LT4; $LT4 ± 0.5 μg/kg/d; #LT4 ± 1 μg/kg/d. (Reprinted with permission from Decallonne B, Bartholomé E, Delvaux V, et al. Thyroid disorders in alemtuzumab-treated multiple sclerosis patients: a Belgian consensus on diagnosis and management. *Acta Neurol Belg.* 2018;118(2):153-159.)

to 48 months after the last dose. Patients with TPO antibodies or prior thyroid history should be watched closely, because of an increased risk of AITD. Women of childbearing potential should use effective contraceptive methods during and up to 4 months after alemtuzumab treatment.

Thyroid dysfunction is not an absolute contraindication to alemtuzumab therapy, as most associated AITDs are mild/self-resolve. It is important for the clinician to be aware of them and perform appropriate clinical and biochemical screening before, during, and after treatment.

Interferon-Related Thyroid Dysfunction

IFN-β therapy is also used in the treatment of MS, and AITD can be a side effect of therapy, occurring in up to 6.2% of patients. The mechanism of action is unknown but is proposed to be due to the result of autoantibodies or immune system dysregulation. Preexisting thyroid antibodies (TPO or TRAbs) are a risk factor, with 70% of the cases with IFN-β-associated AITD occurring in patients with MS with TPO antibodies. Hypothyroidism in general occurred more frequently than hyperthyroidism in treated patients (3.9% vs. 2.3%, respectively). Patients can present with a destructive thyroiditis picture, with early transient hyperthyroidism followed by hypothyroidism. Most thyroid dysfunction was subclinical and found on screening laboratory work. Spontaneous resolution occurred in almost 60% of patients regardless of IFN therapy.[45]

Similar to alemtuzumab, thyroid dysfunction is not an absolute contraindication to therapy, as AITD is usually subclinical or mild and 60% self-resolve. There also does not appear to be a dose-dependent or time-dependent relationship with IFN-β. Nevertheless, it is important for the prescribing clinician to be aware and perform appropriate clinical and biochemical screening during therapy.[45]

Biotin-Associated Thyroid Laboratory Abnormalities

Biotin is a water-soluble vitamin (B7) that is being studied for use in high doses (300-600 mg/d) for the treatment of primary progressive MS. It has been known to interfere with laboratory thyroid assays that use biotin as a test reagent. In competitive binding immunoassays (used for free and total T4 and T3), biotin interference causes a falsely high result. In sandwich immunoassays (used for TSH), excessive biotin can give a falsely low result. This can lead to an inaccurate diagnosis of hyperthyroidism (more common) or hypothyroidism.[46-49]

Studies have shown persistent biotin interference even after 16 hours after the last dose.[47] Therefore, it is recommended that patients stop biotin treatment for at least 2 days before having laboratory tests done.[46] In addition, any abnormal laboratory results should be correlated with clinical signs and symptoms. Of note, biotin has been found to also interfere with assays for parathyroid hormone, dehydroepiandrosterone sulfate, testosterone, thyroglobulin, estradiol, and ferritin. This results in abnormal laboratory data because of assay interference, but the data do not correlate with clinical findings.[46,47,50]

Conclusion

MS is a complex disorder with various treatment modalities. There are endocrine-related complications of both the disease itself as well as side effects from therapy. Patients with MS have a higher rate of osteopenia and osteoporosis, both as a function of the musculoskeletal changes in MS as well as prolonged steroid exposure. Vitamin D deficiency has been reported at higher rates. GC therapy is associated with a multitude of endocrine adverse effects, such as osteoporosis, iatrogenic Cushing syndrome, and secondary adrenal insufficiency. Hyperglycemia can result from T1D, T2D, GCs, or Acthar Gel. Patients are at risk for metabolic syndrome and associated cardiovascular disease. Autoimmune thyroid disorders occur at a higher rate in patients with MS even before taking into account treatment. Alemtuzumab immunotherapy can result in thyroid dysfunction, especially hyperthyroidism. Biotin can interfere with thyroid laboratory assays, resulting in false results. One should be aware of these endocrinopathies when caring for patients with MS.

References

1. Provvedini DM, Tsoukas CD, Deftos LJ, Manolagas SC. 1,25-Dihydroxyvitamin D3 receptors in human leukocytes. *Science.* 1983;221(4616):1181-1183.
2. Munger KL, Levin LI, Hollis BW, Howard NS, Ascherio A. Serum 25-hydroxyvitamin D levels and risk of multiple sclerosis. *JAMA.* 2006;296(23):2832-2838.
3. Salzer J, Hallmans G, Nyström M, Stenlund H, Wadell G, Sundström P. Vitamin D as a protective factor in multiple sclerosis. *Neurology.* 2012;79(21):2140-2145.
4. Mokry LE, Ross S, Ahmad OS, et al. Vitamin D and risk of multiple sclerosis: A Mendelian Randomization Study. *PLoS Med.* 2015;12(8):e1001866.
5. Runia TF, Hop WC, de Rijke YB, Buljevac D, Hintzen RQ. Lower serum vitamin D levels are associated with a higher relapse risk in multiple sclerosis. *Neurology.* 2012;79(3):261-266.
6. Mowry EM, Waubant E, McCulloch CE, et al. Vitamin D status predicts new brain magnetic resonance imaging activity in multiple sclerosis. *Ann Neurol.* 2012;72(2):234-240.
7. Fitzgerald KC, Munger KL, Köchert K, et al. Association of vitamin D levels with multiple sclerosis activity and progression in patients receiving interferon beta-1b. *JAMA Neurol.* 2015;72(12):1458-1465.
8. Soilu-Hänninen M, Aivo J, Lindström BM, et al. A randomised, double blind, placebo controlled trial with vitamin D3 as an add on treatment to interferon β-1b in patients with multiple sclerosis. *J Neurol Neurosurg Psychiatry.* 2012;83(5):565-571.

9. Smolders J, Hupperts R, Vieth R, et al. High dose cholecalciferol (vitamin D3) oil as add-on therapy in subjects with relapsing-remitting multiple sclerosis (RRMS) receiving subcutaneous interferon b-1a (scIFNb-1a). *ECTRIMS Online Libr.* 2016:147013.

10. Holick MF, Binkley NC, Bischoff-Ferrari HA, et al. Evaluation, treatment, and prevention of vitamin D deficiency: An Endocrine Society Clinical Practice Guideline. *J Clin Endocrinol Metab.* 2011;96(7):1911-1930.

11. Shoemaker TJ, Mowry EM. A review of vitamin D supplementation as disease-modifying therapy. *Mult Scler.* 2018;24(1):6-11.

12. Sintzel MB, Rametta M, Reder AT. Vitamin D and multiple sclerosis: a comprehensive review. *Neurol Ther.* 2018;7(1):59-85.

13. Heaney RP, Recker RR, Grote J, Horst RL, Armas LA. Vitamin D(3) is more potent than vitamin D(2) in humans. *J Clin Endocrinol Metab.* 2011;96(3):E447-E452.

14. Kimball SM, Ursell MR, O'Connor P, Vieth R. Safety of vitamin D3 in adults with multiple sclerosis. *Am J Clin Nutr.* 2007;86(3):645-651.

15. Rostami M, Tehrani FR, Simbar M, et al. Effectiveness of prenatal vitamin D deficiency screening and treatment program: a stratified randomized field trial. *J Clin Endocrinol Metab.* 2018;103(8):2936-2948.

16. Burton JM, Kimball S, Vieth R, et al. A phase I/II dose-escalation trial of vitamin D3 and calcium in multiple sclerosis. *Neurology.* 2010;74(23):1852-1859.

17. Smolders J, Peelen E, Thewissen M, et al. Safety and T cell modulating effects of high dose vitamin D3 supplementation in multiple sclerosis. *PLoS One.* 2010;5(12):e15235.

18. Bischoff-Ferrari HA, Dawson-Hughes B, Orav EJ, et al. Monthly high-dose vitamin D treatment for the prevention of functional decline: a randomized clinical trial. *JAMA Intern Med.* 2016;176(2):175-183.

19. Lane NE, Lukert B. The science and therapy of glucocorticoid-induced bone loss. *Endocrinol Metab Clin North Am.* 1998;27(2):465-483.

20. Laan RF, van Riel PL, van de Putte LB, van Erning LJ, van't Hof MA, Lemmens JA. Low-dose prednisone induces rapid reversible axial bone loss in patients with rheumatoid arthritis. A randomized, controlled study. *Ann Intern Med.* 1993;119(10):963-968.

21. Kanis JA, Johansson H, Oden A, McCloskey EV. Guidance for the adjustment of FRAX according to the dose of glucocorticoids. *Osteoporos Int.* 2011;22(3):809-816.

22. Buckley L, Guyatt G, Fink H, McAlindon T. 2017 American College of Rheumatology guideline for the prevention and treatment of glucocorticoid-induced osteoporosis. *Arthritis Care Res (Hoboken).* 2017;69(8):1521-1537.

23. Chan KL, Mok CC. Glucocorticoid-induced avascular bone necrosis: diagnosis and management. *Open Orthop J.* 2012;6:449-457.

24. Streck WF, Lockwood DH. Pituitary adrenal recovery following short-term suppression with corticosteroids. *Am J Med.* 1979;66(6):910-914.

25. Paragliola RM, Papi G, Pontecorvi A, Corsello SM. Treatment with synthetic glucocorticoids and the hypothalamus-pituitary-adrenal Axis. *Int J Mol Sci.* 2017;18(10).

26. Broersen LH, Pereira AM, Jørgensen JO, Dekkers OM. Adrenal insufficiency in corticosteroids use: systematic review and meta-analysis. *J Clin Endocrinol Metab.* 2015;100(6):2171-2180.

27. Felig P, Frohman L, Chrousos GP. *Glucocorticoid therapy.* In: *Endocrinology and Metabolism.* 4th ed. New York: McGraw-Hill; 2001:609-632.

28. Hopkins RL, Leinung MC. Exogenous Cushing's syndrome and glucocorticoid withdrawal. *Endocrinol Metab Clin North Am.* 2005;34(2):371-384, ix.

29. Marrosu MG, Cocco E, Lai M, Spinicci G, Pischedda MP, Contu P. Patients with multiple sclerosis and risk of type 1 diabetes mellitus in Sardinia, Italy: a cohort study. *Lancet.* 2002;359(9316):1461-1465.

30. Bechtold S, Blaschek A, Raile K, et al. Higher relative risk for multiple sclerosis in a pediatric and adolescent diabetic population: analysis from DPV database. *Diabetes Care.* 2014;37(1):96-101.

31. Tettey P, Simpson S, Taylor BV, van der Mei IA. The co-occurrence of multiple sclerosis and type 1 diabetes: shared aetiologic features and clinical implication for MS aetiology. *J Neurol Sci.* 2015;348(1-2):126-131.

32. Pitzalis M, Zavattari P, Murru R, et al. Genetic loci linked to type 1 diabetes and multiple sclerosis families in Sardinia. *BMC Med Genet.* 2008;9:3.

33. Jain N, Bhatti MT. Fingolimod-associated macular edema: incidence, detection, and management. *Neurology.* 2012;78(9):672-680.

34. Pinhas-Hamiel O, Livne M, Harari G, Achiron A. Prevalence of overweight, obesity and metabolic syndrome components in multiple sclerosis patients with significant disability. *Eur J Neurol.* 2015;22(9):1275-1279.

35. Keytsman C, Eijnde BO, Hansen D, Verboven K, Wens I. Elevated cardiovascular risk factors in multiple sclerosis. *Mult Scler Relat Disord.* 2017;17:220-223.

36. Sicras-Mainar A, Ruíz-Beato E, Navarro-Artieda R, Maurino J. Comorbidity and metabolic syndrome in patients with multiple sclerosis from Asturias and Catalonia, Spain. *BMC Neurol.* 2017;17(1):134.

37. Kutz C. H.P. Acthar gel (repository corticotropin injection) treatment of patients with multiple sclerosis and diabetes. *Ther Adv Chronic Dis.* 2016;7(4):190-197.

38. Igel LI, Sinha A, Saunders KH, Apovian CM, Vojta D, Aronne LJ. Metformin: an old therapy that deserves a new indication for the treatment of obesity. *Curr Atheroscler Rep.* 2016;18(4):16.

39. Marrie RA, Reider N, Cohen J, et al. A systematic review of the incidence and prevalence of autoimmune disease in multiple sclerosis. *Mult Scler.* 2015;21(3):282-293.

40. Decallonne B, Bartholomé E, Delvaux V, et al. Thyroid disorders in alemtuzumab-treated multiple sclerosis patients: a Belgian consensus on diagnosis and management. *Acta Neurol Belg.* 2018;118(2):153-159.

41. Daniels GH, Vladic A, Brinar V, et al. Alemtuzumab-related thyroid dysfunction in a phase 2 trial of patients with relapsing-remitting multiple sclerosis. *J Clin Endocrinol Metab.* 2014;99:80-89.

42. Haugen BR, Alexander EK, Bible KC, et al. 2015 American Thyroid Association Management Guidelines for adult patients with thyroid nodules and differentiated thyroid cancer: the American Thyroid Association Guidelines task force on thyroid nodules and differentiated thyroid cancer. *Thyroid.* 2016;26(1):1-133.

43. Rotondi M, Molteni M, Leporati P, Capelli V, Marinò M, Chiovato L. Autoimmune thyroid diseases in patients treated with alemtuzumab for multiple sclerosis: an example of selective anti-TSH-receptor immune response. *Front Endocrinol (Lausanne).* 2017;8:254.

44. Devonshire V, Phillips R, Wass H, Da Roza G, Senior P. Monitoring and management of autoimmunity in multiple sclerosis patients treated with alemtuzumab: practical recommendations. *J Neurol.* 2018;265(11):2494-2505.

45. Monzani F, Caraccio N, Dardano A, Ferrannini E. Thyroid autoimmunity and dysfunction associated with type I interferon therapy. *Clin Exp Med.* 2004;3(4):199-210.

46. De Roeck Y, Philipse E, Twickler TB, Van Gaal L. Misdiagnosis of Graves' hyperthyroidism due to therapeutic biotin intervention. *Acta Clin Belg.* 2018; 73(5):372-376.

47. Elston MS, Sehgal S, Du Toit S, Yarndley T, Conaglen JV. Factitious Graves' disease due to biotin immunoassay interference-A case and review of the literature. *J Clin Endocrinol Metab.* 2016;101(9):3251-3255.

48. Minkovsky A, Lee MN, Dowlatshahi M, et al. High-dose biotin treatment for secondary progressive multiple sclerosis may interfere with thyroid assays. *AACE Clin Case Rep.* 2016;2(4):e370-e373.

49. Kummer S, Hermsen D, Distelmaier F. Biotin treatment mimicking Graves' disease. *N Engl J Med.* 2016;375(7):704-706.

50. Piketty ML, Prie D, Sedel F, et al. High-dose biotin therapy leading to false biochemical endocrine profiles: validation of a simple method to overcome biotin interference. *Clin Chem Lab Med.* 2017;55(6):817-825.

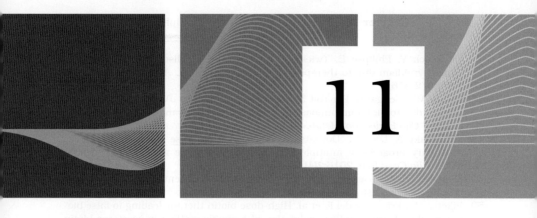

Obesity and Multiple Sclerosis

■ ▨ ▨ ▨ Katherine H. Saunders, Mohini Aras, Louis J. Aronne

Introduction

Obesity affects 39.8% of adults (93.3 million) and 18.5% of children and adolescents (13.7 million) in the United States.[1] Obesity is defined as a body mass index (BMI) of greater than or equal to 30 kg/m^2 in adults and a BMI of greater than or equal to age- and sex-specific 95th percentile of the 2000 Centers for Disease Control and Prevention growth charts in children.[2] The medical costs associated with obesity are tremendous. The latest published estimate was US$147 billion in 2008.[3]

Obesity is a multifactorial, chronic disease characterized by an accumulation of visceral and subcutaneous fat, which leads to a predisposition toward a wide variety of comorbid conditions.[4] Obesity-related comorbidities include many of the leading causes of preventable death, such as heart disease, type 2 diabetes, stroke, and many types of cancer. Mechanisms including abnormalities in lipid metabolism, insulin resistance, inflammation, endothelial function, adipokine balance, and inflammasome activation have been implicated in the development of these weight-related chronic conditions, including multiple sclerosis (MS) among patients with obesity.[4]

Modest weight loss of 5% to 10% body weight is sufficient for significant and clinically relevant improvements in risk factors among patients with overweight and obesity.[5,6] This risk reduction appears to be dose related, as a 10% to 15% reduction in body weight is associated with even greater odds of clinically significant improvements in most risk factors. The magnitude of weight loss at 1 year is strongly associated with improvements in many parameters including blood sugar, blood pressure, triglycerides, and HDL cholesterol.

Most patients have limited success with weight loss because of the body's resistance to the effects of lifestyle modifications. Reduced caloric intake and increased energy expenditure are counteracted by a variety of adaptive physiological responses.[7] Alterations in a range of hormones cause appetite to increase and resting metabolic rate to slow out of proportion to what would be expected based on changes in body composition.[8] This phenomenon, called metabolic adaptation or adaptive thermogenesis, inhibits weight loss and leads to weight regain.[9,10]

As a result, successful treatment of obesity requires a multidisciplinary approach to counteract the body's resistance to weight loss. Although diet, physical activity, and behavioral modifications are the cornerstones of weight management, many patients require additional interventions, such as antiobesity medications and/or bariatric surgery, to achieve and maintain clinically significant weight loss.

In this chapter, we describe how obesity is a risk factor for MS. We also review the available treatment strategies for obesity, including medications and devices approved by the US Food and Drug Administration (FDA), as well as bariatric surgery. Finally, we examine the impact of obesity treatment on MS and present a patient case that illustrates key points.

Obesity as a Risk Factor for Multiple Sclerosis

Epidemiology

MS is a chronic autoimmune disease of the central nervous system (CNS). It is an inflammatory and demyelinating condition that affects both white and gray matter. Symptoms range from fatigue, numbness, and tingling to pain, blindness, spasticity, incontinence, and paralysis. It is estimated that MS affects between 400,000 to 1 million Americans and at least 2.3 million people worldwide.[11-13] MS affects twice as many women as men. According to the World Health Organization, rates of MS have increased over the last few years from 2.1 million in 2008 to 2.3 million in 2011.[12] The medical costs associated with MS are significant and are estimated to be upward of US$52,000 per patient per year.[11]

MS is the second leading cause of neurological disease in young people and leads to a wide range of functional debilities.[12] The most common subtype is relapsing-remitting MS, which is associated with numerous brain and spinal cord lesions that resolve either partially or completely between flares.[14] Pediatric MS, and clinically isolated syndrome, which includes optic neuritis and transverse myelitis, are being reported at increasing rates.[15] Although causes of MS remain unknown, both genetic and environmental factors have been implicated—human leukocyte antigen (HLA)-DRB1*15:01 allele, other non–major histocompatibility complex variants, tobacco exposure, vitamin D deficiency, viral exposures, reproductive history, and obesity.[11]

The prevalence of obesity in MS is estimated to range from 21% to 37%.[16] The increasing prevalence of obesity over the past few decades could account for increased rates of MS. Numerous studies have confirmed an approximately twofold increased risk of developing MS in women who were obese during late adolescence/early adulthood (age 18-25 y) versus women who had a BMI in the normal range during those years.[17,18] This association between adolescent/early adult obesity and MS has not been consistently shown in men.

There is also an association between childhood obesity and MS. In 2013, a Danish prospective study of children in the Copenhagen School Health Records Register found that girls who were ≥95th percentile for BMI had a 1.61- to 1.95-fold increased risk of MS compared with girls <85th percentile.[19] Among boys, this association was attenuated and only significant in particular age groups (e.g., among boys aged 8-10 y). Given the strong association between childhood obesity and adult obesity, treating childhood obesity may be an important initiative to reduce the prevalence of MS in adulthood.

Pathophysiology

Genetics

The HLA-DRB*15:01 allele is the most common genetic marker for the risk of developing MS. This allele carries a 2.9-fold increased risk of developing MS among individuals with a normal BMI. The presence of both obesity and the HLA-DRB1*15 allele confers a 9.1-fold increased risk of developing MS compared with noncarriers of the allele with a normal BMI.[14] These findings suggest that obesity is a significant risk factor for developing MS in genetically predisposed individuals.

Inflammation

Previously, it was believed that adipose tissue was metabolically inactive and its main purpose was storage, thermal regulation, and protection of vital organs. However, we now understand that adipose tissue is metabolically active and highly involved in hormonal and immune functions both locally and systemically.[20] Adipose tissue consists of the adipocyte as well as supporting cells, including fibroblasts, endothelial cells, and immune cells of both innate (macrophages, neutrophils, eosinophils, and mast cells) and adaptive (T and B cells) immunity. The adipocyte secretes a variety of adipokines (signaling proteins specific to adipocytes), including leptin and adiponectin. Under conditions of excess weight, adipocytes secrete proinflammatory cytokines, including tumor necrosis factor alpha, monocyte chemoattractant protein 1, and interleukin 6.[20] As a result, obesity is considered a chronic proinflammatory state. This chronic inflammation has been associated with a variety of disorders including atherosclerosis, diabetes mellitus, many types of cancer, inflammatory bowel disease, and MS.

On a cellular level, the damage that occurs in MS is due to autoreactive T cells entering the CNS and destroying oligodendrocytes, cells that produce myelin to insulate neurons.[21] Furthermore, inflammatory dendritic cells and macrophages promote disease by activating these autoreactive T cells and secreting proinflammatory cytokines. The chronic inflammation associated with obesity leads to unrestricted activation of the inflammasome, a multiprotein intracellular complex that secretes proinflammatory cytokines.[21,22]

Gut Microbiome

The gut microbiome is composed of microbes, such as bacteria, viruses, and fungi, that reside in the bowel.[14,23] These microorganisms contribute to the development of the immune system, protect against pathogens, and even assist in metabolic functions of the body both locally and systemically. Stool samples from patients with MS reveal significantly increased levels of *Methanobrevibacter* and *Akkermansia* and decreased levels of *Butyricimonas* (phylum: *Bacteroidetes*) compared with controls without MS.[14,24] *Methanobrevibacter* and *Akkermansia* are associated with T cell activation and proinflammatory cytokines, whereas *Butyricimonas* are associated with anti-inflammatory cytokines. Patients with obesity have also been found to have elevated levels of *Methanobrevibacter* and reduced levels of *Bacteroidetes*. These correlations in relative levels of microbiome species support an association between the proinflammatory environments among patients with obesity and MS.

Leptin and Adiponectin

Leptin is one of the peptide hormones secreted by adipocytes. It signals satiety, reduces food intake and regulates fat stores. Patients with obesity are relatively resistant to leptin, so levels are often found to be elevated. Interestingly, leptin has strong proinflammatory effects and is also found to be elevated in patients with MS. Although there are conflicting findings on the utility of leptin as a biomarker of MS disease activity, significantly increased levels have been reported in the cerebrospinal fluid (CSF) of patients during MS flares or relapses.[14,25,26] The rise in leptin is thought to be related to either increased leptin synthesis in the CSF or increased movement of leptin through a more permeable blood-brain barrier that might occur during an MS flare. In both obesity and MS, leptin modulates the immune system toward a proinflammatory state by secreting proinflammatory cytokines and downregulating anti-inflammatory cells.[14] There are many other hormones that regulate appetite and fat storage, which may be similarly upregulated in both inflammatory conditions.

In contrast to leptin, adiponectin is a hormone produced by the adipocyte that has anti-inflammatory effects. It has been shown in animal studies to be protective in autoimmune CNS inflammation. Mice without adiponectin have greater disease markers for MS, and when these mice are treated with adiponectin, there is improvement in these markers.[27] Adiponectin is an important regulator of T cells and could potentially have clinical implications for treating MS.

Vitamin D

Vitamin D is one of the fat-soluble vitamins. As it is sequestered in adipose tissue, circulating levels are often lower in patients with obesity. Vitamin D has been found to have many effects on the immune system, and low levels of vitamin D are thought to be a risk factor for the development of MS. New studies implicate the potential role of vitamin D in neuroprotection and myelin repair, and research is underway to determine if vitamin D supplementation among patients with MS can alter disease progression or rate of relapse.[28,29] Whether vitamin D deficiency and obesity are independent risk factors for MS or there are other underlying mechanisms has not yet been elucidated.

Obesity Treatment

Patients with both MS and obesity often suffer more pronounced disabilities than patients with MS who are not obese. In particular, ambulation can be affected early in the disease process and can severely impact quality of life.[30] In addition to physical disabilities, patients with MS and obesity also have higher rates of depression and suicide.[16] As a result, treating obesity in patients with MS should be a priority to improve disability and quality of life.

Lifestyle Modifications and Drug-Induced Weight Gain

Lifestyle interventions, including diet, exercise, and behavioral modifications, are the foundation of obesity treatment. Many dietary strategies can be effective for weight loss. Recommendations should be tailored to a patient's preferences, as adherence to diet is associated with greater weight loss and greater reductions in cardiac risk factors.[31] A Mediterranean diet can be a good option for patients at high cardiovascular risk, as it has been shown to reduce the incidence of major cardiovascular events in this population.[32] A low-glycemic-index diet can curb hunger and decrease cravings by reducing blood sugar fluctuations.[33] All patients trying to lose weight should be counseled to limit sugary drinks, fast food, junk food, and sweets. Registered dietitians can provide dietary education and customize diet plans.

The American College of Sports Medicine recommends 150 minutes of moderate-intensity aerobic physical activity (such as brisk walking or tennis) per week, 75 minutes of vigorous-intensity aerobic physical activity (such as jogging or swimming laps) per week, or an equivalent combination of moderate- and vigorous-intensity aerobic physical activity.[34] Episodes should last at least 10 minutes and, if possible, be spread out through the week. In addition, weight resistance (muscle strengthening) is recommended at least twice weekly. Patients with physical limitations should be encouraged to do what they can even if they cannot meet the recommendations. Exercise physiologists, physical therapists, and trainers can provide additional support for patients.

Behavioral interventions for weight loss include self-monitoring, such as weighing on a scale at regular intervals and keeping a food log to track caloric intake. Stress reduction and adequate sleep can also be helpful for weight loss. Support can be provided to patients by an interdisciplinary team including physicians, dietitians, sports physiologists, physical therapists, psychologists, social workers, and other health care professionals. As weight maintenance can be more difficult than initial weight loss, it is important that patients continue regular follow-up to ensure long-term adherence to their treatment plan.

Medications can have unpredictable and variable effects on a patient's weight, so it is important to balance the benefits of treatment against the probability of weight gain.[35] Multiple medications are associated with weight gain, including certain antidiabetic, antihypertensive, antidepressant, antipsychotic, antiepileptic, and antihistamine agents, as well as steroids, contraceptives, and other hormonal agents.[36] Table 11.1 provides an overview of these medications as well as potential alternative options. When possible, practitioners should utilize weight-neutral or weight-loss-promoting medications. If there are no alternative medications, weight gain can be prevented or lessened by selecting the lowest dose required to produce clinical efficacy for the shortest duration necessary.

TABLE 11.1

MEDICATIONS ASSOCIATED WITH WEIGHT GAIN, WEIGHT NEUTRALITY, AND WEIGHT LOSS

	Weight Gain	Weight Neutral/ Less Weight Gain	Weight Loss
Antidiabetics	Insulin	α-Glucosidase inhibitors	GLP-1 agonists
	Meglitinides	Bromocriptine	Metformin
	Sulfonylureas	Colesevelam	Pramlintide
	Thiazolidinediones	DPP-4 inhibitors	SGLT2 inhibitors
Antihypertensives	α-Adrenergic blockers β-Adrenergic blockers (atenolol, metoprolol, nadolol, propranolol)	ACE inhibitors ARBs β-Adrenergic blockers (carvedilol, nebivolol) Calcium channel blockers Thiazides	
Antidepressants	Lithium MAOIs Mirtazapine SSRIs (paroxetine) Tricyclic antidepressants (amitriptyline, doxepin, imipramine, nortriptyline)	SSRIs (fluoxetine, sertraline)	Bupropion
Antipsychotics	Clozapine Olanzapine Quetiapine Risperidone	Aripiprazole Lurasidone Ziprasidone	
Antiepileptics	Carbamazepine Gabapentin Pregabalin Valproic acid	Lamotrigine Levetiracetam Phenytoin	Topiramate Zonisamide
Contraceptives	Medroxyprogesterone acetate	Barrier methods IUDs Surgical sterilization	
Antihistamines	First-generation antihistamines	Second- and third-generation antihistamines Decongestants = alternatives	

TABLE 11.1

MEDICATIONS ASSOCIATED WITH WEIGHT GAIN, WEIGHT NEUTRALITY, AND WEIGHT LOSS (CONTINUED)

	Weight Gain	Weight Neutral/ Less Weight Gain	Weight Loss
Steroids	Glucocorticoids	Inhaled steroids Topical steroids NSAIDs, DMARDs = alternatives	

Adapted from Igel LI, Kumar RB, Saunders KH, et al. Practical use of pharmacotherapy for obesity. *Gastroenterology.* 2017;152(7):1765-1779. Copyright © 2017 AGA Institute. With permission.

ACE, angiotensin-converting enzyme; ARB, angiotensin II receptor blockers; DMARD, disease-modifying antirheumatic drug; DPP-4, dipeptidyl peptidase-4; GLP-1, glucagon-like peptide-1; IUD, intrauterine device; MAOI, monoamine oxidase inhibitor; NSAID, nonsteroidal anti-inflammatory drug; SGLT2, sodium-glucose cotransporter 2; SSRI, selective serotonin reuptake inhibitor.

Antiobesity Medications

Weight loss achieved by lifestyle modifications alone is often limited and difficult to maintain. As a result, patients may require antiobesity medications, bariatric surgery, devices, or endoscopic bariatric therapies to achieve and maintain clinically significant weight loss.

Antiobesity pharmacotherapy is one strategy to offset the changes in appetite and energy expenditure that occur with weight loss and improve adherence to lifestyle changes. According to the 2013 American College of Cardiology/American Heart Association/The Obesity Society's guideline for the management of overweight and obesity in adults and the Endocrine Society's clinical practice guidelines on the pharmacologic management of obesity, pharmacotherapy for obesity can be considered in patients with a BMI $\geq$ 30 kg/m^2 or a BMI $\geq$ 27 kg/m^2 with weight-related comorbidities, such as hypertension, dyslipidemia, type 2 diabetes, and obstructive sleep apnea.[37,38]

As obesity is a chronic disease, most antiobesity medications are approved for long-term treatment. Many of the antiobesity medications affect appetite mechanisms, signaling through serotonergic, noradrenergic, or dopaminergic pathways. They primarily target the arcuate nucleus of the hypothalamus to stimulate the anorexigenic pro-opiomelanocortin (POMC) neurons, which promote satiety.

Medications approved for weight management should be viewed as useful additions to diet and exercise for patients who have been unsuccessful with lifestyle changes alone *not* substitutions for lifestyle changes. The six most widely prescribed antiobesity medications approved by the FDA are phentermine, orlistat, phentermine/topiramate extended release (ER); lorcaserin; naltrexone sustained release (SR)/bupropion SR; and

TABLE 11.2

MOST COMMONLY USED MEDICATIONS FOR OBESITY APPROVED BY THE FOOD AND DRUG ADMINISTRATION

Medication	Mechanism, Dosage, Available Formulation	Total Body Weight Loss (%)	Initial FDA Approval
Phentermine (Adipex,[43] Ionamin,[44] Lomaira,[46] Suprenza[45])	Adrenergic agonist 8-37.5 mg daily (8 mg dose can be prescribed up to TID) Capsule, tablet	15 mg/d: 6.06 7.5 mg/d: 5.45 Placebo: 1.71 28 wk[42]	1959 Schedule IV controlled substance Approved for short-term use
Orlistat (Alli,[51] Xenical[50])	Lipase inhibitor 60-120 mg TID with meals Capsule	120 mg TID: 9.6 Placebo: 5.61 52 wk[49]	1999
Phentermine/ topiramate extended release (Qsymia[54])	Adrenergic agonist/ neurostabilizer 3.75/23-15/92 mg daily Capsule	15/92 mg daily: 9.8 7.5/46 mg daily: 7.8 Placebo: 1.2 56 wk[53]	2012 Schedule IV controlled substance
Lorcaserin (Belviq, Belviq XR[56])	Serotonin (5-HT)$_{2C}$ receptor agonist 10 mg BID or 20 mg XR daily Tablet	10 mg BID: 5.8 Placebo: 2.2 52 wk[59]	2012 Schedule IV controlled substance
Naltrexone/ bupropion sustained release (Contrave[110])	Opioid receptor antagonist/dopamine and norepinephrine reuptake inhibitor 8/90 mg daily to 16/180 mg BID Tablet	16/180 mg BID: 6.1 8/180 mg BID: 5.0 Placebo: 1.3 56 wk[61]	2014
Liraglutide 3.0 mg (Saxenda[64])	GLP-1 receptor agonist 0.6-3.0 mg daily Prefilled pen for subcutaneous injection	3.0 mg daily: 8.0 Placebo: 2.6 56 wk[63]	2014

Adapted from Saunders KH, Umashanker D, Igel LI, et al. Obesity pharmacotherapy. *Med Clin North Am.* 2018;102(1):135-148. Copyright © 2017 Elsevier. With permission.
BID, twice daily; GLP-1, glucagon-like peptide-1; TID, three times daily; XR, extended release.

liraglutide 3.0 mg.[39-41] Table 11.2 provides an overview of the medications. In addition to producing weight loss, each medication improves metabolic biomarkers, including blood pressure, blood sugar, and lipids. The four agents approved since 2012 have stopping rules, which suggest discontinuing the medication if a certain amount of weight loss has not been achieved after 12 to 16 weeks.

Phentermine

Phentermine was approved by the FDA in 1959 and is the most commonly prescribed antiobesity medication in the United States. It is an adrenergic agonist that suppresses appetite and increases resting energy expenditure. Phentermine is indicated for short-term use (up to 3 mo), as there are no long-term safety trials of phentermine monotherapy; however, it was approved in combination with topiramate ER for long-term therapy, so many providers prescribe phentermine for longer durations as off-label therapy. In a 28-week randomized controlled trial comparing phentermine, topiramate ER, and the combination of the two medications, participants taking phentermine 15 mg daily lost an average of 6.0 kg compared with 1.5 kg among those assigned to placebo.[42]

The recommended dosage of phentermine is up to 37.5 mg daily, but dosage should be individualized to achieve adequate response with the lowest effective dose.[43-45] In 2016, the FDA approved an 8-mg formulation, which can be prescribed up to three times per day.[46] Administration of the last dose late in the day should be avoided to prevent insomnia. Phentermine is a schedule IV controlled substance. There seems to be no advantage of continuous compared with intermittent phentermine treatment.[47] The most common treatment-emergent adverse events (TEAEs) include dry mouth, headache, insomnia, dizziness, irritability, nausea, diarrhea, and constipation. Contraindications include pregnancy, nursing, history of drug abuse or cardiovascular disease, hyperthyroidism, glaucoma, and agitated states.

Orlisat

Orlistat was approved by the FDA in 1999 for long-term weight management. It promotes weight loss by inhibiting pancreatic and gastric lipases, thereby reducing fat absorption from the gastrointestinal tract. At the recommended prescription dose, orlistat blocks absorption of approximately 30% of ingested fat.[48] In a double-blind, prospective study that randomized 3305 patients with a BMI of 30 kg/m^2 or higher to lifestyle changes with either orlistat 120 mg or placebo three times per day, the mean weight loss was significantly greater with orlistat (5.8 kg) than with placebo (3.0 kg) after 4 years.[49]

The recommended dosage of orlistat is one 120-mg capsule (Xenical, prescription strength) or one 60-mg capsule (Alli, over the counter) three times a day with each main meal containing fat.[50,51] Orlistat is not often prescribed for weight management because of the TEAEs of fecal urgency, oily stool, and fecal incontinence; however, it may have a role as an additional agent for patients who are constipated on other antiobesity pharmacotherapy. Side effects can be reduced by the addition of a psyllium fiber supplement. Orlistat should not be used in patients who are pregnant or those who have cholestasis or chronic malabsorption syndromes. Orlistat can decrease the absorption of certain medications such as levothyroxine and warfarin.

Phentermine/Topiramate Extended Release

Phentermine/topiramate ER was approved in 2012 for long-term weight management. As appetite regulation involves multiple pathways, targeting different mechanisms simultaneously with a combination of two low-dose medications can have an additive or synergistic effect on body weight while reducing the risk of TEAEs. Topiramate, which was approved for epilepsy in 1996 and migraine prophylaxis in 2004, reduces caloric intake through inhibition of carbonic anhydrase, antagonism of glutamate, and modulation of gamma-aminobutyric acid receptors.[52] In a double-blind, placebo-controlled trial that randomized 2487 patients with a BMI of 27 to 45 kg/m^2 and two or more weight-related comorbidities (dyslipidemia, hypertension, diabetes or prediabetes, or abdominal obesity), participants taking phentermine/topiramate ER 15/92 mg lost significantly more weight (9.8 kg) than those assigned to the 7.5/46-mg dosage (7.8 kg) or placebo (1.2 kg) after 56 weeks.[53]

Phentermine/topiramate ER is available in four doses (3.75/23, 7.5/46, 11.25/69, and 15.0/92 mg), which should be prescribed using a dose-escalation protocol.[54] Phentermine/topiramate ER is a schedule IV controlled substance. The FDA requires a risk evaluation and mitigation strategy to inform women of reproductive potential and prescribers about the potential increased risk of orofacial clefts in infants exposed to the medication during the first trimester of pregnancy.[55] The most common TEAEs include dry mouth, paresthesias, dizziness, dysgeusia, insomnia, and constipation. Contraindications include pregnancy, hyperthyroidism, glaucoma, and monoamine oxidase inhibitor (MAOI) use.

Lorcaserin

Lorcaserin was the second medication approved by the FDA in 2012 for long-term treatment of obesity. It is a selective agonist of the serotonin-2C receptor in the hypothalamus. It increases satiety and reduces appetite by targeting the POMC neurons in the hypothalamus. In a randomized, double-blind, placebo-controlled trial, 3182 patients received lorcaserin 10 mg twice daily or placebo for 52 weeks.[56] Mean weight loss in the lorcaserin group was 5.8% compared with 2.2% in the placebo group. In the recently published CAMELLIA-TIMI 61 trial, which enrolled a high-risk population of subjects with obesity and overweight, lorcaserin facilitated sustained weight loss without a higher rate of major cardiovascular events compared with placebo.[57]

The recommended dosage of lorcaserin is either 10 mg immediate-release twice daily or 20 mg extended-release tablet once daily.[58,59] Lorcaserin is a schedule IV controlled substance. The most common TEAEs are dry mouth, dizziness, headache, fatigue, nausea, and constipation. Coadministration with other serotonergic drugs could potentially lead to the development of serotonin syndrome or neuroleptic malignant syndrome-like reactions; however, none have been reported.

Naltrexone Sustained Release/Bupropion Sustained Release

Naltrexone SR/bupropion SR was approved for the treatment of obesity in 2014. Bupropion, a dopamine and norepinephrine reuptake inhibitor, was approved as an antidepressant in 1989 and as an aide for smoking cessation in 1997. Naltrexone, an opioid antagonist, was approved to treat opioid dependence in 1984 and alcohol abuse in 1994. The combination reduces both appetite and food cravings by targeting two areas of the brain, the arcuate nucleus of the hypothalamus and the mesolimbic dopamine reward circuit.[60] In a double-blind, placebo-controlled trial that enrolled 1742 subjects who were obese or overweight with at least one weight-related comorbidity, mean change in bodyweight was 6.1% in the group assigned to naltrexone 32 mg + bupropion 360 mg daily compared with 5.0% in the group assigned to naltrexone 16 mg + bupropion 360 mg daily and 1.3% in the placebo group after 56 weeks.[61]

Each tablet of naltrexone SR/bupropion SR contains 8 mg of naltrexone and 90 mg of bupropion. The initial prescription is one tablet daily with instructions to increase by one tablet weekly to a maximum dosage of two tablets twice daily (32/360 mg).[62] The most common TEAEs include headache, dizziness, insomnia, nausea, and constipation. Naltrexone/bupropion is contraindicated in pregnant patients, those taking chronic opioids or MAOIs, and in patients with uncontrolled hypertension, history of seizures, or conditions that predispose one to seizure. Similar to all antidepressants, bupropion carries a black box warning related to a potential increase in suicidality among younger patients during the early phase of treatment.

Liraglutide 3.0 mg

Liraglutide 3.0 mg was also approved by the FDA in 2014 for chronic weight management. It mimics the incretin hormone, glucagonlike peptide-1, which is released following food ingestion. In addition to reducing hunger and energy intake, it delays gastric emptying. Liraglutide was initially approved in 2010 for the treatment of type 2 diabetes under the brand name Victoza at doses up to 1.8 mg daily. In a 56-week, randomized, placebo-controlled, double-blind trial of patients who were overweight or obese, the mean weight loss was 6.0% with liraglutide 3.0 mg daily, 4.7% with 1.8 mg daily, and 2.0% with placebo.[63]

Liraglutide is administered as a subcutaneous injection once per day.[64] The starting dose is 0.6 mg daily for 1 week with instructions to increase by 0.6 mg weekly to a therapeutic dosage of 3.0 mg daily. The most common TEAEs include nausea, dyspepsia, diarrhea, constipation, and abdominal pain. Liraglutide is contraindicated in patients who are pregnant as well as patients with personal or family history of medullary thyroid carcinoma or multiple endocrine neoplasia syndrome type 2. Thyroid C-cell tumors were found in rodents given supratherapeutic doses of liraglutide, but there have been no reports of liraglutide causing C-cell tumors in humans.

Bariatric Surgery

Bariatric surgery is the most effective of the treatments available for obesity.[65] Not only is it associated with significant and sustained weight loss, but it has also been shown to reduce obesity-related comorbidities and improve quality of life.[66] In addition, bariatric surgery is associated with lower incidence of cardiovascular events, a decreased number of cardiovascular deaths, and a reduction in overall mortality compared with usual care.[67-69] The three most common bariatric procedures in the United States are the sleeve gastrectomy (SG), the Roux-en-Y gastric bypass (RYGB), and the and laparoscopic adjustable gastric band (LAGB).[70] Table 11.3 provides an overview of the three procedures. SG and RYGB are performed more frequently than LABG because of greater efficacy and a lower complication rate.

The 2013 American College of Cardiology/American Heart Association/The Obesity Society's guideline for the management of overweight and obesity in adults recommends considering bariatric surgery in patients with a BMI $\geq$ 40 kg/m^2 or a BMI $\geq$ 35 kg/m^2 who have weight-related comorbid conditions and are motivated to lose weight but have not achieved sufficient weight loss for target health goals following behavioral treatment, with or without pharmacotherapy.[37] The American Association of Clinical Endocrinologists and American College of Endocrinology clinical practice guidelines for comprehensive medical care of patients with obesity recommend considering surgery in an expanded population: patients with a BMI $\geq$ 40 kg/m^2, a BMI $\geq$ 35 kg/m^2 with one or more severe obesity-related complications, or a BMI 30 to 34.9 kg/m^2 with diabetes or metabolic syndrome.[71] Evidence for bariatric surgery among patients with a BMI < 35 kg/m^2 is limited.

Long-term lifestyle changes, adherence to a vitamin regimen, and medical follow-up are critical to the success of bariatric surgery; however, some patients have difficulty maintaining weight loss and regain at least some of the lost weight.[37] Contraindications to bariatric surgery include poor cardiac reserve, chronic obstructive pulmonary disease or respiratory

TABLE 11.3
MOST COMMONLY PERFORMED BARIATRIC SURGERIES

Procedure	Description	Total Body Weight Loss at 1 y (%)	Procedures Performed in 2013 (%)
Sleeve gastrec-tomy (SG)	~70% of the stomach removed along the greater curvature	25	43
Roux-en-Y gastric bypass (RYGB)	A small pouch (~<50 mL) is created from the proximal stomach and attached to the jejunum, thus bypassing 95% of the stomach, duodenum, and most of the jejunum	30	49
Laparoscopic adjustable gastric band (LAGB)	An inflatable silicone band is placed around the fundus of the stomach to create a small pouch (~30 mL). The size of the pouch can be adjusted to reg-ulate food intake by increasing or decreasing the amount of saline in the band via a subcu-taneous access port	15-20	6

Data from Heymsfield SB, Wadden TA. Mechanisms, pathophysiology, and management of obesity. *N Engl J Med.* 2017;376:254-266.

dysfunction, severe psychological disorders, and nonadherence to medical treatment.[72]

Sleeve Gastrectomy

Sleeve gastrectomy is a procedure in which approximately 70% of the stomach is removed along the greater curvature. The remaining stomach is shaped like a tube or a sleeve. The pyloric valve and the small intestine remain intact. The fundus of the stomach, which secretes ghrelin, a hormone that stimulates appetite, is removed. SG is associated with approximately 25% total body weight loss (TBWL) after 1 year.[73] As this procedure is mainly restrictive (vs. RYGB, which is also malabsorptive), there is a lower risk of nutritional deficiencies. In general, SG is associated with fewer complications than both RYGB and LAGB. Early adverse events include leaking along the staple line, bleeding, stenosis, gastroesophageal reflux, and vomiting due to excessive eating.[72] Late complications include stomach expansion, leading to decreased restriction. Unlike the other two procedures, SG is not reversible.

Roux-en-Y Gastric Bypass

The Roux-en-Y gastric bypass is a procedure that attaches a small pouch created from the proximal stomach to the jejunum, thus bypassing the remainder of the stomach, duodenum, and most of the jejunum. In addition to the resulting restriction and malabsorption, other potential mechanisms for weight loss associated with the procedure include alteration in levels of endogenous gut hormones, which promote postprandial satiety, and increased bile acids, which affect the gut microbiome intestinal hypertrophy.[74]

RYGB is associated with approximately 30% to 35% TBWL at 2 years and greater improvements in comorbid disease markers compared with the two other procedures.[68,73] RYGB is associated with a lower rate of gastroesophageal reflux than SG and can even alleviate gastroesophageal reflux in patients who have the disease. RYGB is often recommended over SG for patients with mild or moderate type 2 diabetes, as it leads to greater long-term remission; however, both RYBG and SG have low efficacy for type 2 diabetes remission among patients with limited pancreatic beta cell reserve.

Early adverse events associated with RYGB include obstruction, stricture, leak, and failure of the staple partition of the upper stomach.[72] Late adverse events include nutritional deficiencies and anastomosis ulceration. Dumping syndrome can develop at any time. Early dumping results in abdominal cramping and osmotic diarrhea, and late dumping results in reactive hypoglycemia. RYGB is technically a reversible procedure; however, it is generally only reversed in extreme circumstances.

Laparoscopic Adjustable Gastric Band

The laparoscopic adjustable gastric band is an inflatable device that is placed around the fundus of the stomach to create a small pouch. The size of the pouch can be adjusted to regulate food intake by increasing or decreasing the amount of saline in the band. Saline can be added or removed through a subcutaneous access port. LAGB is associated with 15% TBWL at 2 years.[75] As the procedure is purely restrictive, there is a lower risk of nutritional deficiencies compared with RYGB. LAGB is reversible and less invasive than the other two procedures but is associated with more complications than SG and RYGB. The most common adverse events include nausea, vomiting, obstruction, band erosion or migration, and esophageal dysmotility leading to acid reflux.[66] LAGB often requires more postoperative visits than the other procedures to optimize band tightness. A large number of bands are eventually removed because of adverse events, difficulty tolerating the device, and/or inadequate weight loss.[75,76]

Antiobesity Devices

Patients who cannot achieve clinically meaningful weight loss with antiobesity medications and who do not undergo bariatric surgery (because they are not surgical candidates, they do not meet eligibility criteria, or they choose not to) fall into a "treatment gap." Devices and endoscopic procedures are emerging options to address this significant treatment gap in the management of obesity.[77] Not only are these devices and procedures reversible and minimally invasive, but they are also potentially more effective than antiobesity medications, possibly less expensive than bariatric surgery, and often safer for poor surgical candidates. The five FDA-approved devices include three intragastric balloons (Orbera, ReShape, and Obalon), the AspireAssist aspiration device, and the Maestro Rechargeable System intermittent vagal blockade device (vBloc). Table 11.4 provides an overview of the devices. There are also many investigational devices and endoscopic bariatric therapies being developed.

Intragastric Balloons

Intragastric balloons (Orbera; Apollo Endosurgery, Austin, TX, ReShape; ReShape Lifesciences, San Clemente, CA, Obalon; Obalon Theraputics, Inc., Carlsbad, CA) are space-occupying devices, which are deployed in the stomach and expand, thus reducing functional gastric volume. Proposed mechanisms of action include delayed gastric emptying and hormonal alterations affecting appetite and satiety. The balloons were approved in 2015-2016 for patients with a BMI of 30 to 40 kg/m^2.[78-80] Balloons are swallowed or placed endoscopically, filled with gas or fluid, and removed endoscopically after 6 months. Serial balloon placement has demonstrated additional weight loss; however, these protocols are not currently approved. Total body weight loss ranges from 6.6% to 10.2% compared with 3.3% to 3.4% with sham.[81-86] Contraindications include history of gastrointestinal surgery, clotting/ bleeding disorders, large hiatal hernia or other structural abnormality, gastric mass and pregnancy. The most common TEAEs include abdominal pain, nausea, vomiting, intolerance, and early explantation. Migration, deflation, perforation, and gastric ulcers have also been reported.

Aspiration Therapy

The AspireAssist device (Aspire Bariatrics, King of Prussia, PA) is a percutaneous gastrostomy tube that facilitates partial aspiration of each meal after ingestion. It was approved in 2016 for patients with a BMI of 35 to 55 kg/m^2.[87] After the tube is placed endoscopically, an external aspiration port is created at the abdominal surface. After meal ingestion, patients attach an aspiration device to the port for infusion of water followed by aspiration of ~30% of the meal. AspireAssist leads to weight loss not only by direct calorie loss but also by smaller meal portions. Food particles can

TABLE 11.4
DEVICES APPROVED FOR OBESITY BY THE FOOD AND DRUG ADMINISTRATION

Device	Description	Total Body Weight Loss (%)	FDA Approval
Orbera Intragastric Balloon[78]	Endoscopically placed intragastric balloon filled with 400-700 mL saline, removed endoscopically after 6 mo	10.2 Sham: 3.3 6 mo[81,82]	2015 BMI 30-40 kg/m²
ReShape Integrated Dual Balloon (IDB) System[79]	Endoscopically placed balloons (2) attached via a silicone tube and filled with 750-900 mL of saline (total), removed endoscopically after 6 mo	6.8 Sham: 3.3 6 mo[83,84]	2015 BMI 30-40 kg/m² + at least one weight-related comorbid condition
Obalon Balloon System[80]	Sequentially swallowed balloons (3) filled with 250 mL of gas each, removed endoscopically 6 mo after 1st balloon placed	6.6 Sham: 3.4 6 mo[85,86]	2016 BMI 30-40 kg/m²
AspireAssist[87]	Endoscopically placed percutaneous gastrostomy aspiration tube	12.1 Lifestyle alone: 3.5 12 mo[88]	2016 BMI 35-55 kg/m²
vBloc Therapy/ Maestro Rechargeable System[89]	Laparoscopically implanted device providing intermittent vagal blockade	9.2 Sham: 6.0 12 mo[90]	2015 BMI 40-45 kg/m² or 35-40 kg/m² + at least one weight-related comorbid condition

Adapted by permission from Springer: Saunders KH, Igel LI, Saumoy M, Sharaiha RZ, Aronne LJ. Devices and endoscopic bariatric therapies for obesity. *Curr Obes Rep.* 2018;7(2):162-171. Copyright © 2018 Springer Science+Business Media, LLC, part of Springer Nature.
BMI, body mass index; lifestyle, lifestyle counseling (diet + exercise).

flow through the tube only if they are 5 mm or less in diameter and in a slurry, so patients must take time to chew thoroughly and drink sufficient liquid with each meal. AspireAssist is associated with 12.1% total body weight loss compared with 3.5% with lifestyle counseling alone.[88] There has been no evidence of eating disorder development or device overuse and no reported increase in food intake during or between meals to compensate for the aspirated calories. The most frequently reported TEAEs included postoperative abdominal pain, nausea, vomiting, peristomal irritation, and peristomal granulation tissue.[88]

Vagal Blockade

The Maestro Rechargeable System or vBloc (ReShape Lifesciences, San Clemente, CA) is a device that provides intermittent electrical blockade to the vagus nerve. It was approved in 2015 for patients with a BMI of 40 to 45 kg/m² or 35 to 40 kg/m² with at least one weight-related comorbidity.[89] vBloc is implanted laparoscopically. Two leads are placed around the vagal trunks near the gastroesophageal junction, and a rechargeable neuroregulator is placed subcutaneously on the thoracic wall. The device is recharged transcutaneously. The vagus nerve plays a role in weight regulation via effects on appetite, metabolism, and autonomic control of the upper gastrointestinal track. vBloc is associated with 9.2% total body weight loss compared with 6.0% with a sham intervention as well as reductions in hunger and improved food-related cognitive restraint.[90] The most frequently reported TEAEs are dyspepsia, heartburn, and implant site pain.[90,91]

Impact of Obesity Treatment on Multiple Sclerosis

Recently, it has been hypothesized that weight loss can delay the development of MS, so obesity treatment is particularly important among patients with concurrent MS.[92] Furthermore, interferon beta is a cornerstone of disease-modifying treatment for MS that can reduce the number of relapses, delay disability, and limit new disease activity seen on magnetic resonance imaging (MRI). There is a reduction in treatment effect in patients with excess weight, so it is particularly important to treat obesity in patients who would benefit from interferon beta therapy.[93]

Lifestyle Modifications

The National Multiple Sclerosis Society recommends a well-balanced and planned diet for patients with MS.[94] Although there is no "MS diet," it is suggested that patients follow a low-fat, high-fiber diet similar to the diets recommended by the American Heart Association and the American Cancer Society. Sodium is a dietary factor that has been linked to MS. A recent observational study reported that patients who consumed moderate to high amounts of sodium had increased rates of relapse and a greater risk of developing new MRI lesions than patients who consumed a low-sodium diet.[95]

Diet may play an important role in risk of MS, disease progression, and symptom management, especially energy level and bladder and bowel function. Possible mechanisms through which diet can affect MS include direct effect on the immune system or indirectly through changes in a patient's gut microbiome. Currently there is insufficient evidence to recommend particular dietary interventions; however, there are several ongoing pilot studies investigating the role of the Mediterranean diet and other diets in inflammation associated with MS.

Limited animal studies have led to theories that a ketogenic diet could improve the neurodegenerative (vs. inflammatory) component of MS.[96] Ketogenic diets have been shown to promote mitochondrial biogenesis and thus increase antioxidant levels and decrease oxidative damage, which eventually leads to less neuronal damage. Further studies on ketogenic diets among human patients with MS are needed before broad dietary recommendations can be made.

Although physical activity plays an important role in weight loss, weight loss maintenance, and overall metabolic health, exercise can be difficult for patients with MS because of pain and physical limitations. Pain affects quality of life both physically and emotionally. Patients with pain tend to reduce physical activity and, as a result, suffer from worsening stiffness, reduced flexibility, increasing weakness, and overall deconditioning.[97] A recent systemic review and meta-analysis found that exercise has a small to moderate effect size in reducing pain and thereby improving quality of life in patients with MS.[97] Physical therapy, stretching, and low-impact exercise such as swimming can be reasonable options for patients with MS.

Antiobesity Medications

When prescribing antiobesity medications to patients with MS, it is important to consider potential interactions with MS medications as well as possible adverse events that could exacerbate symptoms of MS. There are limited data on the effect of antiobesity medications in patients with MS specifically; however, there is some evidence that several of the antiobesity drugs (or components of combination medications) could provide benefit beyond weight loss to patients with MS.

Among the six most widely prescribed antiobesity agents approved by the FDA—phentermine, orlistat, phentermine/topiramate extended release (ER); lorcaserin, naltrexone sustained release (SR)/bupropion SR, and liraglutide 3.0 mg—there are potential benefits associated with phentermine, topiramate, naltrexone, bupropion, and liraglutide. There are no data on orlistat or lorcaserin.

Phentermine and bupropion are both activating medications that can increase energy. Although there are no studies of phentermine in patients with MS, bupropion has been reported to improve fatigue among patients with MS. Over 80% of patients with MS report symptoms of fatigue, which is a poorly understood interplay between disease, physical fatigue, psychological factors, drug-induced/side effect, and sleep dysfunction.[98] Patients with MS treated with bupropion have shown higher fatigue remission rates and improved reward responsive rates thereby enriching quality of life.[98,99]

Topiramate has been shown to improve cerebellar tremors and dysesthetic pain, both of which can be symptoms of MS. Cerebellar tremors, which are action-mediated tremors that most frequently affect the arms, and can also involve the head, trunk, and voice, are common in patients with MS.[100] These tremors affect 25% to 60% of patients with MS and have been historically difficult to treat pharmacologically. Per a single case report, topiramate was shown to improve symptoms of cerebellar ataxia and tremor in a patient with MS who was followed over a 2-year period.[101]

Dysesthetic pain is a type of neuropathic pain found commonly in patients with MS. It is a constant, mostly burning pain affecting the legs and feet.[102] First-line treatment for this pain includes tricyclic antidepressants (such as amitriptyline) and antiepileptic medications (carbamezapine, gabapentin, and pregabalin), many of which can induce significant weight gain. Although topiramate can sometimes lead to paresthesias, it can also improve such neuropathic pain. One case report described resolution of dysesthetic pain in a patient with MS who had suffered from treatment-resistant pain for over 8 years.[102]

Low-dose naltrexone (LDN) has been used off-label for the treatment of pain and inflammation in many chronic inflammatory diseases, including MS, Crohn disease, and fibromyalgia.[103] It is hypothesized that lower-than-standard doses of naltrexone inhibit cellular proliferation of T and B cells and block Toll-like receptor 4, resulting in analgesia and an anti-inflammatory effect. Numerous studies have explored the effects of LDN on MS. It has been shown to reduce fatigue; however, it has not been shown to alter the disease course in MS.[103]

In addition to treating diabetes and obesity, GLP-1 agonists have demonstrated a range of other physiological effects in the body. In preclinical trials, a substantial body of evidence has shown that these incretin mimetics have neuroprotective and anti-inflammatory effects.[104] In animal models for other neurodegenerative diseases, GLP-1 was found to cross the blood-brain barrier and reduce CNS inflammation. The neuroprotective effect is thought to be secondary to neurogenesis and increased neuronal repair, protection against oxidative stress, and reduction in plaque formation.[104,105] A recent study in animals models of MS found that liraglutide delays disease onset and progression.[105] These preliminary results in animal models are promising for potentially using GLP-1 receptor agonists to concurrently treat obesity and MS.

Finally, metformin is FDA approved for the treatment of type 2 diabetes but is commonly used off-label for other conditions, including type 2 diabetes prevention in patients with prediabetes or impaired fasting glucose, treatment of polycystic ovarian syndrome, and obesity/overweight.[106] Metformin has been shown to reduce disease severity in animal models of MS by downregulating the proinflammatory response in the CNS.[107,108] These benefits observed in animal models have been confirmed in human subjects with both metabolic syndrome and MS: metformin reduces disease activity in these patients as evidenced by fewer MRI lesions.[93]

Bariatric Surgery

Although there are no studies evaluating antiobesity devices and endoscopic bariatric therapies in patients with MS, there are a few studies examining bariatric surgery outcomes. After bariatric surgery, patients with MS experience weight loss similar to that seen in the general population.[109] Small retrospective studies and case reports confirm that bariatric surgery is safe in patients with MS. In general, these patients have improved ambulation from the significant weight loss and do not have worsening disease progression or increased relapse rates when compared with patients with MS and obesity who do not undergo bariatric surgery.[30,109] Following bariatric surgery, patients with MS have improved Patient Health Questionnaire (PHQ-9) depression scores for the first year; however, rates of depression reach the MS control rates after about 3 years post surgery.[16] Although patients with MS are often at higher risk for surgery, preliminary studies show good outcomes in this patient population. Larger studies are necessary to further optimize treatment.

As rates of obesity and MS increase, bariatric surgery may play an important role in a multidimensional treatment plan. It is important that practitioners who follow these patients post surgery have a heightened awareness of nutritional deficiencies. Bariatric patients in the general population are at risk for neurological complications due to deficiencies in vitamin B12, thiamine, and copper. In patients with underlying MS, these deficiencies could lead to more severe symptoms, so long-term monitoring of vitamin levels is necessary. Vitamin D deficiency is also of particular concern for patients following bariatric surgery, as it may be an independent risk factor for the development of MS as well as increased relapse rate, severity of disease, and degree of disease-related disability.

Conclusion

Not only is obesity a risk factor for MS, but obesity can also worsen symptoms of MS and complicate treatment. As a result, it is important to treat obesity in patients with MS. Lifestyle modifications are the cornerstones of weight management; however, such interventions are insufficient for clinically significant weight loss in the majority of patients. Health care providers who treat patients with MS should be familiar with more advanced options for patients with obesity, including antiobesity pharmacotherapy, devices, endoscopic bariatric procedures, and bariatric surgery. The future of obesity treatment is a multidisciplinary approach, as combinations of strategies can lead to additive or synergistic weight loss. This is an area that requires further investigation.

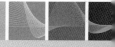

Case Study

A 56-year-old woman presented to our center 2 years ago for weight management. Her BMI was 39 kg/m². She had undergone a Roux-en-Y gastric bypass in 1999 and exceeded her expectations losing 147 lbs (297 → 150 lbs); however, she then regained 61 lbs gradually over the years. Her comorbidities included MS, type 2 diabetes, and hyperlipidemia. MS had been diagnosed 25 years earlier. She required intravenous steroids once years ago and described occasional right arm numbness but did not take an ongoing medication for MS. She noted fatigue, generalized weakness and bilateral lower extremity paresthesias. She had not seen her bariatric surgeon in years.

Laboratory evaluation revealed:

- hemoglobin A1c 8.5%
- comprehensive metabolic panel notable for fasting glucose of 206
- complete blood count notable for mean corpuscular volume 75
- bariatric laboratory tests notable for iron saturation 12%, vitamin B12 93, vitamin D 17

The patient was educated about a low-carbohydrate diet and an exercise regimen and was prescribed metformin, which was titrated up to 1000 mg twice daily by 500 mg per week. She was also prescribed intramuscular vitamin B12, vitamin D 50,000 mg, iron supplements, and a multivitamin.

Over the next 6 months, she lost 30 lbs. Her iron and vitamin levels normalized, and her hemoglobin A1c decreased to 5.7%. Her energy improved and weakness and paresthesias resolved. At this point, she had reached a weight plateau and her hunger was increasing. She was given lorcaserin and was able to lose another 45 lbs over the next few months. She is now maintaining her weight with a low-carbohydrate diet, daily exercise routine, metformin, and lorcaserin.

This case illustrates several important points.

- Patients with obesity and MS can present with symptoms common to both diseases, including fatigue and weakness. Treating a patient's obesity can improve these symptoms.
- Patients who have undergone bariatric surgery and present with neurologic symptoms should be evaluated for vitamin deficiencies (especially iron, thiamine, and vitamin B12). Patients who have undergone bariatric surgery require life-long follow-up, including yearly laboratory tests to evaluate for these deficiencies.

■ The patient had difficulty maintaining her weight loss after surgery and reached a weight plateau a few months after initial presentation because of metabolic adaptation (described in the chapter).

■ Weight-centric diabetes management includes prioritizing medications that can help with weight loss (metformin, GLP-1 agonists, SGLT2 inhibitors) instead of medications that can lead to weight gain. See Table 11.1.

■ Metformin is FDA approved for the treatment of type 2 diabetes but is commonly used off-label for other conditions, including type 2 diabetes prevention in patients with prediabetes or impaired fasting glucose, treatment of polycystic ovarian syndrome, and obesity/overweight.

■ Successful weight loss requires a comprehensive approach including diet, exercise, and behavioral modifications.

■ Antiobesity medications can be used after surgery to help patients lose more weight, maintain weight loss, or lose regained weight.

References

1. Hales CM, Carroll MD, Fryar CD, Ogden CL. Prevalence of obesity among adults and youth: United States, 2015–2016. *NCHS Data Brief*. 2017;(288). Hyattsville, MD: National Center for Health Statistics.
2. Ogden CL, Flegal KM. Changes in terminology for childhood overweight and obesity. *Natl Health Stat Rep*. 2010;(25):1-5.
3. Finkelstein EA, Trogdon JG, Cohen JW, Dietz W. Annual medical spending attributable to obesity: payer-and service-specific estimates. *Health Aff (Millwood)*. 2009;28(5):w822-w831.
4. Lovren F, Teoh H, Verma S. Obesity and atherosclerosis: mechanistic insights. *Can J Cardiol*. 2015;31(2):177-183.
5. Magkos F, Fraterrigo G, Yoshino J. Effects of moderate and subsequent progressive weight loss on metabolic function and adipose tissue biology in humans with obesity. *Cell Metab*. 2016;23(4):591-601. pii:S1550-4131(16):30053-5.
6. Wing RR, Lang W, Wadden TA, et al. Benefits of modest weight loss in improving cardiovascular risk factors in overweight and obese individuals with type 2 diabetes. *Diabetes Care*. 2011;34(7):1481-1486.
7. Sumithran P, Prendergast LA, Delbridge E, et al. Long-term persistence of hormonal adaptations to weight loss. *N Engl J Med*. 2011;365(17):1597-1604.
8. Greenway FL. Physiological adaptations to weight loss and factors favouring weight regain. *Int J Obes (Lond)*. 2015;39(8):1188-1196.
9. Fothergill E, Guo J, Howard L, et al. Persistent metabolic adaptation 6 years after "The Biggest Loser" competition. *Obesity (Silver Spring)*. 2016;24(8):1612-1619.
10. Rosenbaum M, Leibel RL. Adaptive thermogenesis in humans. *Int J Obes (Lond)*. 2010;34:S47-S55.
11. Gianfrancesco MA, Barcellos LF. Obesity and multiple sclerosis susceptibility: a review. *J Neurol Neuromed*. 2016;1(7):1-5.

12. Rasul T, Frederiksen J. Link between overweight/obese in children and youngsters and occurrence of multiple sclerosis. *J Neurol.* 2018;265(12): 2755-2763. [Epub ahead of print]
13. MS Prevalence. National Multiple Sclerosis Society. Available at https:// www.nationalmssociety.org/About-the-Society/MS-Prevalence. Accessed October 12, 2018.
14. Huitema MJD, Schenk GJ. Insights into the mechanisms that may clarify obesity as a risk factor for multiple sclerosis. *Curr Neurol Neurosci Rep.* 2018;18(4):18.
15. Langer-Gould A, Brara SM, Beaber BE, Koebnick C. Childhood obesity and risk of pediatric multiple sclerosis and clinically isolated syndrome. *Neurology.* 2013;80(6):548-552.
16. Fisher CJ, Heinberg LJ, Lapin B, Aminian A, Sullivan AB. Depressive symptoms in bariatric surgery patients with multiple sclerosis. *Obes Surg.* 2018;28(4):1091-1097.
17. Munger KL, Chitnis T, Ascherio A. Body size and risk of MS in two cohorts of US women. *Neurology.* 2009;73(19):1543-1550.
18. Hedström AK, Olsson T, Alfredsson L. High body mass index before age 20 is associated with increased risk for multiple sclerosis in both men and women. *Mult Scler.* 2012;18(9):1334-1336.
19. Munger KL, Bentzen J, Laursen B, et al. Childhood body mass index and multiple sclerosis risk: a long-term cohort study. *Mult Scler.* 2013;19(10):1323-1329.
20. Palavra F, Almeida L, Ambrosio AF, Reis F. Obesity and brain inflammation: a focus on multiple sclerosis. *Obes Rev.* 2016;17(3):211-224.
21. Lukens JR, Dixit VD, Kanneganti TD. Inflammasome activation in obesity-related inflammatory diseases and autoimmunity. *Discov Med.* 2011;12(62):65-74.
22. Heneka MT, McManus RM, Latz E. Inflammasome signalling in brain function and neurodegenerative disease. *Nat Rev Neurosci.* 2018;19(10):610-621. [Epub ahead of print]
23. Shreiner AB, Kao JY, Young VB. The gut microbiome in health and in disease. *Curr Opin Gastroenterol.* 2015;31(1):69-75.
24. Jangi S, Gandhi R, Cox LM, et al. Alterations of the human gut microbiome in multiple sclerosis. *Nat Commun.* 2016;7:12015.
25. Kvistad SS, Myhr KM, Holmøy T, et al. Serum levels of leptin and adiponectin are not associated with disease activity or treatment response in multiple sclerosis. *J Neuroimmunol.* 2018;323:73-77.
26. Matarese G, Carrieri PB, La Cava A, et al. Leptin increase in multiple sclerosis associates with reduced number of CD4+CD25+ regulatory T cells. *Proc Natl Acad Sci USA.* 2005;102(14):5150-5155.
27. Piccio L, Cantoni C, Henderson JG, et al. Lack of adiponectin leads to increased lymphocyte activation and increased disease severity in a mouse model of multiple sclerosis. *Eur J Immunol.* 2013;43(8):2089-2100.
28. Mowry EM, Pelletier D, Gao Z, Howell MD, Zamvil SS, Waubant E. Vitamin D in clinically isolated syndrome: evidence for possible neuroprotection. *Eur J Neurol.* 2016;23(2):327-332.
29. Oveland E, Nystad A, Berven F, Myhr KM, Torkildsen Ø, Wergeland S. 1,25-Dihydroxyvitamin-D3 induces brain proteomic changes in cuprizone mice during remyelination involving calcium proteins. *Neurochem Int.* 2018;112:267-277.

30. Bencsath K, Jammoul A, Aminian A, et al. Outcomes of bariatric surgery in morbidly obese patients with multiple sclerosis. *J Obes.* 2017;2017:1935204.

31. Dansinger ML, Gleason JA, Griffith JL, Selker HP, Schaefer EJ. Comparison of the Atkins, Ornish, Weight Watchers, and Zone diets for weight loss and heart disease risk reduction: a randomized trial. *JAMA.* 2005;293(1): 43-53.

32. Estruch R, Ros E, Salas-Salvadó J, et al. Primary prevention of cardiovascular disease with a Mediterranean diet. *N Engl J Med.* 2013;368(14):1279-1290.

33. Lennerz BS, Alsop DC, Holsen LM, et al. Effects of dietary glycemic index on brain regions related to reward and craving in men. *Am J Clin Nutr.* 2013;98(3):641-647.

34. Physical Activity Guidelines for Americans. US Department of Health and Human Services. https://health.gov/paguidelines/.

35. Saunders KH, Igel LI, Shukla AP, Aronne LJ. Drug-induced weight gain: rethinking our choices. *J Fam Pract.* 2016;65(11):780-788.

36. Igel LI, Kumar RB, Saunders KH, Aronne LJ. Practical use of pharmacotherapy for obesity. *Gastroenterology.* 2017;152(7):1765-1779. pii:S0016-5085(17)30142-7.

37. Jensen MD, Ryan DH, Apovian CM, et al. 2013 AHA/ACC/TOS guideline for the management of overweight and obesity in adults: a report of the American College of Cardiology/American Heart Association Task Force on Practice Guidelines and the Obesity Society. *J Am Coll Cardiol.* 2014;63(25 Pt B):2985-3023.

38. Apovian CM, Aronne LJ, Bessesen DH, et al. Pharmacological management of obesity: an Endocrine Society Clinical Practice Guideline. *J Clin Endocrinol Metab.* 2015;100(2):342-362.

39. Saunders KH, Umashanker D, Igel LI, Kumar RB, Aronne LJ. Obesity pharmacotherapy. *Med Clin North Am.* 2018;102(1):135-148.

40. Saunders KH, Shukla AP, Igel LI, Aronne LJ. Obesity: when to consider medication. *J Fam Pract.* 2017;66(10):608-616.

41. Saunders KH, Kumar RB, Igel LI, Aronne LJ. Pharmacologic approaches to weight management: recent gains and shortfalls in combating obesity. *Curr Atheroscler Rep.* 2016;18(7):36.

42. Aronne LJ, Wadden TA, Peterson C, et al. Evaluation of phentermine and topiramate versus phentermine/topiramate extended-release in obese adults. *Obesity (Silver Spring).* 2013;21(11):2163-2171.

43. *Adipex [package insert].* Tulsa, OK: Physicians Total Care, Inc.; 2012.

44. *Ionamin [package insert].* Rochester, NY: Celltech Pharmaceuticals, Inc.; 2006.

45. *Suprenza [package insert].* Cranford, NJ: Akrimax Pharmaceuticals, LLC; 2013.

46. *Lomaira [package insert].* Newtown, PA: KVK-Tech, Inc.; 2016.

47. Munro JF, MacCuish AC, Wilson EM, Duncan LJ. Comparison of continuous and intermittent anorectic therapy in obesity. *Br Med J.* 1968;1(5588):352-354.

48. Zhi J, Melia AT, Guerciolini R, et al. Retrospective population-based analysis of the dose-response (fecal fat excretion) relationship of orlistat in normal and obese volunteers. *Clin Pharmacol Ther.* 1994;56(1):82-85.

49. Torgerson JS, Hauptman J, Boldrin MN, et al. XENical in the prevention of diabetes in obese subjects (XENDOS) study: a randomized study of orlistat as an adjunct to lifestyle changes for the prevention of type 2 diabetes in obese patients. *Diabetes Care.* 2004;27(1):155-161.

50. *Xenical [package insert].* South San Francisco, CA: Genentech USA, Inc.; 2015.
51. *Alli [package insert].* Moon Township, PA: GlaxoSmithKline Consumer Healthcare, LP; 2015.
52. Kushner RF. Weight loss strategies for treatment of obesity. *Prog Cardiovasc Dis.* 2014;56(4):465-472.
53. Gadde KM, Allison DB, Ryan DH, et al. Effects of low-dose, controlled-release, phentermine plus topiramate combination on weight and associated comorbidities in overweight and obese adults (CONQUER): a randomised, placebo controlled, phase 3 trial. *Lancet.* 2011;377(9774):1341-1352.
54. *Qsymia [package insert].* Mountain View, CA: VIVUS, Inc.; 2012.
55. Qsymia Risk Evaluation and Mitigation Strategy (REMS). VIVUS, Inc. Available athttp://www.qsymiarems.com/. Accessed September 17, 2018.
56. *Belviq [package insert].* Zofingen, Switzerland: Arena Pharmaceuticals; 2012.
57. Bohula EA, Wiviott SD, McGuire DK, et al. Cardiovascular safety of lorcaserin in overweight or obese patients. *N Engl J Med.* 2018;379(12):1107-1117. [Epub ahead of print].
58. *Belviq XR [package insert].* Zofingen, Switzerland: Arena Pharmaceuticals; 2016.
59. Smith SR, Weissman NJ, Anderson CM, et al. Multicenter, placebo-controlled trial of lorcaserin for weight management. *N Engl J Med.* 2010;363(3):245-256.
60. Greenway FL, Whitehouse MJ, Guttadauria M, et al. Rational design of a combination medication for the treatment of obesity. *Obesity (Silver Spring).* 2009;17(1):30-39.
61. Greenway FL, Fujioka K, Plodkowski RA, et al. Effect of naltrexone plus bupropion on weight loss in overweight and obese adults (COR-I): a multicentre, randomised, double-blind, placebo-controlled, phase 3 trial. *Lancet.* 2010;376(9741):595-605.
62. *Contrave [package insert].* La Jolla, CA: Orexigen Therapeutics, Inc.; 2016.
63. Pi-Sunyer X, Astrup A, Fujioka K, et al. A randomized, controlled trial of 3.0 mg of liraglutide in weight management. *N Engl J Med.* 2015;373(1):11-22.
64. *Saxenda [package insert].* Plainsboro, NJ: Novo Nordisk; 2014.
65. Barenbaum SR, Saunders KH, Igel LI, Shukla AP, Aronne LJ. Obesity: when to consider surgery. *J Fam Pract.* 2018;67(10):614;616;618;620.
66. Roux CW, Heneghan HM. Bariatric surgery for obesity. *Med Clin North Am.* 2018; 102: 165-182.
67. Reges O, Greenland P, Dicker D, et al. Association of Bariatric surgery using laparoscopic banding, Roux-en-Y, gastric bypass, or laparoscopic sleeve gastrectomy vs usual care obesity management with all-cause mortality. *JAMA.* 2018;319(3):279-290.
68. Sjostrom L. Review of the key results from the Swedish Obese Subjects (SOS) trial – a prospective controlled intervention study of bariatric surgery. *J Intern Med.* 2013;273:219-234.
69. Sjostrom L, Peltonen M, Jacobson P, et al. Bariatric surgery and long-term cardiovascular events. *JAMA.* 2012;307(1):56-65.
70. Lee JH, Nguyen QN, Le QA. Comparative effectiveness of 3 bariatric surgery procedures: Roux-en-Y gastric bypass, laparoscopic adjustable gastric band, and sleeve gastrectomy. *Surg Obes Relat Dis.* 2016;12:997-1002.
71. Garvey WT, Mechanick JI, Brett EM, et al; Reviewers of the AACE/ACE Obesity Clinical Practice Guidelines. American Association of Clinical Endocrinologists and American College of Endocrinology clinical practice guidelines for comprehensive medical care of patients with obesity. *Endocr Pract.* 2016;22(suppl 3):1-203.

72. Colquitt JL, Pickett K, Loveman E, Frampton GK. Surgery for weight loss in adults. *Cochrane Database Syst Rev.* 2014;(8):CD003641.

73. Heymsfield SB, Wadden TA. Mechanisms, pathophysiology, and management of obesity. *N Engl J Med.* 2017;376:254-266.

74. Abdeen G, le Roux CW. Mechanism underlying the weight loss and complications of Roux-en-Y gastric bypass. *Obes Surg.* 2016;26:410-421.

75. Courcoulas AP, King WC, Belle SH, et al. Seven-year weight trajectories and health outcomes in the longitudinal assessment of bariatric surgery (LABS) study. *JAMA Surg.* 2018;153:427-434.

76. Smetana GW, Jones DB, Wee CC. Beyond the guidelines: should this patient have weight loss surgery? Grand rounds discussion from Beth Israel Deaconess Medical Center. *Ann Intern Med.* 2017;166:808-817.

77. Saunders KH, Igel LI, Saumoy M, Sharaiha RZ, Aronne LJ. Devices and endoscopic bariatric therapies for obesity. *Curr Obes Rep.* 2018;7(2):162-171.

78. *Orbera Intragastric Balloon [package insert].* Austin, TX: Apollo Endosurgery; 2015.

79. *ReShape Integrated Dual Balloon System [package insert].* San Clemente, CA: ReShape Lifesciences; 2015.

80. *Obalon Balloon System [package insert].* Carlsbad, CA: Obalon Theraputics, Inc.; 2016.

81. Courcoulas A, Abu Dayyeh BK, Eaton L, et al. Intragastric balloon as an adjunct to lifestyle intervention: a randomized controlled trial. *Int J Obes (Lond).* 2017;41(3):427-433.

82. U.S. Food and Drug Administration. PMA P140008: FDA Summary of Safety and Effectiveness Data. Available athttps://www.accessdata.fda.gov/cdrh_docs/pdf14/P140008b.pdf. Accessed October 1, 2018.

83. Ponce J, Woodman G, Swain J, et al. The REDUCE pivotal trial: a prospective, randomized controlled pivotal trial of a dual intragastric balloon for the treatment of obesity. *Surg Obes Relat Dis.* 2015;11(4):874-881.

84. PMA P140012: FDA Summary of Safety and Effectiveness Data. Available at https://www.accessdata.fda.gov/cdrh_docs/pdf14/P140012b.pdf. Accessed October 1, 2018.

85. Sullivan S, Swain JM, Woodman G, et al. The obalon swallowable 6-month balloon system is more effective than moderate intensity lifestyle therapy alone: results from a 6-month randomized sham controlled trial. *Gastroenterology.* 2016;150(4 suppl 1):S1267.

86. PMA P160001: FDA Summary of Safety and Effectiveness Data. Available at https://www.accessdata.fda.gov/cdrh_docs/pdf16/P160001b.pdf. Accessed October 1, 2018.

87. *AspireAssist [package insert].* King of Prussia, PA: Aspire Bariatrics; 2016.

88. Thompson CC, Abu Dayyeh BK, Kushner K, et al. The AspireAssist is an effective tool in the treatment of class II and class III obesity: results of a one-year clinical trial. *Gastroenterology.* 2016;4(suppl 1):S86.

89. *Maestro Rechargeable System [package insert].* San Clemente, CA: ReShape Lifesciences; 2015.

90. Ikramuddin S, Blackstone RP, Brancatisano A, et al. Effect of reversible intermittent intra-abdominal vagal nerve blockade on morbid obesity: the ReCharge randomized clinical trial. *JAMA.* 2014;312(9):915-922.

91. Apovian CM, Shah SN, Wolfe BM, et al. Two-year outcomes of vagal nerve blocking (vBloc) for the treatment of obesity in the ReCharge trial. *Obes Surg.* 2017;27(1):169-176.

92. Negrotto L, Farez MF, Correale J. Immunologic effects of metformin and pioglitazone treatment on metabolic syndrome and multiple sclerosis. *JAMA Neurol.* 2016;73(5):520-528.

93. Kvistad SS, Myhr KM, Holmoy T, et al. Body mass index influence interferon-beta treatment response in multiple sclerosis. *J Neuroimmunol.* 2015;288:92-97.

94. Diet and Nutrition. National Multiple Sclerosis Society. Available at https://www.nationalmssociety.org/Living-Well-With-MS/Diet-Exercise-Healthy-Behaviors/Diet-Nutrition. Accessed October 12, 2018.

95. Kleinewietfeld M, Manzel A, Titze J, et al. Sodium chloride drives autoimmune disease by the induction of pathogenic TH17 cells. *Nature.* 2013;496(7446):518-522.

96. Storoni M, Plant GT. The therapeutic potential of the ketogenic diet in treating progressive multiple sclerosis. *Mult Scler Int.* 2015;2015:681289.

97. Demaneuf T, Aitken Z, Karahalios A, et al. The effectiveness of exercise interventions for pain reduction in people with multiple sclerosis: a systematic review and meta-analysis of randomized controlled trials. *Arch Phys Med Rehabil.* 2018. pii:S0003-9993(18)31191-2. [Epub ahead of print].

98. Pardini M, Capello E, Krueger F, Mancardi G, Uccelli A. Reward responsiveness and fatigue in multiple sclerosis. *Mult Scler.* 2013;19(2):233-240.

99. Siniscalchi A, Gallelli L, Tolotta GA, Loiacono D, De Sarro G. Open, uncontrolled, nonrandomized, 9-month, off-label use of bupropion to treat fatigue in a single patient with multiple sclerosis. *Clin Ther.* 2010;32(12):2030-2034.

100. Schneider SA, Deuschl G. The treatment of tremor. *Neurotherapeutics.* 2014;11(1):128-138.

101. Schroeder A, Linker RA, Lukas C, Kraus PH, Gold R. Successful treatment of cerebellar ataxia and tremor in multiple sclerosis with topiramate: a case report. *Clin Neuropharmacol.* 2010;33(6):317-318.

102. Siniscalchi A, Gallelli L, De Sarro G. Effects of topiramate on dysaethetic pain in a patient with multiple sclerosis. *Clin Drug Investig.* 2013;33(2):151-154.

103. Patten DK, Schultz BG, Berlau DJ. The safety and efficacy of low-dose naltrexone in the management of chronic pain and inflammation in multiple sclerosis, fibromyalgia, crohn's disease, and other chronic pain disorders. *Pharmacotherapy.* 2018;38(3):382-389.

104. Holscher C. Potential role of glucagon-like peptide-1 (GLP-1) in neuroprotection. *CNS Drugs.* 2012;26(10):871-882.

105. DellaValle B, Brix GS, Brock B, et al. Glucagon-like peptide-1 analog, liraglutide, delays onset of experimental autoimmune encephalitis in lewis rats. *Front Pharmacol.* 2016;7:433.

106. Igel LI, Sinha A, Saunders KH, Apovian CM, Vojta D, Aronne LJ. Metformin: an old therapy that deserves a new indication for the treatment of obesity. *Curr Atheroscler Rep.* 2016;18(4):16.

107. Nath N, Khan M, Paintlia MK, Hoda MN, Giri S. Metformin attenuated the autoimmune disease of the central nervous system in animal models of multiple sclerosis. *J Immunol.* 2009;182(12):8005-8014.

108. Sun Y, Tian T, Gao J, et al. Metformin ameliorates the development of experimental autoimmune encephalomyelitis by regulating T helper 17 and regulatory T cells in mice. *J Neuroimmunol.* 2016;292:58-67.

109. Burn S, Stone A, Strange S, et al. Outcomes of bariatric surgery in patients with multiple sclerosis. *Am Surg.* 2018;84(3):e104-e105.
110. *Contrave [package insert].* Deerfield, IL: Takeda Pharmaceuticals America, Inc.; 2014.

Rheumatology

■ ▨ ▩ Molly Forlines, Mary Ann Picone, Anthony M. Iuso,
Michael A. Ciaramella

Rheumatoid Arthritis and Systemic Lupus Erythematosus

Rheumatoid arthritis (RA) and systemic lupus erythematosus (SLE) are autoimmune diseases with rheumatologic manifestations that can often mimic the symptoms of multiple sclerosis (MS). Marrie et al recently included RA in a systematic review of epidemiological studies assessing the relation between autoimmune diseases and MS.[1] Their review included three studies (two population based) that addressed the incidence of RA in MS populations and calculated an estimated incidence of 0.21%. Additionally, they included 17 studies assessing the prevalence of RA in MS and calculated an estimated prevalence of 2.92%. Two of the studies included found the prevalence of RA before MS diagnosis to be 0.22% to 1.17%.[2,3] The review also included 11 studies that assessed the relation between MS and SLE and estimated an incidence rate of SLE in MS populations to be 0.02% to 0.35% and a prevalence of 0.14% to 2.90%.[1,4,5]

The analysis by Marrie et al, although not definitive, suggests that the incidence and prevalence of RA and SLE in MS is not significantly different from that of RA and SLE in the general population. However, there have been a number of similar trends found in all three autoimmune diseases. The three conditions share rheumatologic symptoms, and new evidence suggests the possibility of a similar pathogenesis between RA, SLE, and MS. Most notably, all three are significantly more likely to occur in females

229

than in males, particularly females of childbearing age.[6-8] On a cellular level, all three are characterized by excess Th1/Th17 cytokine production, B lymphocyte involvement, and the role of tumor necrosis factor (TNF) and extracellular vesicles.[3,9-11]

For the rheumatologist, there is a great deal of overlap between both the clinical manifestations of RA, SLE, and MS and their subsequent treatment. However, some common RA and SLE treatments can exacerbate MS symptoms and even advance the disease. The following chapter will explore the signs and symptoms of these diseases, their treatments, and the implications of some of these treatments in MS.

Rheumatoid Arthritis

RA is among the most common chronic inflammatory diseases and primarily involves the joints.[12] Like MS, RA has many extra-articular manifestations that must be considered during diagnosis and treatment, such as rheumatoid nodules, pulmonary involvement, vasculitis, and other systemic comorbidities. If left untreated, joint destruction and inflammation can lead to decreased physical function and the inability to carry out basic tasks or maintain employment.[13] The exact etiology of RA is unknown. It appears to involve multiple cell types such as T and B cells and genes such as class II MHC genes.[14]

RA should be suspected if an adult patient presents with inflammatory polyarthritis. The location and duration of morning stiffness can suggest an alternative diagnosis, as patients with RA should report pain and/or stiffness in the peripheral joints (not the low back) for at least 30 minutes, with pain improving with activity.[15,16] If symptoms of arthritis have been present for less than 6 weeks, they may be due to an acute viral polyarthritis rather than RA; the longer the symptoms persist, the more likely an RA diagnosis becomes. In addition to performing a complete physical examination to assess for synovitis and the presence and distribution of swollen or tender joints, the laboratory tests indicated in Table 12.1 should also be considered. Diagnosis is also confirmed by exclusion of similar diseases such as psoriatic arthritis, acute viral polyarthritis, polyarticular gout, and SLE.[13]

Systemic Lupus Erythematosus

SLE is a chronic inflammatory disease of unknown etiology that can impact virtually every organ. Like MS, SLE preferentially affects females of childbearing age and is less prominent in prepubescent and postmenopausal women, suggesting that female sex hormones may play a role in pathogenesis.[8] Physical symptoms include mucosal ulcers, inflammatory polyarthritis, photosensitivity, and, most commonly, acute cutaneous lupus erythema, which presents as erythema in a malar distribution over the cheeks and nose and is commonly referred to as "the butterfly rash."[17] Patients with SLE are at risk for developing neuropsychiatric manifestations, which involves depression, encephalopathy, coma, and psychosis and occurs in approximately 50% of patients with SLE.[18] Like RA, SLE involves T and B cell activity and is associated with class II MHC genes.[19]

SLE is diagnosed based on clinical and laboratory findings, but the clinical heterogeneity and lack of pathognomonic features can deter a definitive diagnosis. Additionally, patients may present with only a few clinical indications of SLE, which often resemble other autoimmune diseases or infections.[19] Demographics should be considered when evaluating a patient for SLE. Like MS, it is more common in women of childbearing age. However, MS is more common in women of European descent, whereas SLE disproportionately affects African Americans, Asians, and Hispanic Americans. In addition to routine laboratories and urinalysis, abnormalities in antinuclear antibodies, antiphospholipid antibodies, C3 and C4 or CH50 complement levels, and erythrocyte sedimentation rate and C-reactive protein levels could support a diagnosis of SLE.

How Do RA and SLE Compare With MS?

Patients with MS present with pain in the extremities but not specifically the joints.[20] MS is classified as an immune-mediated inflammatory demyelinating disease of the central nervous system, and clinical features are far less specific than that of RA or SLE. Patients with MS report migraines, painful tonic spasms, and neuropathic pain.[21] The most useful diagnostic tool in support of an MS diagnosis is magnetic resonance imaging (MRI) and would demonstrate multifocal areas of demyelination with loss of oligodendrocytes and astroglial scarring. Disease progression is monitored through annual MRIs.[22]

A key feature of MS is the presence of oligoclonal bands (OCBs) found in the cerebrospinal fluid (CSF) obtained during a lumbar puncture. OCBs are found in up to 95% of patients with clinically definite MS.[22,23] A positive CSF analysis is based on the presence of OCBs or by an increased immunoglobulin G (IgG) index without an increased IgG index in blood serum; if there is an increased IgG index present in blood serum, alternative diagnoses should be considered. Apart from the presence of OCBs, the CSF appearance and pressure are normal. It should be noted that the presence of OCBs in the CSF alone is not enough to confirm a diagnosis of MS; up to 8% of CSF samples from patients without MS contain the bands.[22] This is especially important given that CSF samples from patients with neuropsychiatric SLE have been shown to contain OCBs.[23] Please refer to Table 12.1 for similarities and differences in the diagnoses of these three diseases.

TABLE 12.1

DIAGNOSTIC RESULTS FOR RHEUMATOID ARTHRITIS (RA), SYSTEMIC LUPUS ERYTHEMATOSUS (SLE), AND MULTIPLE SCLEROSIS (MS)[19,22-25]

Test	RA	SLE	MS
Antinuclear antibody	■ Positive in 40%-45% of patients at a dilution of 1:40 ■ Recommended that tests be run at a dilution of 1:160	■ Positive in virtually all patients at some time during course of disease at all dilutions ■ If negative but suspicion of SLE high, more antibody testing necessary	■ Insignificant at all dilutions
Rheumatoid factor (RF)	■ **Positive 50%-70% of the time** ■ Higher the titer, stronger likelihood of RA	■ **Positive in 20%-30% of patients with SLE**	■ Negative
Anti-cyclic citrullinated peptide (CCP) antibodies	■ Positive in nearly all RA patients (>95%) ■ Specificity for RA increases when both RF and anti-CCP are positive	■ **Negative** in most patients with SLE	■ **Negative**
Plain radiographs	■ Normal early in disease ■ Swollen joints **with** erosions later on	■ Swollen joints without erosions ■ Deformities (also present on physical examination)	■ Unremarkable
Erythrocyte sedimentation rate and serum C-reactive protein	■ **Both elevated in RA**	■ **Both elevated in SLE**	■ Unremarkable
Cerebrospinal fluid (CSF) analysis	■ Unremarkable	■ **Oligoclonal bands** found in patients with neuropsychiatric manifestations of SLE, distinguishable from those found in MS CSF analysis with antibody analysis	■ Presence of **oligoclonal bands** found in 95% of patients with MS

TABLE 12.1
**DIAGNOSTIC RESULTS FOR RHEUMATOID ARTHRITIS (RA),
SYSTEMIC LUPUS ERYTHEMATOSUS (SLE), AND MULTIPLE
SCLEROSIS (MS)**[19,22-25] **(CONTINUED)**

Test	RA	SLE	MS
Magnetic resonance imaging	▪ No established role in RA evaluation ▪ Could be helpful in detecting inflammatory changes or the presence of synovitis	▪ Small punctate hyperintensity focal lesions on T2-weighted images in subcortical and periventricular white matter, usual in frontal parietal regions	▪ Multifocal areas of demyelination with loss of oligodendrocytes and astroglial scarring
Electroencephalography	▪ No established role in RA evaluation	▪ In NPSLE, abnormal (but not specific) in 60%-91% of patients	▪ No established role in RA evaluation

Comorbidities

As demonstrated in Figure 12.1,[26-30] there is a great deal of overlap in the symptoms of these autoimmune diseases. As discussed in the chapter regarding pain in MS, determining the source of pain is necessary to determine which treatment will be the most effective.

Treatment

The primary consideration for managing the comorbidity of RA, SLE, and MS comes from balancing the effects of disease-modifying immunotherapies on each disease. Treating either of these diseases in MS requires extensive communication between the neurologist and rheumatologist regarding treatment to avoid excessive immunosuppression via disease-modifying therapies. This section will discuss both the beneficial and deleterious effects of disease-modifying antirheumatic drugs (DMARDs) and antirheumatic biologics in patients with MS (see Table 12.2 for a complete list of RA AND SLE drugs and their effect in patients with MS).

The most significant consideration in the pharmacologic management of RA in patients with MS concerns the use of anti-TNF therapies. The American College of Rheumatology (ACR) suggests using an anti-TNF therapy either alone or in combination with methotrexate once a primary DMARD (usually methotrexate) alone fails in the treatment of RA.[47]

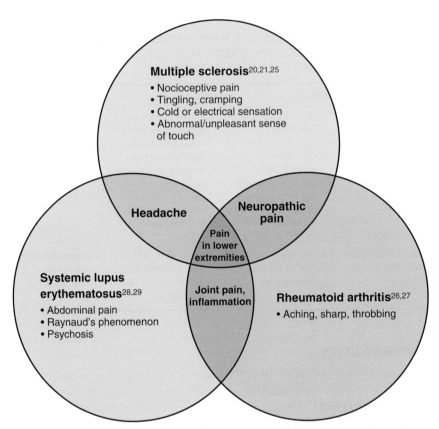

Figure 12.1. Types of pain in multiple sclerosis, systemic lupus erythematosus, and rheumatoid arthritis.

Anti-TNF therapies should not be used in the patient population with MS. Early trials using anti-TNF biologics in the patient population with MS were quickly halted owing to the finding that they worsened myelin lesions and advanced disease progression.[48,49] It is now known that anti-TNF therapies may lead to neuroinflammation and demyelination. Anti-TNF therapies increase immune cell migration to the CNS and impair neuroprotective and regenerative functioning via inhibition of TNFR2.[31-34]

TNF is a cytokine that serves a number of important functions in homeostasis and disease pathology. The importance of TNF stems from its role as an inflammatory mediator and as a trigger of many cellular mechanisms, including induction of tissue repair, organogenesis, and inhibition of tumorigenesis. At normal physiologic levels, TNF signaling contributes to homeostasis and defense against pathogens through these mechanisms. When TNF concentrations exceed normal levels, as seen in many rheumatic diseases and cancers, it can contribute to chronic inflammation and tissue destruction. This section will focus on TNF as a target for the

TABLE 12.2

RHEUMATOID ARTHRITIS (RA) AND SYSTEMIC LUPUS ERYTHEMATOSUS (SLE) DRUGS AND THEIR EFFECT ON MULTIPLE SCLEROSIS (MS) PROGRESSION[31-46]

Drug Class	Drug Names	Effect on MS Progression
Disease-modifying antirheumatic drugs	Methotrexate (Trexall, Rasuvo, Otrexup, Xatmep)	▪ Common treatment for RA ▪ Not proven effective in the treatment of MS
	Hydroxychloroquine (Plaquenil)	▪ Common treatment for SLE ▪ Not proven effective in the treatment of MS
	Leflunomide (Arava)	▪ Common treatment for RA ▪ Cannot take teriflunomide because share same active metabolite
	Sulfasalazine (Azulfidine)	▪ Common treatment for RA, ulcerative colitis
Biologic—TNFi	Adalimumab (Humira) Certolizumab pegol (Cimzia) Etanercept (Enbrel) Golimumab (Simponi) Infliximab (Remicade)	▪ Not recommended in patients with MS (see section on TNFis) ▪ Potential exacerbation of CNS myelin lesions or creation of new lesions because of the inhibitory effect on protective/regenerative function of TNF/TNFR2 in CNS
Biologic—Non-TNFi	Ustekinumab (Stelara)	▪ Treatment for severe cases of psoriatic arthritis ▪ No significant effect
	Tocizumab (Actemra)	▪ No significant effect
	Rituximab (Rituxan)	▪ Potential positive effect in RRMS, but not progressive forms via depletion of B cells[37-39]
Glucocorticoid	Prednisone (or equivalent)	▪ Consult with neurologist before prescribing to avoid adverse events from excess dosage ▪ Main concern is with long-term use—can exacerbate disease progression of SLE ▪ Used to decrease inflammatory response in both RA and MS

CNS, central nervous system; RRMS, relapsing-remitting MS; TNF, tumor necrosis factor; TNFi, TNF inhibitor; TNFR, TNF receptor.

treatment of rheumatic diseases and on the deleterious effect of global TNF inhibitors (TNFi) in patients with both a rheumatic disease and MS.[31]

There are five Food and Drug Administration–approved TNFi biologics that are used in the treatment of RA, inflammatory bowel disease, psoriasis, psoriatic arthritis, and ankylosing spondylitis. Four of these are monoclonal antibodies infliximab (Remicade), adalimumab (Humira), certolizumab pegol (Cimzia), and golimumab (Simponi), and one is a soluble TNF receptor etanercept (Enbrel).[31] Several of these biologics have significantly improved outcomes for rheumatic diseases. A TNFi in combination with methotrexate is the standard of care in the majority of patients with RA (70%-80%) after methotrexate alone fails.[32] Trials for treatment of MS with TNFis were initiated early on in the evolution of anti-TNF therapies. However, these trials were halted because of the surprising effect that, in patients with MS, TNFis caused immune activation and an overall increase in disease activity.[35,48] Even in TNFi trials involving otherwise healthy patients afflicted with rheumatic diseases, demyelinating events were reported.[49]

The contradictory effect of TNFis in MS is likely due to the multiple ways in which TNF receptors carry out an immune response.[33] TNF is initially expressed as a transmembrane cytokine but can be cleaved by TNF converting enzyme (TACE) into a soluble form.[36] The bioactivity of each form of TNF depends on which of two unique cellular receptors it interacts with, TNFR1 (also p55) or TNFR2 (also p75).[37] Outcomes of the two subsequent signaling cascades are considerably different. TNFR1 receptors present on all cells and appear to induce a proinflammatory response. This function can be seen in TNFR1 "knockout" mice, which have a markedly decreased inflammatory response and are subsequently protected from many diseases. TNFR2 is less widely expressed than TNFR1, and its binding with TNF appears to trigger a cascade that results in cellular repair, homeostasis, and survival.[31] The regulation of outcomes stemming from these complexes, and their subsequent effect on physiological and pathological processes, is not well understood and is currently a subject of intensive research. It is believed that outcomes of TNF/TNFR binding are distinct based not only on receptor (TNFR1 vs. TNFR2) and TNF ligand type (soluble vs. transmembrane) but also on local environment and tissue type.[31-34]

Another consideration in the treatment of RA and SLE in patients with MS regards the use of glucocorticoids. The current recommendation from both the ACR and the European League Against Rheumatism is for glucocorticoids to be administered while starting a DMARD or biologic for the management of flare-ups.[21,38] Oral or intravenous glucocorticoids have long been a short-term treatment option for acute manifestations of MS owing to their immunosuppressive and anti-inflammatory properties.[39,40] However, high dosages or long-term usage of glucocorticoids can result in significant side effects.[41] Secondary nociceptive pain due to chronic glucocorticoid usage has been noted as a significant source of pain in the population with MS.[42,43] In SLE, high doses of glucocorticoids can have substantial adverse effects, including infections, osteoporosis, and cardiovascular disorders.[44] Therefore, rheumatologists and neurologists should communicate regarding glucocorticoid usage to ensure that excessive dosage or prolongation of glucocorticoid treatment does not occur.

There are also drugs that have potentially positive off-label effects in the treatment of MS. These drugs capitalize on points of commonality between the complex autoimmune mechanisms found in RA and MS and exert a mutually beneficial effect by inhibiting some part of the shared pathophysiological immune mechanism. For example, rituximab (Rituxan) is often used to treat both RA and MS, and SLE. Rituxan is a genetically engineered chimeric monoclonal antibody that depletes CD20+ B cells through both cytotoxic effects and promotion of apoptosis and has proven effective in treating both MS and SLE.[45,50] Because B cells have been implicated in the pathophysiology of MS through their role in targeted and compartmentalized humoral responses, depletion of B cells by Rituxan has shown preliminary positive results in treating MS, although more clinical trials are needed in this regard.[51-53] A summary of different treatments for RA and SLE and their effect in patients with MS can be seen in Table 12.2.

Psoriasis

Psoriasis is an immune-mediated skin disorder characterized by scaly or silver-appearing erythematous plaques. The risk of incident psoriasis is 54% higher among people with MS than in the general population.[54] Psoriasis and MS seem to share some risk factors; the prevalence of both diseases appears to increase with increasing distance from the equator; obesity and smoking appear to contribute to the pathogenesis.[13,55] Additionally, fumarates have been shown to be effective disease-modifying therapies in both diseases. Treatments for psoriasis include topical corticosteroids and vitamin D analogs, ultraviolet light, and systemic therapies, many of which overlap with MS treatments. Methotrexate, administered in conjunction with a folic acid supplement, is a common treatment for psoriasis.[56]

Psoriatic arthritis develops in 30% of patients with psoriasis and is characterized by a wide range of clinical features, which often results in a delayed diagnosis and treatment.[13] Unlike MS, SLE, and RA, it is equally common in both men and women and primarily manifests as peripheral arthritis, axial disease, enthesitis, dactylitis, and skin and nail disease.[56] Psoriatic arthritis can mimic RA, ankylosing spondylitis, and gout, but these can be ruled out by clinical and laboratory evaluation and imaging in patients who have had the disease for a longer interval.

The treatments for psoriatic arthritis depend on what systems are affected by the disease, and treatment should be coordinated between the rheumatology, general practitioner, and any specialists involved. Patients with mild arthritis (involving fewer than four joints) can take nonsteroidal anti-inflammatories, such as (naproxen sodium) Aleve or (celecoxib)

Celebrex, which can control inflammatory symptoms and lessen pain and stiffness.[57] For patients who have not found relief of their peripheral arthritis without erosions or substantial functional limitations, methotrexate (leflunomide or sulfasalazine can be substituted if the patient is unable to tolerate methotrexate) is suggested.

Because the incidence of psoriasis in MS is 54% higher than in the general population, patients with MS have an increased risk of developing psoriatic arthritis.[15] The treatment for more severe forms of psoriatic arthritis, wherein erosive changes have significantly limited function, is most often a TNF inhibitor.[31] Because TNFis can increase disease activity in patients with MS, it is recommended that biologic disease-modifying antirheumatic drugs (DMARDs) such as Stelara (ustekinumab) or Consentyx (secukinumab) be used instead.[57,58] Glucocorticoids should be avoided in patients with psoriatic arthritis because they have been shown to increase the chances of developing erythroderma or pustular psoriasis, as well as interfering with the effects of other medications.[57]

Sjögren Syndrome, Scleroderma, and Barriers to Drug Absorption

Sjögren syndrome and scleroderma are two autoimmune rheumatologic issues that affect fibrous tissue. Sjögren syndrome is a chronic condition characterized by lymphocytic infiltration and subsequent degeneration of exocrine glands, primarily the salivary and ocular glands, that result in severe dryness in the mouth, eyes, and other mucosal membranes of the body.[59] Scleroderma (or systemic sclerosis) is a complex disease similar to Sjögren syndrome that involves extensive fibrosis, vascular alterations, and autoantibodies proliferation. This disorder is four times more common among women than among men, primarily affecting people from 20 to 50 years old. There are two accepted classifications of scleroderma: limited cutaneous scleroderma and diffuse cutaneous scleroderma.[60] Patients with limited cutaneous scleroderma display fibrosis only on the hands, face, and arms. The majority of these patients suffer from pulmonary hypertension and also a high prevalence of anticentromere antibodies, which can be used to distinguish it from diffuse cutaneous scleroderma.

Patients with either Sjögren syndrome or scleroderma who are also diagnosed with MS face skin issues that may affect drug absorption. For example, Acthar Gel is a subcutaneous adrenocorticotropic hormone injection that helps treat patients with MS by stimulating anti-inflammatory corticosteroids within their bodies.[16] Patients with severe skin disorders, like those with scleroderma, are unable to take Acthar Gel because they are unable to absorb the drug. Thus, these patients with MS may be unable to receive effective and appropriate treatments to treat their MS.[16]

Lyme Disease

Lyme disease is a bacterial infection caused by six species of ticks in the *Borreliaceae* family. It is the most common tick-borne disease in the United States, Canada, and Europe.[16] There is a broad spectrum of disease manifestations, largely because of differences in the infecting species. Lyme disease, or Lyme borreliosis, can mimic the symptoms of MS, particularly headache, fatigue, and muscle aches. About 10% to 15% of patients infected with Lyme disease can develop central nervous system involvement during the early disseminated stage of the disease, and the condition appears similar to MS during CSF analysis and MRI.[61,62]

Symptoms

The clinical manifestations of Lyme disease can be classified into three phases: early localized disease, early disseminated disease, and late Lyme disease. It should be noted that clinical features from these stages can overlap. Refer to Table 12.3 for a comparison of clinical signs and symptoms of Lyme disease and MS.

- Early localized disease: Characterized by the presence of erythema migrans (EM) skin lesion, and usually occurs within 1 month of tick bite

TABLE 12.3

SIGNS AND SYMPTOMS OF LYME DISEASE AND MULTIPLE SCLEROSIS (MS)[22,62]

Signs and Symptoms: Lyme Versus MS	
Lyme Disease	**MS**
Erythema migrans rash (within 3-30 d of tick bite), typically expands over course of days, with central clearing and bulls-eye appearance	No characteristic rashes or lesions
Fatigue	Fatigue (not caused by lack of sleep or exertional exhaustion due to disability)
Joint pain	General pain (not in joints)
Headache	N/A
N/A	Sensory loss
N/A	Motor issues; muscle cramping, spasticity
Eye redness, tearing	Optic neuritis

- Early disseminated disease: Presence of multiple EM lesions (within days to weeks after infection), possibly with the presence of neurologic and/or cardio findings (weeks to months after infection), such as lymphocytic meningitis, facial palsy, radiculoneuropathy, or carditis with heart block
- Late Lyme disease: Associated with intermittent or persistent arthritis involving one or a few large joints (particularly the knee) and/or neurologic problems, such as subtle encephalopathy or polyneuropathy (months to years after initial infection)[16,61,63]

Diagnosis

A diagnosis of early Lyme disease can be determined on clinical findings alone when patients present with EM lesions and live in or have traveled to an endemic area. Patients who present with EM lesions should not be tested for Lyme titers, as they will likely be seronegative, because lesions appear before adaptive immune response.[61] By the time a patient displays symptoms of early disseminated disease, serologic tests are usually positive for both IgM and IgG antibodies.[63]

Clinical presentation should be considered before serologic testing. Indications for Lyme titers are a recent history of living or traveling in an endemic area, exposure to ticks, and symptoms consistent with early disseminated disease or late Lyme disease, such as meningitis, radiculopathy, arthritis, and carditis. Serologic tests should not be conducted if the patient has no EM lesions or does not live in endemic areas or for patients with nonspecific symptoms only (i.e., fatigue, muscle pain).[61]

A two-tier conditional strategy can assist in the diagnosis of Lyme disease. This includes a sensitive enzyme immunoassay, such as enzyme-linked immunosorbent assay (ELISA), followed by a more specific Western blot test.[61]

- Negative ELISA: no further testing needed, patient negative for Lyme disease
- Positive ELISA: should be followed by Western blot
  - □ Negative Western blot: supersedes results of positive ELISA, patient negative for Lyme disease
  - □ Positive Western blot: considered evidence of tick encounter, patient positive for Lyme disease[61]

CSF Analysis

Patients with the disseminating Lyme disease can develop neurologic manifestations, or neuroborreliosis, of the disease, such as meningitis, facial nerve palsy, radiculoneuritis, and focal encephalitis. Lumbar puncture to analyze CSF is useful in determining a definitive diagnosis of Lyme disease as the source of those symptoms and what antibiotic would be the most useful for treatment. For example, oral amoxicillin is appropriate for treating arthritic manifestations of Lyme disease, but not neurologic; however, oral doxycycline could treat both.[61] It should be noted that CSF analysis for patients with neuroborreliosis and MS would yield OCBs, but the OCB antibodies found in the patient with suspected neuroborreliosis binds specifically to a protein from *Borrelia*, and the patient can be differentiated from a patient with MS.[23,64]

Imaging

Persisting Lyme disease often affects the central nervous system with demyelinating lesions, which can be misdiagnosed as MS.[65] MRI may reveal white matter hyperintensities suggestive of inflammation or areas of demyelination. However, antibiotic treatment results in a decrease or disappearance of these hyperintensities. Clinical presentation and blood serology should rule out these regions of hyperintensities in patients with neuroborreliosis.[61,62]

Gout

Pain from gout is often confused with that of MS, when another inflammatory source is gouty arthropathy presenting in a patient with MS. Gout is characterized by acute, intermittent episodes of synovitis caused by the accumulation of monosodium urate crystals in joint fluids, cartilage, bones, tendons, bursae, or other sites.[66,67] Pain from gout is often described as a sharp or burning sensation and commonly presents with considerable erythema, swelling, and increased temperature. It most commonly affects the great toe joint, although it can manifest in any synovial joint. Neuropathic, ongoing extremity pain can overlap with symptoms of gout manifesting in the great toe, ankle, or knee joints. Acute swelling, erythema, or increased temperature, particularly when manifesting in intermittent episodes, enforces gout as a probable differential diagnosis. Additionally, gout interacts with nociceptive pain secondary to musculoskeletal stress in MS and will likely lead to compensational pain as a result of the patient shifting gait to avoid putting weight on the affected joint. The characteristic findings of gout noted earlier can be used to differentiate a manifestation of gout from another source of synovitis in patients with MS.[67]

References

1. Marrie RA, Reider N, Cohen J, et al. A systematic review of the incidence and prevalence of autoimmune disease in multiple sclerosis. *Mult Scler.* 2015;21(3):282-293. doi:10.1177/1352458514564490. Epub 2014/12/24.
2. Marrie RA, Horwitz R, Cutter G, Tyry T, Vollmer T. Association between comorbidity and clinical characteristics of MS. *Acta Neurol Scand.* 2011;124(2): 135-141. doi:10.1111/j.1600-0404.2010.01436.

3. Langer-Gould A, Albers K, Van Den Eeden S, Nelson L. Autoimmune diseases prior to the diagnosis of multiple sclerosis: a population-based case-control study. *Mult Scler.* 2010;16(7):855-861.

4. Marrie RA, Horwitz RI, Cutter G, et al. Smokers with multiple sclerosis are more likely to report comorbid autoimmune diseases. *Neuroepidemiology.* 2011;36:85-90.

5. Fanouriakis A, Mastorodemos V, Pamfil C, et al. Coexistence of systemic lupus erythematosus and multiple sclerosis: prevalence, clinical characteristics, and natural history. *Semin Arthritis Rheum.* 2014;43:751-758.

6. Scott DL, Wolfe F, Huizinga TW. Rheumatoid arthritis. *Lancet.* 2010;376(9746):1094-1108.

7. Wallin M, Kurtzke J. Multiple sclerosis; epidemiology. *Encycl Neurol Sci.* 2014;3:153-160.

8. Lisnevskaia L, Murphy G, Isenberg D. Systemic lupus erythematosus. *Lancet.* 2014;384(9957):1878-1888.

9. Ulivieri C, Baldari CT. Regulation of T Cell activation and differentiation by extracellular vesicles and their pathogenic role in systemic lupus erythematosus and multiple sclerosis. *Molecules.* 2017;22.

10. Buzas EI, György B, Nagy G, Falus A, Gay S. Emerging role of extracellular vesicles in inflammatory diseases. *Nat Rev Rheumatol.* 2014;10(6):356-364.

11. Mantravadi S, Ogdie A, Kraft WK. Tumor necrosis factor inhibitors in psoriatic arthritis. *Expert Rev Clin Pharmacol.* 2017;10(8):899-910. doi:10.1080/17512 433.2017.1329009.

12. Smolen JS, Aletaha D, McInnes IB. Rheumatoid arthritis. *Lancet.* 2016;388(10055):2023-2038. doi:10.1016/s0140-6736(16)30173-8.

13. Ritchlin CT, Colbert RA, Gladman DD. Psoriatic arthritis. *N Engl J Med.* 2017;376:957-970.

14. Veale DJ, Ritchlin C, FitzGerald O. Immunopathology of psoriasis and psoriatic arthritis. *Ann Rheum Dis.* 2005;64(suppl 2):ii26-ii29. doi:10.1136/ard.2004.031740. Epub 2005/02/15. PubMed PMID: 15708930; PubMed Central PMCID: PMCPMC1766860.

15. Marrie RA, Patten SB, Tremlett H, Wolfson C, Leung S, Fisk JD. Increased incidence and prevalence of psoriasis in multiple sclerosis. *Mult Scler Relat Disord.* 2017;13:81-86. doi:10.1016/j.msard.2017.02.012.

16. Steere AC, Strle F, Wormser GP, et al. Lyme borreliosis. *Nat Rev Dis Primers.* 2016;2:16090. doi:10.1038/nrdp.2016.90. Epub 2016/12/16.

17. Gladman DD. *Overview of the Clinical Manifestations of Systemic Lupus Erythematosus in Adults.* In: Curtis MR, ed. UpToDate; 2018. Available at https://www.uptodate.com/contents/overview-of-the-clinical-manifestations-of-systemic-lupus-erythematosus-in-adults?search=lupus%20rash&source=search_result&selectedTitle=2~150&usage_type=default&display_rank=2#H11. Retrieved October 30, 2018.

18. Hirohata S. Epidemiology of neuropsychiatric systemic lupus erythematosus. In: Hirohata S, ed. *Neuropsychiatric Systemic Lupus Erythematosus.* Cham: Springer; 2018.

19. Wallace DJ. *Diagnosis and Differential Diagnosis of Systemic Lupus Erythematosus in Adults.* In: Curtis MR, ed. UpToDate; 2017. Available at https://www.uptodate.com/contents/diagnosis-and-differential-diagnosis-of-systemic-lupus-erythematosus-in-adults?search=systemic%20lupus%20erythematosus&source=search_result&selectedTitle=3~150&usage_type=default&display_rank=3. Retrieved October 28, 2018.

20. Scherder RJ, Kant N, Wolf ET, Pijnenburg BCM, Scherder EJA. Sensory function and chronic pain in multiple sclerosis. *Pain Res Manag.* 2018;2018:1-9.

21. Nick ST, Roberts C, Billiodeaux S, et al. Multiple sclerosis and pain. *Neurol Res.* 2012;34(9):829-841. doi:10.1179/1743132812Y.0000000082.

22. Olek MJ. *Diagnosis of Multiple Sclerosis in Adults.* In: Dashe JF, ed. UpToDate; 2018. Available at https://www.uptodate.com/contents/diagnosis-of-multiple-sclerosis-in-adults?search=multiple%20sclerosis&source=search_result&selectedTitle=2~150&usage_type=default&display_rank=2. Retrieved on October 10, 2018.

23. Farina G, Magliozzi R, Pitteri M, et al. Increased cortical lesion load and intrathecal inflammation is associated with oligoclonal bands in multiple sclerosis patients: a combined CSF and MRI study. *J Neuroinflammation.* 2017;14(1):40. doi:10.1186/s12974-017-0812-y. Epub 2017/02/23.

24. Venables PJW, Maini RN. *Diagnosis and Differential Diagnosis of Rheumatoid Arthritis.* In: Romain PL, ed. UpToDate; 2014. Available at https://www.uptodate.com/contents/diagnosis-and-differential-diagnosis-of-rheumatoid-arthritis?search=rheumatoid%20arthritis&source=search_result&selectedTitle=1~150&usage_type=default&display_rank=1. Retrieved October 28, 2018.

25. Agmon-Levin N, Damoiseaux J, Kallenberg C, et al. International recommendations for the assessment of autoantibodies to cellular antigens referred to as anti-nuclear antibodies. *Ann Rheum Dis.* 2014;73(1):17-23.

26. Ghajarzadeh M, Jalilian R, Sahraian MA, et al. Pain in multiple sclerosis. *Maedica(Buchar).* 2018;13(2):125-130.

27. Walsh DA, McWilliams DF. Pain in rheumatoid arthritis. *Curr Pain Headache Rep.* 2012;16:509-517.

28. Walsh DA, McWilliams DF. Mechanisms, impact and management of pain in rheumatoid arthritis. *Nat Rev Rheumatol.* 2014;10:581-592.

29. Di Franco M, Guzzo M, Spinelli F, et al. Pain and systemic lupus erythematosus. *Reumatismo.* 2014;66(1):33-38.

30. Waldheim E, Ajeganova S, Bergman S, Frostegard J, Welin E. Variation in pain related to systemic lupus erythematosus (SLE): a 7-year follow-up study. *Clin Rheumatol.* 2018;37:1825-1834.

31. Kalliolias GD, Ivashkiv LB. TNF biology, pathogenic mechanisms and emerging therapeutic strategies. *Nat Rev Rheumatol.* 2016;12(1):49-62. doi:10.1038/nrrheum.2015.169. PubMed PMID: 26656660; PubMed Central PMCID: PMCPMC4809675.

32. Kemanetzoglou E, Andreadou E. CNS demyelination with TNF-α blockers. *Curr Neurol Neurosci Rep.* 2017;17(4). doi:10.1007/s11910-017-0742-1. PubMed PMID: 28337644; PubMed Central PMCID: PMCPMC5364240.

33. Mohan N, Edwards ET, Cupps TR, et al. Demyelination occurring during anti–tumor necrosis factor α therapy for inflammatory arthritides. *Arthritis Rheum.* 2001;44(12):2862-2869.

34. Haas TL, Emmerich CH, Gerlach B, et al. Recruitment of the linear ubiquitin chain assembly complex stabilizes the TNF-R1 signaling complex and is required for TNF-mediated gene induction. *Mol Cell.* 2009;36(5):831-844. doi:10.1016/j.molcel.2009.10.013. Epub 2009/12/17. PubMed PMID: 20005846.

35. Monaco C, Nanchahal J, Taylor P, Feldmann M. Anti-TNF therapy: past, present and future. *Int Immunol.* 2014;27(1):55-62.

36. Probert L. TNF and its receptors in the CNS: the essential, the desirable and the deleterious effects. *Neuroscience.* 2015;302:2-22.

37. Locksley RM, Killeen N, Lenardo MJ. The TNF and TNF receptor superfamilies: integrating mammalian biology. *Cell.* 2001;104(4):487-501. Epub 2001/03/10. PubMed PMID: 11239407.

38. Smolen JS, Landewé R, Bijlsma J, et al. EULAR recommendations for the management of rheumatoid arthritis with synthetic and biological disease-modifying antirheumatic drugs: 2016 update. *Ann Rheum Dis.* 2017;76(6). doi:10.1136/annrheumdis-2016-210715.

39. Bowen JD, Qian P. Oral rather than intravenous corticosteroids should be used to treat MS relapses–No. *Mult Scler.* 2017;23(8):1058-1060.

40. Chataway J. *Oral Versus Intravenous Steroids in Multiple Sclerosis Relapses–A Perennial Question?* London, England: Sage Publications; 2014.

41. van der Goes MC, Jacobs JW, Bijlsma JW. The value of glucocorticoid co-therapy in different rheumatic diseases–positive and adverse effects. *Arthritis Res Ther.* 2014;16(suppl 2):S2. doi:10.1186/ar4686.

42. Seixas D, Foley P, Palace J, Lima D, Ramos I, Tracey I. Pain in multiple sclerosis: a systematic review of neuroimaging studies. *Neuroimage Clin.* 2014;5:322-331. doi:10.1016/j.nicl.2014.06.014.

43. O'Connor AB, Schwid SR, Herrmann DN, Markman JD, Dworkin RH. Pain associated with multiple sclerosis: systematic review and proposed classification. *Pain.* 2008;137(1):96-111. doi:10.1016/j.pain.2007.08.024. Epub 2007/10/12. PubMed PMID: 17928147.

44. He J, Li Z. An era of biological treatment in systemic lupus erythematosus. *Clin Rheumatol.* 2018;37(1):1-3. doi:10.1007/s10067-017-3933-x. Epub 2017/12/14. PubMed PMID: 29234909; PubMed Central PMCID: PMCPMC5754454.

45. Reff ME, Carner K, Chambers KS, et al. Depletion of B cells in vivo by a chimeric mouse human monoclonal antibody to CD20. *Blood.* 1994;83(2):435-445. Epub 1994/01/15. PubMed PMID: 7506951.

46. Feldman SR. *Epidemiology, Clinical Manifestations, and Diagnosis of Psoriasis.* In: Ofori AO, ed. UpToDate; 2018. Available at https://www.uptodate.com/contents/epidemiology-clinical-manifestations-and-diagnosis-of-psoriasis?search=risk%20factors%20psoriasis&source=search_result&selectedTitle=1~150&usage_type=default&display_rank=1#H3. Retrieved October 28, 2018.

47. Singh JA, Saag KG, Bridges SL, et al. 2015 American College of Rheumatology guideline for the treatment of rheumatoid arthritis. *Arthritis Rheumatol.* 2016;68(1):1-26.

48. Group TMSS. TNF neutralization in MS. Results of a randomized, placebo-controlled multicenter study. *Neurology.* 1999;53(3):457. doi:10.1212/wnl.53.3.457.

49. van Oosten BW, Barkhof F, Truyen L, et al. Increased MRI activity and immune activation in two multiple sclerosis patients treated with the monoclonal anti-tumor necrosis factor antibody cA2. *Neurology.* 1996;47(6):1531-1534. Epub 1996/12/01. PubMed PMID: 8960740.

50. Aguiar R, Araujo C, Martins-Coelho G, Isenberg D. Use of rituximab in systemic lupus erythematosus: a single center experience over 14 years. *Arthritis Care Res (Hoboken).* 2017;69(2):257-262. doi:10.1002/acr.22921. Epub 2016/04/26. PubMed PMID: 27110698.

51. Castillo-Trivino T, Braithwaite D, Bacchetti P, Waubant E. Rituximab in relapsing and progressive forms of multiple sclerosis: a systematic review. *PLoS One.* 2013;8(7):e66308. doi:10.1371/journal.pone.0066308. Epub 2013/07/12.

52. Owens GP, Bennett JL, Gilden DH, Burgoon MP. The B cell response in multiple sclerosis. *Neurol Res.* 2006;28(3):236-244. doi:10.1179/016164106x98099. Epub 2006/05/12. PubMed PMID: 16687047.

53. Hauser SL, Waubant E, Arnold DL, et al. B-cell depletion with rituximab in relapsing–remitting multiple sclerosis. *N Engl J Med.* 2008;358(7):676-688.

54. Firestein GS, Gabriel SE, McInnes IB, ODell JR. *Kelley and Firesteins Textbook of Rheumatology.* Philadelphia, PA: Elsevier; 2017.

55. Setty AR, Curhan G, Choi HK. Obesity, waist circumference, weight change, and the risk of psoriasis in women: Nurses' Health Study II. *Arch Intern Med.* 2007;167(15):1670-1675.

56. Gladman DD. *Clinical Manifestations and Diagnosis of Psoriatic Arthritis.* In: Romain PL, ed. UpToDate; 2017. Available at https://www.uptodate.com/contents/clinical-manifestations-and-diagnosis-of-psoriatic-arthritis?search=psoriatic%20arthritis&source=search_result&selectedTitle=1~150&usage_type=default&display_rank=1. Retreived October 20, 2018.

57. Gladman DD, Ritchlin C. *Treatment of Psoriatic Arthritis.* In: Romain PL, ed. UpToDate; 2018. Available at https://www.uptodate.com/contents/treatment-of-psoriatic-arthritis?search=psoriatic%20arthritis%20treatment&source=search_result&selectedTitle=1~150&usage_type=default&display_rank=1#H20469265. Retrieved October 30, 2018.

58. Chang S, Chambers CJ, Liu F, Armstrong AW. Successful treatment of psoriasis with ustekinumab in patients with multiple sclerosis. *Dermatol Online J.* 2015;21(7). Available at https://escholarship.org/uc/item/3bs971cr.

59. Nair JJ, Singh TP. Sjogren's syndrome: review of the aetiology, pathophysiology & potential therapeutic interventions. *J Clin Exp Dent.* 2017;9(4):e584.

60. Gabrielli A, Avvedimento EV, Krieg T. Scleroderma. *N Engl J Med.* 2009; 360(19):1989-2003.

61. Schur PH. *Neuropsychiatric Manifestations of Systemic Lupus Erythematosus.* In: Wilterdink JL, ed. UpToDate; 2014. Available at https://www.uptodate.com/contents/neuropsychiatric-manifestations-of-systemic-lupus-erythematosus?search=lupus%20psychosis&source=search_result&selectedTitle=1~150&usage_type=default&display_rank=1. Retrieved October 28, 2018.

62. Toledano M, Weinshenker BG, Solomon AJ. A clinical approach to the differential diagnosis of multiple sclerosis. *Curr Neurol Neurosci Rep.* 2015;15(8):57. doi:10.1007/s11910-015-0576-7. Epub 2015/06/27.

63. Ross Russell AL, Dryden M, Pinto AA, Lovett J. Lyme disease: diagnosis and management. *Pract Neurol.* 2018;18(6):455-464. doi:10.1136/practneurol-2018-001998.

64. Brandle SM, Obermeier B, Senel M, et al. Distinct oligoclonal band antibodies in multiple sclerosis recognize ubiquitous self-proteins. *Proc Natl Acad Sci USA.* 2016;113:7864-7869.

65. Santino I, Comite P, Gandolfo GM. Borrelia burgdorferi, a great chameleon: know it to recognize it! *Neurol Sci.* 2010;31(2):193-196. doi:10.1007/s10072-009-0175-y. Epub 2009/11/07. PubMed PMID: 19894021.

66. Winter DA. Human balance and posture control during standing and walking. *Gait Posture.* 1995;3(4):193-214.

67. Shekelle PG, Newberry SJ, FitzGerald JD, et al. Management of gout: a systematic review in support of an American College of Physicians clinical practice guideline. *Ann Intern Med.* 2017;166(1):37-51. doi:10.7326/M16-0461.

13

Pulmonary Complications in Multiple Sclerosis

■ ■ ■ Priyank Trivedi, Anthony J. Smith, Joseph T. Cooke

Introduction

Pulmonary complications are a significant cause of morbidity and mortality in patients with multiple sclerosis (MS). Symptoms are insidious, and respiratory dysfunction may present as late as 9 years after the onset of neurologic symptoms.[1] The pattern, severity, and morbidity of respiratory failure is related to the size and location of the demyelinating plaques within the central nervous system. The respiratory dysfunction is related to the degree of neurologic involvement and related respiratory muscle weakness. This is manifested as loss of ventilation control, sleep apnea, difficulty swallowing, and an ineffective cough. Current and future treatments for MS may also result in a decreased immune response to infection. The respiratory failure treatment is often supportive, with both invasive and noninvasive mechanical ventilation.

Pulmonary Function Testing

Pulmonary function tests may not be the most sensitive marker of respiratory muscle dysfunction in MS.[2] Common measurements used to measure respiratory function in patients with MS include vital capacity (VC),

247

maximal inspiratory pressure (MIP), maximal expiratory pressure (MEP), and maximal voluntary ventilation (MVV).

Reduction of the VC suggests significant diaphragmatic weakness. Patients often exhibit correlative signs such as paradoxical abdominal breathing. The MIP, MEP, and MVV, in contrast, are more sensitive indicators of respiratory muscle weakness.[3] Similar to other neuromuscular diseases, the decline in MIPmax and MEPmax precede changes in lung volumes. Patients with moderately severe MS on average exhibit a 40% decline in MIP and a 60% decline in MEP.[8] MVV measures the respiratory muscle endurance. This decreases in parallel to the decrease in MEP.[4]

Studies have demonstrated a larger decrease in expiratory muscle strength than in inspiratory muscle strength. Expiratory muscle weakness can occur without inspiratory muscle weakness in patients with mild disease.[5] This pattern can be explained by the progression of paresis in patients with MS. In MS, muscular impairment generally progresses from lower to upper extremities. The abdominal muscles become impaired earlier than the muscles of the diaphragm and intercostal muscles. This results in impaired expiration before inspiration.[6] This can be clinically manifested as an ineffective cough and an inability to clear secretions.

Respiratory muscle weakness occurs both in patients who are ambulatory and wheelchair bound. However, patients who are ambulatory with minimal upper extremity involvement have a much smaller decline in MEP, VC, and MVV and essentially no decline in MIP when compared with patients who are wheelchair bound with significant upper extremity impairment[4] (Figure 13.1). Patients with a mild degree of neurologic impairment rarely show any abnormalities in pulmonary function testing with normal (VC), forced expiratory volume in 1 s (FEV1), total lung capacity (TLC), and residual volume (RV). In contrast, patients with more advanced disease may show lung volume loss with a decreased VC and a preserved FEV1/FVC ratio. This pattern suggests restrictive lung disease; however, the TLC tends to be preserved in MS[5] (Figure 13.2). This is attributable to submaximal inspiratory and expiratory efforts that are expected in patients with whole body muscle weakness, which results in an increase of the residual volume (RV). The rise in the RV correlates with the decline in the MEP.

Although MIPs and MEPs provide for a more useful tool than usual pulmonary function tests, they can be difficult to administer in patients with facial and bulbar muscle weakness.[7] Clinical indices may be the best predictor of expiratory muscle weakness.[5] Activities such as talking, coughing, and upper extremity strength serve as reliable markers of muscle strength. Talking requires complex coordination of upper and lower respiratory muscles, and coughing requires muscle contraction against a closed glottis. Smeltzer et al developed a pulmonary index score that appeared to be the best predictor of expiratory muscle weakness. The score comprised four parameters: patient's report of his or her ability to handle

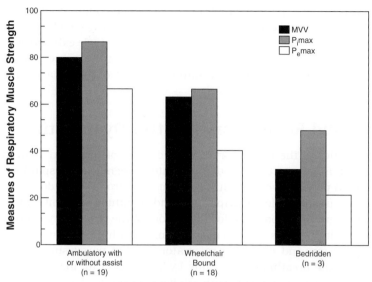

Figure 13.1. Measures of respiratory muscle function by category of neurologic disability expressed as percent predicted. Reproduced with permission from Smeltzer SC, Skurnick JH, Troiano R. Respiratory function in multiple sclerosis: utility of clinical assessment of respiratory muscle function. *Chest.* 1992;101:479-484.

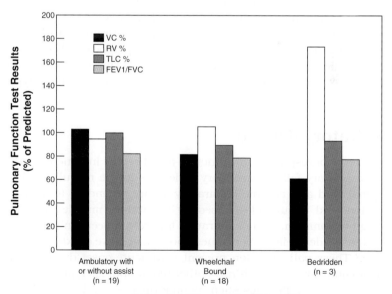

Figure 13.2. Pulmonary function test results by category of neurologic disability expressed as percent predicted. Reproduced with permission from Smeltzer SC, Skurnick JH, Troiano R. Respiratory function in multiple sclerosis: utility of clinical assessment of respiratory muscle function. *Chest.* 1992;101:479-484.

secretions/mucus, patient's report of a weakened cough, examiner's evaluation of a patient's cough when asked to voluntarily cough as forcefully as possible, and the patient's ability to count on a single exhalation. Using stepwise regression analysis it was concluded that the index score, upper extremity weakness, and MVV accounted for 60% of the variance in maximal expiratory muscle strength.[5]

Sleep and Respiratory Control Dysfunction

Abnormalities of the respiratory control centers of the brain stem impair normal breathing patterns and contribute to significant respiratory dysfunction in patients with MS. Involvement of neurons of the dorsal medullary group (responsible for inspiration and breathing rhythm) and ventral medullary group (responsible for expiration) of the respiratory control center located in the pons leads to dysrhythmic breathing. Patients experience loss of voluntary and autonomic respiratory control, paroxysmal ventilation, and apneustic breathing. In a study by Tantucci et al, measuring mouth occlusion pressures, patients with MS were found to have increased baseline respiratory drive when compared with control subjects. Their breathing response to carbon dioxide was preserved but failed to generate an adequate ventilatory response, which may reflect underlying muscle dysfunction.[8]

Patients with MS have more abnormalities in sleep patterns than the general population.[9] They report a greater degree of abnormal sleep initiation and maintenance, snoring, nighttime shortness of breath, sleep adequacy, and higher levels of daytime somnolence. Brainstem involvement increases the risk of developing obstructive sleep apnea and central sleep apnea.[10] Additionally, patients with significant respiratory muscle weakness may also develop nocturnal hypoventilation, although this is typically manifested in very advanced disease in bedridden patients.[6]

Respiratory Failure

Two patterns of respiratory dysfunction are observed in patients with MS: acute respiratory failure secondary to lesions in the medulla and cervical spinal cord and chronic respiratory failure secondary to atelectasis, aspiration, and pneumonia caused by respiratory muscle dysfunction. Although uncommon, acute respiratory failure can occur in patients with new extensive demyelinating plaques and is suggestive of extensive bulbar disease.[2] These patients often present with acute-onset dyspnea, orthopnea, or confusion in the setting of other motor findings typical of patients with MS, including findings such as quadriparesis and spastic paraplegia with upper arm weakness.[1] Commonly reported respiratory symptoms include progressive breathlessness, impaired cough, difficulty handling secretions, orthopnea, and sleep disturbances. When compounded by secondary systemic factors such as dehydration, aspiration pneumonitis, and sepsis, patients in acute respiratory failure often require mechanical ventilatory support and antibiotics.[11]

Chronic respiratory failure develops in the terminal stages of disease. These patients are severely debilitated, often wheelchair bound with significant limb and respiratory muscle weakness. They have recurrent bouts of mucous plugging, atelectasis, aspiration with subsequent pneumonia secondary to respiratory muscle weakness, abnormal control of breathing, and an impaired cough.

Morbidity and Mortality

Respiratory muscle weakness is a known complication of MS and is identified in patients who are both ambulatory and bedbound. Assessment of muscle function is of critical value so that patients who are at high risk are identified early so that measures can be taken to prevent both upper and lower respiratory tract infections. Although demyelination of respiratory motor tracts is the most common cause of muscle weakness, additional causes such as deconditioning, malnutrition, and steroid-induced myopathy may also play a role.

Mortality data in patients with MS have been conflicting, with some reporting only slightly higher mortality than that of the general population,[12] whereas others report rates three times higher than non-MS cohorts[13] (Figure 13.3). Regardless, almost half of MS deaths are related to respiratory disease[14,15] (Table 13.1). Therefore, general supportive measures

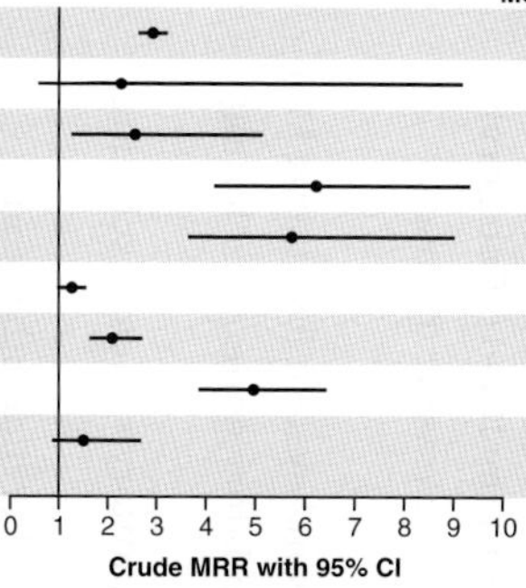

		MR per 1000 patient-years		Crude MRR (95% CI)
		MS cohort	Non-MS cohort	
All causes		10.8	3.7	2.9 (2.7-3.2)
Cardiac/respiratory arrest		0.05	0.02	2.3 (0.6-9.2)
Suicide		0.2	0.07	2.6 (1.3-5.2)
Infections and parasites		0.8	0.1	6.2 (4.2-9.4)
Diseases of the nervous system[a]		0.6	0.1	5.8 (3.7-9.0)
Neoplasms		1.3	1.0	1.2 (1.0-1.6)
Diseases of the circulatory system[b]		1.6	0.8	2.1 (1.7-2.7)
Diseases of the respiratory system[c]		1.9	0.4	5.0 (3.9-6.4)
Injury, poisoning and certain other consequences of external causes[d]		0.3	0.2	1.5 (0.9-2.7)

0 1 2 3 4 5 6 7 8 9 10
Crude MRR with 95% CI

Figure 13.3. Forest plots of crude MRRs for all-cause mortality and selected causes leading to death in the MS cohort versus the non-MS cohort. Error bars indicate 95% confidence intervals (CIs). MR, mortality rate; MRR, mortality rate ratio; MS, multiple sclerosis. [a]excluding MS; [b]excluding cardiac arrest; [c]excluding respiratory arrest; [d]excluding suicide. Reproduced with permission from Capkun G, Dahlke F, Lahoz R, et al. Mortality and comorbidities in patients with multiple sclerosis compared with a population without multiple sclerosis: an observational study using the US Department of Defense administrative claims database. *Mult Scler Relat Disord.* 2015;4(6):546-554. doi:10.1016/j.msard.2015.08.005.

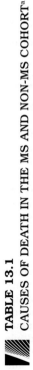

TABLE 13.1
CAUSES OF DEATH IN THE MS AND NON-MS COHORT[a]

	Cause Leading to Death		Primary Underlying Cause of Death		Immediate Cause of Death	
	Mortality Rate Ratio	95% CI	Mortality Rate Ratio	95% CI	Mortality Rate Ratio	95% CI
Causes of Death[b]						
Cardiac/respiratory arrest	2.30	0.58-9.20	1.85	0.58-5.89	3.62	2.76-4.77
Suicide	2.56	1.26-5.16	2.56	1.26-5.16	NA	NA
Other Causes of Death (by ICD-10 Category)[c]						
Certain infectious and parasitic diseases	6.24	4.17-9.36	3.50	1.99-6.16	5.77	3.65-9.13
Neoplasms	1.24	0.97-1.57	1.20	0.96-1.49	1.27	0.99-1.64
Diseases of the nervous system (excluding MS)	5.75	3.66-9.04	6.45	3.68-11.31	2.92	1.67-5.11
Diseases of the circulatory system (excluding cardiac arrest)	2.12	1.68-2.66	1.74	1.36-2.24	1.91	1.48-2.47
Diseases of the respiratory system (excluding respiratory arrest)	4.99	3.86-6.44	2.20	1.47-3.29	4.80	3.64-6.32
Injury, poisoning, and certain other consequences of external causes (excluding suicide)	1.52	0.87-2.68	NA	NA	1.92	1.23-2.97

[a]Of those who died, cause of death data were available for 89.6% of individuals in the MS cohort and 86.6% of individuals in the non-MS cohort. Cause of death data were not available for all patients because of the 2-year delay in NDI reporting.

[b]For MS as a CoD the MRR outcome for each CoD category was NA.

[c]A full list of the conditions in each CoD category is provided in the World Health Organization International Statistical Classification of Diseases and Related Health Problems 10th Revision (World Health Organization, 2010).

Reproduced with permission from Capkun G, Dahlke F, Lahoz R, et al. Mortality and comorbidities in patients with multiple sclerosis compared with a population without multiple sclerosis: an observational study using the US Department of Defense administrative claims database. *Mult Scler Relat Disord.* 2015;4(6):546-554. doi:10.1016/j.msard.2015.08.005.

CI, confidence interval; CoD, cause of death; ICD-10, International Classification of Diseases 10th revision; MRR, mortality rate ratio; MS, multiple sclerosis; NA, not applicable.

such as influenza and pneumococcal vaccinations, cough assist devices, and chest physiotherapy with aggressive suctioning should be instituted early. Additional treatment measures such as respiratory muscle training, although shown to improve respiratory muscle function, have yet to show any clinical benefit such as improved cough efficacy or decreased need for invasive or noninvasive ventilation.[16]

References

1. Howard RS, Wiles CM, Hirsch NP, Loh L. Respiratory involvement in multiple sclerosis. *Brain.* 1992;115:479-494.
2. Gosselink R, Kovacs L, Decramer M. Respiratory muscle involvement in multiple sclerosis. *Eur Respir J.* 1999;13:449e-454e.
3. DeTroyer A, Pride NB. The respiratory system in neuromuscular disorders. In: Roussos C, Macklem PT, eds. *The Thorax: Lung Biology in Health and Disease.* New York: Marcel Dekker; 1985;29:1089-1121.
4. Smeltzer SC, Utell MJ, Rudick RA, Herndon RM. Pulmonary function and dysfunction in multiple sclerosis. *Arch Neurol.* 1988;45:1245-1249.
5. Smeltzer SC, Skurnick JH, Troiano R. Respiratory function in multiple sclerosis: utility of clinical assessment of respiratory muscle function. *Chest.* 1992;101:479-484.
6. Tzelepis G, McCool D. Respiratory dysfunction in multiple sclerosis. *Respir Med.* 2015;109(6):671-679.
7. Man WD, Kyroussis D, Fleming TA, et al. Cough gastric pressure and maximum expiratory mouth pressure in humans. *Am J Respir Crit Care Med.* 2003;168:714e-717e.
8. Tantucci C, Massucci M, Piperno R, Betti L, Grassi V, Sorbini CA. Control of breathing and respiratory muscle strength in patients with multiple sclerosis. *Chest.* 1994;105:1163-1170.
9. Bamer AM, Johnson KL, Amtmann D, et al. Prevalence of sleep problems in individuals with multiple sclerosis. *Mult Scler.* 2008;14:1127e-1130e.
10. Braley TJ, Segal BM, Chervin RD. Sleep-disordered breathing in multiple sclerosis. *Neurology.* 2012;79:929e-936e.
11. Boor JW, Johnson RJ, Canales L. Reversible paralysis of automatic respiration in multiple sclerosis. *Arch Neurol.* 1977;34:686-689.
12. Ragonese P, Aridon P, Salemi G, et al. Mortality in multiple sclerosis: a review. *Eur J Neurol.* 2008;15:123e-127e.
13. Capkun G, Dahlke F, Lahoz R, et al. Mortality and comorbidities in patients with multiple sclerosis compared with a population without multiple sclerosis: an observational study using the US Department of Defense administrative claims database. *Mult Scler Relat Disord.* 2015;4(6):546-554. doi:10.1016/j.msard.2015.08.005.
14. Hirst C, Swingler R, Compston DA, et al. Survival and cause of death in multiple sclerosis: a prospective population-based study. *J Neurol Neurosurg Psychiatry.* 2008;79:1016e-1021e.

15. Phadke JG. Survival pattern and cause of death in patients with multiple sclerosis. *J Neurol Neurosurg Psychiatry*. 1987;50:523-531.
16. Reyes A, Ziman M, Nosaka K. Respiratory muscle training for respiratory deficits in neurodegenerative disorders: a systematic review. *Chest*. 2013;143:1386e-1394e.

14

Public Health Considerations in Multiple Sclerosis

■ ▓ ▓ Nida Naushad, Catherine Stratton, Yetsa A. Tuakli-Wosornu

Introduction

The fundamental goal of public health is to prevent disease; promote physical, mental, and social health; and prolong life at the population level (World Health Organization [WHO]). Chronic diseases such as multiple sclerosis (MS) have wide-reaching population-level impacts, so an understanding of these conditions is a central component of public health science. Today, MS affects approximately 2.5 million people worldwide, and the prevalence of this condition is growing. Given the morbidity and long-term disability associated with MS, which may include weakness, chronic pain, gait disturbance, and bladder dysfunction, it is important to understand the disease from a public health perspective. In this chapter, we discuss:

- Screening and prevention strategies
- Health disparities related to MS
- The socioeconomic impact of MS
- Population-level awareness about MS

Better understanding of these aspects of MS can lead to the creation of programs and policies that promote prevention and early diagnosis,

255

increase access to care and support, and improve overall quality of life for the millions of people living with MS.

Risk Factors

MS is a multifactorial disease, which likely arises as a result of a combination of genetics plus environmental exposures that lead to disease phenotype. Researchers have identified a number of genetic and environmental risk factors, which we also reviewed in our discussion of the epidemiology of MS in Chapter 1 (Table 14.1).

Risk Factors and Interventions

Genetics

In the 1890s, scientists noted a familial aggregation of MS, which led to the question of the role genetic factors played in disease development.[1] It has been concluded that first-degree relatives are at a 15- to 25-fold greater risk of developing MS compared with the general population.[2] A study of half-siblings in Canada found that there was an increased risk of MS among maternal half-siblings versus among paternal half-siblings, which informed how important maternal susceptibility to MS is for inheritance risk.[3] Furthermore, another study investigated a group of

 TABLE 14.1
FACTORS THAT MAY INFLUENCE MS DEVELOPMENT

Genetics (e.g., HLA type)

Gender

Latitude

Month and place of birth

High-salt diet

Gut microbiome

Vitamin D

Psychological or emotional stress

Cigarette smoking

Organic solvents

Obesity

Sex hormones

EBV

Early life infections

EBV, Epstein-Barr virus; HLA, human leukocyte antigen; MS, multiple sclerosis.

interracial marriages in Canada between Caucasians and North American Aboriginals; the study found that index cases with a Caucasian mother and North American Aboriginal father had a higher rate of sibling recurrence versus patients with an Aboriginal mother and a Caucasian father, supporting the role of maternal genetics in MS development.[4]

Sex

Similar to many other autoimmune diseases, MS is more common among women than among men.[5] Incidence rates are rising more quickly among women as well, so recent statistics estimate that the ratio of women to men with MS is 2.3 to 3.5:1.[6] Of note, pregnancy appears to be a protective factor that is associated with lower risk of onset and better prognosis in MS.[7] Despite the greater incidence of disease among women, research suggests that men have an increased likelihood of developing a more severe presentation of disease,[8] follow a more malignant course,[9] and have worse recovery after an initial flare-up in their symptoms.[10]

Epstein-Barr Virus

The Epstein-Barr virus (EBV) is a double-stranded DNA γ-herpesvirus causing lifelong infection in over 90% of the world's adult population.[11] Delayed primary infection with EBV, evidenced by infectious mononucleosis, seems to be an important factor in developing MS.[12] MS is less common among those with early childhood infection, which is often asymptomatic or mild.[13] There is also a low risk of developing MS among those who were never infected.[13] This understanding of EBV has numerous implications for treatment strategies. Studies show that antiviral therapy may reduce relapses or reduce the number of new active brain lesions in some of those affected. One study found that therapy with acyclovir decreased the relapse rate by 34% in patients with relapsing-remitting MS.[11] The apparent relationship between EBV and MS has broader public health implications; researchers have posited the utility of a vaccine against MS or early exposure to EBV as a means of prevention.[13]

Vitamin D Hypothesis

With some exceptions, there is an increased incidence of MS among those living further from the equator. This distribution exists even after accounting for HLA-DRB1 allele frequencies, suggesting that there is an environmental factor associated with latitude, such as ultraviolet (UV) radiation exposure/vitamin D.[14] UV radiation exposure has been associated with reduced MS risk, 20-fold stronger than other environmental factors.[15] However, an unusual relationship is found in northern Scandinavia, where there is a lower MS prevalence in spite of the weak sunlight.[14] Of note, this population has a much higher dietary vitamin D intake than that found in the rest of Europe.[14] A move to encourage increased vitamin D intake (e.g., via supplementation) could be a public health initiative in at-risk populations.

Smoking

Smoking cigarettes and exposure to secondhand smoke have been associated with an increased risk of MS.[16] Duration of exposure to passive smoking was associated with MS risk in a dose-dependent manner among never smokers. Those who reported smoking more than 10 pack-years and exposure to passive smoking for more than 20 years had nearly three times higher risk of developing MS compared with those who reported no exposure to tobacco smoke. Furthermore, smoking is associated with worse MS prognosis, with those who started smoking at a younger age being the most likely to develop progressive disease at an earlier onset.[17] Thus, public health initiatives to decrease rates of smoking may also help improve MS outcomes. The following are examples of programs that promote smoking cessation:

- A multipronged approach, which combines both pharmacotherapy and behavioral support, increases rates of smoking cessation compared with usual care or minimal intervention. A combination intervention seems to increase an individual's chance of quitting by about 10% to 25%.[18]
- Mobile phone–based text message interventions have been shown to reduce smoking rates at 6 months. It should be noted that most of these studies were conducted in high-income countries, and so their generalizability to low-income countries is unclear.[19]
- Programs that utilize incentives appear to increase rates of smoking cessation, while the incentives are in place. Programs that require participants to make a deposit have higher rates of smoking cessation, although they also have lower rates of enrollment.[20]
- Mass media campaigns can be an effective way to promote smoking cessation among the general public. Campaigns that contain information about the negative health effects of smoking seem to be most effective at increasing knowledge, have higher perceived effectiveness ratings, and are most likely to result in quitting behavior.[21]

Obesity

Obesity is associated with an increased MS risk, and that risk is modulated by the level of obesity. There is an increased odds of MS with increasing levels of obesity.[22-24] It is believed that the association between obesity and MS may be stronger among females, as obesity is associated with a significantly increased risk of MS or clinically isolated syndrome in girls but not in boys.[23] The relationship between obesity and MS is particularly important given the childhood obesity epidemic. Thus, initiatives to decrease obesity, such as the following, may also have a positive impact on MS outcomes:

- Behavioral weight management programs that combine both diet and physical activity seem to be more effective in the long term than programs focusing on diet or physical activity alone.[25]
- Programs that aim to prevent childhood obesity are particularly effective if targeting children ages 6 to 12 years.[26] There is moderately strong evidence that school-based interventions are effective for preventing childhood obesity.[27] Programs and policies that may be helpful to reduce childhood obesity include a school curriculum that provides education about healthy eating, physical activity, and body image; increased opportunities for physical activity throughout the school week; more nutrition food in schools; support for teachers and staff to implement health promotion activities; and a home environment that encourages increased activity, more nutritious meals, and less screen time.[26] Community health workers in the home, clinic, school, or community setting may also help improve body mass index among children.[28]
- Modifying the built environment may also positively influence health. Environmental factors that had a greater effect include bans or restriction on unhealthy foods, mandates offering healthier foods, altering rules for food purchased using low-income food vouchers, and improvements to active transportation infrastructure.[29]

Diet

Diet has a significant impact on body weight, cholesterol levels, and other vascular risk factors that affect MS risk and disease course. These include effects mediated by dietary metabolites derived directly from food, dietary induction of metabolite production by gut microbiota, and diet-mediated changes in gut microbial composition. To summarize, some proinflammatory dietary factors that people with MS may want to avoid include saturated fatty acids of animal origin, trans fats, red meat, sweetened drinks, increased dietary salt, cow milk proteins of the milk fat globule membrane (MGFM proteins), and salt.[30] A low-calorie diet rich in vegetables, fruit, legumes, fish, prebiotics, and probiotics is beneficial because it helps upregulate oxidative metabolism, downregulate the synthesis of proinflammatory molecules, and restore or maintain a healthy symbiotic gut microbiota.[30] The Mediterranean diet, which is a diet rich in vegetables, legumes, and fruits; moderate in fish; and low in meat, has been positively correlated with a reduced risk of acquiring MS.[31]

Given this baseline understanding, we have detailed some of the dietary factors that affect MS:

- High salt: It is well established that a diet high in salt increases MS risk. This is because salt can encourage pathogenic T cell responses, which are believed to promote central nervous system autoimmunity.[32] Clinical observations have noted that patients with a high sodium intake tend to present with worse and more frequent radiological disease activity.[33]
- Dairy: The Nurses' Health Study cohorts showed an increased risk for developing MS among women with high intake of whole milk during adolescence.[34] Patients with MS have presented with remarkably heightened T cell responses to milk antigens.[34]
- Fats: The results of studies on the relationship between dietary fat and MS risk are mixed, with one large-scale study showing that dietary fat intake is not linked to an increased risk of MS.[35] In two large cohorts of over 90,000 women enrolled in each study, it was shown that dietary fat intake is not linked to an increased risk of MS. Theoretically, consumption of fatty foods may lead to inflammation, which could lead to worsening MS symptoms.
  - Saturated fats are found in foods such as whole milk, butter, cheese, and meat. They are associated with inflammation and are potentially relevant to MS for this reason.[34] It is also established that saturated fat plays a role in increasing low-density lipoprotein cholesterol, which has been correlated with poor outcomes in MS.[34] Saturated fats directly affect the innate immune system through activation of proinflammatory toll-like receptors.[34]
  - Trans fats were introduced in the 1960s to replace animal fat but are not actually healthy, as they still have deleterious effects on metabolism.[30] Intake is associated with gut inflammation and upregulation of proinflammatory cytokines.
  - Regarding omega 3 fatty acids, a self-reported survey of people with MS has found that those consuming fish more frequently and those taking omega 3 supplements had significantly better quality of life and less disability.[36]
- Fruits and vegetables—Gut microbiota are connected to high-fiber foods. A case control study found protective role for components in plants (fruits/vegetables and grains), including vegetable protein, dietary fiber, cereal fiber, vitamin C, thiamin, riboflavin, calcium, and potassium.[37] This is a public health interest, as it can possibly reduce the incidence and decrease the severity of disease. Among people with MS, healthy consumption of fruit and vegetables and dietary fat predicted better quality of life and less likelihood of higher disability when compared with respondents with a "poor" diet.[38]

Exercise

Exercise can prove to be challenging to patients with MS because of barriers such as pain, frequent medical appointments, and transportation.[39] However, exercise therapy may lead to small but important improvements in walking, balance, cognition, fatigue, depression, and quality of life in MS.[40-42] Given the lack of effective therapeutic strategies for managing the long-term disability associated with MS, exercise training can be an alternative approach.[43]

Air Pollution

There is an association between air pollution and autoimmune diseases, including MS.[44] For example, a cross-sectional study in the state of Georgia found that the best predictive models of MS prevalence in the state included PM-10 for females. Another study found a clustering of prevalence of MS around Atlanta, the largest metropolitan statistical area in Georgia, even after controlling for population distribution, suggesting that another factor such as pollution may be at play.[45] Another study in Tehran, Iran, found that there was a significant difference in exposure to certain air pollutants (PM10, SO_2, NO_2, NO_x) in those with MS compared with controls.[46] The potential relationship between MS and air pollution is important given the urbanization of societies and increased exposure to pollutants. Decreasing exposure to these pollutants has important health implications, including for MS.

Health Disparities

MS causes a host of different problems, including physical disability, fatigue, depression, pain, bladder dysfunction, and more, and requires extensive services. Effective management of MS requires coordination between various medical providers and social services to meet the needs of the patient. However, many people with MS do not receive the appropriate treatment for disease management. For example, when asked about the percentage of qualifying people with MS who received treatment, the average answer was 64% from responding members of the European Union, 45% from Brazil, 50% from Russia, 10% to 15% from Turkey, and less than 5% from India.[47]

There is significant variation in delivery of care based on the resources available locally. Lack of resources is particularly an issue in developing countries, where there may not be a magnetic resonance imaging (MRI) scanner, which is needed for diagnosis; a sufficient number of neurologists; or rehabilitation centers for people with MS.[47] On the bright side, there have been increases in these resources over the years. Between 2008 and 2013, the number of neurologists worldwide increased by 30%, and more emerging countries have acquired MRI machines.[48] However, this increase has not occurred equitably: high-income countries saw an increase of 4.7 new neurologists per 100,000 people, whereas low-income countries only saw 0.4 per 100,000.[48] There are also areas of the United States where it is more difficult to access MS care. Compared with individuals with MS living in urban areas, those living in rural areas are more likely to use a general practitioner rather than a neurologist as their primary physician and they have to travel greater distances to access MS-focused care.[49]

Public health efforts to quantify the resources available in a given region can provide valuable data to motivate governments to initiate change. For example, in 2008, the Multiple Sclerosis Atlas, a joint project of the Multiple Sclerosis International Society and the World Health Organization, found that Ireland had the lowest number of neurologists per head in the European Union. This information was used to advocate for increasing the number of neurologists in the country, and by 2013, the number of neurologists in the country had increased from 14 to 34.[48]

In addition to difficulties accessing MS-specific care, disparities also exist in the management of MS comorbidities. For example:

- Mental health conditions are often underdiagnosed and undertreated among people with MS. This holds particularly true for those with lower socioeconomic status: a lower income is associated with increased odds of depression and increased odds of undiagnosed depression, and a lower education level is associated with increased odds of untreated depression.[50]
- People with MS often have bladder dysfunction that would benefit from special care, although they do not always receive the treatment they need. Those without health insurance have reduced odds of receiving medications for bladder symptoms.[50]
- Individuals with MS commonly have a number of risk factors for osteoporosis, including impaired mobility, limited weight-bearing activity, and low vitamin D levels, which places them at increased risk of fractures. One study of 20 years of a sample of hospital admissions in the United States found that the prevalence of hip fractures among the MS cohort was over two times greater than in the non-MS cohort and those with MS tended to be younger at the time of fracture.[51] Another study found that many people with MS did not take vitamin D or calcium supplements, which are often recommended to improve bone health.[52]

Cost is another source of health disparity among individuals with MS. Those living in low-income countries receive less assistance to fund their MS treatment: 96% of high-income countries partly or fully fund disease-modifying therapies for MS, whereas there is no funding in low-income countries.[48] Even in developed countries, a patient's insurance influences the ability to adhere to recommended treatment. Higher out-of-pocket copayments and coinsurance are associated with less adherence to disease-modifying therapies.[53] Adherence to therapy affects health outcomes, with increased adherence being associated with less risk of relapse, fewer emergency room visits, and fewer inpatient admissions,[54] as well as less medical costs.[55] Thus, strategies that address cost barriers are important to promote the health of those with MS and to reduce cost to the health care system.

Programs that assist patients with managing their therapy may increase treatment adherence. One study showed that a specialty care management program, which consisted of mailed medications, educational materials, and phone calls from a nurse, was associated with increased adherence to therapy, as well as fewer MS-related hospitalizations in the next year and reduced MS-related medical costs.[56]

Additionally, there is a need to better understand the impact of MS on minority populations to deliver better patient-centered care. A persistent challenge in MS treatment is that long-term adherence to treatment is low when compared with other serious, progressive conditions.[57] A more patient-centered approach, which takes into account a patient's cultural beliefs, treatment preferences, and personal values, may help improve patient experience and quality of life among people with MS. Although such information is important, the severity of MS among non-Hispanic African American and Hispanic populations remains grossly underresearched in the literature.[58] Thus, it is necessary to study the experience of MS among minority populations, to address this barrier to providing patient-centered care.

Socioeconomic Disparities

The age of onset for MS is usually between 20 and 40 years; therefore, the disease can result in a substantial loss of productivity for an individual with MS. Many individuals with MS give up their jobs sooner than they would otherwise, and individuals often face a decrease in their standard of living.[59] Factors that influence work capacity include:

- *Symptomatology:* In studies, reported reasons for reducing work hours or becoming unemployed include fatigue, heat sensitivity, cognitive difficulties, and emotional distress.[60,61]
- *Social factors:* A study of 50 individuals with MS found that, compared with those who were unemployed, those who had reduced their work hours had more hours of education and higher occupational prestige.[61]

Caregivers may also face a negative impact on their professional development because of MS.[59]

■ Individuals with MS, both in the United States and globally, face a number of health-related disparities that influence their ability to manage their disease. Certain regions may not have the resources to provide the medical services required to diagnose and treat MS. Even when such resources are available, an individual's socioeconomic and insurance status influence his or her ability to access disease-modifying therapies and treatment for comorbid conditions.

■ Individuals with MS may become underemployed or unemployed as a result of their illness. Programs that provide vocational rehabilitation and training services and employer education regarding MS may be useful.

■ Support organizations provide a variety of services that benefit the individual with MS from advocacy at the government level to support groups to transportation. Currently, there are many countries where no such groups exist, but it would be beneficial to ensure that everyone with MS has access to such groups (see the Appendix for more about patient resources and advocacy).

References

1. Eichhorst H. Über infantile und hereditäre multiple Sklerose. *Arch Pathol Anat Physiol Klin Med.* 1896;146(2):173-192.
2. Dyment DA, Ebers GC, Dessa Sadovnick A. Genetics of multiple sclerosis. *Lancet Neurol.* 2004;3(2):104-110. doi:10.1016/S1474-4422(03)00663-X.
3. Ebers GC, Sadovnick AD, Dyment DA, Yee IML, Willer CJ, Risch N. Parent-of-origin effect in multiple sclerosis: observations in half-siblings. *Lancet.* 2004;363(9423):1773-1774. doi:10.1016/S0140-6736(04)16304-6.
4. Ramagopalan SV, Yee IM, Dyment DA, et al. Parent-of-origin effect in multiple sclerosis. Observations from interracial matings. *Neurology.* 2009;73(8):602-605. doi:10.1212/WNL.0b013e3181af33cf.
5. Compston A, Coles A. Multiple sclerosis. *Lancet.* 2002;359(9313):1221-1231. doi:10.1016/S0140-6736(02)08220-X.
6. Harbo HF, Gold R, Tintoré M. Sex and gender issues in multiple sclerosis. *Ther Adv Neurol Disord.* 2013;6(4):237-248.
7. Runmarker B, Andersen O. Pregnancy is associated with a lower risk of onset and a better prognosis in multiple sclerosis. *Brain.* 1995;118(1):253-261. doi:10.1093/brain/118.1.253.
8. Confavreux C, Compston A. Chapter 4-The natural history of multiple sclerosis. In: Compston A, Confavreux C, Lassmann H, et al, eds. *McAlpine's Multiple Sclerosis.* 4th ed. Edinburgh: Churchill Livingstone; 2006:183-272.
9. Gholipour T, Healy B, Baruch NF, Weiner HL, Chitnis T. Demographic and clinical characteristics of malignant multiple sclerosis. *Neurology.* 2011;76(23):1996-2001. doi:10.1212/WNL.0b013e31821e559d.
10. Scott TF, Schramke CJ. Poor recovery after the first two attacks of multiple sclerosis is associated with poor outcome five years later. *J Neurol Sci.* 2010;292(1):52-56. doi:10.1016/j.jns.2010.02.008.

11. Pender MP, Burrows SR. Epstein-Barr virus and multiple sclerosis: potential opportunities for immunotherapy. *Clin Transl Immunology.* 2014;3(10):e27. doi:10.1038/cti.2014.25.

12. Hernan MA, Zhang SM, Lipworth L, Olek MJ, Ascherio A. Multiple sclerosis and age at infection with common viruses. *Epidemiology.* 2011;12(3):301-306.

13. Thacker EL, Mirzaei F, Ascherio A. Infectious mononucleosis and risk for multiple sclerosis: a meta-analysis. *Ann Neurol.* 2006;59(3):499-503. doi:10.1002/ana.20820.

14. Simpson S, Blizzard L, Otahal P, Van der Mei I, Taylor B. Latitude is significantly associated with the prevalence of multiple sclerosis: a meta-analysis. *J Neurol Neurosurg Psychiatry.* 2011;82(10):1132-1141. doi:10.1136/jnnp.2011.240432.

15. Harandi AA, Harandi AA, Pakdaman H, Sahraian MA. Vitamin D and multiple sclerosis. *Iran J Neurol.* 2014;13(1):1.

16. Hedström AK, Hillert J, Olsson T, Alfredsson L. Smoking and multiple sclerosis susceptibility. *Eur J Epidemiol.* 2013;28(11):867-874.

17. Sundström P, Nyström L. Smoking worsens the prognosis in multiple sclerosis. *Mult Scler.* 2008;14(8):1031-1035.

18. Stead LF, Koilpillai P, Lancaster T. Additional behavioural support as an adjunct to pharmacotherapy for smoking cessation. *Cochrane Database Syst Rev.* 2015;(10).

19. Whittaker R, McRobbie H, Bullen C, Rodgers A, Gu Y. Mobile Phone-based interventions for smoking cessation. *Cochrane Database Syst Rev.* 2016:CD006611.

20. Cahill K, Hartmann-Boyce J, Perera R. Incentives for smoking cessation. *Cochrane Database Syst Rev.* 2015;(5):CD004307.

21. Durkin S, Brennan E, Wakefield M. Mass media campaigns to promote smoking cessation among adults: an integrative review. *Tob Control.* 2012;21(2):127-138.

22. Hedström AK, Olsson T, Alfredsson L. High body mass index before age 20 is associated with increased risk for multiple sclerosis in both men and women. *Mult Scler.* 2012;18(9):1334-1336.

23. Langer-Gould A, Brara SM, Beaber BE, Koebnick C. Childhood obesity and risk of pediatric multiple sclerosis and clinically isolated syndrome. *Neurology.* 2013;80(6):548-552. doi:10.1212/WNL.0b013e31828154f3.

24. Munger KL, Bentzen J, Laursen B, et al. Childhood body mass index and multiple sclerosis risk: a long-term cohort study. *Mult Scler.* 2013; 19(10):1323-1329.

25. Johns DJ, Hartmann-Boyce J, Jebb SA, Aveyard P. Diet or exercise interventions vs combined behavioral weight management programs: a systematic review and meta-analysis of direct comparisons. *J Acad Nutr Diet.* 2014;114(10):1557-1568. doi:10.1016/j.jand.2014.07.005.

26. Waters E, de Silva-Sanigorski A, Burford BJ, et al. Interventions for preventing obesity in children. *Sao Paulo Med J.* 2014;132(2):128-129.

27. Wang Y, Cai L, Wu Y, et al. What childhood obesity prevention programmes work? A systematic review and meta-analysis. *Obes Rev.* 2015;16(7):547-565. doi:10.1111/obr.12277.

28. Schroeder K, McCormick R, Perez A, Lipman T. The role and impact of community health workers in childhood obesity interventions: a systematic review and meta-analysis. *Obes Rev.* 2018;19(10):1371-1384.

29. Mayne SL, Auchincloss AH, Michael YL. Impact of policy and built environment changes on obesity-related outcomes: a systematic review of naturally occurring experiments. *Obes Rev.* 2015;16(5):362-375. doi:10.1111/obr.12269.

30. Riccio P, Rossano R. Nutrition facts in multiple sclerosis. *ASN Neuro.* 2015;7(1):1759091414568185.

31. Sedaghat F, Jessri M, Behrooz M, Mirghotbi M, Rashidkhani B. Mediterranean diet adherence and risk of multiple sclerosis: a case-control study. *Asia Pac J Clin Nutr.* 2016;25(2):377-384.

32. Hucke S, Wiendl H, Klotz L. Implications of dietary salt intake for multiple sclerosis pathogenesis. *Mult Scler.* 2016;22(2):133-139. doi:10.1177/1352458515609431.

33. Farez MF, Fiol MP, Gaitan MI, Quintana FJ, Correale J. Sodium intake is associated with increased disease activity in multiple sclerosis. *J Neurol Neurosurg Psychiatry.* 2015;86(1):26-31. doi:10.1136/jnnp-2014-307928.

34. Katz Sand I. The role of diet in multiple sclerosis: mechanistic connections and current evidence. *Curr Nutr Rep.* 2018;7(3):150-160. doi:10.1007/s13668-018-0236-z.

35. Zhang SM, Willett WC, Hernan MA, Olek MJ, Ascherio A. Dietary fat in relation to risk of multiple sclerosis among two large cohorts of women. *Am J Epidemiol.* 2000;152(11):1056-1064.

36. Jelinek GA, Hadgkiss EJ, Weiland TJ, Pereira NG, Marck CH, van der Meer DM. Association of fish consumption and omega 3 supplementation with quality of life, disability and disease activity in an international cohort of people with multiple sclerosis. *Int J Neurosci.* 2013;123(11):792-801. doi:10.3109/00207454.2013.803104.

37. Ghadirian P, Jain M, Ducic S, Shatenstein B, Morisset R. Nutritional factors in the aetiology of multiple sclerosis: a case-control study in Montreal, Canada. *Int J Epidemiol.* 1998;27(5):845-852.

38. Hadgkiss EJ, Jelinek GA, Weiland TJ, Pereira NG, Marck CH, van der Meer DM. The association of diet with quality of life, disability, and relapse rate in an international sample of people with multiple sclerosis. *Nutr Neurosci.* 2015;18(3):125-136. doi:10.1179/1476830514Y.0000000117.

39. Pilutti LA, Edwards TA. Is exercise training beneficial in progressive multiple sclerosis? *Int J MS Care.* 2017;19(2):105-112.

40. Halabchi F, Alizadeh Z, Sahraian MA, Abolhasani M. Exercise prescription for patients with multiple sclerosis; potential benefits and practical recommendations. *BMC Neurol.* 2017;17(1):185. doi:10.1186/s12883-017-0960-9.

41. Heine M, van de Port I, Rietberg MB, van Wegen EE, Kwakkel G. Exercise therapy for fatigue in multiple sclerosis. *Cochrane Database Syst Rev.* 2015;(9):CD009956. doi:10.1002/14651858.CD009956.pub2.

42. Motl RW, Sandroff BM. Benefits of exercise training in multiple sclerosis. *Curr Neurol Neurosci Rep.* 2015;15(9):62. doi:10.1007/s11910-015-0585-6.

43. Edwards T, Pilutti LA. The effect of exercise training in adults with multiple sclerosis with severe mobility disability: a systematic review and future research directions. *Mult Scler Relat Disord.* 2017;16:31-39. doi:10.1016/j.msard.2017.06.003.

44. Gawda A, Majka G, Nowak B, Marcinkiewicz J. Air pollution, oxidative stress, and exacerbation of autoimmune diseases. *Cent Eur J Immunol.* 2017;42(3):305-312. doi:10.5114/ceji.2017.70975.

45. Gregory AC II, Shendell DG, Okosun IS, Gieseker KE. Multiple sclerosis disease distribution and potential impact of environmental air pollutants in Georgia. *Sci Total Environ.* 2008;396(1):42-51. doi:10.1016/j.scitotenv.2008.01.065.

46. Heydarpour P, Amini H, Khoshkish S, Seidkhani H, Sahraian MA, Yunesian M. Potential impact of air pollution on multiple sclerosis in Tehran, Iran. *Neuroepidemiology.* 2014;43(3-4):233-238. doi:10.1159/000368553.

47. World Health Organization. *European Action Plan for Strengthening Public Health Capacities and Services.* Copenhagen: Regional Committee for Europe; 2012.

48. Browne P, Chandraratna D, Angood C, et al. Atlas of multiple sclerosis 2013: a growing global problem with widespread inequity. *Neurology.* 2014;83(11):1022-1024.

49. Buchanan RJ, Wang S, Stuifbergen A, Chakravorty BJ, Zhu L, Kim M. Urban/rural differences in the use of physician services by people with multiple sclerosis. *NeuroRehabilitation.* 2006;21(3):177-187.

50. Marrie RA, Horwitz R, Cutter G, Tyry T, Campagnolo D, Vollmer T. The burden of mental comorbidity in multiple sclerosis: frequent, underdiagnosed, and undertreated. *Mult Scler.* 2009;15(3):385-392.

51. Bhattacharya RK, Vaishnav N, Dubinsky RM. Is there an increased risk of hip fracture in multiple sclerosis? Analysis of the Nationwide Inpatient Sample. *J Multidiscip Healthc.* 2014;7:119-122. doi:10.2147/JMDH.S54786.

52. Marrie RA, Cutter G, Tyry T, Vollmer T. A cross-sectional study of bone health in multiple sclerosis. *Neurology.* 2009;73(17):1394-1398.

53. Menzin J, Caon C, Nichols C, White LA, Friedman M, Pill MW. Narrative review of the literature on adherence to disease-modifying therapies among patients with multiple sclerosis. *J Manag Care Pharm.* 2013;19(1 suppl A):S24-S40. doi:10.18553/jmcp.2013.19.s1.S24.

54. Steinberg SC, Faris RJ, Chang CF, Chan A, Tankersley MA. Impact of adherence to interferons in the treatment of multiple sclerosis: a non-experimental, retrospective, cohort study. *Clin Drug Investig.* 2010;30(2):89-100. doi:10.2165/11533330-000000000-00000.

55. Tan H, Cai Q, Agarwal S, Stephenson JJ, Kamat S. Impact of adherence to disease-modifying therapies on clinical and economic outcomes among patients with multiple sclerosis. *Adv Ther.* 2011;28(1):51-61. doi:10.1007/s12325-010-0093-7.

56. Tan H, Yu J, Tabby D, Devries A, Singer J. Clinical and economic impact of a specialty care management program among patients with multiple sclerosis: a cohort study. *Mult Scler.* 2010;16(8):956-963. doi:10.1177/1352458510373487.

57. Carlin CS, Higuera L, Anderson S. Improving patient-centered care by assessing patient preferences for multiple sclerosis disease-modifying agents: a stated-choice experiment. *Perm J.* 2017;21.

58. Amezcua L, Rivas E, Joseph S, Zhang J, Liu L. Multiple sclerosis mortality by race/ethnicity, age, sex, and time period in the United States, 1999-2015. *Neuroepidemiology.* 2018;50(1-2):35-40.

59. Hakim EA, Bakheit AM, Bryant TN, et al. The social impact of multiple sclerosis–a study of 305 patients and their relatives. *Disabil Rehabil.* 2000;22(6):288-293.

60. Flensner G, Landtblom AM, Söderhamn O, Ek AC. Work capacity and health-related quality of life among individuals with multiple sclerosis reduced by fatigue: a cross-sectional study. *BMC Public Health.* 2013;13:224.

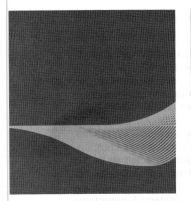
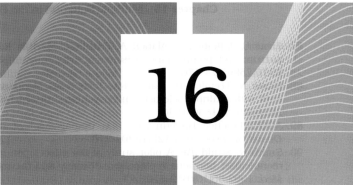

16

Urologic Issues in the Multiple Sclerosis Patient

◼◼◼ Philip J. Aliotta

Introduction

Multiple sclerosis (MS) is an autoimmune inflammatory disease that results in damage to the myelin sheaths of the nerves in the central nervous system.[1] It presents with a broad spectrum of clinical presentations that are time and disease course related. MS plaque (intracranial and/or spinal) location is a key feature in the pathophysiology of disease-related lower urinary tract symptoms (LUTS).[2] It is commonly diagnosed between the ages of 20 and 40 years, with a female predominance of 3:1.[1,2] The prevalence in the United States is 57.8 per 100,000 and is twice as common in the north as compared with the southern United States.[3] About 80% to 96% of all patients with MS will seek urologic care because of bothersome LUTS at some point in their disease course, and as many as 12% have symptoms before the actual diagnosis.[4,5] If a patient has ambulatory difficulties, the prevalence of lower urinary tract complaints is close to 100%.[6,7] The 2005 North American Research Committee on Multiple Sclerosis (NARCOMS) reported that 65% of patient responders experienced at least one moderate to severe urinary symptom.[8] Patients with bladder dysfunction have lower scores on quality-of-life scales.[9] There is also noted to be a greater burden on professional or family caregivers associated with urinary disorders.[10] Access to treatment is uncertain

292

45. Gregory AC II, Shendell DG, Okosun IS, Gieseker KE. Multiple sclerosis disease distribution and potential impact of environmental air pollutants in Georgia. *Sci Total Environ.* 2008;396(1):42-51. doi:10.1016/j.scitotenv.2008.01.065.
46. Heydarpour P, Amini H, Khoshkish S, Seidkhani H, Sahraian MA, Yunesian M. Potential impact of air pollution on multiple sclerosis in Tehran, Iran. *Neuroepidemiology.* 2014;43(3-4):233-238. doi:10.1159/000368553.
47. World Health Organization. *European Action Plan for Strengthening Public Health Capacities and Services.* Copenhagen: Regional Committee for Europe; 2012.
48. Browne P, Chandraratna D, Angood C, et al. Atlas of multiple sclerosis 2013: a growing global problem with widespread inequity. *Neurology.* 2014;83(11):1022-1024.
49. Buchanan RJ, Wang S, Stuifbergen A, Chakravorty BJ, Zhu L, Kim M. Urban/rural differences in the use of physician services by people with multiple sclerosis. *NeuroRehabilitation.* 2006;21(3):177-187.
50. Marrie RA, Horwitz R, Cutter G, Tyry T, Campagnolo D, Vollmer T. The burden of mental comorbidity in multiple sclerosis: frequent, underdiagnosed, and undertreated. *Mult Scler.* 2009;15(3):385-392.
51. Bhattacharya RK, Vaishnav N, Dubinsky RM. Is there an increased risk of hip fracture in multiple sclerosis? Analysis of the Nationwide Inpatient Sample. *J Multidiscip Healthc.* 2014;7:119-122. doi:10.2147/JMDH.S54786.
52. Marrie RA, Cutter G, Tyry T, Vollmer T. A cross-sectional study of bone health in multiple sclerosis. *Neurology.* 2009;73(17):1394-1398.
53. Menzin J, Caon C, Nichols C, White LA, Friedman M, Pill MW. Narrative review of the literature on adherence to disease-modifying therapies among patients with multiple sclerosis. *J Manag Care Pharm.* 2013;19(1 suppl A):S24-S40. doi:10.18553/jmcp.2013.19.s1.S24.
54. Steinberg SC, Faris RJ, Chang CF, Chan A, Tankersley MA. Impact of adherence to interferons in the treatment of multiple sclerosis: a non-experimental, retrospective, cohort study. *Clin Drug Investig.* 2010;30(2):89-100. doi:10.2165/11533330-000000000-00000.
55. Tan H, Cai Q, Agarwal S, Stephenson JJ, Kamat S. Impact of adherence to disease-modifying therapies on clinical and economic outcomes among patients with multiple sclerosis. *Adv Ther.* 2011;28(1):51-61. doi:10.1007/s12325-010-0093-7.
56. Tan H, Yu J, Tabby D, Devries A, Singer J. Clinical and economic impact of a specialty care management program among patients with multiple sclerosis: a cohort study. *Mult Scler.* 2010;16(8):956-963. doi:10.1177/1352458510373487.
57. Carlin CS, Higuera L, Anderson S. Improving patient-centered care by assessing patient preferences for multiple sclerosis disease-modifying agents: a stated-choice experiment. *Perm J.* 2017;21.
58. Amezcua L, Rivas E, Joseph S, Zhang J, Liu L. Multiple sclerosis mortality by race/ethnicity, age, sex, and time period in the United States, 1999-2015. *Neuroepidemiology.* 2018;50(1-2):35-40.
59. Hakim EA, Bakheit AM, Bryant TN, et al. The social impact of multiple sclerosis–a study of 305 patients and their relatives. *Disabil Rehabil.* 2000;22(6):288-293.
60. Flensner G, Landtblom AM, Söderhamn O, Ek AC. Work capacity and health-related quality of life among individuals with multiple sclerosis reduced by fatigue: a cross-sectional study. *BMC Public Health.* 2013;13:224.

61. Smith MM, Arnett PA. Factors related to employment status changes in individuals with multiple sclerosis. *Mult Scler.* 2005;11(5):602-609.
62. Wakefield JR, Bickley S, Sani F. The effects of identification with a support group on the mental health of people with multiple sclerosis. *J Psychosom Res.* 2013;74(5):420-426.

Multiple Sclerosis in the Female Patient

■ ▨ ▧ Tracy B. Grossman, Kathy C. Matthews

A 27-year-old woman presents to you for her yearly gynecologic examinations. She says she has been feeling more tired than usual and sometimes has vision problems. She also mentions that her husband thinks she is clumsier than usual, although she thinks he is exaggerating. She tells you that they have been attempting to conceive over the last year, and although she is trying to be patient, she is concerned that she has not yet gotten pregnant.

Putting together all of her symptoms, you refer her to a neurologist who diagnoses her with multiple sclerosis (MS). She gets placed on medications to help control her disease, and soon enough, she starts feeling much better and her symptoms are mostly resolved. She calls you to ask about getting pregnant. She is scared that the medications she is taking are not safe for pregnancy and also afraid that she will have trouble getting pregnant now that her periods are less regular than they used to be. On top of that, she is worried because most of the time she is not in the mood for sex but is doing it just to try to get pregnant. This is putting a strain on her relationship.

How do you counsel this patient about how MS can affect her fertility, menstrual cycle, pregnancy, and sexual functioning? What medications can she use in pregnancy, and what medications are not considered safe?

271

MS and the Early Reproductive Years

Menses

Many studies have demonstrated important hormonal changes in women with MS. These changes affect the pattern of the menstrual cycle and, subsequently, fertility and sexual functioning. Patients with MS have significantly higher follicle-stimulating hormone and luteinizing hormone levels but lower estrogen levels in the early follicle phase of the menstrual cycle.[1,2] These hormonal changes can cause menstrual cycle irregularities. Additionally, some studies have found that about half of women with MS have worsened symptoms or relapse onset during the premenstrual or menstrual period.[3] Hormonal changes observed in women with MS may account for this exacerbation of symptoms. Specifically, progesterone increases nerve conduction speed by reducing sodium/potassium ATPase,[4] and elevated estrogen and progesterone levels after ovulation cause increased Th-2 anti-inflammatory cytokine production.[5] It has been theorized that the precipitous decline in estrogen and progesterone levels after ovulation, in the premenstrual period, may account for worsening of symptoms and symptom onset.[6] Of note, medications such as cyclophosphamide can cause premature ovarian failure and bring about early menopause in these patients.[7]

Sexual Dysfunction

Women with MS can have complex issues involving psychosocial, sexual, and family relationships, which often happens with chronic illness. They often are taking multiple medications, with side effects that can affect mood and libido and incite physical symptoms such as decreased vaginal lubrication.[1,2,8] One study utilizing a Multiple Sclerosis Intimacy and Sexuality Questionnaire found that 80.4% of the 35 patients with relapsing-remitting MS experienced primary sexual dysfunction, with decreased libido being the most frequent complaint.[8] Another study using the Female Sexual Function Index questionnaire analyzed both hormone levels in relation to sexual dysfunction in patients with MS. Of the 54 women with MS, more than half (57.4%) manifested at least one sexual dysfunction and 36.4% exhibited abnormal hormone alterations, the most common being low 17 beta-estradiol (40%). The study could not find any statistical significance between hormone abnormalities and sexual dysfunction.[2]

Sexual dysfunction among patients with MS can be considered multifactorial, and therefore, it can be very challenging to treat. Sadly, studies have shown that only a small percentage of patients with MS seek treatment for sexual dysfunction.[9] Possible interventions include counseling, psychotherapy, lubricants, and medications. It is important to emphasize that sexual dysfunction can be an inciting cause of, or occur in conjunction with, depression and associated mood disorders. Treatment for mood disorders can also have a side effect of decreasing libido and lubrication, which only exacerbates the problem. Providers should carefully screen for symptoms of sexual dysfunction in patients with MS, because few patients will come forward asking for treatment for this issue, and it can have a major impact on mental health and psychosocial functioning.[10]

Fertility Concerns and Infertility Treatment

Fertility does not appear to be decreased in women with MS.[11] This is evidenced by the fact that pregnant patients with MS, which is an illness typically diagnosed during a woman's reproductive years, are well represented in MS clinical trials.[12] However, international studies have shown that patients with MS have fewer children and are more likely to seek assisted reproductive technology (ART) services.[13,14] This may be at least partially due to higher rates of hyperprolactinemia, decreased estrogen levels, and thyroid disorders, which patients with MS are at increased risk for because these disorders are also typically autoimmune in nature.[1,15,16] Sexual dysfunction, such as decreased libido, vaginal sensory abnormalities, and insufficient lubrication, which can occur early in the course of MS, can also interfere with fertility. Some treatments for MS, such as interferon beta and mitoxantrone, have been associated with menstrual irregularities, which can impact fertility.[8,15,17]

Several studies have shown that ART has been associated with an increased risk of MS relapse, especially in the first 12 weeks after unsuccessful cycle attempts.[17-19] Some studies have shown that the risk of relapse is greater when using gonadotropin-releasing hormone (GnRH) agonists for hormonal downregulation. This may be because GnRH can stimulate the proliferation of immune cells and increase cytokine and endothelial-growth factor production.[20] Rapid hormonal fluctuations, the stress of undergoing fertility treatment, and possibly an interruption in MS therapy owing to the risk of teratogenicity also predispose patients with MS undergoing ART to relapse.[12] One study by Correale et al followed 16 women with relapsing-remitting MS prospectively during 26 ART cycles. There was a ninefold increase in the risk of new brain lesions on magnetic resonance imaging (MRI) and a sevenfold increase in the risk of new brain lesions on MRI in the 3 months after ART.[21] All of the patients in this study were taking GNRH agonists. However, studies analyzing different hormonal treatments during ART cycles have not consistently shown that GNRH agonists have increased rates of MS relapse compared with other hormonal treatments. For example, retrospective case series in Germany did not find a higher rate of relapse in GNRH-agonist ART cycles vs the use of other hormonal treatments,[20,22] whereas reproductive case series performed in France showed increased rates of relapse in the 3 months following ART in patients with MS treated with GNRH-agonists.[21,23]

There is no consensus among ART providers and neurologists as to what hormonal treatments to use and what disease-modifying therapies should be employed or stopped during fertility treatment. Patients with MS should be thoroughly counseled about the risk of relapse with ART treatment, and as with most chronic medical illnesses, disease stabilization before initiating fertility treatment is advisable.[12]

Preconception Management of Medications

As of June 2015, the US Food and Drug Administration (FDA) has removed the categorization of medications in pregnancy and instituted a system of prescription labeling that includes more about the evidenced-based risks of the medication (FDA). Most studies about the safety of disease-modifying treatments in pregnancy are animal studies that use higher doses of medications than are typically used in humans. Medications that have positive safety profiles in pregnancy are interferon beta and glatiramer, which are immunomodulators that are used to prevent the occurrence of relapses and to delay disability.[3,12] These medications, if used before pregnancy, may be continued in pregnancy; however, owing to lack of data with regards their safety in pregnancy, these medications are only used up until the time of conception and then stopped once the patient is pregnant. Natalizumab is a monoclonal antibody that is often used for the treatment of relapsing forms of MS. Current recommendations are that it be discontinued before pregnancy, although it has been used to treat patients during pregnancy in special circumstances.[3,12]

Although there are several disease-modifying drugs for MS, most clinicians recommend discontinuing these medications, if possible, when planning for pregnancy. These medications are discussed in the next section.

MS and Pregnancy

Hormonal Changes in Pregnancy

It is not surprising that the marked hormonal transition and transient immunological tolerance of pregnancy modifies the course and disease activity of MS.

Many animal studies have evaluated the hormonal effects of estrogens (17β-estradiol-E2 and estriol-E3), progesterone, and testosterone in MS. These hormones are thought to provide anti-inflammatory and neuroprotective effects on experimental allergic encephalomyelitis.[24,25] The anti-inflammatory effects appear to be mediated by estrogen nuclear receptors alpha (ERα) and beta (ERβ), which are expressed by regulatory CD4+CD25+ T cells, regulatory B cells, and dendritic cells. E2 neuroprotective effects on experimental allergic encephalomyelitis seem to be mediated by binding to the membrane G-protein-coupled receptor 30 (GPR30). Progesterone appears to play a role in axonal protection and remyelination. Testosterone is thought to work by either binding to androgen receptors or after its conversion to estrogen, through estrogen receptors or GPR30. It can restore synaptic transmission deficits in the hippocampus. Additionally, androgens may induce remyelination by acting on neural androgen receptors.[26-28] As a result, current research efforts are aimed at studying hormones as therapeutic agents, which may have implications for add-on therapy.

MRI During Pregnancy

MRI is widely used for the diagnosis and monitoring of MS. It significantly surpasses other imaging modalities with respect to its positive predictive value.[29-31] MRI is also used in pregnancy for maternal assessment and fetal prenatal diagnosis. Its use is often times avoided in the first trimester because of theoretical risks associated with an increase in body temperature and acoustic noise exposure to a developing fetus. However, when indicated and necessary, MRI should be used regardless of gestational age. The use of gadolinium-contrast agents is generally avoided in pregnancy, mainly because of a lack of safety data in humans.[30]

Vitamin D During Pregnancy

Vitamin D deficiency has been linked to the development of MS in offspring by two distinct mechanisms—autoimmunity with an increase in proinflammatory T cell populations and lipid effect on myelinogenesis.[32] In a recent Finnish study, Munger et al compared maternal vitamin D levels during pregnancy with those of controls. The authors found that offspring of mothers with hypovitaminosis D during their pregnancy had a nearly twofold increase in risk of developing MS when compared with children born to mothers with nondeficient levels. One limitation of this study was the relatively young cohort of children, ranging from 18 to 27 years of age, which may have contributed to an inflated relative risk because the average age of MS diagnosis is 30 years.[33] A dietary study performed in the United States found a similar association, although two smaller Swedish studies did not.[34-36]

Medications During Pregnancy

Fortunately, relapse, which is defined as a worsening of neurologic symptoms lasting more than 24 hours,[12] is less likely to occur in pregnancy.

However, glucocorticoids can be used to reduce the severity and duration of relapses during pregnancy. Corticosteroids, which are often used in pregnancy to treat other autoimmune diseases such as systemic lupus nephritis and rheumatoid arthritis, are generally considered safe in pregnancy. Short-term, high-dose regimens are recommended, because prolonged glucocorticoid exposure can cause neonatal adrenal suppression and maternal glucose intolerance and increase the risk of preterm delivery and premature rupture of membranes.[7] If a relapse occurs in the first trimester, the preferred treatment is prednisolone, as it is inactivated in the placenta and therefore fetal passage is much less than with dexamethasone. Primary or secondary progressive MS was previously treated with immunosuppressants such as cyclophosphamide or methotrexate. These medications are contraindicated in pregnancy because of their teratogenicity and associated adverse pregnancy outcomes and are not commonly used. The only FDA-approved treatment for primary progressive MS is ocrelizumab, which is a monoclonal antibody with limited safety data in pregnancy.[37]

Medications that are not recommended in pregnancy owing to teratogenicity concerns include fingolimod, alemtuzumab, mitoxantrone, ocrelizumab, and teriflunomide. Most physicians recommend that women discontinue treatment with these disease-modifying drugs for MS before attempting to conceive, and often times a "washout" period is recommended before attempting conception. The length of time recommended for these medications to wash out before attempting conception differs according to the medication type. For example, most providers recommend that a patient wait 4 months after alemtuzumab and a 6-month washout period is recommended for rituximab and ocrelizumab. For teriflunomide, patients who are attempting to conceive undergo an elimination procedure, which involves taking cholestyramine or activated charcoal for up to 2 weeks. Of note, men taking teriflunomide and attempting to conceive with a partner are advised not to be on this medication during that period. See Table 15.1 for the washout periods for commonly used medications.

A systematic review of disease-modifying MS therapies during pregnancy, by Lu et al, found associated pregnancy outcomes with several commonly used medications. The study found that interferon beta exposure was associated with lower birthweight and preterm delivery but not with any congenital anomalies. Glatiramer acetate exposure did not have any adverse effects on birthweight or gestational age at delivery and also did not have any associated congenital anomalies. Natalizumab was also not found to have any associated adverse effects on neonates.[41] See Table 15.1 for a list of the most common MS medications and their current pregnancy-related advisories. Importantly, in 2015, the FDA discontinued the use of pregnancy risk categories (A, B, C, D, X) and it has been replaced by the

TABLE 15.1

RECOMMENDED WASHOUT PERIODS FOR VARIOUS DISEASE-MODIFYING THERAPIES BEFORE ATTEMPTING PREGNANCY[38-40]

Disease-Modifying Drug	Washout Period (months)
Glatiramer acetate	0
Interferons	0-1
Dimethyl fumarate	0-1
Natalizumab	1-3
Fingolimod	2
Alemtuzumab	4
Ocrelizumab	6
Rituximab	6
Teriflunomide	Requires a washout protocol using oral cholestyramine or activated charcoal to reduce plasma level to <0.02 mg/L

FDA Pregnancy and Lactation Labeling Rule (PLLR). This rule requires narrative text to describe risk information, clinical considerations, and background data for the drug. Examples of these narratives are included in Table 15.2.[42]

Symptom Management During Pregnancy

Although it is generally recommended that most MS medications be tapered or discontinued in pregnancy, patients may still experience symptoms that interfere with daily life and therefore require treatment. For example, issues with chronic pain, neuropathy, muscle spasticity, and specific neurologic issues such as seizures and trigeminal neuralgia, which is characterized by recurrent episodes of sudden, severe stabbing pain in the distribution of the fifth cranial nerve, may necessitate continuation of medical treatment during pregnancy.[12] Although safety data in pregnancy are limited, chronic pain and neuropathy have been treated during pregnancy with short courses of opioid medications or gabapentin[44-47] and trigeminal neuralgia can be treated with carbamazepine or baclofen.[48] If the patient needs chronic opioid medication, a discussion regarding neonatal concerns, such as need for respiratory support and treatment for neonatal symptoms of withdrawal, as well as prolonged stay in the neonatal intensive care unit, should be had with the patient.[49-52] In case reports, baclofen and tizanidine, which are both muscle relaxants, have been used to treat muscle spasms in pregnant patients[53,54] and no adverse pregnancy outcomes have been reported, although human data largely are unavailable.[55]

TABLE 15.2

PREGNANCY PRECAUTIONS AND MECHANISMS FOR COMMONLY USED DISEASE-MODIFYING MS MEDICATIONS[43]

Medication	Mechanism of Action	Pregnancy Precautions
Glatiramer acetate	T cell activation	Based on animal studies, no increased risk of congenital anomalies. Case reports of successful pregnancies in humans
Interferon-beta-1a, beta-1b	Cytokine that modulates immune responsiveness	Interferons at high exposure levels have been shown to cause adverse pregnancy outcomes in animal studies, but there are case reports of successful pregnancy in humans. Not adequate data in humans
Natalizumab	Monoclonal antibody	Not adequate data in humans, but based on animal data, may cause fetal harm, but not associated with congenital anomalies. May be associated with increased risk of miscarriage
Alemtuzumab	Monoclonal antibody	Not adequate data in humans, but based on animal data, may cause fetal harm
Ocrelizumab	Monoclonal antibody	Not adequate data in humans, but based on animal data, may cause fetal harm. In some humans, has been found to cause lymphocytopenia in neonates
Rituximab	Monoclonal antibody	Not adequate data in humans, but based on animal data, may cause fetal harm. In some humans, has been found to cause lymphocytopenia in neonates and is associated with preterm delivery
Mitoxantrone	Inhibits DNA and RNA synthesis	Not adequate data in humans, but based on animal data, may cause fetal harm. No controlled studies on pregnancy effects
Dimethyl fumarate	Immunomodulator	No adequate human data. Found toxic to animal embryos at very high levels (three times higher than dose used in humans)
Teriflunomide	Immunomodulator, anti-inflammatory	Based on animal data, may cause major birth defects. Contraindicated in pregnancy. However, there are also reports of normal human infants born after exposure

TABLE 15.2

PREGNANCY PRECAUTIONS AND MECHANISMS FOR COMMONLY USED DISEASE-MODIFYING MS MEDICATIONS[43] **(CONTINUED)**

Medication	Mechanism of Action	Pregnancy Precautions
Fingolimod	Anti-inflammatory	Not adequate data in humans, but based on animal data, may cause fetal harm. Associated with decreased fetal viability and caused malformations in animals at doses lower than those used clinically
Cyclophosphamide	Alkylating agent, decreases DNA synthesis	Cyclophosphamide has been associated in experimental animal studies and human case reports with adverse effects on fertility and embryo development
Glucocorticoids (e.g., prednisolone, dexamethasone)	Anti-inflammatory	Considered safe in pregnancy. Small association found with use and fetal facial clefts (OR, 1.16) but not reproduced in all studies
Azathioprine	Blocks DNA synthesis	Most studies did not find azathioprine-associated risk of congenital anomalies after pregnancy exposure; however, one study found an increase in atrial and ventricular septal defects and in preterm delivery. Neonatal hematologic and immune impairment were reported in some exposed infants
IV immunoglobulin	Immunomodulator	Limited human data but based on animal studies, no increased risk of fetal anomalies

IV, intravenous; MS, multiple sclerosis; OR, odds ratio.

There have been case reports of good pregnancy outcomes with intrathecal administration of baclofen in patients with MS.[56] Antiepileptic medications that have been used in pregnancy are lamotrigine, carbamazepine, and levetiracetam, which can also be used to treat other neurologic and psychiatric disorders as well as prevent seizures.[57] Antidepressants that are commonly used in pregnancy but carry an increased risk of persistent pulmonary hypertension of the newborn include selective serotonin reuptake inhibitors (SSRIs), such as citalopram, escitalopram, and fluoxetine, and norepinephrine-dopamine reuptake inhibitors, such as buproprion.[58] There has been a concern about congenital cardiac defects with the use of SSRIs, but studies have shown that the increase in risk of cardiac defects is not substantial.[59] Discontinuation of antiepileptic and antidepressant medications can cause the recurrence of seizures and an exacerbation of depression, respectively, which can be detrimental not only to the pregnant mother but also to the developing fetus. Additionally, owing to an increase in total body fluid volumes and enhanced glomerular filtration in pregnancy, drug levels need to be monitored carefully and doses need to be adjusted accordingly.[60-62]

Treatment of Relapse in Pregnancy

Pregnancy undoubtedly adds a layer of complexity to the management of MS. Women who experience an MS exacerbation during pregnancy typically report progressive neurologic deficit over the course of several days. Optic neuritis, asymmetric numbness, weakness, and ataxia are common presenting symptoms. Pain is very rarely a symptom of an MS relapse.

Generally, interferons can be continued up to attempting pregnancy. However, some routinely used therapies are contraindicated in pregnant women, as they are known to be teratogenic. In fact, many providers avoid using drugs such as teriflunomide in women of childbearing age who are not using reliable contraception. Most physicians suggest that their patients with MS discontinue disease-modifying drugs when they are planning to conceive and during pregnancy.

As with many medications, the risk versus benefit must be weighed for each patient. Although there are only limited data on the safety profile of these therapies in pregnancy, some argue that in the setting of a lower relapse rate in pregnancy, women should strongly consider stopping their medications. Others argue that despite the uncertain fetal risks, there are often times profound benefits to the mother.[41,63]

An acute MS attack during pregnancy is often treated with intravenous glucocorticoids, which are not teratogenic but can be associated with neonatal adrenal suppression, maternal glucose intolerance, and an increased risk of preterm premature rupture of membranes. As a result, most authors recommend high-dose, short-term regimens. Glucocorticoids should be used if indicated and necessary, regardless of gestational age.

Management of MS relapse in pregnancy also includes the consideration of many disease-modifying therapies, particularly if a certain drug has worked successfully for a patient in the past. These include glatiramer acetate, interferons, alemtuzumab, dimethyl fumarate, fingolimod, and natalizumab. A systematic review, published in *Neurology* in 2012, likely provides the highest quality of evidence in regards to the use of disease-modifying therapies for women with MS in pregnancy. Fifteen studies were included in the review and evaluated pregnancies exposed to interferons (n = 761), glatiramer acetate (n = 97), and natalizumab (n = 35). Interferon beta exposure was associated with lower mean neonatal birth weight, shorter mean neonatal birth length, and preterm birth at less than 37 weeks' gestation; however, it was not associated with an increased risk of spontaneous abortion, fetal congenital anomaly, cesarean delivery, or neonatal birth weight less than 2500 g. Glatiramer acetate and natalizumab exposure were not associated with any observed increased risks. Notably, there were no studies reporting exposure to alemtuzumab, dimethyl fumarate, fingolimod, teriflunomide, or mitoxantrone during pregnancy.[41] Fragoso et al later published a study that compared women with MS who were exposed to disease-modifying drugs for at least 8 weeks during pregnancy with those who were not. Although this was a retrospective, nonrandomized study, the authors found that the use of these medications was associated with a significantly lower rate of postpartum relapse and disease progression.[64] Additionally, some authors recommend restarting prophylactic treatment with disease-modifying therapies immediately postpartum and considering the administration of immune globulin in those patients who report a history of severe postpartum exacerbation.[65]

Pregnancy Outcomes

The available data on the effect of MS on pregnancy suggest that maternal disease is associated with an increased rate of cesarean delivery and lower neonatal birth weight. The largest study in the United States analyzed a database with an estimated 15 million deliveries from 2003 to 2006, including 4730 women with MS. MS was associated with a small but statistically significant increase in the risk of cesarean section (odds ratio [OR], 1.3; 95% confidence interval [CI], 1.1-1.4) and fetal growth restriction (OR, 1.7; 95% CI, 1.2-3.3).[66]

A large retrospective study in Norway noted that mothers with MS were more likely to have small for gestational age infants and were more likely to undergo induction of labor with an assisted second stage.[67] Lastly, a report from Taiwan compared women with MS with healthy controls and found that maternal disease was associated with an increased risk for preterm birth and infants who were small for gestational age.[68]

It is important to counsel women with MS that many of them can achieve a healthy full-term pregnancy, often times avoiding the use of any disease-modifying therapies; however, their risk of operative delivery and fetal growth abnormalities is not insignificant.

Anesthesia Considerations

There are limited studies addressing the use of anesthetic techniques for pregnant women with MS. For regional anesthesia, spinal or epidural, the lowest effective concentration is always recommended to minimize any potential risk of local anesthetic crossing into the cerebrospinal fluid with the theoretical risk of neurotoxicity to demyelinated nerves. Although most authors favor the use of epidural when feasible, spinal anesthesia is also thought to be safe in patients with MS. The decision regarding neuraxial anesthesia for labor analgesia and cesarean delivery should be made based on clinical factors, such as coagulopathy and infection, urgency of the situation, and patient preferences.[69]

The literature on the safety of general anesthesia in pregnant women with MS is also sparse; however, current opinion suggests it to be safe. There exists a higher risk of aspiration, lost airway, and desaturation, particularly in patients with bulbar involvement. Antenatal consultation with an obstetric anesthesiologist is of utmost importance so as to make an informed plan for a safe delivery.[69,70]

MS in the Puerperal Period

Contraception

Oral contraceptives contain a form of progesterone with or without a form of estrogen. Studies have found that users of oral contraceptives had a lower incidence of MS than nonusers; however, other studies have not found this relationship.[71,72] Another study found that the incidence of MS was 40% lower in oral contraceptive users compared with nonusers, which further supports the theory that oral contraceptives are protective against MS.[73] Intrauterine devices, intravaginal progesterone rings, subcutaneous progesterone implants, and depoprogesterone injections have not been well studied in MS, but they are not contraindicated for patients with MS. There is also no evidence that oral contraceptives lower the efficacy of disease-modifying therapies; however, modafinil (which is used to treat fatigue in MS) may reduce oral contraceptive efficacy.[74] Patients on disease-modifying therapies are counseled to use contraception to avoid unplanned pregnancy, especially if their disease is not well controlled. Long-acting reversible contraceptives, such as the levonorgestrel-containing intrauterine device (Mirena IUD) or the etonogestrel implant (Implanon), are especially good options for patients with MS.

Breastfeeding

There are imperfect data on breastfeeding in women with MS, with conflicting results regarding disease activity.[75,76] Most studies have suggested either no effect or more commonly suppressed disease activity in women who breastfeed; however, many of these studies did not stratify outcomes based on prepregnancy disease activity and are confounded by mixing patients who exclusively breastfed and those who supplemented with formula.[32,75-79] Exclusive breastfeeding results in a prolonged secondary lactational amenorrhea with ovarian suppression, hyperprolactinemia, and low nonpulsatile luteinizing hormone levels, thereby leading to decrease in disease activity.[80] Exclusive breastfeeding likely lends some protective effect, although it is certainly not clear whether disease suppression is as pronounced as it is with disease-modifying therapies. There are some smaller studies that suggest that breastfeeding may reduce the risk of MS in offspring.[81,82] Overall, the literature suggests that those patients with mild disease are more likely to breastfeed, whereas those with active or severe disease cannot afford to forego treatment and often defer breast-feeding.[83] In general, because breastfeeding has both maternal and neo-natal health benefits, women with MS should not be discouraged from breastfeeding, although they should be supported if they chose not to.

Postpartum Relapse

Several studies have shown that there is a reduced rate of relapse fre-quency during pregnancy, especially in the last trimester, and an increase in the rate of relapse in the postpartum period. The rates of relapse seem to return to baseline starting at about 3 months postpartum.[3] Studies have also shown that women with higher rates of relapse in the year before pregnancy, as well as a higher disease activity, have increased rates of postpartum relapse.[84] Therapies that have been shown to somewhat reduce the risk of postpartum relapse include high-dose glucocorticoids and intravenous immunoglobulins.[3,84] Studies have shown that exclusive breastfeeding can have a modestly protective effect against MS relapse, but this must be weighed against the risk of not reinstituting medications that may be contraindicated in breastfeeding.[85]

There is also an increased rate of relapse after pregnancy termination or spontaneous miscarriage. Studies have shown that abortion induces reactivation of inflammation in relapse-remitting MS, which may be due to dysregulated inflammatory processes that occur in the early stages of pregnancy and then are acutely changed when the pregnancy abruptly ends.[86] The increase in MS symptoms may occur as long as 12 months after miscarriage or termination.[12,86]

Postpartum Depression

There are many psychosocial and physical issues that patients with MS face that can become exponentially increased in the postpartum period. The hormonal shifts accompanying delivery, as well as having to endure childbirth and then care for a newborn infant, can cause distress, fatigue, anxiety, and sometimes depressive symptoms in all postpartum women.[87] This is exacerbated in women with MS, who may be dealing with relapse, have underlying depression, or be on medications causing side effects such as lethargy and mood changes. Not surprisingly, peripartum depression has been found to be significantly more common among patients with MS than patients without MS. Interestingly, some studies have shown an increased rate of psychiatric disorders in the children of parents with MS.[88] Increased social support and psychotherapy, as well as antidepressant and anxiolytic medications, can be used to treat postpartum depression in patients with MS; however, treatment of relapse symptoms should also be used to help decrease both physical and neurocognitive symptoms.

MS During Menopause and Beyond

Menopause

Menopause is defined as the permanent cessation of ovarian functioning, and the average age for this to occur in the United States is 51 years.[89] During the onset of puberty, hormonal shifts occur and the pattern of this shift is associated with an increased risk of MS. However, the hormonal shifts that occur in pregnancy, as previously discussed, typically cause a decrease in MS symptoms. Studies on patient-reported outcomes have been limited. Two small studies have shown that menopause is associated with worsening of MS symptoms in 40% to 54% of women, but these studies differed in how beneficial hormone replacement therapy (HRT) was at relieving these symptoms.[90,91]

The symptoms commonly experienced in menopause include malaise, headache, fatigue, poor sleep, as well as cognitive, emotional, visual, and urogenital symptoms. These symptoms significantly overlap with symptoms of MS and may therefore be very difficult to differentiate. Menopause symptoms may therefore go unrecognized in patients with MS. "Hot flashes" may trigger pseudorelapses in patients with MS, which can be differentiated on physical examination and MRI.[7] Nonpharmacologic interventions for menopausal and perimenopausal symptoms include psychotherapy, changes in diet or clothing, bladder training and biofeedback for urinary symptoms, and lifestyle changes, such as smoking cessation and decrease in alcohol intake. Pharmacologic interventions can include hormone replacement, antispasmodics, tricyclic antidepressants, selective serotonin or norepinephrine reuptake inhibitors, gabapentin, anticonvulsants, benzodiazepines, and sleep aids.[92] An integrated approach to perimenopausal symptom management is recommended.

Hormone Replacement

HRT may be used in postmenopausal women with MS. Studies have shown that symptom severity was improved in postmenopausal patients with MS on HRT therapy.[90] There are risks associated with HRT, such as the increased risk of endometrial cancer with unopposed estrogen in women with an intact uterus. Studies have also implicated some forms of HRT in increasing the risk of breast cancer recurrence, thrombosis, and coronary heart disease.[92] Studies in patients with MS on HRT have shown that it can be neuroprotective; however, it alters immune regulation and can increase the risk of osteoporosis, which is more common in patients with MS in than healthy women. Therefore, the ratio of risks to benefits for HRT in patients with MS may be different than reported for patients without MS, and a multidisciplinary approach is needed in treating patients with MS with HRT. Of concern is that premature ovarian failure is increased in patients with MS because of exposure to medications such as cyclophosphamide and Novantrone (which are now rarely used), and therefore, HRT may be used for longer periods in these patients. Studies analyzing the risks and benefits of long-term HRT use in patients with MS who are taking more commonly used medications, such as monoclonal antibody therapies, are lacking. Owing to the various risks associated with HRT, it is recommended that HRT be used for the shortest possible duration and with the lowest possible dose, in patients with and without MS.[7]

Osteoporosis and Its Treatment

Postmenopausal patients are at increased risk for osteoporosis, which is a condition associated with increased fractures and subsequently increased morbidity and mortality. Patients with MS are at high risk for osteoporosis because they are more likely to have had long-term exposure to steroids and deconditioning from being less physically active. The neurocognitive effects of MS can lead to issues with balance, gait, and impaired cognition, which can predispose these patients to falling and suffering from fractures.

Lifestyle changes, such as increasing calcium and vitamin D intake, smoking cessation, decreasing alcohol intake, and performing aerobic exercise, can improve bone strength and are recommended for all patients at risk for osteoporosis. Physical therapy to improve gait and balance, as well as fall prevention precautions in the home, such as removing loose rugs and improving lighting, can also be implemented to decrease fall risk. Pharmacologic interventions are recommended for postmenopausal women with prior osteoporotic vertebral or hip fracture, postmenopausal women with bone mineral density values consistent with osteoporosis, postmenopausal women with abnormal bone mineral density scores and a 10-year fracture risk of at least 20% of major osteoporotic fracture or of hip fracture risk of at least 3%.[92] First-line therapies include calcium and vitamin D supplementation and bisphosphonates, and second-line therapies include parathyroid hormone, selective estrogen receptor modulators, the monoclonal antibody denosumab, as well as calcitonin. In women with premature ovarian failure and early menopause, hormonal therapy should be considered until they reach menopausal age, which is about 51 years.[93]

Neurologists and other physicians caring for patients with MS should be cognizant of the increased risk of osteoporosis as the woman ages. Early implantation of preventative strategies is recommended to decrease the risk of osteoporotic falls. These include making sure the patient with MS has a proper diet with adequate calcium and vitamin D, starting physical therapy and gait and balance training, encouraging aerobic exercise, and encouraging lifestyle modifications. At the time of this writing, pharmacologic interventions for osteoporosis in patients with MS have not been well studied, so recommendations for their implementation in patients with MS are not different from those in patients without MS.[7,93]

Conclusion

Women affected by MS face a unique set of challenges as they progress through their reproductive years. When treating female patients with MS, medical providers must take into consideration how their disease and medications used to treat it interact with their menstrual cycle, sexual functioning, fertility concerns, pregnancy, and menopausal hormonal shifts. It is important for providers to both counsel female patients with MS thoroughly about the possible risks and side effects of recommended treatments and carefully listen to them when they discuss their concerns, their symptoms, and their reproductive goals and priorities. This often requires the care and treatment coordination of a multidisciplinary team of providers, with the patient being an integral part of this team, and part of their disease management.

References

1. Grinsted L, Heltberg A, Hagen C, Djursing H. Serum sex hormone and gonadotropin concentrations in premenopausal women with multiple sclerosis. *J Intern Med*. 1989;226(4):241-244.
2. Lombardi G, Celso M, Bartelli M, Cilotti A, Del Popolo G. Female sexual dysfunction and hormonal status in multiple sclerosis patients. *J Sex Med*. 2011;8(4):1138-1146.
3. Ghezzi A, Zaffaroni M. Female-specific issues in multiple sclerosis. *Expert Rev Neurother*. 2008;8(6):969-977.
4. Deliconstantinos G. Effects of prostaglandin E2 and progesterone on rat brain synaptosomal plasma membranes. *Ciba Found Symp*. 1990;153:190-199; discussion 9-205.
5. Elenkov IJ, Wilder RL, Bakalov VK, et al. IL-12, TNF-alpha, and hormonal changes during late pregnancy and early postpartum: implications for autoimmune disease activity during these times. *J Clin Endocrinol Metab*. 2001;86(10):4933-4938.

6. Zorgdrager A, De Keyser J. The premenstrual period and exacerbations in multiple sclerosis. *Eur Neurol.* 2002;48(4):204-206.
7. Bove R, Alwan S, Friedman JM, et al. Management of multiple sclerosis during pregnancy and the reproductive years: a systematic review. *Obstet Gynecol.* 2014;124(6):1157-1168.
8. Demirkiran M, Sarica Y, Uguz S, Yerdelen D, Aslan K. Multiple sclerosis patients with and without sexual dysfunction: are there any differences? *Mult Scler.* 2006;12(2):209-214.
9. Orasanu B, Frasure H, Wyman A, Mahajan ST. Sexual dysfunction in patients with multiple sclerosis. *Mult Scler Relat Disord.* 2013;2(2):117-123.
10. Zavoreo I, Gržinčić T, Preksavec M, Madžar T, Bašić Kes V. Sexual dysfunction and incidence of depression in multiple sclerosis patients. *Acta Clin Croat.* 2016;55(3):402-406.
11. Cavalla P, Rovei V, Masera S, et al. Fertility in patients with multiple sclerosis: current knowledge and future perspectives. *Neurol Sci.* 2006;27(4):231-239.
12. Hellwig K. Pregnancy in multiple sclerosis. *Eur Neurol.* 2014;72(suppl 1):39-42.
13. Jalkanen A, Alanen A, Airas L. Finnish Multiple Sclerosis and Pregnancy Study Group. Pregnancy outcome in women with multiple sclerosis: results from a prospective nationwide study in Finland. *Mult Scler.* 2010;16(8):950-955.
14. Hellwig K, Haghikia A, Rockhoff M, Gold R. Multiple sclerosis and pregnancy: experience from a nationwide database in Germany. *Ther Adv Neurol Disord.* 2012;5(5):247-253.
15. Niedziela N, Adamczyk-Sowa M, Pierzchała K. Epidemiology and clinical record of multiple sclerosis in selected countries: a systematic review. *Int J Neurosci.* 2014;124(5):322-330.
16. Sloka JS, Phillips PW, Stefanelli M, Joyce C. Co-occurrence of autoimmune thyroid disease in a multiple sclerosis cohort. *J Autoimmune Dis.* 2005;2:9.
17. Lublin FD, Reingold SC. Defining the clinical course of multiple sclerosis: results of an international survey. National Multiple Sclerosis Society (USA) Advisory Committee on Clinical Trials of New Agents in Multiple Sclerosis. *Neurology.* 1996;46(4):907-911.
18. Lublin FD, Reingold SC, Cohen JA, et al. Defining the clinical course of multiple sclerosis: the 2013 revisions. *Neurology.* 2014;83(3):278-286.
19. Hellwig K, Correale J. Artificial reproductive techniques in multiple sclerosis. *Clin Immunol.* 2013;149(2):219-224.
20. Hellwig K, Beste C, Brune N, et al. Increased MS relapse rate during assisted reproduction technique. *J Neurol.* 2008;255(4):592-593.
21. Correale J, Farez MF, Ysrraelit MC. Increase in multiple sclerosis activity after assisted reproduction technology. *Ann Neurol.* 2012;72(5):682-694.
22. Hellwig K, Schimrigk S, Beste C, Muller T, Gold R. Increase in relapse rate during assisted reproduction technique in patients with multiple sclerosis. *Eur Neurol.* 2009;61(2):65-68.
23. Michel L, Foucher Y, Vukusic S, et al. Increased risk of multiple sclerosis relapse after in vitro fertilisation. *J Neurol Neurosurg Psychiatry.* 2012;83(8):796-802.
24. Spence RD, Voskuhl RR. Neuroprotective effects of estrogens and androgens in CNS inflammation and neurodegeneration. *Front Neuroendocrinol.* 2012;33(1):105-115.
25. Voskuhl RR, Gold SM. Sex-related factors in multiple sclerosis susceptibility and progression. *Nat Rev Neurol.* 2012;8(5):255-263.
26. Bodhankar S, Offner H. GPR30 forms an integral part of e2-protective pathway in experimental autoimmune encephalomyelitis. *Immunol Endocr Metab Agents Med Chem.* 2011;11(4):262-274.

27. Matejuk A, Hopke C, Vandenbark AA, Hurn PD, Offner H. Middle-age male mice have increased severity of experimental autoimmune encephalomyelitis and are unresponsive to testosterone therapy. *J Immunol.* 2005;174(4):2387-2395.

28. Hussain R, Ghoumari AM, Bielecki B, et al. The neural androgen receptor: a therapeutic target for myelin repair in chronic demyelination. *Brain.* 2013;136(Pt 1):132-146.

29. Igra MS, Paling D, Wattjes MP, Connolly DJA, Hoggard N. Multiple sclerosis update: use of MRI for early diagnosis, disease monitoring and assessment of treatment related complications. *Br J Radiol.* 2017;90(1074):20160721.

30. Kaunzner UW, Gauthier SA. MRI in the assessment and monitoring of multiple sclerosis: an update on best practice. *Ther Adv Neurol Disord.* 2017;10(6):247-261.

31. Wattjes MP, Steenwijk MD, Stangel M. MRI in the diagnosis and monitoring of multiple sclerosis: an update. *Clin Neuroradiol.* 2015;25(suppl 2):157-165.

32. Pakpoor J, Disanto G, Lacey MV, Hellwig K, Giovannoni G, Ramagopalan SV. Breastfeeding and multiple sclerosis relapses: a meta-analysis. *J Neurol.* 2012;259(10):2246-2248.

33. Munger KL, Åivo J, Hongell K, Soilu-Hänninen M, Surcel HM, Ascherio A. Vitamin D status during pregnancy and risk of multiple sclerosis in offspring of women in the Finnish maternity cohort. *JAMA Neurol.* 2016;73(5):515-519.

34. Bove R, Chua AS, Xia Z, Chibnik L, De Jager PL, Chitnis T. Complex relation of HLA-DRB1*1501, age at menarche, and age at multiple sclerosis onset. *Neurol Genet.* 2016;2(4):e88.

35. Kavak KS, Teter BE, Hagemeier J, Zakalik K, Weinstock-Guttman B; New York State Multiple Sclerosis Consortium. Higher weight in adolescence and young adulthood is associated with an earlier age at multiple sclerosis onset. *Mult Scler.* 2015;21(7):858-865.

36. Sloka JS, Pryse-Phillips WE, Stefanelli M. The relation between menarche and the age of first symptoms in a multiple sclerosis cohort. *Mult Scler.* 2006;12(3):333-339.

37. Juanatey A, Blanco-Garcia L, Tellez N. Ocrelizumab: its efficacy and safety in multiple sclerosis. *Rev Neurol.* 2018;66(12):423-433.

38. Coyle PK. Multiple sclerosis and pregnancy prescriptions. *Expert Opin Drug Saf.* 2014;13(12):1565-1568.

39. Coyle PK. Disease-modifying agents in multiple sclerosis. *Ann Indian Acad Neurol.* 2009;12(4):273-282.

40. Ghezzi A, Annovazzi P, Portaccio E, Cesari E, Amato MP. Current recommendations for multiple sclerosis treatment in pregnancy and puerperium. *Expert Rev Clin Immunol.* 2013;9(7):683-691; quiz 92.

41. Lu E, Wang BW, Guimond C, Synnes A, Sadovnick D, Tremlett H. Disease-modifying drugs for multiple sclerosis in pregnancy: a systematic review. *Neurology.* 2012;79(11):1130-1135.

42. Brucker MC, King TL. The 2015 US Food and Drug Administration pregnancy and lactation labeling rule. *J Midwifery Womens Health.* 2017;62(3):308-316.

43. Center TRT. Available at https://reprotox.org/.

44. Pritham UA, McKay L. Safe management of chronic pain in pregnancy in an era of opioid misuse and abuse. *J Obstet Gynecol Neonatal Nurs.* 2014;43(5):554-567.

45. Guille C, Barth KS, Mateus J, McCauley JL, Brady KT. Treatment of prescription opioid use disorder in pregnant women. *Am J Psychiatry.* 2017;174(3):208-214.

46. Guttuso T, Robinson LK, Amankwah KS. Gabapentin use in hyperemesis gravidarum: a pilot study. *Early Hum Dev.* 2010;86(1):65-66.

47. Guttuso T, Shaman M, Thornburg LL. Potential maternal symptomatic benefit of gabapentin and review of its safety in pregnancy. *Eur J Obstet Gynecol Reprod Biol.* 2014;181:280-283.
48. Fromm GH, Terrence CF, Chattha AS. Baclofen in the treatment of trigeminal neuralgia: double-blind study and long-term follow-up. *Ann Neurol.* 1984;15(3):240-244.
49. Wang MJ, Kuper SG, Sims B, et al. Opioid detoxification in pregnancy: systematic review and meta-analysis of perinatal outcomes. *Am J Perinatol.* 2018. doi:10.1055/s-0038-1670680.
50. Brar B, Jackson D, Nat M, Patil P, Iriye B, Planinic P. Antenatal interventions based upon fetal surveillance of the daily opioid exposed fetus: a descriptive analysis. *J Matern Fetal Neonatal Med.* 2018:1-11.
51. Lacaze-Masmonteil T, O'Flaherty P. Managing infants born to mothers who have used opioids during pregnancy. *Paediatr Child Health.* 2018;23(3):220-226.
52. Johnson AJ, Jones CW. Opioid use disorders and pregnancy. *Obstet Gynecol Clin North Am.* 2018;45(2):201-216.
53. Weatherby SJM, Woolner P, Clarke CE. Pregnancy in stiff-limb syndrome. *Mov Disord.* 2004;19(7):852-854.
54. Goldkamp J, Blaskiewicz R, Myles T. Stiff person syndrome and pregnancy. *Obstet Gynecol.* 2011;118(2 Pt 2):454-457.
55. Moran LR, Almeida PG, Worden S, Huttner KM. Intrauterine baclofen exposure: a multidisciplinary approach. *Pediatrics.* 2004;114(2):e267-e269.
56. Dalton CM, Keenan E, Jarrett L, Buckley L, Stevenson VL. The safety of baclofen in pregnancy: intrathecal therapy in multiple sclerosis. *Mult Scler.* 2008;14(4):571-572.
57. Harden CL, Hopp J, Ting TY, Pennell PB, French JA, Hauser WA, et al. Practice parameter update: management issues for women with epilepsy–focus on pregnancy (an evidence-based review): obstetrical complications and change in seizure frequency: report of the Quality Standards Subcommittee and Therapeutics and Technology Assessment Subcommittee of the American Academy of Neurology and American Epilepsy Society. *Neurology.* 2009;73(2):126-132.
58. Masarwa R, Bar-Oz B, Gorelik E, Reif S, Perlman A, Matok I. Prenatal exposure to SSRIs and SNRIs and risk for persistent pulmonary hypertension of the newborn: a systematic review, meta-analysis and network meta-analysis. *Am J Obstet Gynecol.* 2019;220(1):57.e1-57.e13.
59. Huybrechts KF, Hernández-Díaz S, Avorn J. Antidepressant use in pregnancy and the risk of cardiac defects. *N Engl J Med.* 2014;371(12):1168-1169.
60. Wegner I, Edelbroek P, de Haan GJ, Lindhout D, Sander JW. Drug monitoring of lamotrigine and oxcarbazepine combination during pregnancy. *Epilepsia.* 2010;51(12):2500-2502.
61. Voinescu PE, Park S, Chen LQ, et al. Antiepileptic drug clearances during pregnancy and clinical implications for women with epilepsy. *Neurology.* 2018;91(13):e1228-e1236.
62. Johnson EL, Stowe ZN, Ritchie JC, et al. Carbamazepine clearance and seizure stability during pregnancy. *Epilepsy Behav.* 2014;33:49-53.
63. Coyle PK, Sinclair SM, Scheuerle AE, Thorp JM, Albano JD, Rametta MJ. Final results from the Betaseron (interferon β-1b) pregnancy registry: a prospective observational study of birth defects and pregnancy-related adverse events. *BMJ Open.* 2014;4(5):e004536.
64. Fragoso YD, Boggild M, Macias-Islas MA, et al. The effects of long-term exposure to disease-modifying drugs during pregnancy in multiple sclerosis. *Clin Neurol Neurosurg.* 2013;115(2):154-159.

65. Achiron A, Rotstein Z, Noy S, Mashiach S, Dulitzky M, Achiron R. Intravenous immunoglobulin treatment in the prevention of childbirth-associated acute exacerbations in multiple sclerosis: a pilot study. *J Neurol.* 1996;243(1):25-28.

66. Kelly VM, Nelson LM, Chakravarty EF. Obstetric outcomes in women with multiple sclerosis and epilepsy. *Neurology.* 2009;73(22):1831-1836.

67. Mueller BA, Zhang J, Critchlow CW. Birth outcomes and need for hospitalization after delivery among women with multiple sclerosis. *Am J Obstet Gynecol.* 2002;186(3):446-452.

68. Chen YH, Lin HL, Lin HC. Does multiple sclerosis increase risk of adverse pregnancy outcomes? A population-based study. *Mult Scler.* 2009;15(5):606-612.

69. Bader AM, Hunt CO, Datta S, Naulty JS, Ostheimer GW. Anesthesia for the obstetric patient with multiple sclerosis. *J Clin Anesth.* 1988;1(1):21-24.

70. Hopkins AN, Alshaeri T, Akst SA, Berger JS. Neurologic disease with pregnancy and considerations for the obstetric anesthesiologist. *Semin Perinatol.* 2014;38(6):359-369.

71. Villard-Mackintosh L, Vessey MP. Oral contraceptives and reproductive factors in multiple sclerosis incidence. *Contraception.* 1993;47(2):161-168.

72. Thorogood M, Hannaford PC. The influence of oral contraceptives on the risk of multiple sclerosis. *Br J Obstet Gynaecol.* 1998;105(12):1296-1299.

73. Alonso A, Jick SS, Olek MJ, Ascherio A, Jick H, Hernán MA. Recent use of oral contraceptives and the risk of multiple sclerosis. *Arch Neurol.* 2005;62(9):1362-1365.

74. Robertson P, Hellriegel ET. Clinical pharmacokinetic profile of modafinil. *Clin Pharmacokinet.* 2003;42(2):123-137.

75. Langer-Gould A, Hellwig K. One can prevent post-partum MS relapses by exclusive breast feeding: yes. *Mult Scler.* 2013;19(12):1567-1568.

76. Vukusic S, Confavreux C. One can prevent post-partum MS relapses by exclusive breast feeding: no. *Mult Scler.* 2013;19(12):1565-1566.

77. Hutchinson M. One can prevent post-partum MS relapses by exclusive breast feeding: commentary. *Mult Scler.* 2013;19(12):1569-1570.

78. Langer-Gould A, Huang S, Van Den Eeden SK, et al. Vitamin D, pregnancy, breastfeeding, and postpartum multiple sclerosis relapses. *Arch Neurol.* 2011;68(3):310-313.

79. Langer-Gould A, Beaber BE. Effects of pregnancy and breastfeeding on the multiple sclerosis disease course. *Clin Immunol.* 2013;149(2):244-250.

80. Coyle PK. Management of women with multiple sclerosis through pregnancy and after childbirth. *Ther Adv Neurol Disord.* 2016;9(3):198-210.

81. Conradi S, Malzahn U, Paul F, et al. Breastfeeding is associated with lower risk for multiple sclerosis. *Mult Scler.* 2013;19(5):553-558.

82. Ragnedda G, Leoni S, Parpinel M, et al. Reduced duration of breastfeeding is associated with a higher risk of multiple sclerosis in both Italian and Norwegian adult males: the EnvIMS study. *J Neurol.* 2015;262(5):1271-1277.

83. Kieseier BC, Wiendl H. Postpartum disease activity and breastfeeding in multiple sclerosis revisited. *Neurology.* 2010;75(5):392-393.

84. Vukusic S, Hutchinson M, Hours M, et al. Pregnancy and multiple sclerosis (the PRIMS study): clinical predictors of post-partum relapse. *Brain.* 2004;127(Pt 6):1353-1360.

85. Hellwig K, Rockhoff M, Herbstritt S, et al. Exclusive breastfeeding and the effect on postpartum multiple sclerosis relapses. *JAMA Neurol.* 2015;72(10):1132-1138.

86. Landi D, Ragonese P, Prosperini L, et al. Abortion induces reactivation of inflammation in relapsing-remitting multiple sclerosis. *J Neurol Neurosurg Psychiatry.* 2018;89(12):1272-1278.

87. Airas L, Jalkanen A, Alanen A, Pirttilä T, Marttila RJ. Breast-feeding, post-partum and prepregnancy disease activity in multiple sclerosis. *Neurology.* 2010;75(5):474-476.

88. Razaz N, Tremlett H, Marrie RA, Joseph KS. Peripartum depression in parents with multiple sclerosis and psychiatric disorders in children. *Mult Scler.* 2016;22(14):1830-1840.

89. ACOG Practice Bulletin No. 141: management of menopausal symptoms. *Obstet Gynecol.* 2014;123(1):202-216.

90. Smith R, Studd JW. A pilot study of the effect upon multiple sclerosis of the menopause, hormone replacement therapy and the menstrual cycle. *J R Soc Med.* 1992;85(10):612-613.

91. Holmqvist P, Wallberg M, Hammar M, Landtblom AM, Brynhildsen J. Symptoms of multiple sclerosis in women in relation to sex steroid exposure. *Maturitas.* 2006;54(2):149-153.

92. Practice bulletin No. 141: management of menopausal symptoms: Correction. *Obstet Gynecol.* 2018;131(3):604.

93. Bove R, Chitnis T, Houtchens M. Menopause in multiple sclerosis: therapeutic considerations. *J Neurol.* 2014;261(7):1257-1268.

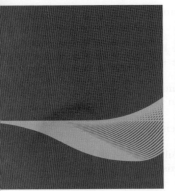
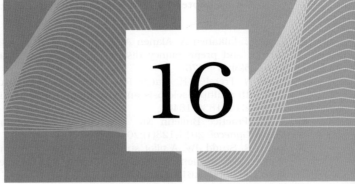

Urologic Issues in the Multiple Sclerosis Patient

■ ■ ■ Philip J. Aliotta

Introduction

Multiple sclerosis (MS) is an autoimmune inflammatory disease that results in damage to the myelin sheaths of the nerves in the central nervous system.[1] It presents with a broad spectrum of clinical presentations that are time and disease course related. MS plaque (intracranial and/or spinal) location is a key feature in the pathophysiology of disease-related lower urinary tract symptoms (LUTS).[2] It is commonly diagnosed between the ages of 20 and 40 years, with a female predominance of 3:1.[1,2] The prevalence in the United States is 57.8 per 100,000 and is twice as common in the north as compared with the southern United States.[3] About 80% to 96% of all patients with MS will seek urologic care because of bothersome LUTS at some point in their disease course, and as many as 12% have symptoms before the actual diagnosis.[4,5] If a patient has ambulatory difficulties, the prevalence of lower urinary tract complaints is close to 100%.[6,7] The 2005 North American Research Committee on Multiple Sclerosis (NARCOMS) reported that 65% of patient responders experienced at least one moderate to severe urinary symptom.[8] Patients with bladder dysfunction have lower scores on quality-of-life scales.[9] There is also noted to be a greater burden on professional or family caregivers associated with urinary disorders.[10] Access to treatment is uncertain

292

and varies from country to country.[11] The MS Barometer 2015—European Multiple Sclerosis Platform,[12] which has measured and compared well-being and quality of life for people living with MS in 33 European countries, including 26 EU member states, shows huge disparities in terms of access to treatment, therapies, and employment. Furthermore, according to the MS Barometer 2015, the average percentage of the total costs for symptomatic treatments and therapies reimbursed over a period of 12 months vary; the Western countries enjoy a generally high level of reimbursement, whereas the Eastern ones reported very different national policies on this topic.

Only 50% of the 9702 patients of the NARCOMS cohort used medications despite severe symptomatology; 47% benefitted from urological evaluation.[7,8,13]

Physiology of Micturition

Bladder storage (Figure 16.1A) occurs through sympathetic nervous system stimulation of alpha adrenergic receptors, which results in closure of the bladder neck, and beta-adrenergic receptor stimulation, which relaxes the detrusor muscle.[14] Bladder contraction and emptying occurs by parasympathetic muscarinic receptor stimulation.[15] Sensory afferent information is carried through myelinated A-delta and unmyelinated C fibers through pelvic and pudendal nerves at S2 to S4 nerve roots.[16] The spinothalamic tract sends sensory impulses to the periaqueductal gray (PAG) region in the midbrain. The PAG inhibits the pontine micturition center in the brainstem allowing for bladder filling. Sympathetic nerve fibers from T10 to L2 via the hypogastric nerve cause the bladder to relax and the bladder neck to close.[17] Awareness of bladder fullness occurs through medial prefrontal cortex and hypothalamic modulation of the PAG area (Figure 16.1).

Bladder emptying (Figure 16.1B) occurs through parasympathetic nervous system efferent activation of the pelvic nerve from sacral nerve roots S2 to S4. Increased parasympathetic activity inhibits sympathetic stimulation, and the bladder neck relaxes. The pelvic plexus ganglia stimulate the detrusor muscle, and voiding occurs.[18] MS plaques occur in the cortex, brainstem, and spinal cord. Corticospinal and reticulospinal tract plaques (innervate bladder detrusor muscle and external sphincter) affect voiding. Sacral plaque involvement has been reported to be 18%, but the exact pathologic role is uncertain owing to imaging limitations and the concomitant presence of multiple plaque lesions throughout the nervous system. Suprasacral lesions occur in 80% of cases and are seen most commonly in cervical lesions and are associated with detrusor hyperreflexia due to loss of descending inhibition. Reticulospinal tract involvement is associated with detrusor-sphincter dyssynergia, incomplete sphincteric relaxation, or sphincter paralysis. Intracranial plaques are commonly encountered in patients with MS, but their clinical significance is unclear. Pontine lesions have been reported to be associated.[19]

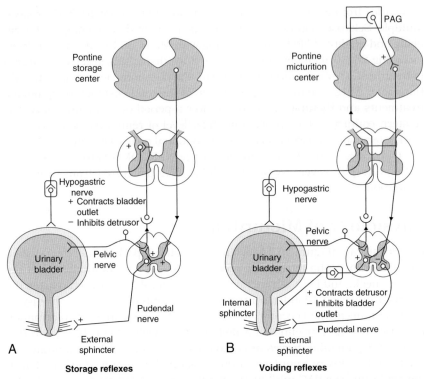

Figure 16.1. Mechanism of storage (A) and voiding reflexes (B). Reprinted from Chai TC, Birder LA. Physiology and Pharmacology of the Bladder and Urethra. In: Wein AJ, ed. *Campbell-Walsh Urology.* 11th ed. Philadelphia, PA: Saunders; 2016:1631-1684. Copyright © 2016 Elsevier. With permission.

Clinical Presentation

Case Study

A 37-year-old white female was diagnosed with Relapsing Remitting MS 1.5 years ago after initially presenting with visual problems and lower extremity weakness and gait disturbance over a 6-month period. She presents with complaints of frequency, urgency, urge incontinence, and complaints of suprapubic pressure making her believe she has a full bladder but is only voiding small-volume voids with an erratic weak stream. She has nocturia ×4. There are no stress- or activity-related complaints of incontinence. Before the diagnosis of MS, there was no history of urinary tract infections, but since the diagnosis, she has had at least three infections, the last one severe enough to exacerbate her MS symptoms requiring hospital admission. She has irregular bowel habits, suffering constipation with associated bowel movements as long as 5 to 6 days apart, culminating in the occurrence of uncontrollable large bowel movements with fecal incontinence occurring occasionally. Oftentimes, after a bout of severe constipation, she will experience frequent loose stools and diarrhea. After one such occurrence, she developed a urinary tract infection, which was treated effectively with an antibiotic.

Between 50% and 90% of patients with MS report LUTS with the prevalence of incontinence as low as 37% and as high as 72%.[20-22] Lower urinary tract symptomatology is directly related to the severity of the disability caused by the MS. Up to 15% of patients who go on to be diagnosed with MS have as an initial presentation symptom attributable to lower urinary tract involvement, that is, acute urinary retention or as an acute onset of urgency and frequency.[20] The most common urinary tract symptom in patients with MS is urgency, as part of the overactive bladder syndrome comprising urgency, urinary frequency, and/or urge incontinence.[21]

LUTS fall into two categories, irritative and obstructive. Irritative symptoms include frequency, urgency, nocturia, and urge incontinence, and obstructive symptoms include hesitancy or difficulty initiating the stream, straining to void, a reduced flow, an intermittent stream, or a sensation of incomplete emptying. However, the presence or absence of symptoms remains an unreliable indicator of the extent or type of bladder dysfunction.[23]

The bladder has two functions, to store urine without leaking and to empty/void without a residual.[24,25] Bladder storage requires low intravesical pressures, a compliant viscoelastic bladder with intact sensation. Efficient and effective bladder emptying requires no evidence of pathologic outlet obstruction (benign prostatic hypertrophy and bladder outlet obstruction), urethral stricture, meatal stenosis, etc., and relaxation of the external striated sphincter with coordinated relaxation of the smooth muscle sphincter at the bladder neck and proximal urethra leading to opening and funneling of the bladder neck, accompanied by the simultaneous coordinated bladder contraction.[25]

Overactive bladder (OAB)—The Standardization Subcommittee of the International Continence Society now recognizes *OAB* as a "symptom syndrome suggestive of lower urinary tract dysfunction." It is specifically defined as "urgency, with or without urge incontinence, usually with frequency and nocturia, in the absence of proven infection or other obvious pathology." *When neurological conditions affect the OAB, it is called* **neurogenic bladder** (NGB).[26,27]

The presence of an indwelling catheter, high-detrusor/intravesical filling pressures, and striated sphincter dyssynergia in men, are causes of serious urologic complications experienced by patients with MS.[28]

Storage Symptoms Experienced During the Storage Phase of the Bladder[29]

Increased daytime frequency is the complaint by the patient who considers that he or she voids too often by day. This term is equivalent to *pollakisuria* used in many countries.

Nocturia is the complaint that the individual has to wake at night one or more times to void. The term nighttime frequency differs from that for nocturia, as it includes voids that occur after the individual has gone to bed but before he or she has gone to sleep and voids that occur in the early morning, which prevent the individual from getting back to sleep as he or she wishes.

Urgency is the complaint of a sudden compelling desire to pass urine that is difficult to defer.

Urinary incontinence is the complaint of any involuntary leakage of urine (Table 16.1).

Voiding Symptoms Experienced During the Voiding Phase[29]

Slow stream is reported by the individual as his or her perception of reduced urine flow, usually compared with previous performance or in comparison with others.

Splitting or spraying of the urine stream may be reported.

Intermittent stream (intermittency) is the term used when the individual describes urine flow that stops and starts, on one or more occasions, during micturition.

Hesitancy is the term used when an individual describes difficulty in initiating micturition resulting in a delay in the onset of voiding after the individual is ready to pass urine.

Straining to void describes the muscular effort used to either initiate, maintain, or improve the urinary stream.

Terminal dribble is the term used when an individual describes a prolonged final part of micturition, when the flow has slowed to a trickle/dribble.

Postmicturition Symptoms Experienced Immediately After Micturition[29]

Feeling of incomplete emptying is a self-explanatory term for a feeling experienced by the individual after passing urine.

TABLE 16.1
TYPES OF INCONTINENCE[29,30]

Stress urinary incontinence	Involuntary leakage on effort, exertion, or sneezing or coughing
Urge urinary incontinence	The complaint of involuntary leakage accompanied by or immediately preceded by urgency
Mixed urinary incontinence	The complaint of involuntary leakage associated with urgency and with exertion, effort, sneezing or coughing
Enuresis	Any involuntary loss of urine If it is used to denote incontinence during sleep, it should always be qualified with the adjective "nocturnal"
Continuous urinary incontinence	The complaint of continuous leakage
Functional incontinence	Occurs when physical disabilities, external obstacles, or cognitive and/or communication problems prevent the person from getting to the bathroom to urinate
Transient incontinence	A temporary form of incontinence, usually caused by a short-lived medical condition—or the treatment for the condition
Reflex incontinence/unconscious incontinence	Occurs when a person is unaware of the need to urinate

Postmicturition dribble is the term used when an individual describes the involuntary loss of urine immediately after he or she has finished passing urine, usually after leaving the toilet in men or after rising from the toilet in women.

Symptoms Associated With Sexual Intercourse[29]

Dyspareunia, vaginal dryness, and incontinence are among the symptoms women may describe during or after intercourse.

These symptoms should be described as fully as possible. Define urine leakage as during penetration, during intercourse, or at orgasm.

Symptoms Associated With Pelvic Organ Prolapse[29]

The feeling of a lump ("something coming down"), low backache, heaviness, dragging sensation, or the need to digitally replace the prolapse to defecate or micturate, are among the symptoms women may describe who have a prolapse.

The Goals of Managing the Multiple Sclerosis Neurogenic Bladder[25]

1. Upper urinary tract preservation or improvement
2. Absence or control of infection
3. Adequate storage at low intravesical pressure
4. Adequate emptying at low intravesical pressure
5. Adequate control
6. No catheter or stoma (depending on the degree of disability)
7. Social acceptability and adaptability
8. Vocational acceptability and adaptability

Urologic Evaluation[20,21,29-33]

Patient assessment should include the following:

History[31]

1. Mental status/cognitive function
2. Functional status activities of daily living, walking, transfer ability
3. Diet
4. Fluid intake habits and bladder diary
5. Bowel habits
   a. Constipation
   b. Diarrhea
   c. Irritable bowel syndrome
6. Type of incontinence
   a. Stress
   b. Urge
   c. Mixed
   d. Functional
7. Recurrent urinary tract infections
8. Postvoid residual (PVR)
9. Urinary frequency and urgency
10. Concurrent medical history
11. Surgical history
    a. Gynecologic history—pelvic surgeries: cystocele, rectocele, sacro-spinous fixation, vaginal vault surgery; pelvic malignancy, pelvic radiation, bladder cancer surgery, bowel surgery
    b. Obstetric history—parity, C-sections
    c. Male pelvic history—urethral surgery or history of stricture disease, benign prostate surgery (transurethral resection prostate), radical prostatectomy, radiation therapy for pelvic malignancy, bowel surgery
12. Associated medications, over the counter, homeopathic, and/or phyto-therapeutic products/remedies[30] (Table 16.2)

TABLE 16.2

MEDICATIONS USED IN MULTIPLE SCLEROSIS MANAGEMENT WITH POTENTIAL UROLOGIC ADVERSE EFFECTS[54]

Type of Medication	Examples	Potential Effects on Continence
Sedatives/hypnotics	Long-acting benzodiazepines (e.g., diazepam, flurazepam)	Sedation, delirium, immobility
Beta receptor agonists	Terbutaline, isoproterenol, Myrbetriq	Urinary retention
Anticholinergics	Dicyclomine, oxybutynin, antihistamines	Urinary retention, overflow incontinence, delirium, fecal impaction
Antipsychotics	Thioridazine, haloperidol	Anticholinergic actions, sedation, rigidity, immobility
Antidepressants	Amitriptyline, desipramine	Anticholinergic actions, sedation
Corticosteroids	Prednisone	Increased urinary tract infections
Narcotic analgesics	Opiates	Urinary retention, fecal impaction, sedation, delirium
α-Adrenergic antagonists	Prazosin, terazosin, tamsulosin, etc.	Urethral relaxation may precipitate stress incontinence in women
α-Adrenergic agonists	Nasal decongestants	Urinary retention in men
Calcium-channel blockers	All, i.e., nifedipine, nicardipine, felodipine	Urinary retention: nocturnal diuresis owing to fluid retention
Potent diuretics	Furosemide, bumetanide	Polyuria, frequency, urgency
Angiotensin-converting enzyme inhibitors	Captopril, enalapril, lisinopril	Drug-induced cough can precipitate stress incontinence in women and in some men with previous prostatectomy
Chemotherapy	Cyclophosphamide (Cytoxan) Vincristine	Bladder cancer risk Urinary retention

Modified from Resnick NM. Geriatric incontinence. *Urol Clin North Am.* 1996;23(1):55-74.

Bladder Sensation Can Be Defined During History Taking by Five Categories[29]

1. Normal

The individual is aware of bladder filling and increasing sensation up to a strong desire to void.

2. Increased

The individual feels an early and persistent desire to void.

3. Reduced

The individual is aware of bladder filling but does not feel a definite desire to void.

4. Absent

The individual reports no sensation of bladder filling or desire to void.

5. Nonspecific

The individual reports no specific bladder sensation but may perceive bladder filling as abdominal fullness, vegetative symptoms, or spasticity.

Physical Examination[6,25,28,29]

MS involvement in the cervical spinal cord is associated with lower extremity spasticity evidenced by hyperactive reflexes and bladder detrusor overactivity (DO) with or without detrusor external sphincter dyssynergia (DESD).[6] General examination with urologic- and neurourologic-focused examination includes the following.[28]

1. Abdominal/pelvic examination/genital examination—prostate examination in men, vaginal vault examination in women
2. A sensorimotor assessment of L1 to S4 cord segments
3. Rectal tone—S2 to S4 sacral reflex assessment
4. Bulbocavernosus reflex—S2 to S4 sacral reflex assessment
5. Plantar response—pyramidal tract integrity
6. Cremasteric reflex—L1 root integrity
7. Deep tendon reflexes—reflect the integrity of the upper motor neuron and lower motor neuron function

Diagnostic Evaluation

The common causes of transient urinary incontinence can be easily remembered by the term **"DIAPPERS"** (Table 16.3).

Patients should undergo microscopic urinalysis, which is more accurate than dipstick testing in that it can detect upper tract pathology by detecting

▨ **TABLE 16.3**
TREATABLE TRANSIENT CAUSES OF INCONTINENCE[31-33,48,54,55]

Delirium (confusional state)

Infection-urinary (only symptomatic)

Atrophic urethritis, vaginitis

Pharmaceuticals

Psychological, especially severe depression (rare)

Excess urine output (e.g., congestive heart failure, hyperglycemia)

Restricted mobility

Stool impaction

---

for protein, hematuria, glucose, ketones, bilirubin, and acid/base status; baseline basic metabolic profile to assess electrolyte status, serum glucose level as a diabetes screen, serum creatinine, and estimated glomerular filtration rate as a measure of kidney function; hemoglobin A1C to assess for diabetes; And prostate-specific antigen to assess for prostate cancer in men.[32]

Radiographic Assessment

Upper tract radiographic studies demonstrating upper tract pathology (elevation in creatinine, caliectasis, stone, renal scarring, hydroureteronephrosis) in patients with MS are limited in number and have been reported to be as low as 0.34% to 16.7%. Patients at risk for upper tract disease progression have been reported (1) to be older patients or as having (2) detrusor sphincter dyssynergia in the male, (3) poor bladder compliance, (4) Expanded Disability Status Scale (EDSS) >5, and (5) indwelling catheter. These at-risk patients should be followed with serum creatinine levels routinely. With respect to the lower urinary tract assessment, a voiding cystourethrogram alone or as part of urodynamic evaluation can be performed to assess concomitant stress urinary incontinence.[1,28]

Postvoid Residual

Checking with handheld ultrasound or straight catheter aids in differentiating between OAB (characterized by minimal to no residual) and a failure to empty either due to one or both an underactive bladder and/or, in men, outlet obstruction from enlarged prostate. A normal PVR is <150 mL.[32]

Voiding Diary

A voiding diary is a record of the timed volumetric oral intake over a 24-hour to 3-day interval with timed documentation of episodes with degree of severity of urgency with urge incontinence and severity of incontinence with physical activities.[33]

Screening Questionnaires

Urogenital Distress Inventory (UDI-6),[34] geriatric self-efficacy scale for urinary incontinence (GSE-UI),[35] incontinence impact questionnaire—short form IIQ-7,[36] and the pelvic floor impact questionnaire (PFIQ)[37] are just a few of urinary and pelvic floor questionnaires used to assess urinary, bowel, and pelvic floor dysfunction. No MS-specific urinary questionnaires are available.

Urodynamics

A cystometrogram (Figure 16.2) measures the ability of the bladder to accommodate urine. It measures changes in bladder pressure with filling, stability, and defines capacity. The normal cystometrogram has two phases:

1. Filling storage phase
   a. Phase I: Initial compliance: represents the initial response to filling
   b. Phase II: Tonus limb
   c. Phase III: Terminal compliance: viscoelastic
2. Voiding phase (Figure 16.3):
   a. Flow rate (Q): Volume of fluid expelled via the urethra per unit time (mL/s)
   b. Voided volume (V_{void}): Total volume expelled via the urethra (mL)
   c. Maximum flow rate (Q_{max}): Maximum measured value of the flow rate after correction for artifacts
   d. Voiding time: Total duration of micturition (s)
   e. Flow time: Time over which measurable flow actually occurs
   f. Average flow rate (Q_{ave}): Voided volume divided by the flow time
   g. Time to maximum flow: Elapsed time from onset of flow to maximum flow

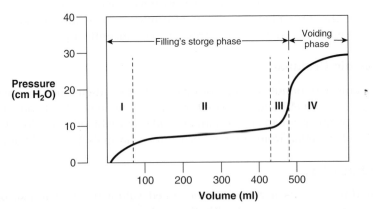

Figure 16.2. Classic cystometrogram. Reprinted from Wein AJ, English WS, Whitmore KE. Office urodynamics. *Urol Clin North Am.* 1988;15(4):609-623. Copyright © 1988 Elsevier. With permission.

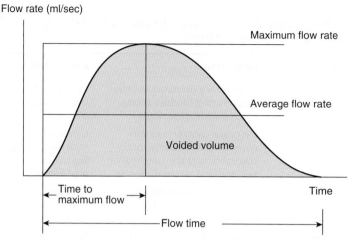

Figure 16.3. Normal uroflow. Reprinted from Wein AJ, English WS, Whitmore KE. Office urodynamics. *Urol Clin North Am.* 1988;15(4):609-623. Copyright © 1988 Elsevier. With permission.

It is the author's practice to perform urodynamics on all patients with MS who present with urologic symptoms. However, others withhold urodynamics until patients present with an elevated PVR of >150 mL and have failed two courses of empiric medical management, with obstructive symptoms and any evidence of upper urinary tract pathology.[1] Female patients with MS may have concomitant stress urinary incontinence and require urodynamic evaluation.[1]

Common Findings on Urodynamic Testing and Associated Symptoms[29,33]

See Table 16.4.

Urodynamic Risk Factors

The following are dangerous and require intervention to prevent upper and lower urinary tract decompensation:

1. Impaired compliance
2. Detrusor-external sphincter dyssynergia (DESD)
3. Detrusor-intrinsic sphincter dyssynergia (DISD)
4. High-pressure detrusor overactivity (DO) present throughout bladder filling
5. Elevated detrusor leak point pressure (DLPP) >40 cm H_2O
6. Poor emptying with high storage pressures

TABLE 16.4
COMMON FINDINGS ON URODYNAMIC TESTING AND
ASSOCIATED SYMPTOMS[29,33]

Urodynamic Finding	Definition	Associated Symptoms
Detrusor overactivity without obstruction	Involuntary detrusor contractions during bladder filling with or without leakage	Urgency, frequency, urge incontinence, and nocturia
Detrusor sphincter dyssynergia	Detrusor contraction concurrent with an involuntary contraction of the urethral or periurethral striated muscle	Urinary hesitancy, straining, stuttering urination, or obstruction
Detrusor overactivity with outlet obstruction	Detrusor overactivity plus detrusor sphincter dyssynergia may obstruct urine flow	Urinary urgency with hesitancy, straining, or obstruction
Detrusor overactivity with impaired contractility	Detrusor overactivity with reduced strength and/or duration of bladder contraction, resulting in prolonged bladder emptying or incomplete emptying	Slow bladder emptying and/or urinary retention
Detrusor areflexia	Inability of the bladder to contract with routine filling at normal physiological volumes to elicit bladder emptying	Urinary retention

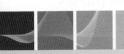

Case Study

The patient underwent complex urodynamics, which demonstrated a small-capacity bladder (298 mL), detrusor overactivity (at 267 mL) leading to uninhibited spontaneous void, abnormal uroflow with low maximum flow (6.4 mL/s) and low average flow (4.1 mL/s), prolonged voiding time, incomplete emptying with a PVR of 165 mL, and evidence of pelvic floor muscle dysfunction during voiding phase (DESD) and subsequent pelvic floor spasm post void.

The patient was treated with pelvic floor therapy, anticholinergic (±beta 3 receptor agonist to further reduce urgency and frequency and help restore bladder capacity without adverse side effects associated with increased doses of anticholinergics), and an alpha blocker. Intermittent clean catheterization was also discussed pending outcome from the above-mentioned interventions.

Cystoscopy

Cystoscopy is used in the evaluation of recurrent urinary tract infection, cystolithiasis, bladder outlet obstruction, and incontinence.

Treatment/Therapies

Treatment is tailored based on the effect of concurrent medications (Table 16.2), patient factors profile (Table 16.5), symptom complex (Table 16.3), urodynamic profile (Figure 16.4), lower urinary tract assessment, medical therapies (Tables 16.6 and 16.7), and additional therapies (Table 16.8) as per symptom/therapy algorithm (Table 16.9 and Figure 16.5).

The reasons to change or augment a given regimen are (1) evidence of upper tract deterioration, (2) recurrent sepsis or fever of urinary tract origin, (3) lower urinary tract deterioration, (4) inadequate storage, (5) inadequate emptying, (6) inadequate control, (8) unacceptable side effects, and (9) skin changes secondary to incontinence or collecting device.[20]

Take alpha blocker with dinner; not at bedtime (hs), as this may cause increased nocturia. Risks associated with alpha blockade are orthostatic hypotension, especially when taken on an empty stomach or in combination with other antihypertensive medications, asthenia, and incontinence.

TABLE 16.5
PATIENT FACTORS TO CONSIDER IN CHOOSING THERAPY[25,32]

---

1. Prognosis of underlying disease, especially if progressive or malignant
2. General health
3. Limiting factors: hand dexterity, body habitus, ability to transfer, ambulatory status
4. Activities of daily living
5. Mental status
6. Motivation
7. Desire to be catheter free (willingness to do intermittent catheterization)
8. Desire to avoid surgery
9. Sexual activity status
10. Reliability
11. Educability
12. Psychosocial environment, family support and cooperation
13. Economic resources

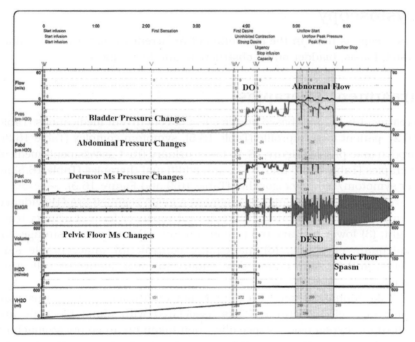

Figure 16.4. Clinical vignette urodynamics. Reproduced from Aliotta PJ. *Personal communications.* 2018. See eBook for color figure.

TABLE 16.6
MEDICATIONS USED TO TREAT BLADDER DYSFUNCTION IN MULTIPLE SCLEROSIS: BLADDER STORAGE

Antimuscarinics/Anticholinergics

- Fesoterodine: Toviaz
- Oxybutynin: Ditropan/Ditropan XL/Oxytrol Patch/Gelnique
- Solifenacin: Vesicare
- Trospium chloride: Sanctura/Sanctura XR
- Darifenacin: Enablex
- Tolterodine: Detrol/Detrol LA
- Hyoscamine: Levsin SL/Levsinex

Beta-3 Agonist

- Miragebron: Myrbetriq

From Orasanu B, Mahajan ST. *Bladder and Bowel Dysfunction in Multiple Sclerosis. Multiple Sclerosis and Related Disorders: Clinical Guide to Diagnosis, Medical Management, and Rehabilitation.* New York: Demos Medical Publishing 2013.

TABLE 16.7

MEDICATIONS USED TO TREAT BLADDER DYSFUNCTION IN MULTIPLE SCLEROSIS: IMPAIRED BLADDER

Alpha Adrenergic Blockers

■ Prazosin: Minipres

■ Doxazosin: Cardura/Cardura XL

■ Terazosin: Hytrin

Uroselective Alpha Blockers

■ Specific to smooth muscle receptors at the bladder neck, approved by the FDA for use in men, but used in females with evidence for bladder neck dysfunction
  □ Tamsulosin: Flomax
  □ Alfuzosin: Uroxatral
  □ Silodosin: Rapaflo

Hormonal Therapy

Desmopressin: DDAVP: Desmopressin works by limiting the amount of water that is eliminated in the urine, acting as an "antidiuretic." Utilized for MS-related nocturia 0.5-1.5 episodes per night, reduces urinary frequency in the first 6-8 h after delivery, and is associated with an increase in uninterrupted sleep by a mean of 2 h

FDA, US Food and Drug Administration.

Refractive Neurogenic Bladder Treatments

Injection of BTX-A in the detrusor muscle has an important direct effect on the motor function of the urinary bladder and an indirect effect on the sensory regulation of bladder function. BTX-A inhibits acetylcholine exocytosis. Parasympathetic postganglionic nerves release acetylcholine in the neuromuscular synapse. Acetylcholine then binds with the M2 and M3 muscarinic receptor in the detrusor muscle, leading to contraction.[17]

BTX-A exerts its inhibition of exocytosis at the neural side of the neuromuscular junction. When the vesicles cannot anchor to the cell membrane, no acetylcholine is shed into the synaptic cleft and the contraction is blocked. The heavy chain of the BTX-A toxin facilitates toxin entry into the nerve cells via endocytosis.[38]

The second effect of intradetrusor injections of BTX-A is via the afferent, sensory pathway. Afferent output from the bladder is normally conducted by myelinated Aδ-fibers that carry the signals to the higher brain regions. When these pathways are damaged by neurological disease, a spinal reflex arc consisting of small, unmyelinated C-fibers arises. This involuntary reflex arc leads to uncontrolled bladder contractions and neurogenic detrusor overactivity (NDO).[17,39] BTX-A injections reduce sensory receptor levels in the bladder suburothelium. In its turn, this may reduce the sensitivity of aberrant C-fibers to mechanical stimulation.[39]

TABLE 16.8

BEHAVIORAL MODIFICATIONS FOR URINARY TRACT SYMPTOMS IN MULTIPLE SCLEROSIS[25,32]

Fluid titration	Moderate fluid intake not to exceed 4-6 oz/h
Reduce bladder irritant consumption	Moderate alcohol, fruit juices, caffeine, chocolate, artificial sweeteners, acidic foods/sauces
Stop oral intake 2-3 h before bedtime	Reduces nocturia, nocturnal enuresis risk
Change medication timing	Avoid diuretics in the evening and take medications 2-3 h before bedtime
Timed voiding	Void at regular intervals vs. voiding when urgency creates demand→reduces urge incontinence risk
Bladder retraining/Kegel exercises	Pelvic floor physical therapy controls urge, extends voiding intervals, promotes efficient voiding
Avoid constipation	Regular bowel movement promotes efficient bladder emptying and reduces risk of urinary tract infection

It is generally accepted that a dosage of 200 to 300 U of onabotulinum toxin is comparable with 500 to 750 U of abobotulinum toxin.[38] These are considered the optimal doses for intradetrusor injections in NDO.[40-42]

Percutaneous Tibial Nerve Stimulation

This type of neuromodulation provides stimulation from the posterior tibial nerve to the sacral nerve plexus and controls for urgency, urge incontinence, and fecal incontinence. A patient sits comfortably with the treatment leg elevated. A fine needle electrode is inserted into the lower, inner aspect of the leg, slightly *cephalad/rostral* to the medial malleolus. As the goal is to send stimulation through the tibial nerve, it is important to have the needle electrode near (but not on) the *tibial nerve*. A surface electrode (grounding pad) is placed over the medial aspect of the *calcaneus* on the same leg. The needle electrode is then connected to an external pulse generator which delivers an adjustable electrical pulse that travels to the sacral plexus via the tibial nerve. Among other functions, the sacral nerve plexus regulates bladder and pelvic floor function. With correct placement of the needle electrode and level of electrical impulse, there is often an involuntary toe flex or fan, or an extension of the entire foot. However, for some patients, the correct placement and stimulation may only result in a mild sensation in the ankle area or across the sole of the foot. The treatment protocol requires once-a-week treatments for 12 weeks, 30 minutes per session. Many patients begin to see improvements

---

TABLE 16.9
CONSORTIUM OF MS CENTERS TREATMENT
RECOMMENDATIONS AND ALGORITHM[32]

Urinary bladder symptoms in multiple sclerosis (*from the algorithm*):

■ Assess for treatable causes: DIAPPERS
■ Check postvoid residual (PVR): <150 mL
  □ No Rx
  □ Observation

■ Symptom complex: urge, frequency, urge incontinence (UI) with *no* voiding complaints and PVR<100 mL
  □ Rx: Anticholinergic, beta-3 agonist, pelvic floor muscle therapy (PFMT) (optional)
    ● No improvement: Refer to urology
    ● Improvement: Continue Rx; genitourinary (GU) referral

■ Symptom complex: urge, frequency, UI, voiding complaints, and PVR > 100 mL
  □ Anticholinergic, beta-3 agonist, PFMT (optional)
  □ No improvement: Refer to urology
  □ Improvement: Continue Rx; GU referral

■ Symptom complex: PVR > 150 mL, urgency, UI, stop-and-go "stuttering" urine flow, incomplete emptying with incontinence: suspect detrusor external sphincter dyssynergia (DSD/DESD)
  □ Anticholinergic + alpha blocker ± skeletal muscle relaxant, trial with B-3 agonist; optional PFMT
    ● If reduction in urge and frequency with elevated PVR: GU referral for CIC ± BTXA; S/P tube ± BTXA
    ● If clinically improved, continue Rx; GU referral

■ Symptom complex: PVR > 150 mL, absent sensory urge or awareness of need to void, no UI; overflow incontinence suspected, abnormal uroflow
  □ Trial to void with alpha blocker and timed voids, PFMT. Check PVR; still elevated—cannot r/o areflexia or underactive bladder ± DESD
    ● Catheterization indwelling vs. CIC; GU referral

■ Stress incontinence only
  □ Urology/urogynecology referral

■ Mixed incontinence
  □ Urology/urogynecology referral

CIC, clean intermittent catheterization.

---

by the 6th treatment. Patients who respond to treatment may require occasional treatments (~ once every 3 weeks) to sustain improvements.[32,43]

InterStim Neuromodulation

This procedure provides an electrical charge to an area near the S3 sacral nerve, altering neural activity. The stimulations cause nerve depolarization, producing an action potential. The signal propagates along the axon and alters abnormal sensory inputs from the bladder. Efferent pathways are

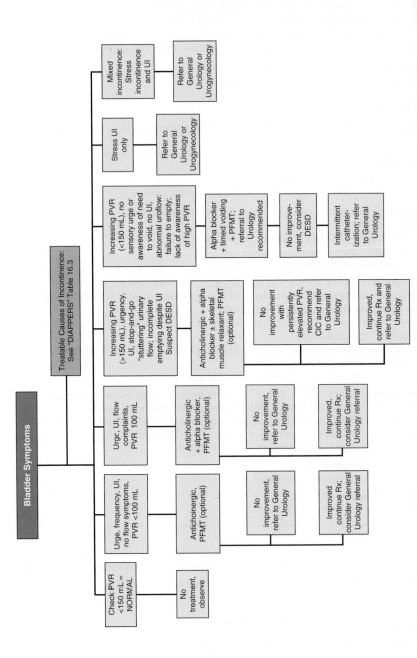

Figure 16.5. Consortium of MS centers bladder symptom and treatment algorithm.[32] DESD, detrusor external sphincter dyssynergia; PFMT, pelvic floor muscle therapy; PVR, postvoid residual; UI, urge incontinence. With permission from CMSC.

uninhibited and do not suppress voluntary voiding.[32,43,44] Full-body magnetic resonance imaging (MRI) can be done safely in all but orthopedic and neurological pathologies, and therefore until such time full-body MRI-safe neurostimulators are developed, sacral nerve stimulation is not recommended.[43,45-47]

Other Treatment Options[32,43,45-52]

Other options include long-term Foley catheter in patients with areflexic NGB and NGB with NDO±DESD (Tables 16.10 and 16.11).

TABLE 16.10
URETHRAL VS. SUPRAPUBIC CATHETERIZATION[50-52,56]

Urethral Catheter	Suprapubic Catheter
■ Urethritis, or inflammation of the urethral meatus	■ Hematuria
■ Balanitis	■ Bladder stones
■ Phimosis	■ Pain
■ Urethral fistula: Vesicovaginal fistula; perineoscrotal abscess and urethrocutaneous fistula	■ Bowel perforation
■ Scrotal abscesses seen in men	■ Latex allergy
■ Epididymitis, orchitis, scrotal abscess, prostatitis, and prostatic abscess	■ Cutaneous infection at cystotomy site
■ Hematuria	■ Urinary tract infection, urosepsis (as a result, MS exacerbation)
■ Bladder stones	■ Bladder spasm requiring anticholinergic therapy, Botox injections
■ Latex allergy	■ Bladder cancer
■ Urethral erosion-hypospadias in men; Urethral decompensation in women with incompetent bladder neck (patulous urethra) requiring urinary diversion	■ Easy catheter changes
■ Pain	■ Urethral encrustation (associated with alkaline urine)
■ Urinary tract infection, urosepsis	■ Requires anesthesia (local, IV sedation, general anesthesia)
■ Bladder spasm requiring anticholinergic therapy, Botox injections	■ Traumatic extraction less commonly occurs
■ Bladder cancer	■ If a suprapubic catheter becomes blocked, urine can drain via the urethra (an alternative option)
■ Difficult catheter passage, especially in men with a large prostate	■ A suprapubic catheter leaves the genitals free for sexual activity
■ Creation of urethral false passage	■ Hygienic maintenance is easier
■ Urethral stricture, bladder neck contracture	■ The procedure is reversible. When a catheter is removed permanently, the hole heals quickly
■ Urethral encrustation	■ Variable-sized catheters can be used, reducing the risk of a blocked catheter without increased pain
■ Injury to external sphincter	■ Urinary diversion
■ Difficult to maintain healthy hygiene	
■ Trauma, traumatic extraction	
■ Prohibited sexual activity	
■ Obstruction of catheter	
■ Urinary diversion	

TABLE 16.11

RECOMMENDATIONS FOR CARE OF THE PATIENT WITH LONG-TERM CATHETERIZATION[49-52,56]

1. Provide for adequate and efficient drainage; prevent kinking

2. Regular bladder irrigations with the appropriate volume of irrigating solution utilizing piston syringe irrigations to break up and aspirate bladder mucus and loose encrustations

3. Persistent blockage and drainage problems should alert treating health care providers to assess for bladder stone by x-Rry and/or cystoscopy

4. Acidification (cranberry pills, vitamin C)

5. Change catheter monthly and as needed

6. Teach willing family and/or health care giver catheter management

7. When symptomatic for infection or exacerbation of MS: perform urine c+s and treat accordingly

c+s, culture and sensitivity.

Urinary Diversion[53]

Most patients undergoing surgical intervention have secondary progressive/primary progressive disease, have failed nonsurgical therapies, and have a higher EDSS (Tables 16.12–16.14).

Tables 16.12– 16.14 describe the indications for urinary diversion, contraindications to urinary diversion, and identifies the various types of urinary diversion.[53,57]

Because bladder dysfunction can often be associated with bowel and sexual dysfunction, the following chapter will focus on these two areas that significantly affect patients' quality of life.

TABLE 16.12

INDICATIONS FOR URINARY DIVERSION[53]

- Chronic urinary tract infections due to retained urine/failure to empty
- Chronic urinary tract infection due to chronic catheter with or without incontinence due to detrusor overactivity
- Bladder cancer (associated with chronic infection)
- Cathctcr-associatcd crosions
- Renal compromise from low bladder compliance and increased intravesical pressures
- Vesicoureteral reflux with nephropathy
- Refractory urinary incontinence causing tissue breakdown with skin complications

TABLE 16.13
ABSOLUTE AND RELATIVE CONTRAINDICATIONS TO URINARY DIVERSION[57]

Absolute Contraindications:	Relative Contraindications:
Renal insufficiency	Advanced age
Hepatic insufficiency	Multiple comorbidities
Inability in the case of continent urinary diversion, to perform clean intermittent stoma catheterization (CISC)	Prior pelvic radiation
	Inflammatory or malignant bowel disease
Unwillingness to do CISC in the case of continent diversion surgery	Need for adjuvant chemotherapy

TABLE 16.14
SURGICAL PROCEDURES IN THE ADULT PATIENT WITH MULTIPLE SCLEROSIS[53]

Ileovesicostomy: A noncontinent diversion in which a loop of small bowel ileum is anastomosed to the bladder dome. This loop of ileum is brought out through the abdominal wall as a stomal urostomy. Often called, "ileal chimney"

Ileal cystoplasty: Bladder wall reconstruction using a segment of ileum to augment bladder capacity

Bladder autoaugmentation: A technique in which detrusor muscle over the entire dome of the bladder is excised while leaving the bladder epithelium intact. The bladder epithelium distends with bladder filling, augmenting bladder capacity. No bowel is used

Ileal conduit diversion: An isolated segment of *ileum* serving as a substitution for the urinary bladder, into which ureters can be implanted, the lumen of which is connected to the skin. The bladder can be removed or left in situ

Continent catheterizable stoma diversion: The creation of an intestinal reservoir with a catheterizable channel that is brought from the reservoir to the skin with creation of a stoma. The channel can be catheterized several times a day to empty the reservoir

References

1. Dillon B, Lemack G. Urodynamics in the evaluation of the patient with multiple sclerosis: when are they helpful and how do we use them? *Urol Clin North Am.* 2014;41(3):439-444.
2. Aharony S, Lam O, Corcos J. Evaluation of lower urinary tract symptoms in multiple sclerosis patients: review of the literature and current guidelines. *Can J Urol.* 2017;11(1-2):61-64.
3. Calabresi P, Newsome S. Multiple sclerosis. In: Weiner J, Goetz CG, Shin RK, Lewis SL, eds. *Neurology for the Non-Neurologist.* Wolters Kluwer/Lippincott Williams & Wilkins; 2010:192-221:chap 11.
4. Eikelenboom M, Killestein J, Krajt J, et al. Gender differences in multiple sclerosis: cytokines and vitamin D. *J Neurol Sci.* 2009;286(1-2):40-42.

5. Radzisewski P, Crayton R, Zaborski J, et al. Multiple sclerosis produces significant changes in urinary bladder innervation which are partially reflected in the lower urinary tract functional status-sensory nerve fibers role in detrusor overactivity. *Mult Scler.* 2009;15(7):860-868.

6. Hinson J, Boone T. Urodynamics and multiple sclerosis. *Clin Urol North Am.* 1996;23:475-481.

7. Denys P, Even A, Chartier-Kastler E. Therapeutic strategies of urinary disorders in MS. Practice and algorithms. *Ann Phys Rehabil Med.* 2014;57(5):297-301.

8. Mahajan S, Patel P, Marie R. Undertreatment of overactive bladder symptoms in patients with multiple sclerosis: an ancillary analysis of the NARCOMS patient registry. *J Urol.* 2010;183(4):1432-1437.

9. Nortvedt M, Riise T, Frugaard J, et al. Prevalence of bladder, bowel and sexual problems among multiple sclerosis patients two to five years after diagnosis. *Mult Scler.* 2007;13:106-112.

10. Buchanan R, Radin D, Huang C. Caregiver burden among informal caregivers assisting people with multiple sclerosis. *Int J MS Care.* 2011;13:76-83.

11. Rivera V, Macias M. Access and barriers to MS care in Latin America. *Mult Scler J Exp Transl Clin.* 2017;3(1):1-7.

12. MS Barometer 2015 – European Multiple Sclerosis Platform. Available at http://www.emsp.org/projects/ms-barometer/. Accessed January 1, 2018.

13. Brichetto G, Messmer Uccelli M, Mancardi GL, Solaro C. Symptomatic medication use in multiple sclerosis. *Mult Scler.* 2003;9:458-460.

14. Gu B, Reiter JP, Schwinn DA, et al. Effects of alpha 1-adrebergic receptor subtype selective antagonists on lower urinary tract function in rats with bladder outlet obstruction. *J Urol.* 2004;172(2):758-762.

15. Clemons JQ. Basic bladder neurophysiology. *Clin Urol North Am.* 2010;37(4):487-494.

16. Birder LA. Nervous network for lower urinary tract function. *Int J Urol.* 2013;20(1):4-12.

17. Fowler C, Griffiths D, deGroat W. The neural control of micturition, *Natl Rev Neurosci.* 2008;9(6):453-466.

18. Araki I, deGroat W. Unitary excitatory synaptic currents in preganglionic neurons mediated by two distinct groups of interneurons in neonatal rat sacral parasympathetic nucleus. *J Neurophysiol.* 1996;76(1):215-226.

19. Isao A, Makoto M, Kyoko O, Masayuki T, Sadako K. Relationship of bladder dysfunction to lesion site in multiple sclerosis. *J Urol.* 2003;169:1384-1387.

20. Wein AJ, Dmochowski R. Neuromuscular dysfunction of the lower urinary tract. In: Wein AJ, Kavoussi LR, Partin AW, Peters CA, eds. *Campbell-Walsh Urology.* 12th ed. Philadelphia: Saunders; 2012:1761-1795.

21. de Seze M, Ruffion A, Denys P, et al. The neurogenic bladder in multiple sclerosis: review of the literature and proposal of management guidelines. *Mult Scler.* 2007;13:915-928.

22. Fowler C. Neurological disorders of micturition and their treatment. *Brain J.* 1999;122:1213-1231.

23. Rao S, Leo G, Haughton V, et al. Correlation of magnetic resonance imaging with neuropsychological testing in multiple sclerosis. *Neurology.* 2004;63:161-166.

24. Wein A, Barrett D. *Normal lower urinary tract filling/storage and emptying: simple overview, extrapolation, and application of the two-phase concept.* In: *Voiding Function and Dysfunction: A Logical and Practical Approach.* Chicago: Year Book Medical Publishers; 1988:114-136.

25. Wein A. Pathophysiology and classification of lower urinary tract dysfunction: overview. In: Wein AJ, Kavoussi LR, Partin AW, Peters CA, eds. *Campbell-Walsh Urology.* 12th ed. Philadelphia: Saunders; 2012:1685-1696.

26. Wein A, Rovner E. Definition and epidemiology of overactive bladder. *Urology.* 2002;60(5 suppl 1):7-12; discussion 12.

27. Drake M. Overactive bladder. In Wein AJ, Kavoussi LR, Partin AW, Peters CA, eds. *Campbell-Walsh Urology.* 12th ed. Philadelphia: Saunders; 2012:1796-1806.

28. Frost N, Szpak J, Litwillerr S, Rae-Grant A. Management of bladder and sexual dysfunction in multiple sclerosis. In: Cohen JA, Rudick RA, eds. *Multiple Sclerosis Therapeutics.* 4th ed. New York: Cambridge University Press; 2011:676-695;chap 58.

29. Abrams P, Cardozo L, Fall M, et al. The standardization of terminology of lower urinary tract function: report for the standardization subcommittee of the International Continence Society. *Neurol Urodyn.* 2002;21:167-178.

30. Sirls LT, Choe JM. The incontinence history and physical examination. In O'Donnell PD (Ed). *Urinary Incontinence.* St. Louis: Mosby-Year Book; 1997:54-63;chap 8.

31. Newsome S, Aliotta P, Bainbridge J, et al. A framework of care in multiple sclerosis. Part 2 symptomatic care and beyond. *Int J MS Care.* 2017;19:42-56.

32. Namey M, Halper J, Aliotta P, et al. Elimination dysfunction in multiple sclerosis. *Int J MS Care.* 2012;14(suppl 1):1-26.

33. Orasanu B, Mahajan S. Bladder and bowel dysfunction in multiple sclerosis. In Rae-Grant AD, Fox RJ, Bthoux F, eds. *Multiple Sclerosis and Related Disorders.* 1st ed. New York: Demos Medical Publishing; 2013:200-210.

34. Utomo E, Korfage I, Wildhagen M, Steensma A, Bangma C, Blok B. Validation of the Urogenital Distress Inventory (UDI-6) and Incontinence Impact Questionnaire (IIQ-7) in a Dutch population. *Neurourol Urodyn.* 2015;34(1):24-31.

35. Tannenbaum C, Brouillette J, Korner-Bitensky N, et al. Creation and testing of the geriatric self-efficacy index for urinary incontinence. *J Am Geriatr Soc.* 2008;56(3):542-547.

36. Uebersax J, Wyman J, Shumaker S, McClish D, Fantl J, The Continence Program for Women Research Group. 1995. Short forms to assess life quality and symptom distress for urinary incontinence in women: the Incontinence Impact Questionnaire and the Urogenital Distress Inventory. *Neurourol Urodyn.* 1995;14:131-139.

37. Barber M, Walters M, Bump R. Short forms of two condition-specific quality-of-life questionnaires for women with pelvic floor disorders (PFDI-20 and PFIQ-7). *Am J Obstet Gynecol.* 2005;193:103-113.

38. Aoki KR, Guyer B. Botulinum toxin type A and other botulinum toxin serotypes: a comparative review of biochemical and pharmacological actions. *Eur J Neurol.* 2001;8(suppl 5):21-29.

39. Tanagho EA, McAninch JW, eds. *Smith's General Urology.* 17th ed. New York: The McGraw-Hill Companies, Inc.; 2008:438-453.

40. Grise P, Ruffion A, Denys P, et al. Efficacy and tolerability of botulinum toxin type A in patients with neurogenic detrusor overactivity and without concomitant anticholinergic therapy: comparison of two doses. *J Eur Urol.* 2010;58:759-766.

41. Cruz F, Herschorn S, Aliotta P, et al. Efficacy and safety of onabotulinumtoxinA in patients with urinary incontinence due to neurogenic detrusor overactivity: a randomized, double-blind, placebo-controlled trial. *Eur Urol J.* 2011;60:742-750.

42. Ginsberg D, Gousse A, Keppene V, et al. Phase 3 efficacy and tolerability study of onabotulinumtoxinA for urinary incontinence from neurogenic detrusor overactivity. *J Urol.* 2012;187:2131.

43. MacDiarmid S, Peters K, Shobeiri S, et al. Long-term durability of percutaneous tibial nerve stimulation for the treatment of overactive bladder. *J Urol*. 2010;183(1):234-240.

44. Schurch B, De Seze M, Denys P, et al. Botulinum toxin type A is a safe and effective treatment for neurogenic urinary incontinence: results of a single treatment, randomized, placebo controlled 6-month study. *J Urol*. 2005;174:196-200.

45. Neuromodulation: Chancellor MB. How sacral nerve stimulation neuromodulation works. *Clin Urol North Am*. 2005;32:11-18.

46. Siegel SW. Selecting patients for sacral nerve stimulation. *Clin Urol North Am*. 2005;32:19.

47. Wein AJ, English WS, Whitmore KE. Office urodynamics. *Clin Urol North Am*. 1988;15(4):609-623.

48. Pannil FC, Williamsm TF, Davis R. Evaluation and treatment of urinary incontinence in long term care. *J Am Geriatr Soc*. 1988;36:902-910.

49. Lloyd J, Gill B, Pizarro-Berdichevsky, et al. Removal of sacral nerve stimulation devices for magnetic resonance imaging: what happens next. Abstract PD54-02. *J Urol*. 2017;197(4S):1046.

50. Drinka PJ. Complications of chronic indwelling urinary catheters. *J Am Med Dir Assoc*. 2006;7(6):388-392.

51. Warren JW, Muncie HL, Hebel JR, Hall-Craggs M. Long-term urethral catheterization increases risk of chronic pyelonephritis and renal inflammation. *J Am Geriatr Soc*. 1994;42(12):1286-1290.

52. Ouslander JG, Greengold B, Chen S. Complications of chronic indwelling urinary catheters among male nursing home patients: a prospective study. *J Urol*. 1987;138(5):1191-1195.

53. Stoffel JT. Contemporary management of the neurogenic bladder for multiple sclerosis patients. *Clin Urol North Am*. 2010;37:547-557.

54. Resnick N. Geriatric incontinence. *Clin Urol North Am*. 1996;23:55.

55. Resnick N. Urinary incontinence in the elderly. *Med Grand Rounds*. 1984;3:281.

56. Igawa Y, Wyndaele JJ, Nishizawa O. Catheterization: possible complications and their prevention and treatment. *Int J Urol*. 2008;15:481-485.

57. Spencer ES, Lyons MD, Pruthi RS. Patient selection and counseling for urinary diversion. *Uro Clin N Am*. 2018;45:1-9.

Bowel and Sexual Dysfunction in the Multiple Sclerosis Patient

■■■ Philip J. Aliotta

Elimination Issues in Multiple Sclerosis: Bowel Disorders

In the population with multiple sclerosis (MS), bowel dysfunction is under-reported. When investigated, 60% of patients with MS experience some form of bowel dysfunction.[1] Constipation is reported to predate diagnosis in many cases and may be an early nonspecific symptom of the disease.[2,3] Upper gut symptoms, such as difficulty swallowing, are also widespread.[2] NARCOMS identifies three types of bowel complaints experienced by patients with MS: 39% have constipation, 11% have fecal incontinence, and 36% have both.[4] The Bowel Function Questionnaire for MS helps differentiate the three types of bowel dysfunction and comprises 15 items pertaining to constipation, 13 items for fecal incontinence, and 20 items for both constipation and fecal incontinence. It is self-administered. Other questionnaires are Brief Fecal Incontinence Questionnaire, Quality of Life Scoring Tool Relating to Bowel Management (QOL-BM), and the Constipation Symptom Assessment Instrument (PAC-SYM).[5,6] Das Gupta and Fowler categorized symptoms associated with bowel dysfunction into disorders of elimination (constipation) or storage (incontinence) or a combination of both.[7,8] Constipation is caused by slow colonic transit, abnormal rectal function, and intussusception. It is the most common bowel complaint of people with MS.[9] Rectal overload and overflow with impaired sensation due to neurogenic bowel in the patient with constipation can lead to fecal incontinence.[10,11]

Owing to the variable range of related symptoms and the timing of their occurrence, the term constipation has different meanings for different individuals.[12] Constipation is defined as less than or equal to two bowel movements per week or the need for stimulation (digitally or with the use of laxatives, enemas, or suppositories) more often than once per week.[13]

Fecal incontinence is less difficult to characterize, as it can present with solid or liquid stool or flatus alone. It may be passive, occurring without the patient' awareness, or urgent (Table 17.1).[14] Bowel problems have been found to be associated with more severe disability, disease progression, genitourinary symptoms, and depression but not necessarily with gender. The bowel problems associated with specific subtypes of MS have not been identified.[15,16] Time spent on bowel management affects daily activities. It has been reported that 23% of patients spend 16 to 30 minutes per day and approximately 30% spend anywhere form 16 minutes to over 1 hour daily attending to bowel issues. Thirty-five percent of patients with MS report that their bowel management problems stops them from working outside of the home. Fifteen percent identify bowel issues as interfering with personal intimacy.[3] The cause of the bowel dysfunction can be multifactorial: due to disease progression, secondary to drug therapies for MS and its associated comorbidities, behavioral problems, or concurrent medical problems.[7]

From a neurological perspective, bulbar and spinal involvement can affect bowel regulation by interfering with afferent sensory or efferent motor pathways. Patients with MS with constipation or fecal incontinence are reported to have delayed somatosensory evoked potentials when

TABLE 17.1
SYMPTOM PRESENTATION RELATED TO CONSTIPATION[13]

No stool	Distended abdomen
Decreased bowel movements	Palpable mass
Hard, formed stools	Headache
Severe flatus	Anorexia
Rectal fullness	Nausea and/or vomiting
Decreased bowel sounds	Diarrhea related to fecal impaction
	Increased fatigue

TABLE 17.2
SYMPTOM PRESENTATION OF FECAL INCONTINENCE[14]

Presentation	Timing/Occurrence
Solid with or without flatus	Passive/urgent
Liquid with or without flatus	Passive/urgent
Flatus alone	Passive/urgent

recorded from the brain but normal potentials at the lumbar spine, suggesting higher spinal or cerebral involvement in these patients.[17] Motor spinal pathways show prolongation in cortex to lumbar spine and cortex to pelvic floor striated muscle conduction times. Altered large bowel compliance and prolonged colonic transit time have been associated with demyelinating lesions of the conus medullaris.[18]

Presentation

As stated, the cause of bowel problems in MS is often multifactorial. Patients present with variable complaints and symptoms (Table 17.1). The presence of constipation correlated strongly with the duration of illness, presence of genitourinary symptoms, and use of medications.[14]

Chronic constipation accounts for exacerbation and persistence of the presenting symptoms (Table 17.2) and is a source of complications (Table 17.3).

Evaluation

Bowel problems in MS are multifactorial, and aside from the presentation of constipation with or without flatus, fecal incontinence with or without liquid stools, or flatus alone, assessment should include an assessment of the physical limitations, psychosocial challenges, work environment assessment, dietary habits, fluid hydration, as well as an evaluation of bladder control.

TABLE 17.3
COMPLICATIONS OF CONSTIPATION[11]

Hemorrhoidal irritation
Rectal prolapse
Anal fissures
Pain
Bleeding
Excessive secretion of mucus

TABLE 17.4
ASSESSMENT OF BOWEL FUNCTION[13]

Muscle tone and Strength	Environment
Cognitive and communication abilities	Personal assistance
Ability to chew and swallow	Medication
Past bowel history	Bladder management
Eating habits	Patient's perception of the problem
Motor skills and degree of independence	

Various scales exist to assess for fecal incontinence. These scales, i.e., Pescatori,[19] Wexner,[20] American Medical Systems Score,[21] correlate well with careful clinical impression and severity.[14] The application of questionnaires for fecal incontinence and quality-of-life assessment has a positive impact because they include the improvement not only of individual clinical practice but also of evaluating the effectiveness of treatments and the functioning of health services.[22]

In addition to the general assessment of bowel habits and function (Table 17.4), measurement of gut transit time provides a measure of large bowel function. Radiopaque markers can be used to evaluate gut transit. Other tests include anorectal manometry, balloon expulsion testing, and electrical rectal sensory testing, and evacuation proctography has been used to assess pelvic floor coordination and distal colonic innervation, to rule out megarectum, and to assess slow or incomplete rectal emptying and sphincter function.[12]

Medications must be reviewed, as most medications used for bladder overactivity, i.e., anticholinergics, can cause and or exacerbate bowel problems (Table 17.5).

Past medical and surgical history must be obtained and reviewed. Previous bowel surgeries, pelvic surgeries, radiation therapy, underlying medical disease of the colon, i.e., Crohn disease, diverticulosis with or without diverticulitis, ulcerative colitis, and irritable bowel syndrome must be evaluated. If diarrhea is the chief complaint, a search for the causes of diarrhea is required (Table 17.6). In women, obstetric history may contribute to bowel disturbances. A focused physical examination should be performed, including abdominal examination, pelvic/perineal assessment, and rectal examination. A rectal examination assesses external sphincter pressure and resting anal tone. Stool for occult blood can be obtained. Laboratory assessment includes blood glucose, electrolytes, calcium, and thyroid function tests.[5] Emotional factors and behavioral changes may influence toileting habits directly or through altered autonomic control of gut function.[12] As part of the history, diet and lifestyle play an important role in understanding bowel dysfunction. Having a poor diet is often cited as the reason why people have constipation, but there are many factors that can contribute to the development of this problem.

TABLE 17.5
AGENTS THAT CAUSE CONSTIPATION[23]

- Oral contraceptives
- Opioid pain relievers
- Anticholinergic agents
- Antispasmodics
- Tricyclic antidepressants
- Calcium channel blockers
- Sympathomimetics
- Antipsychotics
- Diuretics
- Antihypertensives
- Antihistamines
- Antacids (containing calcium and aluminum)
- Calcium supplements
- Iron supplements
- Antidiarrheal agents (loperamide, attapulgite)
- Anticonvulsants
- Nonsteroidal anti-inflammatory drugs
- Miscellaneous compounds, including octreotide, polystyrene resins, cholestyramine

Measurement of gut transit time provides a measure of large bowel function. Radiopaque markers can be used to evaluate gut transit. Anorectal manometry, balloon expulsion testing, and electrical rectal sensory testing, and evacuation proctography has been used to assess pelvic floor coordination and distal colonic innervation, to rule out megarectum, and to assess slow or incomplete rectal emptying and sphincter function.[12]

The **Bristol stool scale** (Figure 17.1) is a diagnostic medical tool designed to classify the form of human feces into seven categories. It is used in both clinical and experimental fields. It is sometimes also referred to as the Bristol stool chart (BSC), Bristol stool form scale, or BSF scale.[24]

TABLE 17.6
CAUSES OF DIARRHEA[13]

Fecal impaction
Diet/irritating foods-dietary intolerance
Inflammatory bowel disease
Stress/anxiety
Medications
Overuse of laxatives/stool softeners
Interruption in the neural pathways
Impaired cortical awareness of urge to defecate
Sensory loss in perineum and rectum

It was developed as a clinical assessment tool and is widely used as a research tool to evaluate the effectiveness of treatments for various diseases of the bowel, as well as a clinical communication aid.[25]

Constipation

Rome IV Criteria for Constipation. This is used in patients with complaints of constipation for at least 3 months with symptoms onset >6 months.

Do not use in patients with gastrointestinal (GI) bleeding, unexplained iron deficiency anemia, unintentional weight loss, palpable abdominal mass, family history of colon cancer, or symptom onset >5 years and not yet screened for colon cancer, or sudden/acute inset of new change in bowel habit.

Rome IV criteria define constipation as any two of the following criteria[24,26,27]:

- Straining: for greater than one-fourth (25%) of defecations
- Lumpy or hard stools: type 1 or 2 on the Bristol Stool Form Scale; for greater than one-fourth (25%) of defecations

Type 1		Separate hard lumps, like nuts (hard to pass)
Type 2		Sausage-shaped but lumpy
Type 3		Like a sausage but with cracks on the surface
Type 4		Like a sausage or snake, smooth and soft
Type 5		Soft blobs with clear-cut edges
Type 6		Fluffy pieces with ragged edges, a mushy stool
Type 7		Water, no solid pieces, **Entirely Liquid**

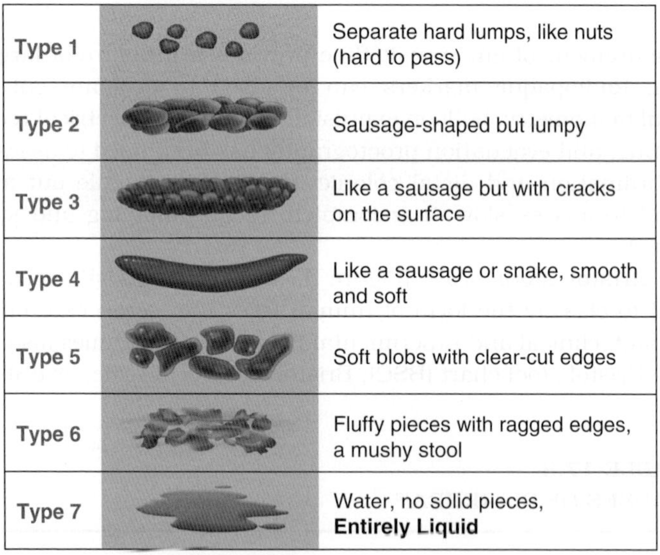

Figure 17.1. Bristol Stool Chart. See eBook for color figure.

Interpretation:

- **Types 1–2** indicate constipation,
- **Types 3–4** are ideal stools as they are easier to pass, and
- **Types 5–7** may indicate diarrhea and urgency.

Reprinted with permission from Baskin LS. *Handbook of Pediatric Urology*. 3rd ed. Philadelphia, PA: Wolters Kluwer; 2018. Figure 10-1.

- Sensation of incomplete evacuation: for greater than one-fourth (25%) of defecations
- Sensation of anorectal obstruction/blockage: for greater than one-fourth (25%) of defecations
- Manual maneuvers to facilitate defecation, that is, digital evacuation, pelvic floor support; for greater than one-fourth (25%) of defecations
- Less than three spontaneous bowel movements per week

The lifestyle factors that increase chances of becoming constipated include:

- Not eating enough foods that are high in fiber
- Not drinking enough liquids
- Not getting enough exercise
- Not maintaining a healthy weight

Fecal Incontinence

Demyelinating lesions and reflexive activity cause frequent diarrhea leading to recurrent emptying of the rectum.[28] Patients need to be assessed for their ability to sense rectal fullness and when they need to defecate.[10]

Fecal incontinence is caused by a reduced sensation of rectal filling, poor pelvic floor muscle control, reduced rectal compliance, and weakness of the anal sphincter.[7-9]

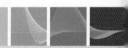

Case Study

A patient with a neurogenic bladder in follow-up presented with the lower GI complaints of bowel irregularities now exacerbated by the bladder therapy. Her symptoms included severe constipation of up to 6 to 7 days longer then her initial presentation with flatulence, cramping, and increasing malaise, culminating with massive, often unexpected, bowel movements. Stools were described as a mix of hard lumps both large and medium seen initially with lumps and formed stool. There is no hematochezia. Her stool pattern is consistent with Bristol types 1 and 2 (Figure 17.1). These episodes of constipation were followed by intermittent attacks of diarrhea, which could last 1 to 2 days before "settling down to my normal routine." Laboratory data reviewed were normal. Medications were re-evaluated. On pelvic examination, a small rectocele and fecal impaction was noted. Abdominal flat plate x-ray demonstrated severe constipation (Figure 17.2). Neurological examination was intact.

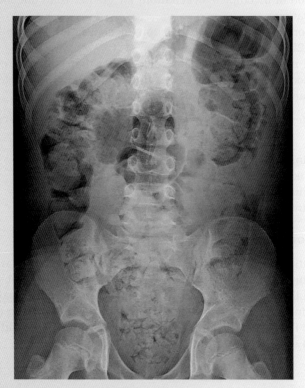

Figure 17.2. Abdominal flat plate x-ray: severe constipation.

Treatment

An important aspect of treating bowel disturbances in the patient with MS is to recognize that, with MS, disease progression, exacerbations, and remissions affect bowel function. Revisiting the problem at regular intervals is necessary to best maintain consistency and predictable outcomes for the patient, reduce unwanted secondary effects of medications on bowel regularity and adequacy of bowel movements, and reduce secondary effects from constipation, fecal incontinence, or both. The first line of treatment for constipation with incontinence is lifestyle modification (Table 17.7) or a bowel training program.

A bowel training program should:

- Normalize stool consistency
- Establish a regular pattern of defecation

TABLE 17.7

BOWEL DYSFUNCTION IN MULTIPLE SCLEROSIS: TREATMENT— LIFESTYLE MODIFICATIONS[5]

- High-fiber diet: 25 g/d young females; 21 g/d for women >50 y; 38 g/d males
- Avoid gas-producing aliments such as sugar substitutes, caffeine, and alcohol
- Total fluid intake should be 2000 mL per day
- Digital rectal stimulation
- Daily abdominal massages
- Exercise: CMSC Consensus Panel recommends walking 10-30 min per day or more intense activity if patient mobility allows
- PT/OT: to optimize mobility and upper and lower body strength and enhance ADL functioning
- Eat regular meals and try to have a bowel movement 15-30 min after a warm meal
- In an upright seated position with feet on the floor/stool, attempt at defecation with abdominal Credé maneuver to facilitate the bowel movement

ADL, activity of daily living; CMSC, Consortium of Multiple Sclerosis Centers; PT/OT, physical therapy/occupational therapy.

- Stimulate rectal emptying before rectal overload and overflow leading to incontinence
- Avoid diarrhea, constipation, and incontinence as side effects
- Improve quality of life

Bowel training program is reported to take 3 to 4 weeks to establish.[13] Exercise:

- Improves digestion
- Stimulates the contraction of intestinal muscles
- Speeds transit time

It lessens the amount of water absorbed from the stool into the body, which reduces the occurrence of hard, dry, painful stools.

For patients with MS who are immobile, a home exercise program can be devised by a physical therapist.

The role of timing elimination:

Patients should be recommended to eat at regular intervals and choose a time about 20 to 30 minutes after a warm meal or beverage, when the gastrocolic reflex produces an urge to defecate, to try and have a bowel movement. Timed voiding and bowel movements are useful in patients who do not sense the urge to eliminate.[13]

If lifestyle modifications do not result in effective elimination, nonprescription stool softeners, stimulants, or osmotically active laxatives that cause rhythmic contractions can be used (Tables 17.8 and 17.9).

TABLE 17.8
BOWEL DYSFUNCTION IN MULTIPLE SCLEROSIS (MS):
MEDICATIONS THAT RELIEVE CONSTIPATION[11]

Stimulant Laxatives
Fleet Bisacodyl enema/Cascara sagrada/Senekot

Fiber Supplements/Bulk Formers
Benefiber/Citrucel/Fiberall/FiberCon/Metamucil/Naturacil/Perdiem

Stool Softeners
Colace/Chronulac syrup/Surfak

Osmotically Active and Saline Laxatives
MiraLAX/Milk of Magnesia/Modane/Pericolace

Harsh Products to be Avoided in Patients with MS:
Castor Oil
Correctol
Dulcolax tablets
Ex-Lax
Feen-a-Mint

TABLE 17.9
BOWEL DYSFUNCTION IN MULTIPLE SCLEROSIS: MEDICATIONS
THAT RELIEVE DIARRHEA[11]

Antidiarrheals (Loperamide)
Imodium and Imodium AD
Kaopectate II
Maalox Antidiarrheal
Pepto Diarrhea Control

Bulking Agents
Natural Bran
Benefiber
Citrucel
Fiberall/FiberCon
Metamucil
Perdiem

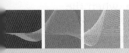

Case Study

The patient was counseled in lifestyle modifications, given a PT/OT refer-ral, and treated successfully with osmotically active laxative, Miralax.

The Consortium of MS Centers Consensus Panel on Elimination Disorders divided patients with MS-related bowel dysfunction into two groups: constipation with incontinence and incontinence only. These two groups were further divided on the basis of mobility status, mobile and immobile (Figure 17.3). A minimum trial period of at least 4 weeks is recommended for each treatment regimen to determine efficacy of care.[5,13]

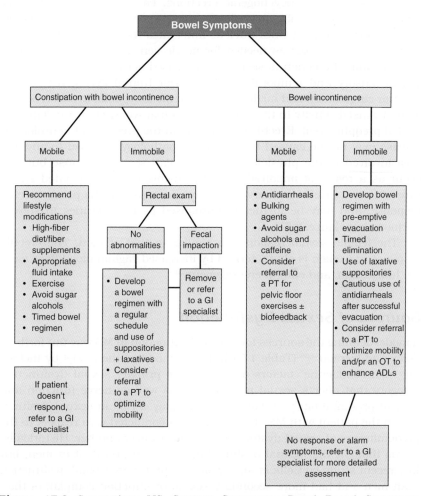

Figure 17.3. Consortium MS Centers Consensus Panel Bowel Symptoms Algorithm. ADL, activity of daily living; GI, gastrointestinal; OT, occupational therapy; PT, physical therapy. Reprinted with permission from Namey M, Halper J, Aliotta P, et al. Elimination dysfunction in multiple sclerosis. *Int J MS Care.* 2012;14(Suppl 1):1-26. Copyright © 2012 by the Consortium of Multiple Sclerosis Centers and Rehabilitation in Multiple Sclerosis.

Sexual Dysfunction in Multiple Sclerosis

In the patient with MS, sexual dysfunction is reported to affect 80% to 90% of men and 40% to 80% of women.[4,29]

Neurogenic erectile dysfunction is the inability to obtain and maintain a penile erection to the mutual satisfaction of both partners because of existing neurological disease.[30] It involves the central nervous system or the peripheral neural pathway. Sympathetic innervation from T10 to L2 is responsible for psychogenic erections. Parasympathetic S2 to S4 innervation is responsible for reflexogenic erections. Somatic innervation S2 to S4 originating in Onuf nucleus innervates the ischiocavernous and bulbocavernosus muscles needed for penile sensation and penile rigidity.[31] Sustained erection is seen with increased activity in the secondary somatosensory and temporal cortex, inferior frontal gyrus, the insula, anterior cingulatem, and medial nucleus of the amygdala. Erection occurs with increased activity in the hypothalamus (paraventricular nucleus and medial preoptic area). Erectile dysfunction in the presence of neurological disease may not be caused by damage or pathology confined to any one area involved in the physiology of the human sexual response but can occur as a result of impaired neural transmission to associated structures, afferent or efferent nerve pathways necessary in the penile erectile response, and may be further compromised by irregularities in steroid hormone imbalance.[30-32]

The female sexual response is similar to that of men. The erectile response in women is characterized by increased vaginal blood flow, vaginal lubrication, and clitoral engorgement.[33]

Sources of Sexual Dysfunction

A model defining the sources for sexual dysfunction in MS was put forth by Foley and Iverson[34,35] (Table 17.10). I have modified the model by including "neuroendocrine" factors as part of the primary sexual dysfunction category that affects sexual performance as well as nerve function and clinical presentation.[34-37,48] Gender issues play a role in sexual dysfunction in the patient with MS. The literature is conflicted with respect to the predominance of sexual dysfunction in one sex over another. Historically, it was thought that sexual dysfunction was more prevalent in men, but in a recent study by Celik et al.,[49] women report more sexual dysfunction than men and had more secondary sexual dysfunction complaints than men.[38,39,49,50] Although sexual dysfunction is more prevalent in women, the prognosis is better for women than for men.[51,52]

Conflicting data exist as to the effect of age, disease duration, and occurrence. Symptoms severity of sexual dysfunction in MS is reported by Foley and by Zorzon et al. to be related to disability and duration of

TABLE 17.10

SOURCES OF SEXUAL DYSFUNCTION IN MULTIPLE SCLEROSIS (MS)[34-47]

Primary Sexual Dysfunction: Neurological	Physiologic impairments due to demyelinating lesions in the spinal cord and/or brain	Numbness, sensory paresthesia in genitalia, erectile dysfunction, loss of vaginal lubrication
Primary Sexual Dysfunction: Neuroendocrine	Physiologic impairment involving: **Hypothalamic-pituitary-adrenal axis (HPA) Hypothalamic-pituitary-gonadal axis**	HPA hyperactivity: increased cortisol, adrenocorticotropic hormone (ACTH), dehydroepiandrosterone sulfate (DHEAS) The HPA hyperactivity is accompanied with progressive disease and global neurodegeneration MS disturbs steroid hormone metabolism and damages the hypothalamus, affecting sex hormone levels MS interferes with the protective role of estrogen and progesterone in myelin metabolism and by preventing neuron apoptosis interfering with intracellular neuron cell death cascades Menstrual cycle changes: Lower levels of progesterone are associated with more frequent MS relapses/exacerbations. Demyelination and cytokine release are associated with lower testosterone levels, hypogonadism, and impaired semen parameters
Secondary Sexual Dysfunction	Nonsexual physiological changes affecting sexual response	Fatigue, spasticity, bladder-bowel pelvic floor dysfunction, and pain
Tertiary Sexual Dysfunction	Psychosocial and cultural issues that interfere with sexual satisfaction or performance	Role changes that stem from MS, low self-esteem, depression, demoralization, communication difficulties, family support network, fear of rejection, fear of dependency, anger

MS.[53,54] Greer et al. reported that age, time since diagnosis of MS, and the Expanded Disability Status Scale score were not correlated with the incidence or severity of sexual dysfunction.[55]

Sexual dysfunction is a major cause of distress,[56] and patients with bladder and sexual dysfunction have poorer quality of life, as measured by the Short-Form 36 survey.[57]

Normal sexual functions require the integrity of the nervous system.[33] MS lesions on the occipital cortex compromise female sexual arousal. Left insular cortex lesions impair vaginal lubrication.

Arousal and lubrication issues are not affected by age, severity of disease, time since diagnosis, cord involvement, or depression.[58]

Sexual Arousal Models

Masters and Johnson identified four stages of physiologic response to sexual stimulation: (1) sexual desire, (2) sexual arousal, (3) sexual orgasm, and (4) the resolution phase. These phases of the sexual response cycle were originally proposed as a linear model, meaning that desire must precede arousal, arousal must precede orgasm, and so on, in a fixed linear sequence. This model appears to work for men but is felt to not be representative of women.[59]

As evidenced from the many models put forward (Table 17.11),[28,40-43,59-64] gender differences in sex drive, sexual motivation, sexual concordance, and capacity for orgasm exist. Acknowledging the four phases in the Masters and Johnson model, Basson postulated that the female cycle begins with women feeling a need for intimacy, which leads her to seek out and be receptive to sexual stimuli; women then feel sexual arousal, in addition to sexual desire, resulting in an enhanced feeling of intimacy; many women experience sexual arousal and responsive desire simultaneously when they are engaged in sexual activity. Kaplan in the three-phase

TABLE 17.11
SEXUAL AROUSAL SEXUAL RESPONSE MODELS

Male Sexual Response Cycle Models	Female Sexual Response Cycle Models
Masters and Johnson four-stage linear model of sexual arousal and response	Masters and Johnson four-stage linear model of sexual arousal and response
Kaplan triphasic linear model of sexual response	Kaplan triphasic linear model of sexual response
Singer's three sequential phase model of sexual arousal	Singer's three sequential phase model of sexual arousal
Toates incentive-motivation model of sexual response	Whipple and Brash-McGreer circular model of sexual arousal
	Toates incentive-motivation model of sexual response
	Basson's nonlinear model of sexual response

TABLE 17.12

MOST COMMON SEXUAL DYSFUNCTION SYMPTOM PRESENTATION IN MULTIPLE SCLEROSIS BY GENDER

Male	Female
Erectile Dysfunction	Loss of libido
■ Inability to achieve and maintain erection	Fatigue
	Decreased tactile sensation
■ Able to achieve but not maintain an erection	Decreased or absent orgasm
	Arousal issues
Ejaculatory Dysfunction	Reduced enjoyment
■ Premature ejaculation	Depression
■ Retrograde ejaculation	Frequent urinary tract infection
■ Anejaculation	Vaginal dryness
■ Delayed ejaculation	Dyspareunia
Reduced libido	
Anorgasmia	
Dyspareunia	

model defined the psychological aspect of desire as driving the two physiological responses of arousal and orgasm.[28,40-43,60-64]

In men, erectile dysfunction (Table 17.12)[33] is the most commonly reported sexual problem that directly affects quality of life. Cord involvement in MS may initially result in partial erections and erections on morning waking. This presents a diagnostic dilemma in that practitioners erroneously equate morning erections and intermittent successful erectile response to be diagnostic of psychogenic erectile dysfunction. As the neurological disability progresses, men will experience complete erectile failure as well as ejaculatory dysfunction.[33]

In females, (Table 17.12) sexual dysfunction occurs in all subtypes of MS. Sexual dysfunction occurs irrespective of the type of MS. The most common symptom complaint of females is impaired or absent genital sensations, vaginal dryness, orgasmic dysfunction, loss of libido, and dyspareunia. Other symptoms are present but to a lesser extent reported.[33]

Time since the diagnosis of MS is not a predictor of sexual dysfunction. The main difference between male and female sexual dysfunction is the role the loss of libido plays in the quality-of-life issues. In females, the loss of libido is associated with relationship/intimacy issues, whereas in males, libido is associated with sexual function. Libido is negatively affected by increasing age equally in both sexes.[44]

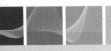

Case Study

A 47-year-old white male with relapsing remitting MS presents with complaints of erectile dysfunction (ED). Before his ED presentation, he complained of urge incontinence, bladder pain from detrusor overactivity, and bladder neck dysfunction manifested as incomplete bladder emptying and a slow stream. These lower urinary tract complaints distracted and interfered with his attempts at intimacy. These symptoms were being successfully managed with an anticholinergic and an alpha blocker.

His erectile dysfunction is characterized by inconsistent morning erections, intact libido, a "partial erection," which at times is "barely capable of vaginal penetration," or as he stated, "the erection was stuffable." The clear majority of time, the erection is not adequate for vaginal penetration. When he can penetrate, he reaches orgasm quickly and loses the erection. He is not able to satisfy not only himself but more importantly to him, his partner. There is significant performance anxiety, relationship fears, and depression. The depression was managed with a selective serotonin reuptake inhibitor. His medical history is significant for hypertension, controlled with thiazide diuretics and beta blockers, and hypertriglyceridemia managed by fenofibrate therapy. There is no family history of urologic malignancy. He complains of late day fatigue. He had a former tobacco use of one-half pack per day for 10 years. He quit smoking 12 years ago. Alcohol consumption is limited to 2 to 3 beers or 1 to 2 mixed cocktails on weekends. He is 20 pounds overweight.

Comorbid factors affecting his erectile function are obesity, hypertriglyceridemia, antihypertensive medications, past history of tobacco use, anxiety/depression, and psychotropic medication.

Evaluation

In the patient with MS, sexual dysfunction can be the presenting symptom of other shared comorbid diseases (Table 17.13).[37,65] It can occur because of patient exposures to medications (Table 17.14),[66,67] medical therapy, radiotherapy, or surgical therapies. A thorough history and focused physical assessing medical, surgical, and psychosocial issues along with requisite laboratory testing is initiated (Tables 17.15 and 17.16).

TABLE 17.13

MEDICAL CONDITIONS ASSOCIATED WITH ERECTILE DYSFUNCTION IN MALES AND FEMALES

Male	Female
Diabetes mellitus	Increasing age
Hypertension	Menopause
Cardiovascular disease	Age of partner
Hypercholesterolemia	Partner sexual dysfunction
Benign prostate enlargement	Bladder control issues
Obstructive urinary symptoms	Depression
BMI > 30	Tobacco use
Physical inactivity	HIV infection
Cigarette abuse	Diabetes mellitus
Antidepressant drug use	Sleep panes
Antihypertensive medications	Hypothyroidism
Psychosocial issues	Poor general health

BMI, body mass index; HIV, human immunodeficiency virus.

TABLE 17.14

MEDICATIONS ASSOCIATED WITH SEXUAL DYSFUNCTION

Male	Female
Antihypertensives	Antiandrogens: spironolactone
■ Diuretics	Anticonvulsants
■ Beta blockers	Anticholinergics
	Antiestrogens
Antiandrogens	Antihistamines
■ 5-alpha reductase inhibitors	Corticosteroids
■ LHRH agonists	
	Antihypertensives
Opiates	■ Diuretics
Alcohol	■ Beta blockers
Tobacco use/abuse	■ Calcium channel blockers
Antiretroviral agents	
Antipsychotics	Contraceptives
SSRI	Metoclopramide
Baclofen	Metronidazole
H-2 receptor antagonists	Alcohol
	Amphetamines
	Opiates

LHRH, luteinizing hormone-releasing hormone; SSRI, selective serotonin reuptake inhibitor.

TABLE 17.15
SPECIALIZED TESTING FOR SEXUAL DYSFUNCTION[66,67,75,76]

Male	Female
Specialist testing: Nocturnal penile tumescence, sacral evoked potential, intracavernosal injection separately or with color duplex Doppler ultrasound, penile brachial index, dynamic cavernosometry/cavernosography, internal pudendal arteriography, bulbocavernosus reflex latency, biothesiometry-vibratory thresholds	**Specialist testing:** sacral evoked potential, pudendal evoked potential, genital sensation: vibration perception thresholds; temperature perceptions, pressure volume changes—vaginal compliance/elasticity, vaginal lubrication measurements, genital blood flow

TABLE 17.16
SEXUAL FUNCTION/QUALITY OF LIFE QUESTIONNAIRES[68-74]

Male	Female
Questionnaires: International Index of Erectile Function (IIEF), Multiple Sclerosis Intimacy and Sexuality Questionnaire (MSISQ-19), Sexual Quality of Life Questionnaire-Male Version (SQoL-M)	**Questionnaires:** Multiple Sclerosis Intimacy and Sexuality Questionnaire (MSISQ-19), Sexual Quality of Life Questionnaire-Female Version (SQoL-F), Female Sexual Function Index (FSFI)

Case Study

Referral to a urologic specialist for sexual dysfunction disease management was made. The patient's hormonal profile assessment was normal and neurourologic examination was normal. The International Index of Erectile Function was abnormal. The nerve conduction sacral evoked potential study showed prolonged bulbocavernosus reflex nerve responses bilaterally, indicating a neurological etiology for his erectile dysfunction. Nocturnal penile tumescence studies were abnormal.

Treatment[36,37,65-67,75]

1. **Patient education**
2. **Aggressive symptom management**
   a. Identify MS symptoms that interfere with intimacy
   b. Assess MS therapies for unintended effect on sexual function
   c. Planning for sexual activities
   d. Altering medications and/or catheterization schedules
3. **Counseling with focus on communication skills**
   a. **Body mapping** exercise: identifies sensory patterns that have been altered by MS, alters patterns of thinking and behaving that contribute to sexual problems
   b. **Cognitive behavioral therapy with focus on communication skills training**
      i. Three phases
         1. Educational: teaches the educational framework for understanding sexual and communicative problems
         2. Rehearsal phase: teaches the patient with MS skills that improve and correct communication problems
         3. Application phase: teaches applying those learned communication skills in the affairs of day-to-day life
4. **Gender-specific therapies**
   a. **Male**
      i. Psychotherapy
      ii. PDE5 inhibitors: sildenafil, vardenafil, tadalafil, avanafil
      iii. Muse intraurethral alprostadil
      iv. Intracavernosal injection therapies
         1. PGE-1 (alprostadil)
         2. Trimix: alprostadil + papaverine + phentolamine
      v. Vacuum erection device
      vi. Hormonal replacement: testosterone replacement
      vii. Vibratory stimulation
      viii. Dopamine agonists, apomorphine
      ix. Ejaculatory dysfunction: yohimbine and midodrine
      x. Penile prosthesis: semirigid, two-piece/three-piece inflatable prosthesis
   b. **Female**
      i. Psychotherapy
      ii. Lubricants
      iii. Hormonal therapy: estrogen replacement; testosterone therapy
      iv. PDE5 inhibitor: sildenafil (limited benefit)
      v. EROS-CTD vacuum device
      vi. Vibratory stimulation

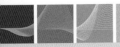

Case Study

The patient was treated with referral to a nutritionist to help with weight loss, a change in antihypertensives with angiotensin II receptor blockers added to the alpha blocker prescribed for bladder neck dysfunction, and a selective serotonin reuptake inhibitor with minimal sexual side effects. Couple therapy and personal counseling were recommended.

Therapeutic options for this patient were identified and discussed in a shared decision-making format. Referral to a urologic specialist for sexual dysfunction disease management was made. Treatment options available were vacuum erection device, 5-phosphodiesterase inhibitor (5PDEi) therapy, intraurethral alprostadil intracavernosal injection (ICI) therapy, and penile prosthesis implantation. He failed first-line 5PDEi therapy but responded to ICI therapy, which he chose to reestablish his intimate life with.

Sexual dysfunction is a challenging part of the MS disease process affecting both men and women. It exerts its primary effect through identifiable and measurable lesions affecting neural pathways (neurological primary sexual dysfunction), identifiable physiologic impairments due to demyelinating lesions in the spinal cord and/or brain, measurable physiologic impairment involving the hypothalamic-pituitary-adrenal axis and hypothalamic-pituitary-gonadal axis (neuroendocrine primary sexual dysfunction), nonsexual physiological changes affecting sexual response (secondary sexual dysfunction), and psychosocial and cultural issues that interfere with sexual satisfaction or performance (tertiary sexual dysfunction). An integrated plan of treatment should include all respective care stakeholders in the care and management of the patient with MS.[33]

References

1. Bennett SE, Belhoux F, Weinstock-Guttman B. Comorbidities breakout group discussion. *Int J MS Care.* 2014;16(suppl 1):19-24.
2. Hinds J P, Wald A. Colonic and anorectal dysfunction associated with multiple sclerosis. *Am J Gastroenterol.* 1989;84(6):587-595.
3. Norton C, Chelvanayagam S. Bowel problems and coping strategies in people with multiuplesclerosis. *Brit J Nurs.* 2010;19(4):220-226.
4. Namey M, Halper J. Elimination dysfunction in multiple sclerosis. *Int J MS Care.* 2012;14(suppl 1):1-26.]

5. Orasanu B, Mahajan ST. Bladder and bowel dysfunction in multiple sclerosis. In: Rae-Grant AD, Fox RJ, Bethoux F, eds. *Multiple Sclerosis and Related Disorders*. 1st ed. New York: Demos Medical Publishing; 2013:200-210.

6. Gullick E, Namey M. Bowel dysfunction in persons with multiple sclerosis. In: Catto-Smith A, ed. *Constipation – Causes Diagnosis and Treatment*: In Tech; 2012.

7. DasGupta R, Fowler C. Bladder, bowel and sexual dysfunction in multiple sclerosis. Management strategies. *Drugs*. 2003;63(2):153-166.

8. Fowler C. Neurological disorders of micturition and their treatment. *Brain*. 1999;122:1213-1231.

9. Fowler CJ, Henry MM. Gastrointestinal dysfunction in multiple sclerosis. *Semin Neurol*. 1977;16:277-279.

10. Kim J-H. Management of urinary and bowel dysfunction in multiple sclerosis. In: Halper J, Holland NJ, eds. *Comprehensive Nursing Care in Multiple Sclerosis*. 3rd ed. New York: Springer Publishing Company; 2010:197-209.

11. Namey M, Halper J, Aliotta PJ, et al. Elimination dysfunction in multiple sclerosis. Proceedings of a consensus conference. *Int J MS Care*. 2011;14:1-26.

12. Wiesel PH, Norton C, Glickman S, Kamm MA. Pathophysiology and management of bowel dysfunction in multiple sclerosis. *Eur J Gastroenterol Hepatol*. 2001;13(4):441-448.

13. Namey MA, Halper J. Bowel disturbance. In: Burks J, Johnson K, eds. *Multiple Sclerosis Diagnosis, Medical Management, and Rehabilitation*. New York, NY: Demos Publishing; 2000:453-459.

14. Vaizey CJ, Carapeti E, Cahill JA, Kamm MA. Prospective comparison of faecal incontinence grading systems. *Gut*. 1999;44:77-80.

15. Bakke A, Myhr KM, Gronning M, Nyland H. Bladder, bowel and sexual dysfunction in patients with multiple sclerosis – a cohort study. *Scand J Urol Nephrol Suppl*. 1996;179:61-66.

16. Bauer H J, Firnhaber W, Winkler W. Prognostic criteria in multiple sclerosis. *Ann N Y Acad Sci*. 1965;122:542-551.

17. Glick ME, Meshkinpour H, Haldeman S, et al. Colonic dysfunction in multiple sclerosis. *Gastroenterology*. 1982;83:1002-1007.

18. Taylor MC, Bradley WE, Bhatia N, et al. The conus demyelination syndrome in multiple sclerosis. *Acta Neurol Scand*. 1984;69:80-89.

19. Pescatori M, Anastasio G, Bottini, et al. New grading system and scoring for anal incontinence. Evaluation of 335 patients. *Dis Colon Rectum*. 1992;35: 482-487.

20. Jorge JMN, Wexner SD. Etiology and management of fecal incontinence. *Dis Colon Rectum*. 1993;36:77-97.

21. American Medical Systems. *Fecal Incontinence Scoring System*. Minnetonka: American Medical Systems; 1996.

22. Silva Rodrigues BD, Nogueira Reis IG, de Oliveira Coelho FM, de Lacerda Rodrigues Buzatti KC. Fecal incontinence and quality of life assessment through questionnaires. *J Coloproctol (Rio J)*. 2017;37(4):341-348.

23. Adyad A, Murad F. Constipation in the elderly: diagnosis and management strategies. *Geriatrics*. 1996;51:28-36.

24. Riegler G, Esposito I. Bristol scale stool form. A still valid help in medical practice and clinical research. *Tech Cololproctology*. 2001;5(3):163-164.

25. Heaton KW. Radvan J. Cripps H. Mountford RA. Braddon FE. Hughes AO. Defecation frequency and timing, and stool form in the general population: a prospective study. *Gut*. 1992;33(6):818-824.

26. Drossman DA. Functional gastrointestinal disorders: history, pathophysiology, clinical features, and Rome IV. *Gastroenterology*. 2016;150(6):1481-1491.

27. Chumpitazi BP, Self MM, Czyzewski DI, Cejka S, Swank PR, Shulman RJ. Bristol stool form scale reliability and agreement decreases when determining Rome III stool form designations. *Neurogastroenterol Motil.* 2016;28(3):443-448.

28. Basson R. Women's sexual dysfunction: revised and expanded definitions. *CMAJ.* 2005;172(10):1327-1333.

29. Hinds J P, Eidelman B H, Wald A. Prevalence of bowel dysfunction in multiple sclerosis. A population survey. *Gastroenterology.* 1990;98(6):1538-1542.

30. Lue TF. Neurogenic erectile dysfunction. *Clin Auton Res.* 2001;11:285-294.

31. Lombardi G, Nelli F, Celso M, et al. Treating erectile dysfunction and central neurological diseases with oral phosphodiesterase type 5 inhibitors. Review of the literature. *J Sex Med.* 2012;9:970-985.

32. Rees PM, Fowler CJ, Maas CP. Sexual function in men and women with neurological disorders. *Lancet.* 2007;369:512-525.

33. Kessler TM, Fowler CJ, Panicker JN. Sexual dysfunction in multiple sclerosis. *Expert Rev Neurotherapy.* 2009;9(3):341-350.

34. Foley FW, Iverson. Multiple Sclerosis and the Family. In: Kalb RC, Scheinberg LC, eds. New York: Demos Publications; 1992.

35. Foley FW, LaRocca NG, Zemon V. Rehabilitation of intimacy and sexual dysfunction in couples with multiple sclerosis. *Mult Scler.* 2001;7:417-421.

36. Kipp M, Berger K, Clarner T, Dang J, Beyer C. Sex steroids control neuroinflammatory processes in the brain: relevance for acute ischemia and degeneration demyelination. *J Neuroendocrinol.* 2012;24:62-70.

37. Micevych P, Sinchak K. Estradiol regulation of progesterone synthesis in the brain. *Mol Cell Endocrinol J.* 2008;290:44-50.

38. Voumvourakis KI, Tsiodras S, Kitsos DK, Stamboulis E. Gender hormones: role in the pathogenesis of central nervous system disease and demyelination. *Curr Neurovascular Resource.* 2008;5:1353-1360.

39. Safarinejad MR. Evaluation of endocrine profile, hypothalamic-pituitary-testis axis and semen quality in multiple sclerosis. *J Neuroendocrinol.* 2008;20:1368-1375.

40. Basson R, Leiblum S, Brotto L, et al. Definitions of women's sexual dysfunctions reconsidered: advocating expansion and revision. *J Psychosomatic Obstetrics Gynecol.* 2003;24:221-229.

41. Basson R. Recent advances in women's sexual function and dysfunction. *Menopause.* 2004;11(6 Pt 2):714-725.

42. Singer B. Conceptualizing sexual arousal and attraction. *J Sex Res.* 1984;20:230-240.

43. Toates F. An integrative theoretical framework for understanding sexual motivation, arousal, and behavior. *J Sex Res.* 2009;46(2-3):168-193.

44. Starowicz ML, Rola R. Sexual dysfunctions and sexual quality of life in men with multiple sclerosis. *J Sex Med.* 2014;11:1294-1301.

45. Winder K, Linker RA, Seifert F, et al. Neuroanatomic correlates of female sexual dysfunction in multiple sclerosis. *Ann Neurol.* 2016;80:490-498.

46. Ysrraelit MC, Gaitan MI, Lopez AS, Correlae J. Impaired hypothalamic-pituitary-adrenal axis activity in patients with multiple sclerosis. *Neurology.* 2008;71:1948-1954.

47. Goldstein I, Traish A, Kim N, Munarriz R. The role of sex steroid hormones in female sexual function and dysfunction. *Curr Opinions Urol.* 2002;12:503-507.

48. Acs P, Kipp M, Norkute A, et al. 17beta-estradiol and progesterone prevent cuprizone provoked demyelination of corpus callosum in male mice. *Glia.* 2009;57:807-814.

49. Celik DB, Poyraz EC, Bingol A, et al. Sexual dysfunction in multiple sclerosis: gender differences. *J Neurosci.* 2013;324:17-20.

50. Valleroy MI, Kraft GH. Sexual dysfunction in multiple sclerosis. *Arch Phys Med Rehabil.* 1984;65:125-128.
51. Schindel AW, Goldstein I. Sexual function and dysfunction in the female. In: Wein AJ, Kavoussi LR, Partin AW, Peters CA, eds. Campbell-Walsh Urology. 11th ed. Philadelphia, PA: Elsevier; 2015:749-764:chap 32.
52. Zivadinov R, Zorzon M, Bosco A, et al. Sexual dysfunction in multiple sclerosis: II. correlation analysis. *Mult Scler J.* 1999;5:428-431.
53. Foley FW, Sanders A. Sexuality, multiple sclerosis and women. *Mult Scler Manage.* 1997;1:1-9.
54. Zorzon M, Zivadinov R, Monti Bragadin L, et al. Sexual dysfunction in multiple sclerosis: a 2-year follow-up study. *J Neurol Sci.* 2001;187(1-2):1-5.
55. Greer JM, McCombe PA. Role of gender in multiple sclerosis: clinical effects and potential molecular mechanisms. *J Neuroimmunol.* 2011;234:7-18.
56. DasGupta R, Fowler CJ. Sexual and urological dysfunction in multiple sclerosis: better understanding and improved therapies. *Curr Opin Neurol.* 2002;15(3):271-278.
57. Nortvedt MW, Riise T, Myhr KM, et al. Reduced quality of life among multiple sclerosis patients with sexual disturbance and bladder dysfunction. *Mult Scler.* 2001;7(4):231-235.
58. Jobin C, Laroochelle C, Parpal H, Coyle P., Duquette P. Gender issues in multiple sclerosis: an update. *Womens Health (Lond).* 2010;6:797-820.
59. Masters WH, Johnson VE. *Human Sexual Response.* Toronto; NY: Bantam Books; 1966. ISBN:0-553-20429-7.
60. JBarnatt. Kaplan Triphasic Model. Available at https://sexual-communica-tion.wikispaces.com/Kaplan%E2%80%99s+Triphasic+Model. Accessed May 26, 2018.
61. Whipple B, Brash-McGreer K. Management of female sexual dysfunction. Sipski ML, Alexander CJ, eds. *Sexual Function in People with Disability and Chronic Illness. A Health Professional's Guide.* Gaithersburg, MD: Aspen Publishers Inc; 1997:509-534.
62. Basson R. The female sexual response: a different model. *J Sex Marital Ther.* 2000;26:51-65.
63. Mark K. What we can learn from sexual response cycles. *Psychol Today.* November 19, 2012. Available at https://www.psychologytoday.com/us/blog/the-power-pleasure/20211/what-we-can-learn-sexual-response-cycles.
64. Basson R, Althof S, Davis S, et al. Summary of the recommendations on sexual dysfunctions in women. *J Sex Med.* 2004;1:24-34.
65. Burnett A II. Evaluation and management of erectile dysfunction. In: Wein AJ, Kavoussi LR, Partin AW, Peters CA, eds. Campbell-Walsh Urology. 11th ed. Philadelphia, PA: Elsevier; 2015:643-668:chap 27.
66. Lue TF. Erectile dysfunction. *New Engl J Med.* 2000;342(24):1802-1813.
67. Berman JR. Physiology of female sexual function. *Int J Impot Res.* 2005;17:S44-S51.
68. Rosen RC, Riley A, Wagner G, et al. The International Index of Erectile Function (IIEF): a multidimensional self-report instrument for the assessment of erectile function. *Urology.* 1997;49(6):822-830.
69. Rosen RC, Brown C, Heiman J, et al. The Female sexual function Index (FSFI): a multidimensional self-report instrument for the assessment of female sexual function. *J Sex Marital Ther.* 2000;26(2):191-208.
70. Foley FW, Zemon V, Campagnolo D, et al. Multiple sclerosis intimacy and sexuality questionnaire re-evaluation and development of a 15-item version with a large US sample. *Mult Scler.* 2013;19:1197-1203.

71. Sanders AS, Foley FW, LaRocca NG, et al. Multiple sclerosis intimacy and sexuality questionnaire 19 (MSISQ-19). *Sex Disabil.* 2000;18:3-24.

72. Quirk FH, Heiman JR, Rosen RC, Laan E, Smith MD, Boolell MD. Development of the sexual function questionnaire for clinical trials of female sexual dysfunction. *J Womens Health Gend Based Med.* 2002;11:277-289.

73. Abraham L, Symonds T, Morris MF. Psychometric validation of a sexual quality of life questionnaire for use in men with premature ejaculation or erectile dysfunction. *J Sex Med.* 2008;5:595-601.

74. Symonds T, Boolell M, Quirk F. Development of a questionnaire on sexual quality of life in women. *J Sex Marital Ther.* 2005;31:385-397.

75. Frank JE, Mistretta P, Will J. Diagnosis and treatment of female sexual dysfunction. *Am Fam Pract.* 2008;77(5):635-642.

76. Kandeel FR, Koussa VKT, Swerdloff RS. Male sexual function and its disorders: physiology, pathophysiology, clinical investigation, and treatment. *Endocr Rev.* 2001;22(3):342-388.

Cognitive Function in Multiple Sclerosis

■ ▨ ▨ Jeffrey G. Portnoy, Frederick W. Foley

Introduction

Cognitive dysfunction is a common and impactful manifestation of multiple sclerosis (MS). For decades, it has been known that, despite the frequency with which cognitive deficits tend to occur in the MS population, cognition is not formally assessed as often as is necessary, leading to under-diagnosis of this critical disabling symptom.[1] Estimates of the prevalence of cognitive impairment have fluctuated alongside changes in diagnostic criteria, methodological approaches in research, and instruments used to assess cognitive functioning. Nonetheless, a general consensus has emerged that approximately half of MS patients experience clinically meaningful changes in cognition, with recent appraisals ranging from 40% to 65%.[2-4]

Impaired cognitive ability is one facet of the broader neuropsychiatric symptomatology present in MS, which also includes high comorbidity with depression, anxiety, and other forms of mood disturbance. Multifactorial neuropsychiatric disability is a primary detractor from health-related quality of life in MS patients[5,6] and an important consideration when planning treatment around patients' changes in function and ability to maintain their routines when disease status worsens.

Psychosocial Impact and Quality of Life

Patients and their caregivers frequently describe changes in cognitive function as a particularly intrusive element of the MS disability profile, and its functional consequences can be severe and far-reaching. The trend in diagnosing presence and severity of neurocognitive disorders has shifted to emphasize the impact of cognitive change on the performance of everyday functions. It is therefore important to consider the manner in which cognitive changes may negatively impact patients' normal activities in order to help them retain high quality of life.

MS patients with cognitive impairment often experience numerous changes in life circumstance that can present additional sources of medical, emotional, and financial hardship. Loss of employment occurs frequently, and although physical disability undoubtedly plays a large role, patients also frequently complain of reduced ability to complete work-related tasks at the cognitive level preceding the onset and worsening of their MS. It may be difficult for individuals to pinpoint what exactly is different about their cognition or when their changes in thinking began. Nonetheless, patients and their families, friends, and coworkers may still implicitly perceive neurocognitive changes. This potential salience of patients' deficits, despite the uncertainty of their origin or nature, makes them an especially meaningful chronic stressor, particularly when these yield changes in ability to work, engage in normal social activities, or function independently.

Employment

Vocational status holds a central role as an element of patients' self-efficacy, quality of life, and general sense of well-being. Employment is notably disrupted among individuals with MS, with cross-sectional and longitudinal studies estimating unemployment upwards of 50% and documenting significant trends in loss of employment over time.[7,8] Although the complex nature of disability in MS suggests that multiple etiological considerations are in play to explain change in work status, cognition has been shown to be a strong independent predictor of employment among MS patients.

Instruments such as the Multiple Sclerosis Work Difficulties Questionnaire can be used to examine the origin of patients' employment-related concerns and their risk for change in work status.[9] Both subjective and objective measures of cognitive impairment have been shown to predict employment status among MS patients.[10] In-depth examination of barriers to maintenance of employment shows that patients relate the changes in their cognitive functioning to specific aspects of their ability to complete tasks at work and follow standard protocols in line with company policy.[11] Unemployed individuals perform worse than their employed counterparts on neuropsychological tests,[12,13] and while general increase in age and worsening of disease status are associated with both cognitive decline and loss of employment, the results of cognitive testing exist as independent predictors of change in employment.[14] By contrast, patients with relative stability in cognitive functioning and other elements of disease progression show a significant ability to retain employment, even in the context of the numerous life challenges associated with managing a severe disease.[15]

Social Functioning

Following diagnosis of an incurable disease, patients will have an increased need for coping methods and mentally healthy ways to consider the role of their illness. These new demands can present inherent challenges to the maintenance of interpersonal relationships. Social isolation can occur due to physical and psychological barriers associated with primary and secondary aspects of any chronic illness. In MS, this is further complicated by the presence of cognitive risk factors that may detract from patients' ability to remain socially involved. Given high rates of depression and the reliance of MS patients on caregivers for functional and emotional support, the consequences of loss of social relationships can be devastating.

Research has related self-reported and objectively measured cognitive functioning to various aspects of community integration. Subjective impairment is associated with reduced participation in social activities both inside and outside the home, and poorer performance on tests of cognition has been linked to decreased social involvement.[16] Core cognitive deficits in MS have been tied to difficulty participating in important domestic events, such as the preparation of meals.[17]

The influence of cognitive symptomatology on social functioning is not limited to the patient. Cognitive decline is accompanied by a decrease in maintenance of social contacts and leisure activities, both among individuals with MS and their caregivers.[18] Cognitive changes may prompt increased levels of social isolation and lead to dissatisfaction and conflict with family members.[19] Social relations can misinterpret patients' cognitive changes as emotional instability or lack of desire to socially relate. This can be compounded by the genuine neurobehavioral change sometimes found in patients with certain forms of cognitive dysfunction, including diminished motivation.[20] The erroneous attribution of decreased social ability to volitional changes in attitude, emotional dysregulation, or altered personality can lead to a breakdown in social connectedness that originates from the social contact rather than the MS patient.

Overt dysfunction of social cognitive processes can also occur, producing an expected set of problems with social relatedness. Social cognitive deficits, such as decreased emotion recognition and theory of mind, can be a manifestation of MS.[21] Deficits of this variety have been associated with disease status and duration,[22] raising additional concerns about implications on psychosocial health for more disabled individuals. Alexithymia has been known to occur and progress in MS[23,24] and is associated with higher levels of personal distress and emotional reactivity, as well as difficulty relating to others empathetically.[25] Alexithymia tends to occur in the presence of poorer performance on other cognitive tasks, further adding to the list of social challenges that cognitively impaired patients with MS may be forced to endure.[26]

Independence

The loss of independence associated with MS can be a source of frustration for patients and caregivers, as well as a threat to patient safety. Cognitively impaired MS patients have difficulty completing instrumental activities of daily living (IADLs) in real time compared with healthy individuals and are frequently unable to participate in common daily activities due to cognitive limitations.[17,27] Deficits in executive functioning, such as organization and planning ability, directly impact capacity to perform everyday activities and overall functional status.[28] Longitudinally, a significant effect of declining cognitive performance emerges as a predictor of functional status independent of physical disability.[29]

Increased reliance on others is an important social and emotional change. Research has recommended preparing patients and their caregivers for changes in independence through education and awareness to aid transitions in daily living and promote safety by helping patients understand and acknowledge their limitations.[30] This includes monitoring of changes in patients' ability to drive[31]; clean, organize, and manage the home[32,33]; handle finances[34,35]; and make appropriate medical decisions.[36]

Nature of Cognitive Change

As might be expected in a disease that presents as heterogeneously as MS, patients' degree and type of cognitive dysfunction varies widely. Many patients, even those who have had MS for many years, may be cognitively asymptomatic. Those with complaints may experience mild changes in a single area of thinking or report significant impairment across multiple domains. While some cognitive functions are more frequently affected than others, the MS disease process and its sequelae have the potential to manifest in the form of cognitive impairment in effectively any area.

There is undoubtedly a connection between central nervous system disease activity and cognitive changes, but the link is not always clear-cut. Patients can have intact cognition even when disease is active in the areas of the brain corresponding to those cognitive domains. By contrast, they can show highly specific cognitive deficits associated with brain regions in which there is little or no radiological evidence of inflammation, demyelination, or volume loss.

Formal methods of assessing cognition in MS will be discussed later in this chapter, but broadly, the neurocognitive profile in MS is often subtle and difficult for the layperson, including the patient, to identify or describe with accuracy.[6] Attempts to develop valid self-report measures of cognition have not been successful to this point.[37] General intellectual functioning and conversational language ability are relatively preserved, emphasizing the need for increased awareness and vigilance on the part of patients, clinicians, and family members toward the possibility of cognitive changes. When dysfunction is suspected, formal neuropsychological evaluation is the best way to rule out or clarify the nature of cognitive dysfunction. Examples of patient complaints in relation to types of cognitive dysfunction are shown in Table 18.1.

TABLE 18.1

COMMON SYMPTOMS REPORTED BY PATIENTS IN RELATION TO COGNITIVE DOMAINS AFFECTED BY MULTIPLE SCLEROSIS (MS)

Cognitive Domain Affected	Examples of Reported Symptoms
Processing speed	■ Decreased speed of thinking ■ Taking longer to finish projects at work or home ■ Trouble understanding others or following conversations ■ Difficulty with word-finding or fluent speech ■ Poor ability to learn new information ■ Forgetfulness, or being told that they are repeating questions
Attention	■ Distractibility ■ Decreased ability to multitask ■ Trouble keeping track of information at prior level ■ Difficulty sustaining effort ■ Requiring more frequent breaks ■ Changes in memory
Executive functioning	■ Difficulty starting tasks or initiating behaviors ■ Problems following through once a task is started ■ Becoming stuck or fixated easily ■ Trouble performing routine functions at work ■ Inability to plan activities or efficiently solve problems ■ Demonstrating poor judgment or self-control
Visual-spatial processing	■ Trouble navigating ■ Concerns about ability to drive, voiced by the patient or by others ■ Failing to notice visual details in the environment ■ Difficulty recognizing objects or other visual information

(Continued)

TABLE 18.1

COMMON SYMPTOMS REPORTED BY PATIENTS IN RELATION TO COGNITIVE DOMAINS AFFECTED BY MULTIPLE SCLEROSIS (MS)   (CONTINUED)

Cognitive Domain Affected	Examples of Reported Symptoms
Memory	■ Problems learning new information at work ■ Being told they agreed to complete a task or chore but failing to do so ■ Starting an activity but forgetting what they were doing, or being unable to recall steps to routine activities ■ Forgetting information shortly after reading it, or needing to reread information multiple times ■ Requiring additional time and effort to recall things
Language	■ Problems with word-finding ■ Circumlocution, verbosity, or inefficient communication of ideas ■ Stopping mid-sentence to gather thoughts ■ Problems producing language, including tripping over words ■ Incomplete or inaccurate understanding of others ■ Difficulty following conversations

Processing Speed

Information processing speed is the rate at which patients can apply cognitive ability in real time. Dysfunction in processing speed has implications for functional ability across many areas of cognition.[38] Over the course of an individual's life, he or she naturally develops an internal cognitive rhythm that enables effective employment of cognitive processes. Even slight changes in the rate at which individuals can think or react in certain areas can give the patient the feeling of considerable alteration in overall cognition. In many respects, decreased processing speed is the core cognitive deficit in MS, where demyelination and reduced white matter integrity directly affect the speed of neural signal propagation and transduction.[39-41]

While many individuals with MS will endorse reduced speed of thinking when it is presented as an option, few will consider this independently as an explanation for changes they have noticed or volunteer it in discussions with a clinician. More often, patients may report the functional cognitive symptoms that exist secondary to slowed processing, including the following: difficulty sustaining attention, as patients can no longer keep pace with externally presented information at their prior level of ability; memory problems, which can occur in the context of diminished attention and learning of information; difficulty understanding others, as normal rate of speech is now faster than they can adequately process and comprehend; or trouble finding words, as the formation of a thought process representing an idea is no longer occurring in lockstep with the retrieval of words and formation of language output. This loss of synchronization is of particular relevance in MS given the presence of focal white matter changes, which can manifest such that cognitive slowing does not occur evenly throughout the brain.[42]

Attention

Simple attention can be disrupted in MS, with some patients endorsing changes in their ability to focus either in short bursts or for extended periods of time. Patients also may complain that they have become easily distractible. More typical and specific to MS, however, are changes in complex attention and working memory, defined as the ability to mentally hold and interact with information. Patients may also report difficulty with multitasking that becomes noticeable when engaging in complicated multistep activities, such as driving or cooking. Diminished ability to multitask has been specifically related to patients experiencing difficulties at work.[43]

MS patients with late-onset changes in attention may not recognize the nature of their deficits and subsequently frame them as novel memory complaints. An individual given a request or new piece of information will not have the opportunity to consolidate that information to memory if attentional processes fail to engage. The patient may subsequently be told by others that they have forgotten something, when in reality they never learned it. Patients who begin an activity but lose focus may also feel that they have forgotten why they intended to do something, although this too is less a genuine memory deficit than a reflection of impaired attention.

Executive Functioning

Executive functions are a broad set of complex thinking abilities, including behavioral initiation, self-monitoring and control, cognitive flexibility, planning, organization, and judgment. Because of the intricacy of these functions, assessing them independent of other MS-related deficits is a challenge. Patients often complain of the functional manifestations of executive dysfunction, although depression and processing speed have been implicated as potential confounding variables.[44-46] Nonetheless, patients do demonstrate impairments in objective and subjective executive measures, particularly at higher levels of overall disability or in the presence of frontal lobe change.[47-49] As executive deficits can be reflected prominently in everyday life, they are an important consideration within the cognitive disability profile.

Visual-Spatial Processing

The ability to accurately perceive and interpret visual and spatial information can be disrupted in MS for several reasons. Patients with visual disturbance originating in the eyes, optic nerve, or ocular muscles may present with visual deficits.[50,51] Cortical change, particularly in occipital or posterior parietal regions, can impact navigation, driving ability, visual recognition, or simple visual-spatial perception. Because of the reliance on vision for many daily activities, evaluation of dysfunction in this area is of clear importance.

Memory

Memory complaints are perhaps the most common subjective complaint among MS patients concerned about their cognitive function. This is unsurprising, as there is a strong tendency among patients with neurological conditions to describe changes in cognition in terms of practical memory, which may be most apparent to them and to others. While other cognitive functions can produce what appears to be changes in memory, as has been discussed, organic changes in verbal and visual memory have been observed in MS. Disruption of hippocampal circuitry is heavily implicated in memory dysfunction,[52-54] although other limbic and frontal lobe connections likely play a role as well.[55,56]

Language

Many patients describe difficulties with word-finding, particularly in real time, and trouble keeping up during conversations. Processing speed and executive control are thought to be a considerable part of practical language dysfunction. Significant damage to language cortex is not especially pervasive among MS patients, and while isolated cases of aphasic disorders have been observed, they are not considered typical.[57] Patients who describe difficulties with speech output should also be evaluated for dysarthria and speech apraxia, which may impact language production but are not necessarily suggestive of a language deficit at the cognitive level.

Case Study

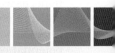

Deficits in Processing Speed and Executive Functioning

A 44-year-old right-handed man with a 13-year history of MS was referred for neuropsychological evaluation owing to progressive cognitive complaints. Specifically, he reported periods of "brain fog" beginning around the time of his MS diagnosis, accompanied by a gradual decrease in his speed of thinking. He also reported difficulty with planning and adapting to changes; he had become confused and flustered by minor deviations from his routine at work and had difficulty navigating even familiar roads if he needed to adjust his route due to traffic or road conditions. A series of significant errors at his job, dating back several years, was discovered and ultimately resulted in loss of employment.

Before his dismissal, he had been told by coworkers that he had become more irritable and abrupt, and his wife reportedly informed him of subtle personality changes and behavior that seemed uncharacteristic for him. Neuroimaging had showed gradual progression of MS, with multiple T2 hyperintensities present in supratentorial white matter at the time of his latest magnetic resonance imaging (MRI).

Several months prior to this evaluation, he had been started on a serotonin and norepinephrine reuptake inhibitor (SNRI), which he reported was of some benefit to his mood. Nonetheless, he presented as anxious, and when queried, he endorsed multiple symptoms of depression and significant fatigue. Speech was of normal rate, rhythm, and volume, and he had no difficulty understanding questions or instructions. However, thought process during the evaluation appeared mildly disorganized, and he was tangential at times.

Estimates of premorbid functioning based on educational background, vocational history, and crystallized ability testing suggested cognition had been well above average at baseline. On neuropsychological testing, aspects of executive functioning were impaired, including planning, complex problem-solving, and pattern recognition. Processing speed was below expectation. Auditory attention and working memory were mildly weak for age. Memory was generally intact; while learning of new information was mildly weak, likely as a consequence of diminished attentional capacity, he was able to accurately recall most of what he had initially acquired. Language functions were broadly normal, but phonemic verbal fluency was considerably weaker than semantic fluency. Simple visuospatial processing was normal.

Commentary: Neurocognitive profiles of the pattern seen in this patient are not uncommon among those suffering from diseases primarily affecting white matter integrity such as MS. In particular, the gradual onset of slowed processing speed and executive dysfunction, accompanied by mild and insidious changes in mood and behavior, is frequently seen in the context of disruption to frontal-subcortical circuitry. A large discrepancy between phonemic verbal fluency (which relies heavily on frontal lobe function) and semantic verbal fluency (which uses many of the same neural pathways, but with greater dependence on functioning temporal cortex) is strongly suggestive of abnormalities in efficient frontal lobe use.

Quite typically, the cognitive changes in this patient were of the variety not readily noticed by others. General intellect and language ability were not considerably altered, and the lack of overt suspicion about his cognitive performance allowed his mistakes at work to go unnoticed for years. A relatively young patient with a high level of baseline functioning such as this could effectively compensate for, or at least minimize, many cognitive and behavioral changes up until a point at which they became too disruptive to ignore.

Neurocognitive Assessment

The cognitive and behavioral presentation of MS patients is defined by many diverse features. This adds a degree of difficulty to the application of many standard test batteries to neuropsychological evaluation in MS.[2] In addition to basic psychometric validity, examination of deficits requires accounting for confounding variables that may interfere with the results of neuropsychological testing, such as fatigue, physical difficulty completing tests requiring fine motor dexterity, and problems affecting speech or vision. In consideration of the fact that MS usually worsens over time, ideal instruments would be relatively short and easy to repeat so as to enable longitudinal assessment of patients' functioning. Neuropsychological methodology often uses a comparison of patients' level of performance to a normative sample matched in features such as age and education. However, intraindividual comparison at multiple time points allows for the most effective and precise long-term tracking of cognition. This can be of great benefit in assessing whether meaningful change has occurred and in distinguishing normal age-related alterations in cognitive function from those suggestive of active disease pathology.

Many brief cognitive assessments such as the Mini-Mental State Examination (MMSE)[58] have been shown to lack the necessary sensitivity to cognitive impairment in MS (as low as 28%) and are not recommended.[59-61] The Montreal Cognitive Assessment (MoCA),[62] which contains measures of attention and executive functioning, has somewhat more clinical use, with a recommended cutoff of 26 points in MS,[63] although there are still questions regarding its advanced diagnostic value and correlation with lesion volume.[64] Work on developing computerized tests in MS has begun, although further research is needed in this area.[65-68]

Generally, the best practice in cases of suspected cognitive impairment is a formal neuropsychological evaluation. Fortunately, the past several decades have seen an increase in research and development of neuropsychological batteries designed to assess and monitor cognition in MS. These include the Brief Repeatable Battery of Neuropsychological Tests (BRB-N),[69] the Minimal Assessment of Cognitive Function in MS (MACFIMS),[70] and the Brief International Cognitive Assessment for MS (BICAMS).[71] Some of the tests appearing in these batteries are discussed below, and are further described in Table 18.2.

The most extensively studied and empirically validated single measure of cognitive function in MS is the Symbol Digit Modalities Test (SDMT).[72-75] The SDMT is a 90-second task that measures processing speed, visual working memory, and sustained attention. It is a valid longitudinal instrument,[76] and it can be administered as a traditional paper-and-pencil measure or orally to accommodate patients with upper motor dysfunction. Processing speed and working memory in the auditory modality can be measured with the Paced Auditory Serial Addition Test (PASAT).[77]

TABLE 18.2

COMMON NEUROPSYCHOLOGICAL TESTS ADMINISTERED IN MULTIPLE SCLEROSIS (MS)

Neuropsychological Test	Cognitive Abilities Required	Description
Symbol Digit Modalities Test (SDMT)	■ Processing speed ■ Attention ■ Behavioral initiation ■ Ability to sustain performance ■ Visual working memory	Patients use a response key to identify number-symbol pairings as quickly as possible. Successful performance requires several of the cognitive functions that are frequently affected by MS, making it an effective screening and monitoring tool. Normative data are available for written or oral administration to allow for assessment of patients with physical disability.
Paced Auditory Serial Addition Test (PASAT)	■ Attention ■ Auditory working memory ■ Ability to sustain performance	Patients hear single-digit numbers read at consistent intervals and must add each new number to the number preceding it. Two difficulty levels, determined by the length of the interval between numbers, can be administered independently or together.
California Verbal Learning Test, Second Edition (CVLT-II)	■ Verbal learning and memory ■ Use of cues to consolidate and retrieve information	Patients are read a list of words to learn and recall. Subsequent trials assess how patients benefit from repetition and reminder cues, susceptibility to learning interference, and maintenance of memory after a delay.
Selective Reminding Test (SRT)	■ Verbal learning and memory ■ Attention and self-monitoring	Patients are presented with a list of words and asked to recall them. On successive trials, they are reminded only of the words that they did not provide during the preceding trial, measuring efficiency of learning and memory.

(Continued)

TABLE 18.2

COMMON NEUROPSYCHOLOGICAL TESTS ADMINISTERED IN MULTIPLE SCLEROSIS (MS)   (CONTINUED)

Neuropsychological Test	Cognitive Abilities Required	Description
Brief Visuospatial Memory Test—Revised (BVMT-R)	■ Visual learning and memory ■ Graphomotor functioning	Patients are shown an array of simple figures and required to memorize their shapes and relative locations. The test is repeated several times and is subsequently followed by delayed recall and recognition trials.
Spatial Recall Test (SPART)	■ Visual learning and memory ■ Spatial awareness	Patients are shown a visual pattern of shapes on a square board and must then reproduce the arrangement from memory, immediately and again after a delay.
Controlled Oral Word Association Test (COWAT)	■ Word-finding using phonetic cues ■ Behavioral initiation and fluency ■ Processing speed	Patients are asked to rapidly generate words beginning with specified letters. This test can be administered with one trial using a single letter or by combining the total score across multiple letter trials.
Word List Generation (WLG)	■ Word-finding using semantic cues ■ Ability to sustain performance ■ Processing speed	Patients are asked to quickly name as many items as possible within a specified category, such as types of animals. Normative data are available for numerous semantic categories, and for various demographic populations.

Neuropsychological tests of memory are traditionally dichotomized into verbal and visual modalities. Verbal memory can be measured with a list-learning task over repeated trials, such as the California Verbal Learning Test, Second Edition (CVLT-II)[78] or Selective Reminding Test (SRT).[79] Visual memory is assessed with the Brief Visuospatial Memory Test—Revised (BVMT-R)[80] or Spatial Recall Test (SPART).[69] These tests allow for distinct measurement of both short-term learning and long-term retention of information.

Word retrieval and language production can be measured using the Controlled Oral Word Association Test (COWAT), in which patients are tasked with generating words rapidly according to phonemic cues. In addition to language, this test also requires behavioral initiation and processing speed, making it a valuable tool for MS evaluations.[81] Other common tests measure visual-spatial processing and executive functions such as concept formation.

Recent efforts to reduce administration time of cognitive screening measures have revealed that abbreviated versions of many of these instruments are often sufficient to produce sensitive and specific conclusions about cognitive functioning.[82] This is a promising finding for future development of neurocognitive screeners in MS and has already produced an abbreviated MACFIMS battery (aMACFIMS), which reduces administration time to under 10 minutes while accurately screening for dysfunction in processing speed, attention, memory, language, and executive functioning.[83] A summary of neurocognitive screening and assessment batteries used with the MS population is provided in Table 18.3.

Other Etiological Considerations

The complexity of MS is reflected in the many possible etiologies of cognitive dysfunction. As described previously, MS-related central nervous system damage can directly influence cognitive ability,[84,85] but other precipitants should be considered. Fatigue is highly prevalent and can impact functional use of cognitive resources. Psychiatric dysfunction is also common, and the acute effects of stress may prevent an individual from applying cognition in an optimal manner. Additional medical risk factors, including many conditions that commonly occur alongside MS, also place patients at risk for cognitive impairment.

Fatigue and Stress

Fatigue is highly prevalent and disabling in MS,[86,87] and it can result in cognitive performance well below peak ability. Fatigue has been found to be related to diminished executive control in MS but not in matched healthy controls.[88] The phenomenon of cognitive fatigue is an area of ongoing research, but it is thought that exhaustion of cognitive resources can occur independently of physical fatigue, although the two are strongly related.[3,89] Neurophysiological correlates of cognitive fatigue have also been described.[90-92] Sleep disturbance is known to impact cognition in MS,[93] and fatigue effects can be exacerbated by commonly prescribed medications, including MS disease-modifying therapies, corticosteroids, muscle relaxants, and opioid pain medication.

Life stressors and psychiatric disorders also occur frequently. Psychological factors play a considerable role in both performance on cognitive tests and the ability to apply otherwise intact cognitive abilities in a real-world environment. The presence of acute and chronic stressors should be evaluated as a potential causative factor in patients who report cognitive concerns.

TABLE 18.3

COGNITIVE SCREENERS AND NEUROPSYCHOLOGICAL TEST BATTERIES USED IN MULTIPLE SCLEROSIS (MS) EVALUATION

	Length of Administration	Clinical Notes
Minimal Assessment of Cognitive Function in MS (MACFIMS)	90 min (<10 min for abbreviated version)	■ Comprehensive standardized assessment of cognition in MS, including processing speed, attention, working memory, executive functioning, memory, language, and visuospatial processing ■ Tests function extensively in both verbal and nonverbal modalities ■ Abbreviated form (aMACFIMS) has been validated as a screening measure and allows for intraindividual comparison over time against shortened or full battery
Brief Repeatable Battery of Neuropsychological Tests (BRB-N)	30 min	■ Short neuropsychological battery containing measures of attention and working memory, memory, and verbal fluency ■ Alternate form available to allow retesting of patients
Brief International Cognitive Assessment for MS (BICAMS)	15 min	■ Three-test screening battery validated in MS cross-culturally ■ Assessment of processing speed and memory ■ Indicated for screening and monitoring
Montreal Cognitive Assessment (MoCA)	10 min	■ Short evaluation of executive functions, attention, memory, language, and construction ■ Demonstrates some use in MS as a screener, but not valid as a formal diagnostic instrument
Mini-Mental State Examination (MMSE)	10–15 min	■ Brief screening of memory, language, and construction ■ Poor sensitivity due to inadequate assessment of cognitive functions typically affected by MS

Other Medical Disorders

Patients with MS are certainly not immune to other maladies that carry cognitive risk factors. White matter change on neuroimaging in a patient with diagnosed MS is usually assumed to be a product of the disease, making it easy to overlook the potential contribution of vascular risk factors to changes in a patient's neurocognitive profile. Hypertension, hyperlipidemia, and diabetes are common among individuals with MS, and patients are at elevated risk of congestive heart failure and ischemic heart and cerebrovascular disease.[94]

Chronic small vessel ischemic disease yields subtle white matter degradation that can be difficult to distinguish from low-grade MS-related inflammation both radiologically and cognitively. In both cases, MRI can show periventricular white matter change, and patients tend to present cognitively with mildly slowed information processing speed and subtle forms of executive dysfunction. Widespread cerebral hypoperfusion has been implicated as a possible mechanism for cognitive dysfunction in MS as well.[95]

With advances in effective disease-modifying therapies, MS patients continue to live longer. Older adults with MS must contend with normal age-related cognitive change and disorders such as Alzheimer disease (AD). The public awareness of AD makes it a source of concern for many individuals, particularly those perceiving cognitive changes in themselves or family members. To conclusively rule in or out an AD diagnosis, there is no substitute for complete neurological evaluation, aided by structural/functional neuroimaging and neuropsychological testing. Nonetheless, there are several identifying features which can help the clinician determine whether AD is likely, and put the patient's mind at ease when it is not.

Age is the most significant AD risk factor, with incidence highest after age 65 years and increasing dramatically with each subsequent decade of life. Genetic factors also play a role, and several primary genes have been identified in association with AD development. Nonetheless, greater than 95% of AD cases are of the sporadic variant and tend to follow a later-onset course.[96] Early-onset AD, defined alternately in research by presentation before either age 60 or 65 years, is uncommon and is strongly associated with mutation in three specific genes, rarely occurring in the absence of such familial risk.[97] Accordingly, MS patients under the age of 60 years should be counseled that their cognitive complaints are not likely indicative of AD. Furthermore, even patients with a family history of AD should know that this only slightly increases their risk of AD development and is by no means a guarantee that they will eventually develop a dementia.

The MS neurocognitive profile, involving subcortical dysfunction, also tends to be more subtle and less specific than the cortical disruption seen in AD. While MS patients demonstrate reduced processing speed and difficulties learning new information, the hallmarks of AD are reductions in language and retrieval of both recent and distant memories. While both MS and AD cognitive dysfunction may lead to complaints by patients, the overt loss of language and generally poor memory in AD can be more noticeable to friends, family, and coworkers.

Severity of cognitive impairment is often defined by the extent to which it interferes with a patient's day-to-day functioning. However, loss of independence due to physical disability, as is common in MS, should not be conflated with inability to perform essential cognitive tasks. Although the latter does occur in MS, patients often maintain the ability to care for themselves given appropriate compensatory aids. By contrast, patients with AD frequently progress to a point where they cannot safely engage in self-care due to their cognitive impairment.

Finally, the course of onset is important clinical evidence. AD pathology is insidious and progressive, and associated cognitive deficits emerge in the same manner. As noted previously, MS-related cognitive dysfunction is often linked to the presence of new inflammatory events or other signs of increased disease activity. For patients with the relapsing-remitting MS subtype, the presence of stepwise cognitive changes, particularly when temporally related to inflammatory events, represents a considerable distinction from the consistent worsening of cognition over time in AD and other progressive dementias. Furthermore, cognitive changes do not remit after onset in AD but may do so partially or fully in MS, particularly during quiescent periods of disease or in direct response to MS treatment. In general, a second diagnosis of AD or another progressive dementia should only be made when there is sufficient evidence of an additional disease process beyond MS; otherwise, it is more likely that cognitive changes can be attributed to a preexisting MS diagnosis.

Numerous other medical conditions with high comorbidity to MS are associated with onset or exacerbation of cognitive symptoms. Seizure disorders occur in approximately three percent of MS patients,[98] and presence of seizures is associated with higher rate of subcortical white matter lesions.[99] Autoimmune thyroid disease, associated with fluctuations in cognitive performance and energy level, occurs in more than six percent of MS patients.[100] This list is by no means exhaustive, and the presence of any other significant medical comorbidities should be taken into account when assessing the etiology of cognitive complaints in patients with MS.

Treatment and Intervention

Development and validation of empirical treatments for MS-related cognitive dysfunction is an active area of research, but it remains a work in progress. Early monitoring of cognitive impairment should be considered a priority, as research suggests that cognitive decline may accelerate after an initial period, providing a window for intervention to begin promptly.[37,101]

Adherence to disease-modifying therapy and prevention of MS progression may be the best way to prevent cognitive decline, as pharmacological interventions targeted specifically at cognitive symptoms have not yet demonstrated significant effectiveness.[102-104] Cognitive rehabilitation protocols are under development, with mixed initial results. Several systematic reviews have found limited evidence for cognitive rehabilitation programs, though statistical comparisons were made difficult by heterogeneous research methodology across studies.[105-108] There are two class I randomized controlled trials (RCTs) providing good evidence that verbal learning and memory can be improved in MS.[109,110] Both studies demonstrated accompanying functional MRI (fMRI) cerebral activation data as supporting evidence.[110,111] Improvements in the former study were maintained at 6-month follow-up. In addition, there is some mixed evidence that attention can be improved with computerized cognitive rehabilitation program.[112]

An important theoretical basis of cognitive training programs is enhancement of cognitive reserve, the resilience of the mind to brain disease. Patients with stronger cognitive ability before the onset of disease are not only less likely to fall below the threshold for normal cognition but are generally more resistant to experiencing significant decline from their personal cognitive baseline.[113,114] Level of education is the best-known predictor of cognitive reserve,[115] although vocational status and premorbid engagement in intellectually stimulating leisure activities also appear relevant.[116-118] Additional research is needed to determine whether these links are solely correlational and manifest only in the premorbid phase of illness or whether behavioral changes can induce greater cognitive resilience after disease onset.[119]

Physical exercise programs have general health benefits, and there is preliminary evidence that aerobic exercise may improve memory in MS patients.[120,121] To encourage safety, driving evaluations may be indicated in patients with deficits in processing speed, attention, or visual-spatial ability, which can impact driving ability.[122] Addressing fatigue, mood, and physical health can also be beneficial to functional cognitive performance. Pending the outcome of further intervention trials, current best practices include using evidence-based interventions for memory and attention, as well as provision of supportive therapy and teaching of compensatory strategies for impaired cognitive functions in general.[123]

Summary

Cognitive dysfunction is highly prevalent among MS patients and is a prominent aspect of the MS disability profile. Changes in cognition are associated with poorer quality of life, decreased capacity to work and engage socially, and loss of independence. Processing speed is the primary cognitive deficit in MS, but it can manifest in ways other than generalized slowing. Patients may also complain of problems with memory, attention, language, visual-spatial processing, or executive functioning, and the heterogeneity of disease progression and focal nature of central nervous system lesions allow for the possibility of impairment in any cognitive domain. The best way to elucidate the nature and severity of cognitive deficits is through formal neuropsychological evaluation, and recent developments in MS-specific cognitive assessment have improved methods for screening and longitudinal monitoring of cognition.

Etiological considerations for cognitive impairment in MS are multifactorial and include the direct consequences of disease activity, fatigue, medication effects, psychological stressors, and other medical conditions that may influence cognitive ability. Efforts to develop effective cognitive rehabilitation protocols are ongoing. There is some class I evidence for improvements in verbal memory, preliminary evidence for improvements in attention, and evidence in favor of supportive therapy and teaching of compensatory skills for cognitive impairment in general. More importantly, educating patients, clinicians, and caregivers about the frequency and impact of cognitive change in MS is an important step toward addressing this critical area of disability.

References

1. Peyser JM, Edwards KR, Poser CM, Filskov SB. Cognitive function in patients with multiple sclerosis. *Arch Neurol.* 1980;37(9):577-579.
2. Korakas N, Tsolaki M. Cognitive impairment in multiple sclerosis: a review of neuropsychological assessments. *Cogn Behav Neurol.* 2016;29(2):55-67.
3. Jongen PJ, Ter Horst AT, Brands AM. Cognitive impairment in multiple sclerosis. *Minerva Med.* 2012;103(2):73-96.
4. Amato MP, Zipoli V, Portaccio E. Multiple sclerosis-related cognitive changes: a review of cross-sectional and longitudinal studies. *J Neurol Sci.* 2006;245(1-2):41-46.
5. Wynia K, Middel B, van Dijk JP, De Keyser JHA, Reijneveld SA. The impact of disabilities on quality of life in people with multiple sclerosis. *Mult Scler.* 2008;14(7):972-980.
6. Chiaravalloti ND, DeLuca J. Cognitive impairment in multiple sclerosis. *Lancet Neurol.* 2008;7(12):1139-1151.
7. Julian LJ, Vella L, Vollmer T, Hadjimichael O, Mohr DC. Employment in multiple sclerosis. Exiting and re-entering the work force. *J Neurol.* 2008;255(9):1354-1360.
8. Simmons RD, Tribe KL, McDonald EA. Living with multiple sclerosis: longitudinal changes in employment and the importance of symptom management. *J Neurol.* 2010;257(6):926-936.
9. Honan CA, Brown RF, Hine DW, et al. The multiple sclerosis work difficulties questionnaire. *Mult Scler.* 2012;18(6):871-880.
10. Honan CA, Brown RF, Batchelor J. Perceived cognitive difficulties and cognitive test performance as predictors of employment outcomes in people with multiple sclerosis. *J Int Neuropsychol Soc.* 2015;21(2):156-168.

11. Carrieri L, Sgaramella TM, Bortolon F, et al. Determinants of on-the-job-barriers in employed persons with multiple sclerosis: the role of disability severity and cognitive indices. *Work Read Mass.* 2014;47(4):509-520.

12. Strober L, Chiaravalloti N, Moore N, DeLuca J. Unemployment in multiple sclerosis (MS): utility of the MS functional composite and cognitive testing. *Mult Scler.* 2014;20(1):112-115.

13. Campbell J, Rashid W, Cercignani M, Langdon D. Cognitive impairment among patients with multiple sclerosis: associations with employment and quality of life. *Postgrad Med J.* 2017;93(1097):143-147.

14. Krause I, Kern S, Horntrich A, Ziemssen T. Employment status in multiple sclerosis: impact of disease-specific and non-disease-specific factors. *Mult Scler.* 2013;19(13):1792-1799.

15. Sayao AL, Bueno AM, Devonshire V, Tremlett H, UBC MS Clinic Neurologists. The psychosocial and cognitive impact of longstanding "benign" multiple sclerosis. *Mult Scler.* 2011;17(11):1375-1383.

16. Hughes AJ, Hartoonian N, Parmenter B, et al. Cognitive impairment and community integration outcomes in individuals living with multiple sclerosis. *Arch Phys Med Rehabil.* 2015;96(11):1973-1979.

17. Goverover Y, Strober L, Chiaravalloti N, DeLuca J. Factors that moderate activity limitation and participation restriction in people with multiple sclerosis. *Am J Occup Ther.* 2015;69(2):6902260020p1-69022600209.

18. Hakim EA, Bakheit AM, Bryant TN, et al. The social impact of multiple sclerosis – a study of 305 patients and their relatives. *Disabil Rehabil.* 2000;22(6):288-293.

19. Lysandropoulos AP, Havrdova E, ParadigMS Group. "Hidden" factors influencing quality of life in patients with multiple sclerosis. *Eur J Neurol.* 2015;22(suppl 2):28-33.

20. Rao SM, Leo GJ, Ellington L, Nauertz T, Bernardin L, Unverzagt F. Cognitive dysfunction in multiple sclerosis. II. Impact on employment and social functioning. *Neurology.* 1991;41(5):692-696.

21. Cotter J, Firth J, Enzinger C, et al. Social cognition in multiple sclerosis: a systematic review and meta-analysis. *Neurology.* 2016;87(16):1727-1736.

22. Banati M, Sandor J, Mike A, et al. Social cognition and theory of mind in patients with relapsing-remitting multiple sclerosis. *Eur J Neurol.* 2010;17(3):426-433.

23. Chahraoui K, Duchene C, Rollot F, Bonin B, Moreau T. Longitudinal study of alexithymia and multiple sclerosis. *Brain Behav.* 2014;4(1):75-82.

24. Prochnow D, Donell J, Schäfer R, et al. Alexithymia and impaired facial affect recognition in multiple sclerosis. *J Neurol.* 2011;258(9):1683-1688.

25. Gleichgerrcht E, Tomashitis B, Sinay V. The relationship between alexithymia, empathy and moral judgment in patients with multiple sclerosis. *Eur J Neurol.* 2015;22(9):1295-1303.

26. Cecchetto C, Aiello M, D'Amico D, et al. Facial and bodily emotion recognition in multiple sclerosis: the role of alexithymia and other characteristics of the disease. *J Int Neuropsychol Soc.* 2014;20(10):1004-1014.

27. Goverover Y, Genova HM, Hillary FG, DeLuca J. The relationship between neuropsychological measures and the timed instrumental activities of daily living task in multiple sclerosis. *Mult Scler.* 2007;13(5):636-644.

28. Kalmar JH, Gaudino EA, Moore NB, Halper J, Deluca J. The relationship between cognitive deficits and everyday functional activities in multiple sclerosis. *Neuropsychology.* 2008;22(4):442-449.

64. Ashrafi F, Behnam B, Arab Ahmadi M, et al. Correlation of MRI findings and cognitive function in multiple sclerosis patients using montreal cognitive assessment test. *Med J Islam Repub Iran.* 2016;30:357.

65. Lapshin H, Audet B, Feinstein A. Detecting cognitive dysfunction in a busy multiple sclerosis clinical setting: a computer generated approach. *Eur J Neurol.* 2014;21(2):281-286.

66. Papathanasiou A, Messinis L, Georgiou VL, Papathanasopoulos P. Cognitive impairment in relapsing remitting and secondary progressive multiple sclerosis patients: efficacy of a computerized cognitive screening battery. *ISRN Neurol.* 2014;2014:151379.

67. Lapshin H, O'Connor P, Lanctôt KL, Feinstein A. Computerized cognitive testing for patients with multiple sclerosis. *Mult Scler Relat Disord.* 2012;1(4):196-201.

68. Lapshin H, Lanctôt KL, O'Connor P, Feinstein A. Assessing the validity of a computer-generated cognitive screening instrument for patients with multiple sclerosis. *Mult Scler.* 2013;19(14):1905-1912.

69. Rao SM. *A Manual for the Brief, Repeatable Battery of Neuropsychological Tests in Multiple Sclerosis.* National Multiple Sclerosis Society; 1991.

70. Benedict RHB, Cookfair D, Gavett R, et al. Validity of the minimal assessment of cognitive function in multiple sclerosis (MACFIMS). *J Int Neuropsychol Soc.* 2006;12(4):549-558.

71. Langdon DW, Amato MP, Boringa J, et al. Recommendations for a brief international cognitive assessment for multiple sclerosis (BICAMS). *Mult Scler.* 2012;18(6):891-898.

72. Benedict RH, DeLuca J, Phillips G, et al. Validity of the Symbol Digit Modalities Test as a cognition performance outcome measure for multiple sclerosis. *Mult Scler.* 2017;23(5):721-733.

73. Kim S, Zemon V, Rath JF, et al. Screening instruments for the early detection of cognitive impairment in patients with multiple sclerosis. *Int J MS Care.* 2017;19(1):1-10.

74. Sonder JM, Burggraaff J, Knol DL, Polman CH, Uitdehaag BMJ. Comparing long-term results of PASAT and SDMT scores in relation to neuropsychological testing in multiple sclerosis. *Mult Scler.* 2014;20(4):481-488.

75. Van Schependom J, D'hooghe MB, Cleynhens K, et al. The Symbol Digit Modalities Test as sentinel test for cognitive impairment in multiple sclerosis. *Eur J Neurol.* 2014;21(9):1219-1225, e71-72.

76. López-Góngora M, Querol L, Escartín A. A one-year follow-up study of the Symbol Digit Modalities Test (SDMT) and the Paced Auditory Serial Addition Test (PASAT) in relapsing-remitting multiple sclerosis: an appraisal of comparative longitudinal sensitivity. *BMC Neurol.* 2015;15:40.

77. Gronwall DM. Paced auditory serial-addition task: a measure of recovery from concussion. *Percept Mot Skills.* 1977;44(2):367-373.

78. Stegen S, Stepanov I, Cookfair D, et al. Validity of the California Verbal Learning Test-II in multiple sclerosis. *Clin Neuropsychol.* 2010;24(2):189-202.

79. Buschke H. Selective reminding for analysis of memory and learning. *J Verbal Learn Verbal Behav.* 1973;12(5):543-550.

80. Benedict R. *Brief Visuospatial Memory Test – Revised: Professional Manual.* Odessa, FL: Psychological Assessment Resources; 1997.

81. Connick P, Kolappan M, Bak TH, Chandran S. Verbal fluency as a rapid screening test for cognitive impairment in progressive multiple sclerosis. *J Neurol Neurosurg Psychiatry.* 2012;83(3):346-347.

82. Gromisch ES, Zemon V, Holtzer R, et al. Assessing the criterion validity of four highly abbreviated measures from the minimal assessment of cognitive function in multiple sclerosis (MACFIMS). *Clin Neuropsychol.* 2016;30(7):1032-1049.

83. Gromisch ES, Portnoy JG, Foley FW. Comparison of the abbreviated minimal assessment of cognitive function in multiple sclerosis (aMACFIMS) and the brief international cognitive assessment for multiple sclerosis (BICAMS). *J Neurol Sci.* 2018;388:70-75.

84. Yildiz M, Tettenborn B, Radue EW, Bendfeldt K, Borgwardt S. Association of cognitive impairment and lesion volumes in multiple sclerosis – a MRI study. *Clin Neurol Neurosurg.* 2014;127:54-58.

85. Calabrese M, Poretto V, Favaretto A, et al. Cortical lesion load associates with progression of disability in multiple sclerosis. *Brain J Neurol.* 2012;135(Pt 10):2952-2961.

86. Khan F, Amatya B, Galea M. Management of fatigue in persons with multiple sclerosis. *Front Neurol.* 2014;5:177.

87. Induruwa I, Constantinescu CS, Gran B. Fatigue in multiple sclerosis - a brief review. *J Neurol Sci.* 2012;323(1-2):9-15.

88. Holtzer R, Foley F. The relationship between subjective reports of fatigue and executive control in multiple sclerosis. *J Neurol Sci.* 2009;281(1-2):46-50.

89. Holtzer R, Foley F, D'Orio V, Spat J, Shuman M, Wang C. Learning and cognitive fatigue trajectories in multiple sclerosis defined using a burst measurement design. *Mult Scler.* 2013;19(11):1518-1525.

90. Hanken K, Eling P, Kastrup A, Klein J, Hildebrandt H. Integrity of hypothalamic fibers and cognitive fatigue in multiple sclerosis. *Mult Scler Relat Disord.* 2015;4(1):39-46.

91. Yaldizli Ö, Penner IK, Frontzek K, et al. The relationship between total and regional corpus callosum atrophy, cognitive impairment and fatigue in multiple sclerosis patients. *Mult Scler.* 2014;20(3):356-364.

92. Genova HM, Rajagopalan V, Deluca J, et al. Examination of cognitive fatigue in multiple sclerosis using functional magnetic resonance imaging and diffusion tensor imaging. *PLoS One.* 2013;8(11):e78811.

93. Hughes AJ, Dunn KM, Chaffee T. Sleep disturbance and cognitive dysfunction in multiple sclerosis: a systematic review. *Curr Neurol Neurosci Rep.* 2018;18(1):2.

94. Marrie RA, Reider N, Cohen J, et al. A systematic review of the incidence and prevalence of cardiac, cerebrovascular, and peripheral vascular disease in multiple sclerosis. *Mult Scler.* 2015;21(3):318-331.

95. D'haeseleer M, Cambron M, Vanopdenbosch L, De Keyser J. Vascular aspects of multiple sclerosis. *Lancet Neurol.* 2011;10(7):657-666.

96. Masters CL, Bateman R, Blennow K, Rowe CC, Sperling RA, Cummings JL. Alzheimer's disease. *Nat Rev Dis Primer.* 2015;1:15056.

97. Jiang T, Yu JT, Tian Y, Tan L. Epidemiology and etiology of Alzheimer's disease: from genetic to non-genetic factors. *Curr Alzheimer Res.* 2013;10(8): 852-867.

98. Marrie RA, Reider N, Cohen J, et al. A systematic review of the incidence and prevalence of sleep disorders and seizure disorders in multiple sclerosis. *Mult Scler.* 2015;21(3):342-349.

99. Shaygannejad V, Ashtari F, Zare M, Ghasemi M, Norouzi R, Maghzi H. Seizure characteristics in multiple sclerosis patients. *J Res Med Sci.* 2013;18(suppl 1):S74-S77.

100. Marrie RA, Reider N, Cohen J, et al. A systematic review of the incidence and prevalence of autoimmune disease in multiple sclerosis. *Mult Scler.* 2015;21(3):282-293.

101. Achiron A, Chapman J, Magalashvili D, et al. Modeling of cognitive impairment by disease duration in multiple sclerosis: a cross-sectional study. *PLoS One.* 2013;8(8).

102. Amato MP, Langdon D, Montalban X, et al. Treatment of cognitive impairment in multiple sclerosis: position paper. *J Neurol.* 2013;260(6):1452-1468.

103. He D, Zhang Y, Dong S, Wang D, Gao X, Zhou H. Pharmacological treatment for memory disorder in multiple sclerosis. *Cochrane Database Syst Rev.* 2013;(12):CD008876.

104. Lacy M, Hauser M, Pliskin N, Assuras S, Valentine MO, Reder A. The effects of long-term interferon-beta-1b treatment on cognitive functioning in multiple sclerosis: a 16-year longitudinal study. *Mult Scler.* 2013;19(13):1765-1772.

105. Patti F. Treatment of cognitive impairment in patients with multiple sclerosis. *Expert Opin Investig Drugs.* 2012;21(11):1679-1699.

106. Mitolo M, Venneri A, Wilkinson ID, Sharrack B. Cognitive rehabilitation in multiple sclerosis: a systematic review. *J Neurol Sci.* 2015;354(1-2):1-9.

107. Rosti-Otajärvi EM, Hämäläinen PI. Neuropsychological rehabilitation for multiple sclerosis. *Cochrane Database Syst Rev.* 2014;(2):CD009131.

108. Hämäläinen P, Rosti-Otajärvi E. Is neuropsychological rehabilitation effective in multiple sclerosis? *Neurodegener Dis Manag.* 2014;4(2):147-154.

109. Chiaravalloti ND, Moore NB, Nikelshpur OM, DeLuca J. An RCT to treat learning impairment in multiple sclerosis. *Neurology.* 2013;81(24):2066-2072.

110. Thaut MH, Peterson DA, McIntosh GC, Hoemberg V. Music mnemonics aid verbal memory and induce learning-related brain plasticity in multiple sclerosis. *Front Hum Neurosci.* 2014;8.

111. Leavitt VM, Wylie GR, Girgis PA, DeLuca J, Chiaravalloti ND. Increased functional connectivity within memory networks following memory rehabilitation in multiple sclerosis. *Brain Imaging Behav.* 2014;8(3):394-402.

112. Cerasa A, Gioia MC, Valentino P, et al. Computer-assisted cognitive rehabilitation of attention deficits for multiple sclerosis: a randomized trial with fMRI correlates. *Neurorehabil Neural Repair.* 2013;27(4):284-295.

113. Sumowski JF, Rocca MA, Leavitt VM, et al. Brain reserve and cognitive reserve protect against cognitive decline over 4.5 years in MS. *Neurology.* 2014;82(20):1776-1783.

114. Sumowski JF, Leavitt VM. Cognitive reserve in multiple sclerosis. *Mult Scler.* 2013;19(9):1122-1127.

115. Martins Da Silva A, Cavaco S, Moreira I, et al. Cognitive reserve in multiple sclerosis: protective effects of education. *Mult Scler.* 2015;21(10):1312-1321.

116. Della Corte M, Santangelo G, Bisecco A, et al. A simple measure of cognitive reserve is relevant for cognitive performance in MS patients. *Neurol Sci.* 2018;39(7):1267-1273.

117. Nunnari D, De Cola MC, Costa A, Rifici C, Bramanti P, Marino S. Exploring cognitive reserve in multiple sclerosis: new findings from a cross-sectional study. *J Clin Exp Neuropsychol.* 2016;38(10):1158-1167.

118. Sumowski JF, Rocca MA, Leavitt VM, et al. Reading, writing, and reserve: literacy activities are linked to hippocampal volume and memory in multiple sclerosis. *Mult Scler.* 2016;22(12):1621-1625.

119. Sumowski JF. Cognitive reserve as a useful concept for early intervention research in multiple sclerosis. *Front Neurol.* 2015;6:176.

120. Motl RW, Sandroff BM, DeLuca J. Exercise training and cognitive rehabilitation: a symbiotic approach for rehabilitating walking and cognitive functions in multiple sclerosis? *Neurorehabil Neural Repair.* 2016;30(6):499-511.

121. Leavitt VM, Cirnigliaro C, Cohen A, et al. Aerobic exercise increases hippocampal volume and improves memory in multiple sclerosis: preliminary findings. *Neurocase.* 2014;20(6):695-697.

122. Schultheis MT, Weisser V, Ang J, et al. Examining the relationship between cognition and driving performance in multiple sclerosis. *Arch Phys Med Rehabil.* 2010;91(3):465-473.

123. Stuifbergen AK, Becker H, Perez F, Morison J, Kullberg V, Todd A. A randomized controlled trial of a cognitive rehabilitation intervention for persons with multiple sclerosis. *Clin Rehabil.* 2012;26(10):882-893.

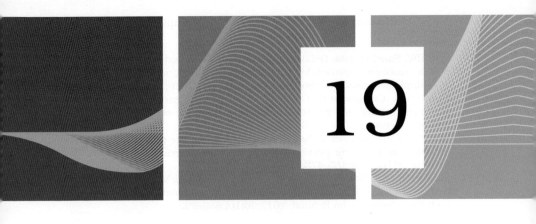

19

Mood Disorders in Multiple Sclerosis

■ ■ ■ Jagriti "Jackie" Bhattarai, Jeffrey G. Portnoy, Frederick W. Foley, Meghan Beier

Introduction

Mood disorders, such as depression, anxiety, and bipolar disorder are substantially more common among individuals with multiple sclerosis (MS) compared with the general population.[1] Mood symptoms can impact quality of life, reduce adherence to disease-modifying medications, and increase risk of suicide, pain, fatigue, cognitive impairment, and poor health behaviors, such as excessive alcohol use and smoking.[2,3] The prevalence of mood disorders, as well as their impact on functional activity, necessitates the medical provider to assess, monitor, and adequately treat these symptoms in their patients with MS. The following chapter introduces the prevalence and typical presentation of common mood disorders found in multiple sclerosis. Options for assessment, treatment, and exemplifying case examples are also described.

Depression

Depression is a disorder characterized by low mood and anhedonia (the loss of interest or pleasure in ones normal activities).[4] The presentation of depression symptoms may vary from individual to individual and can include any of the following (as presented in Table 19.1): observed and/or

366

TABLE 19.1

FEATURES OF DEPRESSION BASED ON THE *DIAGNOSTIC AND STATISTICAL MANUAL OF MENTAL DISORDERS*, **FIFTH EDITION** *(DSM-5)* **OF THE AMERICAN PSYCHIATRIC ASSOCIATION (APA; 2013)**[4]

298.0 (F32.3) Major Depressive Disorder (MDD)

1. Five or more symptoms (with at least one of the symptoms being number 1 or 2) must be present in the same 2-wk period
2. Single or recurrent episodes (2 consecutive months between single episodes)

1. Depressed mood most of the day (subjective or observed)
2. Loss of interest or pleasure in usual activities
3. Significant change in weight or appetite
4. Insomnia or hypersomnia
5. Psychomotor agitation (observed)
6. Loss of energy or fatigue
7. Worthlessness or excessive guilt
8. Diminished concentration or indecisiveness
9. Thoughts of death, suicidal ideation, or suicidal attempt

300.4 (F34.1) Persistent Depressive Disorder (Dysthymia)

1. Depressed mood on most days for at least 2 y
2. Two or more (of six) symptoms present for at least 2 y
3. Criteria for MDD may be met for 2 y

1. Poor appetite or overeating
2. Insomnia or hypersomnia
3. Low energy or fatigue
4. Low self-esteem
5. Poor concentration or difficulty making decisions
6. Feelings of hopelessness

V62.82 (Z63.4) Uncomplicated Bereavement is a normal reaction to a significant loss during which some individuals present with symptoms of depression. This should be differentiated from depressive disorders during assessment.

reported depressed mood, anhedonia, feelings of excessive guilt or worthlessness, loss of interest in usual activities, sleep or diet changes, fatigue or an increase in existing fatigue, and difficulty with cognitive functioning, particularly in terms of attention/concentration and decision-making.

22% to 54% of individuals with MS will experience depression during their lifetime.[1,5-7] One might presume that depressive symptoms arise as an emotional reaction to the negative impact MS symptoms have on a person's life. However, research suggests that biological and neuroimmunological factors may also be at play. In other words, depression may be a psychosocial response to difficult life circumstances, including living with a chronic progressive medical condition; a direct consequence of physiological changes caused by MS; or both.[8,9] The stability of depressive symptoms over time lends support to the notion that MS-related depression is not always reactionary. One longitudinal study found that depressive symptoms remained relatively stable over 4 years, suggesting that depression in MS may resemble persistent depressive disorder, a chronic low-grade level of depressed mood, unlike the waxing and waning episodes seen in major depressive disorder (MDD; see Table 19.1).[5] Additionally, structural brain changes have been observed in depressed persons with MS, including hippocampal atrophy, temporal lobe atrophy, and decreased right hemisphere brain volume.[10-12]

In the event that patients or their families report symptoms of depression, it is advisable to administer brief screener to assess for the presence and severity of symptoms as well as the potential need for intervention. Repeat use of the following screening tools is advisable, as higher rates of depressive symptomatology have been observed during relapses/exacerbations.[13] There are several validated self-report questionnaires for assessing depressive symptoms in persons with MS: the 9-item and 2-item forms of Patient Health Questionnaire (PHQ-9 and PHQ-2, respectively); Beck Depression Inventory Fast Screen (BDI-FS); Hospital Anxiety and Depression Scale (HADS); and the Center for Epidemiological Studies Depression Scale (CES-D).[3,14-19] Consisting of two questions pertaining to the primary symptoms of MDD, depressed mood and anhedonia, the PHQ-2 is the most practical to administer. Tools such as these are especially critical for detecting depression symptoms in individuals with MS.

Therapeutic Options for Depression in MS

Several behavioral and pharmacological treatments for depression have been recommended for individuals with MS. There are a limited number of randomized controlled trials of antidepressant medications in this population, but open-label trials of duloxetine, fluoxetine, sertraline, moclobemide, imipramine, and tranylcypromine concluded efficacy for patients with MS. Both a Cochrane review and an American Academy of Neurology 2014 consensus paper described insufficient evidence to advocate use of one pharmacologic agent over another without head-to-head trials.[6,9,14]

Use of psychotropic pharmacotherapy in MS is widespread, and while further study is needed to improve the efficacy of first-line therapies and better tailor treatments to patients' needs, best practices do currently support the use of antidepressant medications for the treatment of depression in MS.[5] The choice of which medication to prescribe for depressive symptoms often involves some degree of trial and error, and ideally the initiation and management of a psychotropic medication regimen would be aided by the expertise of a psychiatrist or other prescribing mental health practitioner. In MS, prescriptive decisions are further complicated by the variety of additional symptoms that patients experience and the potential for interaction with other prescribed medications, including disease-modifying agents. The risk of noncompliance due to adverse events should be monitored closely by the prescriber. However, patients should also be counseled that side effects may lessen or abate entirely once they have adjusted to the antidepressant medication and that they should persist with medication trials past the initiation phase if possible to determine long-term efficacy and tolerability.

Sexual dysfunction is widespread in MS, and antidepressants acting broadly on serotonergic systems, including selective serotonin reuptake inhibitors (SSRIs), serotonin-norepinephrine reuptake inhibitors (SNRIs), tricyclic antidepressants (TCAs), and monoamine oxidase inhibitors (MAOIs) can exacerbate sexual symptoms. Atypical antidepressants, such as mirtazapine and bupropion, are options for these patients, although the latter is contraindicated in MS patients who experience seizures. Mirtazapine may also be considered in patients who regularly experience nausea or suffer from poor appetite; SSRIs and SNRIs can increase these symptoms, and mirtazapine not only carries a lower risk of nausea but may reduce such symptoms and promote weight gain in patients with these difficulties. Mirtazapine's sedative effect can also be beneficial in patients with sleep disorders. It should be noted that while these efficacy profiles have been described generally, there have been few studies evaluating mirtazapine specifically in MS.

Fatigue is a highly prevalent MS symptom, and there is limited evidence that bupropion can reduce fatigue symptoms while treating depression. Further studies are needed to explore the best treatments for patients with comorbid fatigue and mood disturbance, particularly those taking other stimulant medications for fatigue, which can exacerbate mood dysfunction.

TCAs are generally not tolerated as well as newer antidepressants but should be considered in patients with neuropathic pain, insomnia, or urinary incontinence. The risk of anticholinergic side effects should be monitored, and patients may experience cognitive disturbance, dizziness, dry mouth, visual changes, and constipation. Orthostatic hypotension and weight gain are also possible side effects and are an important consideration in prescribing TCAs to patients who are overweight or possess other cardiovascular risk factors. SNRIs, including duloxetine and venlafaxine, should be considered in patients with nerve pain, migraine, or other headache disorder.[3,14]

Individuals on antidepressants that can prolong the QT interval may be at risk for torsades de pointes when starting fingolimod, a disease-modifying medication that can result in decreased heart rate upon initiation. If unable to switch antidepressants or take a break from the medication during initiation of fingolimod, these individuals should be monitored overnight.

For patients with preexisting medication adherence difficulties, antidepressants with longer half-lives should be considered, as they carry a lower risk of adverse events if doses are missed. Fluoxetine is dosed such that patients need only take a single pill, and missed doses are less harmful than in paroxetine, a comparable SSRI.[3]

In addition, there is considerable evidence supporting the use of behavioral interventions for depressive symptoms in MS. Both in-person and telephone-based randomized controlled trials of cognitive behavioral therapy (CBT) have shown decreased depressive symptomatology, with the benefits of psychotherapy persisting over time.[9,20,21]

The Overlap of Depression and Fatigue

Fatigue is commonly found alongside, or in the midst of, depressive symptoms in individuals with MS. Fatigue alone affects up to 90% of this population.[22,23] Etiology thought to be multifactorial (physiological, cognitive, and behavioral), and the underlying mechanisms are not yet fully understood.[23,24] Fatigue is considered either primary (caused by the MS disease process, including immunological factors, demyelination, and axonal loss in the central nervous system [CNS]) or secondary, resulting from conditions comorbid with MS such as sleep disturbance and depression.[22,23,25,26]

The association between MS-related depression and fatigue is complex.[27,28] While some individuals will experience fatigue independent of depression, in many cases there is a mutual relationship (see Figure 19.1).[18,19,29] Shared symptoms between the two conditions include anergia,

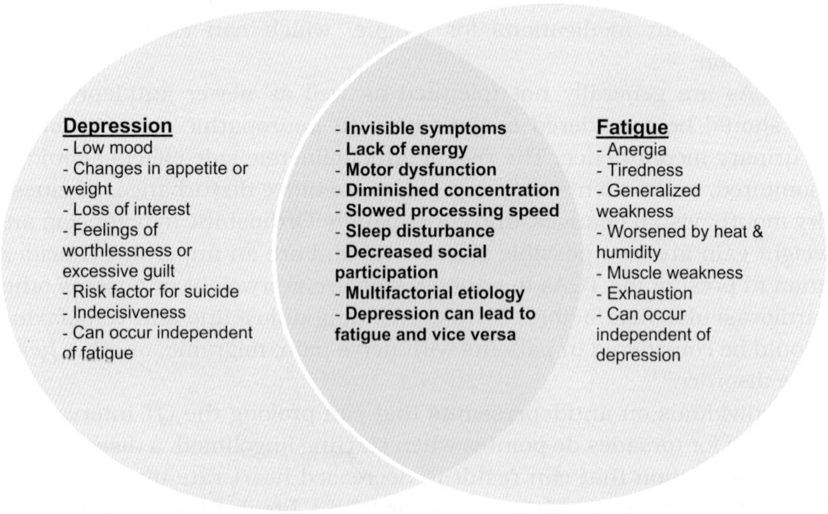

Depression
- Low mood
- Changes in appetite or weight
- Loss of interest
- Feelings of worthlessness or excessive guilt
- Risk factor for suicide
- Indecisiveness
- Can occur independent of fatigue

- **Invisible symptoms**
- **Lack of energy**
- **Motor dysfunction**
- **Diminished concentration**
- **Slowed processing speed**
- **Sleep disturbance**
- **Decreased social participation**
- **Multifactorial etiology**
- **Depression can lead to fatigue and vice versa**

Fatigue
- Anergia
- Tiredness
- Generalized weakness
- Worsened by heat & humidity
- Muscle weakness
- Exhaustion
- Can occur independent of depression

Figure 19.1. Comparison of depressive symptoms and fatigue in individuals with multiple sclerosis (MS).

diminished attention/concentration, slowed processing speed, sleep disturbance, and decreased social participation. When patients present with these shared symptoms, validated fatigue measures should be administered alongside validated depression measures (see recommendations described above). Providers are advised to be vigilant regarding the presence of both conditions in younger patients with higher levels of disability, as these groups are the most vulnerable to concurrent depression and fatigue.[30]

Fatigue can be assessed using the Fatigue Severity Scale (FSS), the Modified Fatigue Index Scale (MFIS), and the Neurological Fatigue Index for MS (NFI-MS), all of which have been validated for use in individuals with MS.[31-33] The FSS is a 9-item self-report measure of fatigue *severity* in individuals with chronic medical conditions like MS and lupus (see Table 19.2). The MFIS is a self-report measure of fatigue *interference* (i.e., how much fatigue interferes with daily activities) that consists of 21 items divided into physical, cognitive, and psychosocial subscales. The NFI-MS is a 10-item outcome measure that assesses the presence of physical and cognitive fatigue.[31,34-36]

When depression and fatigue are both present, interventions that are empirically supported for both conditions should be considered. Pharmacological and behavioral interventions can be effective for groups of people with MS. For example, stimulants and wakefulness-promoting

TABLE 19.2
FATIGUE SEVERITY SCALE (FSS)

Please circle the number between 1 and 7 which you feel best fits the following statements. This refers to your usual way of life within the last week. 1 Indicates "strongly disagree" and 7 indicates "strongly agree."

Read and Circle a Number	Strongly Disagree → Strongly Agree						
1. My motivation is lower when I am fatigued	1	2	3	4	5	6	7
2. Exercise brings on my fatigue	1	2	3	4	5	6	7
3. I am easily fatigued	1	2	3	4	5	6	7
4. Fatigue interferes with my physical functioning	1	2	3	4	5	6	7
5. Fatigue causes frequent problems for me	1	2	3	4	5	6	7
6. My fatigue prevents sustained physical functioning	1	2	3	4	5	6	7
7. Fatigue is among my most disabling symptoms	1	2	3	4	5	6	7
8. Fatigue interferes with my work, family, or social life	1	2	3	4	5	6	7

medications commonly used to treat similar conditions such as chronic fatigue syndrome, attention-deficit/hyperactivity disorder (ADHD), narcolepsy, etc. are also commonly used to treat MS-related fatigue.[37] Behavioral interventions such as energy conservation can make a significant impact on a person's quality of life.[38] Most promising, a number of studies found that psychological interventions, such as CBT, are effective for treating MS-related fatigue symptoms, again suggesting a common etiology.[39,40]

Depression: A Risk Factor for Suicide

A potential consequence of untreated depression is suicide. There are a number of reviews examining rates of suicidal ideation, suicide attempts, and successful suicides in persons with MS. While the rates vary by method of inquiry, the consensus is that death due to suicide is significantly elevated in persons with MS (up to three times higher than in the general population).[41,42] As with the general population, suicide attempts are more common in females with MS, but more likely to be fatal in males with MS.[43] Suicidal ideation is even more common; one study found that up to 22% of persons with MS endorse suicidal thoughts at any one time and 29% endorsed transient suicidal thoughts over the course of 6 months. Ideation was associated with

- depression
- age (both younger and older)
- inability to drive
- lower income
- single relationship status
- alcohol use
- bowel and bladder dysfunction
- swallowing difficulties
- speech impairment
- progressive disease subtype
- higher level of physical disability
- earlier disease course[41,44]

It is important to note that depression was the only predictor of persistent suicidal ideation.[41,45,46]

There have been concerns that suicide, suicide attempts, and/or suicidal ideation could be linked to disease-modifying therapies, particularly interferon β. In the first relapsing-remitting MS interferon β-1b trial, there was one suicide and several unsuccessful suicide attempts in the treatment arms, but none in the placebo group. However, subsequent research has not demonstrated a connection between disease-modifying agents and suicide. Secondary analyses of the original trial suggest that premorbid mood symptoms and family history of mood disturbance were not adequately controlled a priori. Therefore, depression and depressive symptoms are not thought to be a contraindication to interferon β treatment.[47-49]

Anxiety

Anxiety disorders are found in approximately 14% to 45% of individuals living with MS.[30,50] Although detrimental to quality of life, anxiety remains substantially underresearched when compared with depression in individuals with MS.[51] Anxiety—specifically its most common clinical variant, generalized anxiety disorder (GAD)—is characterized by excessive and persistent worry. GAD is associated with an increase in confirmed MS exacerbations, pseudoexacerbations, overutilization of health care services, poor treatment adherence, and increased risk of suicide.[52]

Approximately half of depressed individuals with MS also experience anxiety.[9] Therefore, it is recommended that standardized anxiety assessments are used in MS patients with known depression. The 7-item Generalized Anxiety Disorder Scale (GAD-7) and the Hospital Anxiety and Depression Scale (HADS) are two validated measures for persons with MS.[16,52] The HADS measures both anxiety and depression simultaneously and may therefore be an efficient measure in persons with suspected comorbidity.

At present, there are few evidence-based treatments for MS-related anxiety. Intervention studies of mindfulness-based stress reduction, biofeedback, relaxation training, and an internet-delivered behavioral intervention found indirect effects on anxiety.[53] Further research is needed to support and develop behavioral and pharmacologic interventions for anxiety among those with MS.

Bipolar Disorder

Bipolar disorder is a serious chronic mood disorder characterized by repeated episodes of depressed mood, mania, hypomania, or a mixture of these states. Bipolar disorder is associated with reduced quality of life, unemployment, higher medical utilization, and increased risk of suicide. In the general population, symptom onset typically occurs in the late teenage years, between the ages of 15 and 19 years. General prevalence of bipolar I disorder, the variant involving manic episodes, is up to 2%, while the prevalence of bipolar II disorder, involving hypomanic episodes, has been reported as high as 4%. Generally, bipolar disorder is thought to be twice as common in MS. However, rates varied considerably, from 0% to 16%, depending on methods of data collection. Not unlike MS itself, female gender seems to carry a higher risk of bipolar disorder, existing in approximately 5% of women, compared with 3.9% of men.[42]

As might be expected, bipolar disorder has a significant impact on quality of life and mental health. Compared with depression, bipolar disorder has a significantly greater impact on quality of life, as well as an increased risk of suicide. Up to 50% of individuals with bipolar disorder report at least one suicide attempt, and one-fifth die by suicide.[54,55]

Population-based data from Sweden examined possible causes of the increased prevalence of bipolar disorder in MS, including genetic and biological factors and history of emotional trauma. Temporal data ruled out the development of bipolar disorder due to trauma. Familial studies of siblings ruled out the increased risk due to genetics. Therefore, it was hypothesized that a biological and possibly inflammatory mechanism was responsible for the presence of bipolar disorder in persons with MS.[56]

If bipolar disorder is suspected, the Mood Disorders Questionnaire has been used successfully in persons with MS.[54,57] However, it should be noted that the instrument is prone to high false-positive rates. Therefore, if used, it should prompt a more in-depth assessment by a mental health provider rather than a documented diagnosis of bipolar disorder.

There are no known clinical trials or treatment trials of pharmacologic or behavioral interventions for bipolar disorder in multiple sclerosis. However, available case studies provide a possible starting point for treatment options. Consistent with the inflammatory theory, a female patient was admitted for manic episode with psychotic features and found to have three new T2 gadolinium-enhancing lesions on magnetic resonance imaging (MRI). She was successfully treated with intravenous methylprednisolone and risperidone.[58]

Pseudobulbar Affective Disorder

The estimated prevalence rates of pseudobulbar affect (PBA) in persons with MS range from 7% to 46%.[2,9,59,60] PBA is characterized by affective disinhibition with labile, excessive, and uncontrollable emotional expression. There is often rapid shifting from laughing to crying in a relatively short period of time. In addition to sudden laughter and crying, the majority of individuals with PBA also experience labile anger/frustration.[59] The condition can impact multiple aspects of an individual's psychosocial functioning, including interpersonal relationships, depressive symptoms, self-esteem, and overall psychological health, and can also lead to increased disability.[59,61]

The American Neuropsychiatric Association Committee on Research identified lesions in the frontal lobe, cerebral hemispheres, diencephalon, brainstem, and cerebellum to be involved in PBA symptoms.[62] When PBA is suspected, measures such as the Pathological Laughing and Crying Scale (PLACS) and the Center for Neurologic Study-Lability Scale (CNS-LS) are among the most commonly used instruments.[12,63,64] The PLACS is an interviewer-rated instrument that assesses severity of PBA symptoms and has been successfully used in MS.[25,29,65] The CNS-LS is the first self-reported measure developed to assess pathological laughing and crying (PLC), and it has also been validated in patients with MS.[65,66]

A combination of dextromethorphan and quinidine (Nuedexta) is approved by the U.S. Food and Drug Administration (FDA) for treatment of PBA.[6] However, additional medications such as SSRIs (e.g., fluoxetine, citalopram, sertraline, paroxetine), tricyclics (amitriptyline, nortriptyline), and valproic acid (Depakote) may also be effective for PBA symptoms in persons with MS.[60,61] As described above in relation to depression, potential side effects and drug interactions should be considered before initiating and during maintenance of treatment.

Conclusions

Mood disorders impact individuals living with MS at higher rates than those in the general population, and can emerge both as a psychological response to the difficulties of living with MS and as the direct product of inflammation and physiological disruption of CNS function. However, there are relatively few comprehensive MS-specific treatment guidelines for affective disorders compared with what exists in the general population and many other chronic disease populations. Further research is needed to inform optimal first-line treatments and to develop additional therapy regimens better targeted to the complex, multifactorial psychiatric presentation of the MS patient.

Untreated mood disorders have serious implications for patients' ability to function and their overall quality of life. Many short-form self-report inventories are available for screening and monitoring of mood symptoms, which is essential for identifying patients in need of psychiatric and other mental health services. Current best evidence supports a handful of behavioral and pharmacological interventions for mood disorders in MS, including cognitive behavioral therapy and SSRIs and SNRIs with longer half-lives.

Take Away Points

Mood symptoms can substantially lower the quality of life in individuals with MS.

Education on mood symptoms in MS is crucial for clinicians, patients, and their families to be able to recognize symptoms of depression, anxiety, and other common mood symptoms.

Suicidal ideation is up to three times more common in the MS population compared with the general population. The following factors are associated with greater suicide risk: depression, young or old age, inability to drive, lower income, alcohol use, progressive disease subtype, and higher level of physical disability.

Brief mood symptom screening assessment is highly recommended to identify and track symptoms, particularly given that depressive symptoms can be more prevalent during an exacerbation.

Effective interventions for mood symptoms should include both behavioral and pharmaceutical options.

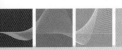

Case Study

- A 34-year-old, engaged, college-educated, full-time employed female, diagnosed with relapsing-remitting MS 1.5 years prior, who presented to clinic for follow-up with her neurologist.
- MS symptoms included difficulty walking long distances (although she ambulates without assistance), mild dysesthesia in both feet, mild cognitive impairment, and fatigue.
- Patient also reported a history of episodic depression preceding her MS diagnosis by 2 years; she had been prescribed low-dose bupropion by her primary care physician, which was well-tolerated and of benefit to her mood.
- Other medications included fingolimod and dalfampridine.
- Patient was observed crying in the clinic and referred for psychological evaluation, which revealed worsening depression for 3 months.
- Patient met criteria for current major depressive episode with fleeting suicidal ideation.
- She previously had no history of alcohol use but reported that she had recently started drinking alcohol daily to cope with depression; she also reported poor adherence to disease-modifying therapy over the prior 3 months.
- Although the patient had no history of seizures, recent onset of alcohol abuse rendered her at greater risk of seizures in the context of MS and treatment with dalfampridine and bupropion.
- Patient was switched from bupropion to 50 mg sertraline, titrated up over 6 weeks to 200 mg.
- She was referred for cognitive behavioral psychotherapy (CBT) twice per week with a health psychologist experienced in MS.
- Psychotherapy initially targeted depression and alcohol abuse, as well as improvement of adherence to fingolimod; other issues addressed included the patient's concerns that her fiancé would leave her due to her MS.

■ Her fiancé attended several sessions with her and reassured the patient that he was committed to their relationship and plans for marriage.

■ Within 5 months of beginning CBT, her major depressive episode was largely in remission.

■ She continued psychotherapy to target residual mood symptoms, adapt to her MS diagnosis and accompanying physical disability, and learn healthier ways of coping with stress and was successfully maintained on 200 mg sertraline.

References

1. Marrie RA, Cutter G, Tyry T, Vollmer T, Campagnolo D. Does multiple sclerosis–associated disability differ between races? *Neurology*. 2006;66(8):1235-1240.

2. Patten SB, Marrie RA, Carta MG. Depression in multiple sclerosis. *Int Rev Psychiatry*. 2017;29:463-472. doi:10.1080/09540261.2017.1322555.

3. Nathoo N, Mackie A. Treating depression in multiple sclerosis with antidepressants: a brief review of clinical trials and exploration of clinical symptoms to guide treatment decisions. *Mult Scler Relat Disord*. 2017;18:177-180. doi:10.1016/j.msard.2017.10.004.

4. American Psychiatric Association (APA). *Diagnostic and Statistical Manual of Mental Disorders*. 5th ed. Arlington, VA: American Psychiatric Association; 2013.

5. Koch MW, Patten S, Berzins S, et al. Depression in multiple sclerosis: a long-term longitudinal study. *Mult Scler J*. 2015;21:76-82. doi:10.1177/1352458514536086.

6. Minden SL, Feinstein A, Kalb RC, et al. Evidence-based guideline: assessment and management of psychiatric disorders in individuals with MS: report of the Guideline Development Subcommittee of the American Academy of Neurology. *Neurology*. 2014;82(2):174-181. doi:10.1212/WNL.0000000000000013.

7. Sadovnick AD, Remick RA, Allen J, et al. Depression and multiple sclerosis. *Neurology*. 1996;46(3):628. doi:10.1212/WNL.46.3.628.

8. Solaro C, Gamberini G, Masuccio FG. Depression in multiple sclerosis: epidemiology, aetiology, diagnosis and treatment. *CNS Drugs*. 2018;32(2):117-133. doi:10.1007/s40263-018-0489-5.

9. Feinstein A, Magalhaes S, Richard J-F, Audet B, Moore C. The link between multiple sclerosis and depression. *Nat Rev Neurol*. 2014;10(9):507-517. doi:10.1038/nrneurol.2014.139.

10. Zorzon M, Zivadinov R, Nasuelli D, et al. Depressive symptoms and MRI changes in multiple sclerosis. *Eur J Neurol*. 2002;9(5):491-496.

11. Gold SM, O'Connor M, Gill R, et al. Detection of altered hippocampal morphology in multiple sclerosis-associated depression using automated surface mesh modeling. *Hum Brain Mapp*. 2014;35(1):30-37.

12. Kiy G, Lehmann P, Hahn HK, Eling P, Kastrup A, Hildebrandt H. Decreased hippocampal volume, indirectly measured, is associated with depressive symptoms and consolidation deficits in multiple sclerosis. *Mult Scler J*. 2011;17(9):1088-1097.

13. Moore P, Hirst C, Harding KE, Clarkson H, Pickersgill TP, Robertson NP. Multiple sclerosis relapses and depression. *J Psychosom Res*. 2012;73(4):272-276.

14. Koch MW, Glazenborg A, Uyttenboogaart M, Mostert J, De Keyser J. Pharmacologic treatment of depression in multiple sclerosis. *Cochrane Database Syst Rev*. 2011;(2):CD007295. doi:10.1002/14651858.CD007295.pub2.

15. Beck A, Ward C, Mendelson M, Mock J, Erbaugh J. An inventory for measuring depression. *Arch Gen Psychiatry.* 1961;4:561-571.
16. Honarmand K, Feinstein A. Validation of the hospital anxiety and depression scale for use with multiple sclerosis patients. *Mult Scler J.* 2009;15(12):1518-1524.
17. Snaith R, Zigmond A. The hospital anxiety and depression scale. *Br Med J (Clin Res Ed).* 1986;292(6516):344.
18. Lewinsohn PM, Seeley JR, Roberts RE, Allen NB. Center for epidemiologic studies depression scale (CES-D) as a screening instrument for depression among community-residing older adults. *Psychol Aging.* 1997;12(2):277.
19. Verdier-Taillefer M-H, Gourlet V, Fuhrer R, Alperovitch A. Psychometric properties of the center for epidemiologic studies-depression scale in multiple sclerosis. *Neuroepidemiology.* 2001;20(4):262-267.
20. Hind D, Cotter J, Thake A, et al. Cognitive behavioural therapy for the treatment of depression in people with multiple sclerosis: a systematic review and meta-analysis. *BMC Psychiatry.* 2014;14:5. doi:10.1186/1471-244X-14-5.
21. Ehde DM, Kraft GH, Chwastiak L, et al. Efficacy of paroxetine in treating major depressive disorder in persons with multiple sclerosis. *Gen Hosp Psychiatry.* 2008;30(1):40-48. doi:10.1016/j.genhosppsych.2007.08.002.
22. Freal JE, Kraft GH, Coryell JK. Symptomatic fatigue in multiple sclerosis. *Arch Phys Med Rehabil.* 1984;65(3):135-138.
23. Strober LB. Fatigue in multiple sclerosis: a look at the role of poor sleep. *Front Neurol.* 2015;6:21. doi:10.3389/fneur.2015.00021.
24. Veauthier C, Gaede G, Radbruch H, Gottschalk S, Wernecke KD, Paul F. Treatment of sleep disorders may improve fatigue in multiple sclerosis. *Clin Neurol Neurosurg.* 2013;115(9):1826-1830. doi:10.1016/j.clineuro.2013.05.018.
25. Strober LB, Arnett PA. An examination of four models predicting fatigue in multiple sclerosis. *Arch Clin Neuropsychol.* 2005;20(5):631-646. doi:10.1016/j.acn.2005.04.002.
26. Attarian HP, Brown KM, Duntley SP, Carter JD, Cross AH. The relationship of sleep disturbances and fatigue in multiple sclerosis. *Arch Neurol.* 2004;61(4):525-528.
27. Kinsinger SW, Lattie E, Mohr DC. Relationship between depression, fatigue, subjective cognitive impairment, and objective neuropsychological functioning in patients with multiple sclerosis. *Neuropsychology.* 2010;24:573-580. doi:10.1037/a0019222.
28. Niino M, Mifune N, Kohriyama T, et al. Apathy/depression, but not subjective fatigue, is related with cognitive dysfunction in patients with multiple sclerosis. *BMC Neurol.* 2014;14(1):3. doi:10.1186/1471-2377-14-3.
29. Greeke EE, Chua AS, Healy BC, Rintell DJ, Chitnis T, Glanz BI. Depression and fatigue in patients with multiple sclerosis. *J Neurol Sci.* 2017;380:236-241. doi:10.1016/j.jns.2017.07.047.
30. Wood B, van der Mei IAF, Ponsonby AL, et al. Prevalence and concurrence of anxiety, depression and fatigue over time in multiple sclerosis. *Mult Scler J.* 2013;19(2):217-224. doi:10.1177/1352458512450351.
31. Mills RJ, Young CA, Pallant JF, Tennant A. Development of a patient reported outcome scale for fatigue in multiple sclerosis: the Neurological Fatigue Index (NFI-MS). *Health Qual Life Outcomes.* 2010;8(1):22.
32. Mills RJ, Young CA, Pallant JF, Tennant A. Rasch analysis of the modified fatigue impact scale (MFIS) in multiple sclerosis. *J Neurol Neurosurg Psychiatry.* 2010;81(9):1049-1051. doi:10.1136/jnnp.2008.151340.
33. Krupp LB. The fatigue severity scale: application to patients with multiple sclerosis and systemic lupus erythematosus. *Arch Neurol.* 1989;46(10):1121. doi:10.1001/archneur.1989.00520460115022.

34. Rosti-Otajärvi E, Hämäläinen P, Wiksten A, Hakkarainen T, Ruutiainen J. Validity and reliability of the fatigue severity scale in Finnish multiple sclerosis patients. *Brain Behav.* 2017;7(7):e00743. doi:10.1002/brb3.743.
35. Amtmann D, Bamer AM, Noonan V, Lang N, Kim J, Cook KF. Comparison of the psychometric properties of two fatigue scales in multiple sclerosis. *Rehabil Psychol.* 2012;57(2):159-166. doi:10.1037/a0027890.
36. Learmonth YC, Dlugonski D, Pilutti LA, Sandroff BM, Klaren R, Motl RW. Psychometric properties of the fatigue severity scale and the modified fatigue impact scale. *J Neurol Sci.* 2013;331(1–2):102-107. doi:10.1016/j.jns.2013.05.023.
37. Rammohan K, Rosenberg J, Lynn D, Blumenfeld A, Pollak C, Nagaraja H. Efficacy and safety of modafinil (Provigil®) for the treatment of fatigue in multiple sclerosis: a two centre phase 2 study. *J Neurol Neurosurg Psychiatry.* 2002;72(2):179-183. doi:10.1136/jnnp.72.2.179.
38. Blikman LJ, Huisstede BM, Kooijmans H, Stam HJ, Bussmann JB, van Meeteren J. Effectiveness of energy conservation treatment in reducing fatigue in multiple sclerosis: a systematic review and meta-analysis. *Arch Phys Med Rehabil.* 2013;94(7):1360-1376. doi:10.1016/j.apmr.2013.01.025.
39. van den Akker LE, Beckerman H, Collette EH, et al. Cognitive behavioral therapy positively affects fatigue in patients with multiple sclerosis: results of a randomized controlled trial. *Mult Scler.* 2017;23(11):1542-1553. doi:10.1177/1352458517709361.
40. Phyo AZZ, Demaneuf T, De Livera AM, et al. The efficacy of psychological interventions for managing fatigue in people with multiple sclerosis: a systematic review and meta-analysis. *Front Neurol.* 2018;9:149. doi:10.3389/fneur.2018.00149.
41. Feinstein A, Pavisian B. Multiple sclerosis and suicide. *Mult Scler J.* 2017;23(7):923-927. doi:10.1177/1352458517702553.
42. Marrie RA, Fisk JD, Tremlett H, et al. Differences in the burden of psychiatric comorbidity in MS vs the general population. *Neurology.* 2015;85(22):1972-1979. doi:10.1212/WNL.0000000000002174.
43. Brenner P, Burkill S, Jokinen J, Hillert J, Bahmanyar S, Montgomery S. Multiple sclerosis and risk of attempted and completed suicide – a cohort study. *Eur J Neurol.* 2016;23(8):1329-1336. doi:10.1111/ene.13029.
44. Pompili M, Forte A, Palermo M, et al. Suicide risk in multiple sclerosis: a systematic review of current literature. *J Psychosom Res.* 2012;73(6):411-417.
45. Viner R, Patten SB, Berzins S, Bulloch AGM, Fiest KM. Prevalence and risk factors for suicidal ideation in a multiple sclerosis population. *J Psychosom Res.* 2014;76(4):312-316. doi:10.1016/j.jpsychores.2013.12.010.
46. Turner AP, Williams RM, Bowen JD, Kivlahan DR, Haselkorn JK. Suicidal ideation in multiple sclerosis. *Arch Phys Med Rehabil.* 2006;87(8):1073-1078. doi:10.1016/j.apmr.2006.04.021.
47. Stenager EN, Jensen B, Stenager M, Stenager K, Stenager E. Suicide attempts in multiple sclerosis. *Mult Scler.* 2011;17(10):1265-1268. doi:10.1177/1352458511401942.
48. Patten SB, Francis G, Metz LM, Lopez-Bresnahan M, Chang P, Curtin F. The relationship between depression and interferon beta-1a therapy in patients with multiple sclerosis. *Mult Scler.* 2005;11(2):175-181. doi:10.1191/1352458505ms1144oa.
49. Feinstein A, O'Connor P, Feinstein K. Multiple sclerosis, interferon beta-1b and depression A prospective investigation. *J Neurol.* 2002;249(7):815-820. doi:10.1007/s00415-002-0725-0.
50. Korostil M, Feinstein A. Anxiety disorders and their clinical correlates in multiple sclerosis patients. *Mult Scler.* 2007;13(1):67-72. doi:10.1177/1352458506071161.

51. Boeschoten RE, Braamse AMJ, Beekman ATF, et al. Prevalence of depression and anxiety in multiple sclerosis: a systematic review and meta-analysis. *J Neurol Sci*. 2016;372:331-341. doi:10.1016/j.jns.2016.11.067.

52. Terrill AL, Hartoonian N, Beier M, Salem R, Alschuler K. The 7-item generalized anxiety disorder scale as a tool for measuring generalized anxiety in multiple sclerosis. *Int J MS Care*. 2015;17(2):49-56. doi:10.7224/1537-2073.2014-008.

53. Turner AP, Alschuler KN, Hughes AJ, et al. Mental health comorbidity in MS: depression, anxiety, and bipolar disorder. *Curr Neurol Neurosci Rep*. 2016;16(12):106. doi:10.1007/s11910-016-0706-x.

54. Carta MG, Moro MF, Lorefice L, et al. Multiple sclerosis and bipolar disorders: the burden of comorbidity and its consequences on quality of life. *J Affect Disord*. 2014;167:192-197. doi:10.1016/j.jad.2014.05.024.

55. Sajatovic M. Bipolar disorder: disease burden. *Am J Manag Care*. 2005;11(3 suppl):S80-S84.

56. Johansson V, Lundholm C, Hillert J, et al. Multiple sclerosis and psychiatric disorders: comorbidity and sibling risk in a nationwide Swedish cohort. *Mult Scler*. 2014;20(14):1881-1891. doi:10.1177/1352458514540970.

57. Hirschfeld RM, Williams JB, Spitzer RL, et al. Development and validation of a screening instrument for bipolar spectrum disorder: the Mood Disorder Questionnaire. *Am J Psychiatry*. 2000;157(11):1873-1875. doi:10.1176/appi.ajp.157.11.1873.

58. Hotier S, Maltete D, Bourre B, Jegouzo X, Bourgeois V, Guillin O. A manic episode with psychotic features improved by methylprednisolone in a patient with multiple sclerosis. *Gen Hosp Psychiatry*. 2015;37(6):621. e1-2. doi:10.1016/j.genhosppsych.2015.07.002.

59. Work SS, Colamonico JA, Bradley WG, Kaye RE. Pseudobulbar affect: an under-recognized and under-treated neurological disorder. *Adv Ther*. 2011;28(7):586-601. doi:10.1007/s12325-011-0031-3.

60. Johnson B, Nichols S. Crying and suicidal, but not depressed. Pseudobulbar affect in multiple sclerosis successfully treated with valproic acid: case report and literature review. *Palliat Support Care*. 2015;13(06):1797-1801. doi:10.1017/S1478951514000376.

61. Feinstein A, Feinstein K, Gray T, O'connor P. Prevalence and neurobehavioral correlates of pathological laughing and crying in multiple sclerosis. *Arch Neurol*. 1997;54(9):1116-1121. doi:10.1001/archneur.1997.00550210050012.

62. Parvizi J, Coburn KL, Shillcutt SD, Coffey CE, Lauterbach EC, Mendez MF. Neuroanatomy of pathological laughing and crying: a report of the American Neuropsychiatric Association Committee on Research. *J Neuropsychiatry Clin Neurosci*. 2009;21(1):75-87. doi:10.1176/jnp.2009.21.1.75.

63. Kroenke K, Spitzer R. The PHQ-9: a new depression diagnostic and severity measure. *Psychiatr Ann*. 2002;32:509-515.

64. Robinson RG, Parikh RM, Lipsey JR, Starkstein SE, Price TR. Pathological laughing and crying following stroke: validation of a measurement scale and a double-blind treatment study. *Am J Psychiatry*. 1993;150(2):286.

65. Moore SR, Gresham LS, Bromberg MB, Kasarkis EJ, Smith RA. A self report measure of affective lability. *J Neurol Neurosurg Psychiatry*. 1997;63(1):89-93.

66. Smith RA, Berg JE, Pope LE, Callahan JD, Wynn D, Thisted RA. Validation of the CNS emotional lability scale for pseudobulbar affect (pathological laughing and crying) in multiple sclerosis patients. *Mult Scler*. 2004;10(6):679-685. doi:10.1191/1352458504ms1106oa.

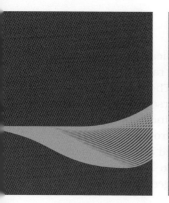

Multiple Sclerosis in Adolescents and Children

■ ▦ ▦ Tanuja Chitnis

Introduction

There has been an increasing awareness of the occurrence of multiple sclerosis (MS) in children and adolescents since approximately 2004. Whether this is due to a true increase in incidence or improved diagnostic criteria and dedicated pediatric MS centers is still unclear. However, it is clear that children can get MS and that this form of disease requires specialized treatment and management.

Pediatric MS is defined as MS with an onset younger than age 18 years. There are some variances in the literature, using a cutoff of age 16 years; however, for practical purposes, most studies including treatment trials use age 18 years as the cutoff.[1]

There have been reports of children as young as 2.5 to 3 years old at the time of the first attack of MS; however, the vast majority of patients are 11 years or older, with a mean age at onset of 15 years in the US Network of Pediatric MS Centers at the first symptom. Puberty seems to be an important transition time for the onset of pediatric MS,[2] with 80% to 85% of children being peripubertal or postpubertal at the time of the first symptoms in a large US cohort.[3] Approximately 3% to 5% of all MS patients are pediatric at the time of first symptoms.[4]

Reports from many centers around the world indicate that the pediatric MS occurs in many regions. Higher prevalence rates are generally reported from regions more distal to the equator. The estimated incidence is approximately 0.51 per 100,000 insured persons less than age 18 years[5] in a California study, and 2009 to 2011 incidence was estimated at 0.64 per 100,000 in an incidence study from Germany.[3,6] A recent report from Canada found the age-standardized annual incidence of MS in the pediatric population ranged from 0.99 to 1.24 per 100,000 population, and the age-standardized prevalence ranged from 4.03 to 6.8 per 100,000 population.[7]

The diagnosis of pediatric MS rests on clinical and magnetic resonance imaging (MRI) features, and the updated diagnostic criteria published in 2013 from the International Pediatric MS Study Group[8] have been the general standard for diagnosis. However, these criteria are updated every 4 to 5 years as more information regarding MRI features and differential diagnosis becomes available. The diagnostic criteria for pediatric MS are listed in Table 20.1.

Typical MRIs from a pediatric patient with MS are shown in Figure 20.1.

Differential Diagnosis

The differential diagnosis of pediatric MS is similar to that of adult MS, with the following caveats. Acute disseminated encephalomyelitis (ADEM) occurs mainly in children[9] and is an important differential diagnosis of pediatric MS. Rarely, ADEM events are the first event of pediatric MS, and for this reason, children with ADEM should be followed longitudinally by a neurologist. Some differentiating features of ADEM and pediatric MS are listed in Table 20.2.

Other similarly appearing white matter disorders include neuromyelitis optica-spectrum disorder[6,10] and myelin oligodendrocyte glycoprotein (MOG)-antibody-associated disorders.[11-13] Testing for Aquaporin-4 antibody and MOG antibodies should be sent in any child with an acute demyelinating syndrome (ADS), and if negative, consider repeating within a year or again for highly suspicious cases.

The differential diagnosis of pediatric MS is broad and includes infectious, metabolic, and other autoimmune disorders (Table 20.3). Red flags for a diagnosis other than pediatric MS include a progressive disease course from onset, prominent seizures, rapid cognitive decline and headaches, multisystemic involvement, onset before age 2 years, and family history of severe neurological deficits.

TABLE 20.1

SUMMARY OF PROPOSED DEFINITIONS OF PEDIATRIC ACQUIRED DEMYELINATING SYNDROMES (IPMSSG CRITERIA): DIAGNOSIS OF PEDIATRIC MS MUST MEET CRITERIA FOR BOTH DISSEMINATION IN TIME AND DISSEMINATION IN SPACE

Dissemination in Time (DIT)	Dissemination in Space (DIS)
One of the following DIT criteria must be met: 1. Two or more nonencephalopathic (e.g., non-acute disseminated encephalomyelitis [ADEM]) clinical CNS events with presumed inflammatory cause separated by more than 30 d involving more than one area of the CNS 2. One nonencephalopathic episode typical of MS that is associated with MRI findings consistent with 2010 Revised McDonald criteria for DIS and in which a follow-up MRI shows at least one new enhancing or nonenhancing lesion consistent with DIT MS criteria (irrespective of its timing with reference to a baseline scan) 3. One ADEM attack followed by a nonencephalopathic clinical event, 3 or more months after symptom onset, that is associated with new MRI lesions that fulfill 2010 Revised McDonald DIS criteria (at least one T2 lesion in two of the following areas: periventricular. juxtacortical, infratentorial, and spinal cord) 4. A first, single acute event that does not meet ADEM criteria and whose MRI findings are consistent with the 2010 Revised McDonald criteria for DIS and DIT (simultaneous presence of asymptomatic gadolinium-enhancing and nonenhancing lesions at any time). These criteria apply only to children <12 y old	2010 Revised McDonald criteria for DIS; at least one T2 lesion in two of the following areas: ■ Periventricular ■ Juxtacortical ■ Infratentorial ■ Spinal cord

Reprinted with permission from Krupp LB, Tardieu M, Amato MP, et al. International Pediatric Multiple Sclerosis Study Group criteria for pediatric multiple sclerosis and immune-mediated central nervous system demyelinating disorders: revisions to the 2007 definitions. *Mult Scler.* 2013;19:1261-1267. Copyright © 2013 SAGE Publications.

CNS, central nervous system; MRI, magnetic resonance imaging.

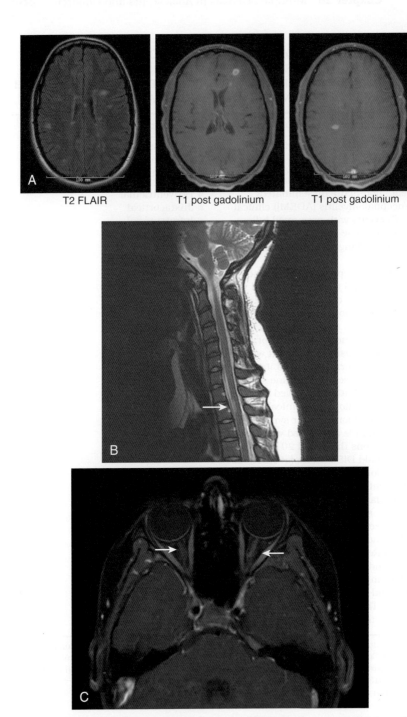

T2 FLAIR   T1 post gadolinium   T1 post gadolinium

Figure 20.1. (A) Magnetic resonance imaging (MRI) findings in pediatric multiple sclerosis. (B) MRI cervical-thoracic spine. (C) MRI orbits.

TABLE 20.2
DIFFERENTIAL FEATURES OF PEDIATRIC MS AND ADEM

	ADEM	Pediatric MS
Age at onset	3-7 y	12-15 y
Female:male ratio	1:1	3:1
Symptoms	Encephalopathy (lethargy, obtundation, coma), polyfocal neurological symptoms	Monofocal or polyfocal neurological symptoms (such as optic neuritis, transverse myelitis, brainstem syndromes) without encephalopathy
Disease course	Symptoms can fluctuate/appear within a 3-mo period. Then generally remits and remains monophasic	Polyphasic—new attacks or new MRI lesions occurring with separation in time by at least 1 mo
CSF features	WBC 50-70 (60%-70% lymphocytes); no oligoclonal bands	WBC 15-30 (90%-95% lymphocytes); positive oligoclonal bands in 70%-85%
MRI features	Fluffy, diffuse lesions in the subcortical white matter or thalamus/basal ganglia. Lesions can occur in other areas including optic nerve, brainstem, spinal cord	Periventricular lesions ovoid discrete lesions. Involvement of the corpus callosum. Lesions can occur in other areas including optic nerve, brainstem, spinal cord

ADEM, acute disseminated encephalomyelitis; CSF, cerebrospinal fluid; MRI, magnetic resonance imaging; MS, multiple sclerosis; WBC, white blood cell.

TABLE 20.3
DIFFERENTIAL DIAGNOSIS OF PEDIATRIC MS

Category	Specific Diseases
Autoimmune conditions	Systemic lupus erythematosus Behçet disease Neurosarcoidosis Isolated or primary angiitis of the CNS Hemophagocytic lymphohistiocytosis Autoimmune encephalitis (NMDAR antibody syndrome) Hashimoto encephalopathy
Immunodeficiency syndromes	XLP, NK
Infections	Neuroborelliosis, progressive multifocal leukoencephalopathy
Tumors	Lymphoma, astrocytoma, glioma, oligodendroglioma, ependymoma
Metabolic diseases of the CNS	Leber hereditary optic neuropathy mitochondrial syndromes biotin-responsive basal ganglia disease
Leukodystrophy	ALD Leukoencephalopathy with brainstem and spinal cord involvement and lactate elevation (LSBL)

ALD, adrenoleukodystrophy; CNS, central nervous system; NK, natural killer; NMDAR, N-Methyl D-aspartate receptor antibody syndrome; XLP, X linked lymphoproliferative syndrome.

Clinical Course of Pediatric MS

General Course

Over 95% of pediatric patients with MS present the relapsing-remitting form of MS. The clinical course of children with MS varies from patient to patient.[5] In general, children with MS experience a higher relapse rate than most adult patients with MS, with 2 to 3 times as many relapses.[14,15]

Acute Attacks

Relapses or attacks in pediatric MS include optic neuritis, transverse myelitis, brainstem attacks, and cerebral attacks. These can affect vision, cognition, motor function, sensation, and bladder/bowel function, as well as pain and spasticity. Relapses should be addressed promptly, and part of the challenge in children can be recognition or reporting of a relapse. Encouraging the patients to develop a good rapport with parents and care-givers to alert them of new symptoms is critical. Pseudorelapses, or those due to overheating, can mimic a true relapse. General advice is that, if symptoms do not remit with cooling down with cold drinks, air condition-ing, or antipyretics, then report to the neurologist or physician immediately. Relapses are generally treated with a course of intravenous steroids, which can reduce the severity and duration of symptoms. Functional relapses in children with MS have been reported. It is essential for the neurologist to ascertain the consistency of relapse symptomatology and consider this in the differential.[16] Most common preparations are methylprednisolone at a dose of 15 to 30 mg/kg for 5 days on average, but courses can range from 3 to 7 days depending on symptom severity. Children may be admitted to the hospital for a course of steroids, or if feasible and available, outpatient infusion units or home infusion administration through a visiting nurse can be used. Although studies have found high-dose prednisone to be effi-cacious for relapse-treatment in adults, this approach has not been stud-ied in children. An oral prednisone taper is generally administered after the first attack of ADS, including in pediatric MS cases; however, it may not be required for every attack, because avoidance of chronic steroids can reduce steroid-related side effects.

Chronic Symptoms

More insidious or chronic symptoms include fatigue, depression,[17] anxiety, cognitive decline, pain, spasticity, and bladder/bowel dysfunction. These should be questioned and addressed at each clinical visit. Treatment of fatigue can include methylphenidate, modafinil, armodafinil, or amanta-dine. Depression and anxiety should be addressed with both counseling and potentially medicinal therapy. Referral for bladder issues may require a referral to a urologist. Pain may be addressed with physical therapy or medical therapies.

Cognitive Deficits

Between one-third to two-thirds of pediatric patients with MS may have significant cognitive deficits, including issues with processing speed, information processing, memory deficits, executive dysfunction, and lowered intelligence quotients, as well as deficits in social cognition.[18,19] Evaluation and monitoring by a neuropsychologist shortly after diagnosis is important for evaluating for the presence of cognitive dysfunction. A 504 or an individualized education plan (IEP) plan should be instituted to address cognitive deficits and ensure appropriate programming at school. This requires interaction with the school and testing neuropsychologist/ neurologist. A guideline for a comprehensive neuropsychological battery can be found in the International Pediatric Multiple Sclerosis Study Group (IPMSSG) publication.

General Management

Periodic visits to the neurologist every 4 to 6 months are recommended to follow symptoms, response to treatment, and psychosocial issues. These may be more frequent, or acute visits may be needed at the time of a relapse. Additional support from a pediatric psychologist/psychiatrist may be required. Neuropsychological testing every 1 to 2 years is generally recommended and can be used to inform the need and details of an IEP. Symptomatic issues may require referral to a pediatric physical therapist, physiatrist, urologist, and other subspecialties as needed. Neuro-ophthalmology examination may be required for evaluation and monitoring of optic neuritis or ophthalmoplegias.[20] Visual rehabilitation may be needed for children with severe visual deficits. MRI scans of the brain, orbits, and spine should be completed at baseline and repeated annually.

Treatment

The treatment of pediatric patients with MS follows the following tenets[21-24]:

1. Institute a disease-modifying treatment (DMT) as soon as the diagnosis of pediatric MS is confirmed. This is a highly relapsing form of disease, and early effective treatment may prevent relapses and relapse-associated disability (Table 20.4). Consideration of a highly effective DMT balancing safety and tolerability is important in this population.

TABLE 20.4

OPTIONS FOR DISEASE-MODIFYING TREATMENTS IN PEDIATRIC MS

	Level of Evidence	Potential Side Effects
Fingolimod (oral)	FDA approved for pediatric MS (2018) based on phase II randomized controlled trial (Chitnis, *NEJM* in press)	Bradycardia, macular edema, infections
Beta-interferon-1a and beta-interferon-1b (im or sc injections)	EMA approval for children >12 y of age. Retrospective observational studies[29,30]	Injection site reactions, flulike symptoms, depression
Glatiramer acetate (sc injections)	Retrospective observational studies	Injection site reactions, postinjection tachycardia
Natalizumab (intravenous infusion)	Prospective observational studies[31,32]	Progressive multifocal leukoencephalopathy, infusion reactions
Rituximab (intravenous infusion)	Observational studies[33-35]	Infusion reactions, infections, hypogammaglobulinemia

EMA, European Medicines Agency; FDA, US Food and Drug Administration; MS, multiple sclerosis.

2. Monitor DMT response clinically and with annual MRI scans.[25] Appropriate bloodwork, screening, and monitoring tests may be required for each DMT.
3. Monitor adherence to therapy continually. Adherence may be challenging in the setting of miseducation about the expectations for DMTs, unaddressed side effects, busy family schedules, and travel/college.[26] In the case of nonadherence, schedule a visit to discuss and address contributing issues and consider switching if not addressable.
4. Switch treatment if there is evidence of intractable nonadherence, intolerance, or treatment failure.[27] Treatment failure may be defined 1 to 2 new lesions or attacks occurring within a 12-month period. One must account for an approximately 3-month period for a new DMT to take effect, and consider a rebaselined MRI at that time. The tolerance for new lesions or attacks versus switching is a discussion between the neurologist and family, with an informed discussion about the risks or benefits of either approach.
5. Consider symptomatic treatments as needed. These may include antidepressants, fatigue medications, and bladder management.
6. Consider contraceptives in sexually active teenagers. This may be a challenging conversation, but important, because many DMTs may have adverse effects on a pregnancy and some are teratogens.

There are additional drugs under study for the treatment of pediatric MS, including dimethyl fumarate, teriflunomide, and alemtuzumab, with results anticipated in 2019 to 2020.[24,28]

Transitional Care and College Planning

Most children with MS will receive a diagnosis during their teenage years and thus may be eligible to transition to adult care within a few years after diagnosis. Our practice is to continue to follow these patients in the pediatric setting up to age 20 to 23 years to provide educational and psychosocial support during this critical period. Transitions to an adult neurologist should include continuation or transition of key support services including school support, psychosocial care, and subspecialty care (urology, physical therapy). Often, meeting with the adult neurologist before transition helps to ease the anxiety of a new clinical setting. Young adults are encouraged to start to participate in their own care early onset and includes making appointments, monitoring medication adherence, and filling prescriptions.

Transition to college requires preparation and consideration of the specific needs of a young adult with MS. Discussion with the patient and family should include consideration of college location, proximity to medical/neurological care, dormitory conditions including privacy, temperature control, and the ability to administer medications. Most colleges have an American for Disabilities Act (ADA) office on campus, and patients with MS should be encouraged to establish a relationship with the ADA office, which can provide academic and legal support.

Resources for Families

There are a number of organizations that offer resources to assist and support children and families affected by pediatric MS. These include the International Pediatric MS Study Group (www.ipmssg.org), the National MS Society (www.nmss.org), and other national organizations.

References

1. Belman AL, Krupp LB, Olsen CS, et al. Characteristics of children and adolescents with multiple sclerosis. *Pediatrics*. 2016;138(1):e20160120.
2. Chitnis T. Role of puberty in multiple sclerosis risk and course. *Clin Immunol.* 2013;149:192-200.
3. Chitnis T, Graves J, Weinstock-Guttman B, et al. Distinct effects of obesity and puberty on risk and age at onset of pediatric MS. *Ann Clin Transl Neurol.* 2016;3:897-907.
4. Chitnis T, Glanz B, Jaffin S, Healy B. Demographics of pediatric-onset multiple sclerosis in an MS center population from the Northeastern United States. *Mult Scler.* 2009;15:627-631.

5. Waldman A, Ness J, Pohl D, et al. Pediatric multiple sclerosis: clinical features and outcome. *Neurology.* 2016;87:S74-S81.

6. Wingerchuk DM, Banwell B, Bennett JL, et al. International consensus diagnostic criteria for neuromyelitis optica spectrum disorders. *Neurology.* 2015;85:177-189.

7. Marrie RA, O'Mahony J, Maxwell C, et al. Incidence and prevalence of MS in children: a population-based study in Ontario, Canada. *Neurology.* 2018;91(17):e1579-e1590.

8. Krupp LB, Tardieu M, Amato MP, et al. International Pediatric Multiple Sclerosis Study Group criteria for pediatric multiple sclerosis and immune-mediated central nervous system demyelinating disorders: revisions to the 2007 definitions. *Mult Scler.* 2013;19:1261-1267.

9. Pohl D, Alper G, Van Haren K, et al. Acute disseminated encephalomyelitis: updates on an inflammatory CNS syndrome. *Neurology.* 2016;87:S38-S45.

10. Chitnis T, Ness J, Krupp L, et al. Clinical features of neuromyelitis optica in children: US Network of Pediatric MS Centers report. *Neurology.* 2016;86:245-252.

11. Fernandez-Carbonell C, Vargas-Lowy D, Musallam A, et al. Clinical and MRI phenotype of children with MOG antibodies. *Mult Scler.* 2016;22:174-184.

12. Ramanathan S, Dale RC, Brilot F. Anti-MOG antibody: the history, clinical phenotype, and pathogenicity of a serum biomarker for demyelination. *Autoimmun Rev.* 2016;15:307-324.

13. Probstel AK, Dornmair K, Bittner R, et al. Antibodies to MOG are transient in childhood acute disseminated encephalomyelitis. *Neurology.* 2011;77:580-588.

14. Benson LA, Healy BC, Gorman MP, et al. Elevated relapse rates in pediatric compared to adult MS persist for at least 6 years. *Mult Scler Relat Disord.* 2014;3:186-193.

15. Gorman MP, Healy BC, Polgar-Turcsanyi M, Chitnis T. Increased relapse rate in pediatric-onset compared with adult-onset multiple sclerosis. *Arch Neurol.* 2009;66:54-59.

16. Fernandez Carbonell C, Benson L, Rintell D, Prince J, Chitnis T. Functional relapses in pediatric multiple sclerosis. *J Child Neurol.* 2014;29:943-946.

17. Pakpoor J, Goldacre R, Schmierer K, Giovannoni G, Waubant E, Goldacre MJ. Psychiatric disorders in children with demyelinating diseases of the central nervous system. *Mult Scler.* 2017. doi:10.1177/1352458517719150.

18. Amato MP, Krupp LB, Charvet LE, Penner I, Till C. Pediatric multiple sclerosis: cognition and mood. *Neurology.* 2016;87:S82-S87.

19. Charvet LE, Cleary RE, Vazquez K, Belman AL, Krupp LB; MS USNfP. Social cognition in pediatric-onset multiple sclerosis (MS). *Mult Scler.* 2014;20:1478-1484.

20. Waldman AT, Hiremath G, Avery RA, et al. Monocular and binocular low-contrast visual acuity and optical coherence tomography in pediatric multiple sclerosis. *Mult Scler Relat Disord.* 2013;3:326-334.

21. Chitnis T. Disease-modifying therapy of pediatric multiple sclerosis. *Neurotherapeutics.* 2013;10:89-96.

22. Chitnis T, Ghezzi A, Bajer-Kornek B, Boyko A, Giovannoni G, Pohl D. Pediatric multiple sclerosis: escalation and emerging treatments. *Neurology.* 2016;87:S103-S109.

23. Chitnis T, Krupp L, Yeh A, et al. Pediatric multiple sclerosis. *Neurol Clin.* 2011;29:481-505.

24. Simone M, Chitnis T. Use of disease-modifying therapies in pediatric MS. *Curr Treat Options Neurol.* 2016;18:36.

25. Banwell B, Arnold DL, Tillema JM, et al. MRI in the evaluation of pediatric multiple sclerosis. *Neurology.* 2016;87:S88-S96.

26. Schwartz CE, Grover SA, Powell VE, et al. Risk factors for non-adherence to disease-modifying therapy in pediatric multiple sclerosis. *Mult Scler.* 2018;24:175-185.

27. Yeh EA, Waubant E, Krupp LB, et al. Multiple sclerosis therapies in pediatric patients with refractory multiple sclerosis. *Arch Neurol.* 2011;68:437-444.

28. Chitnis T, Tardieu M, Amato MP, et al. International pediatric MS study group clinical trials summit: meeting report. *Neurology.* 2013;80:1161-1168.

29. Tenembaum SN, Banwell B, Pohl D, et al. Subcutaneous interferon Beta-1a in pediatric multiple sclerosis: a retrospective study. *J Child Neurol.* 2013;28:849-856.

30. Krupp LB, Pohl D, Ghezzi A, et al. Subcutaneous interferon beta-1a in pediatric patients with multiple sclerosis: regional differences in clinical features, disease management, and treatment outcomes in an international retrospective study. *J Neurol Sci.* 2016;363:33-38.

31. Ghezzi A, Moiola L, Pozzilli C, et al. Natalizumab in the pediatric MS population: results of the Italian registry. *BMC Neurol.* 2015;15:174.

32. Ghezzi A, Pozzilli C, Grimaldi LM, et al. Natalizumab in pediatric multiple sclerosis: results of a cohort of 55 cases. *Mult Scler.* 2013;19:1106-1112.

33. Nosadini M, Alper G, Riney CJ, et al. Rituximab monitoring and redosing in pediatric neuromyelitis optica spectrum disorder. *Neurol Neuroimmunol Neuroinflamm.* 2016;3:e188.

34. Dale RC, Brilot F, Duffy LV, et al. Utility and safety of rituximab in pediatric autoimmune and inflammatory CNS disease. *Neurology.* 2014;83:142-150.

35. Chitnis T, Waubant E. B-cell depletion in children with neuroimmunologic conditions: the learning curve. *Neurology.* 2014;83:111-112.

TABLE 21.1

CONSIDERATIONS IN PREVENTION AND MANAGEMENT OF PATIENTS WITH MULTIPLE SCLEROSIS (MS)

Physical challenges in oral hygiene	■ Customized toothbrush handles from dental acrylic or silicone impression putty to improve grip[7,8] ■ Use of electric toothbrush (Sonicare®, Oral B), power flosser (AirFloss®, Waterpik®) ■ Recommend patient to sit down, rest arms on commode while brushing if fatigued ■ Instruct family member or caretaker on assistance with hygiene when needed
Caries risk prevention	■ Fluoride supplementation in the form of trays, 1.1% sodium fluoride (PreviDent®, Colgate) paste or gel ■ Diet counseling including recommendations for reduction of acidic/sugary beverages and awareness of hidden sugars ■ Use of products with xylitol substitutes (Spry®) ■ Frequent recalls (q3-4 mo)
Xerostomia	■ Sialagogues ■ Muscarinic acetylcholine agonists (pilocarpine and cevimeline) ■ Postmeal rinses with 8 oz water and ½ tsp baking soda ■ Smoking cessation ■ Saliva substitutes (Biotene Oral balance Moisturizing Gel®, Xylimelts®)
Hypersalivation/ inability to control saliva	■ Portable Yankauer suction at home in the more debilitated patient ■ Botox injections at the parotid gland
Increase incidence of herpes simplex virus, candidiasis, angular cheilitis	■ Common findings related to immunosuppression and xerostomia. Prescribe proper antiviral or antifungal medication for fungal or viral infections

Infections in MS Exacerbation of Symptoms

There is sufficient evidence that infection can add to the underlying abnormal immunological response of these patients, which can increase the risk of exacerbation of symptoms.[9,10] No studies have been conducted on the association between dental infections and relapse specifically; however, the activation of the innate immune system by microbial products in MS patients has been proposed to be linked to the induction of MS relapse.[11] Systemic infection increases T-cell proliferation and proflammatory interleukins, leading to higher levels of inflammatory response.[11,12] A number of bacterial and viral strains have been suggested to have a correlation on worsening some MS activity. *Staphylococcus aureus* enterotoxin A, for example, has been suggested to be one risk factor for exacerbations

TABLE 21.2

CONSIDERATIONS IN TREATMENT AND IMPROVING ACCESS TO CARE OF PATIENTS WITH MULTIPLE SCLEROSIS (MS)

Provide wheelchair accessibility and staff assistance from the entrance to the operatories

Provide bathroom breaks before and during procedures for those with urinary incontinence

Provide sources of transportation assistance

Schedule morning visits as fatigue tends to be more pronounced in the afternoon

Consider shorter appointments for more symptomatic patients and more frequent recalls

Consider different levels of sedation for treatment depending on anxiety, neurological symptoms, or severity of the disease

Careful use of isolation methods and adequate evacuation as respiratory muscle and gag reflex impairment become more pronounced. Use a rubber dam for proper isolation if patient can adequately breathe through the nose. Use a bite block. Treat these patients in a semisitting position

Understand existing trigeminal neuralgia or facial anesthesia and avoid triggering episode

Consider dental implants for fixed prosthesis or to improve function of removable prosthesis

Use of resin-modified glass ionomers (RMGI) restorations and cements for biocompatibility and fluoride-releasing properties

---

through activation of disease modulating T-cells.[13] Evidence has also demonstrated that upper respiratory infections have been linked to subsequent relapses.[12,14]

Relapses are a distinctive characteristic of MS, and although they are usually followed by a period of clinical inactivity, residual side effects cause persistent functional impairment, impacting the quality of life of these individuals. Management and reduction of potential causes associated with MS relapses is important, as it may help to shorten and lessen the disability. Furthermore, patients on steroids or disease-modifying drugs may have a decreased ability to fight opportunistic infections or dental infections. Oral-facial infections should be identified and prevented early on. Patients with maxillary tooth and sinus pain or ear pain of nondental origin should be referred for evaluation if an upper respiratory infection is suspected. Antibiotics, antivirals, and/or antifungals should be judiciously prescribed as needed, and necessary treatment should be carried out early on. Patients with any suspicion of infection should be followed up with.

Multiple Sclerosis Treatment Medications and Oral Health

Although there is no cure for MS, the focus of treatment is to reduce the number of relapses and slow the disease process. The most common medications are steroids for treatment of acute attacks, disease-modifying therapies to suppress the activity of the disease, and symptomatic therapy for MS side effects, such as muscle relaxants, antidepressants, and anticholinergics. It is important to be aware of drug interactions when using medications in dentistry, and knowledge of the most common oral side effects of medications used to manage MS can positively impact the education and treatment planning of the patient.

Frequently seen side effects of MS medications that may be encountered include xerostomia, mucositis, ulcerative stomatitis, angular cheilitis, candida, dysgeusia, herpes simplex, and vomiting. See Table 21.3 for an overview.

TABLE 21.3

MEDICATIONS COMMONLY USED TO MANAGE MULTIPLE SCLEROSIS (MS) AND POTENTIAL SIDE EFFECTS[15,16]

	Medications	**Potential side effects**
Disease-modifying therapies	Interferon beta-1a and beta-1b (Avonex®, Betaseron®, Rebif®) Glatiramer acetate (Copaxone®) Monoclonal antibody (Lemtrada®, Ocrevus®)	Immunosuppression (more so with the monoclonal antibodies which can cause lymphopenia), increased risk of infection (fungal, bacterial, or viral), fatigue, myalgia, headache, arthralgia, mucositis, glossitis, dysgeusia, xerostomia, salivary gland enlargement, elevated liver enzymes
Management of relapses	Corticosteroids (Solu-Medrol®, Deltasone®) Adrenocorticotropic hormone (H.P. Acthar Gel®)	Immunosuppression, increased risk of infection (fungal, bacterial, or viral), delayed wound healing, nausea, vomiting, GERD (gastroesophageal reflux disease), osteoporosis, risk of hepatotoxicity
Treatment of tremor, spasticity	Muscle relaxants (Lioresal®, Zanaflex®), Benzodiazepine (Valium®, Klonopin®)	Central nervous system (CNS) depression, hypotension, xerostomia
Treatment of depression, neuropathic pain	Tricyclic antidepressants, selective serotonin and norepinephrine reuptake inhibitors, anticonvulsants (Tegretol®, Dilantin®, Gabapentin)	Anticholinergic effects (i.e., xerostomia), CNS depression, cardiovascular effects, gingival hyperplasia
Treatment of frequent urination	Anticholinergics (Oxybutynin®), antimuscarinic	Xerostomia, dry eyes, CNS depression, constipation

Treatment of Xerostomia

One of the most common issues patients face as a consequence of the medications used to treat MS and depression, as discussed above, is dry mouth. Saliva is beneficial in protecting the dental cavity by diluting, clearing, and buffering acids and by supplying the necessary calcium and phosphorus needed for tooth demineralization. Depending on the extent of hyposalivation, saliva substitutes, gustatory or tactile stimulants, and pharmacologic sialagogues can promote salivation and lubrication of the oral cavity for these patients. The following are suggestions for treatment of xerostomia.

1. Frequent use of plain noncarbonated water.
2. Postmeal rinses with 8 oz. water and ½ tsp. baking soda to neutralize pH.
3. Salivary-stimulating lozenges such as topical pilocarpine lozenges and lozenges containing anhydrous crystalline maltose.[17]
4. Use of xylitol-containing chewing gum immediately after meal for 5 minutes. Xylitol is documented in protecting root caries and erosion, can stimulate salivary flow rates, and can cause mutation of *Streptococcus mutans* to a less acidic form.
5. Use of saliva substitute gels.
6. Treatment with pilocarpine or cevimeline in consultation with the physician. Get a baseline on the flow rates before initiating therapy; hyposalivation is when the stimulated flow rate is approximately below 0.7 mL/min and the unstimulated rate is <0.1 mL/min.[18] Oral administration of pilocarpine HCl is typically 5 mg three to four times daily for 3 months, and cevimeline is prescribed at 30 mg three times daily for 3 month.[19] Both of these medications are contraindicated in patients with uncontrolled asthma, COPD, or patients taking β-adrenergic blockers; the use of these medications should also be advised with caution in patients with cardiovascular disease. Pilocarpine is also contraindicated in patients with narrow-angle glaucoma and iritis.

Trigeminal Neuralgia in the Multiple Sclerosis

Trigeminal neuralgia (TN) is described as a recurrent unilateral brief electric shock–like pain with abrupt onset and termination, limited to distribution of one or more divisions of the trigeminal nerve often triggered by innocuous stimuli.[20] The incidence of TN in MS according to a meta-analysis of 28 articles including 7101 subjects published in 2013 is 3.8%. The symptoms of TN often precede the first MS symptoms.[21,22] The mean age at diagnosis of TN was 45.4 years in a cohort of patients examined by Fallata et al.[22]

Pathophysiology

There are many existing theories that explain the pathophysiology behind TN. TN in absence of MS is thought to be a slowly evolving process where compression may be exerted on the trigeminal nerve by a blood vessel or tumor. However, TN in the presence of MS is thought to be due to the alteration of neural functions by an MS plaque at the level of the dorsal root entry zone, which may lead to excitability in some trigeminal afferents.[23]

Distinguishing Dental Pain From Trigeminal Neuralgia

TN in MS presents as repetitive episodes of sharp pain along the second or third divisions of the trigeminal nerve either unilateral or bilateral which can be triggered by masticating or manipulating the gingiva. Like TN, dental pain can also occur as repetitive episodes of sharp shooting pain along the second or third division of the trigeminal nerve. Patients are likely to seek consultation with their dentist when the symptoms first develop. Some patients with TN have undergone invasive dental procedures such as root canals or extractions owing to the belief that the pain was of dental origin. It is important for the dental providers to be familiar with TN in its presentation, pathophysiology, and association with MS to avoid recommendation of unnecessary treatment (Case Study 1). To distinguish dental pain from TN, a careful physical and radiographic examination of the dentoalveolar and gingival structures must be performed. If there is still a question as to the source of the pain, a trial of medical therapy for TN (i.e., carbamazepine or oxcarbazepine) may be indicated. These medications may alleviate TN pain; however, they will not improve dental pain. Conversely, a course of an antibiotic such as amoxicillin or clindamycin may improve dental pain; however, it will not lessen TN pain.

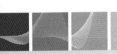

Case Study 1

55-Year-Old Presenting With Left Mandibular Pain Without Prior Diagnosis of Trigeminal Neuralgia

A 55-year-old African American female presented with a complaint of left mandibular pain of 11.5 years. Over the past several years, the patient reports that she sought the care of multiple dental professionals. She received multiple endodontic treatments and dental extractions of the left mandibular teeth which did not alleviate her pain. She reported that the inferior alveolar nerve block given before the dental treatment was the only time of relief for her pain. She was subsequently started on oxcarbazepine, and her symptoms resolved (see Figure 21.1).

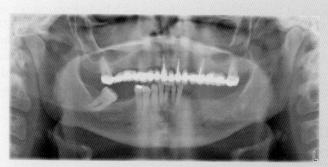

Figure 21.1. Panorex radiograph of a 57-year-old female with left mandible pain who suffered from undiagnosed trigeminal neuralgia affecting the left V3 distribution which subsequently led to extraction of all the left mandibular posterior teeth before diagnosis of trigeminal neuralgia.

Clinical Implications of Trigeminal Neuralgia

In contrast to the patient with undiagnosed TN who may seek dental care, patients with known TN may avoid dental procedures owing to fear or true exacerbation of their current pain or symptoms. TN is often associated with a perioral and/or intraoral trigger zone whereby nontraumatic stimuli such as light touch provoke severe paroxysmal pain.[24] Many patients may fear that perioral/intraoral triggers such as dental work will amplify their pain. Avoidance of oral health may lead to oral disease requiring more invasive dental treatments which further complicates their treatment.[25] The importance of prevention and appropriate oral hygiene should be emphasized to limit invasive dental procedures which can exacerbate a patient's symptoms of TN.

When dental treatment is required in a patient who suffers from TN, treatment approaches should be tailored to minimize any exacerbations of neuropathic pain. The concept of preemptive anesthesia through systemic control of the disease and adequate regional anesthesia has been shown to prevent chronic neuropathic pain.[26] Dental or oral surgical procedures should be scheduled during times of disease control. TN treatment should be optimized whenever possible before dental treatment, as dental work can trigger severe paroxysmal pain.[25] Adequate systemic analgesia achieved through treatment of TN can limit further exacerbation of neuralgic pains. When performing procedures under local anesthesia, careful attention should be made to avoid irritating the trigeminal nerve. The administration of local anesthetics given in the routine course of dental treatment can cause trigeminal nerve injury either by means of direct trauma from the needle contact or neurotoxicity from the local anesthetic. It may be prudent to avoid local anesthetics with higher neurotoxic and ischemic potential for block anesthesia such as 4% articaine 1:100,000 ratio epinephrine.[27] In addition, the clinician should administer a long-acting anesthetic at the end of the procedure to delay postoperative discomfort. When procedures are performed under general anesthesia, the addition of a local anesthetic will reduce peripheral and central sensitization.[26]

Anesthesia Considerations With Multiple Sclerosis

Management of anesthesia in patients with MS must consider the impact of surgical stress on the natural progression of the disease. There are four broad categories of anesthesia given to patients: general anesthesia, conscious sedation, regional anesthesia, and local anesthetics. Regardless of the anesthetic technique or drugs chosen, the manifestations of the disease can be exacerbated by conditions such as infection, inflammation, or fever.[28] The majority of office-based dental procedures are performed under local anesthesia with or without the addition of IV sedation or nitrous oxide.

Local Anesthesia

Historically, the use of peripheral blocks in patients with MS has been regarded as safe, as these blocks are delivered distantly from the main pathogenic demyelination and scarring process occurring with the central nervous system (CNS).[29] There is evidence of peripheral nervous system involvement in MS, whereby peripheral nerves may show evidence of demyelination.[30] The demyelination of peripheral nerves may make them more susceptible to nerve damage with local anesthesia toxicity. The evidence that a substantial share of patients with MS may suffer from subclinical peripheral neuropathy is inconsistent, and therefore, peripheral nerve blocks are probably safe in patients with MS.[29] If a peripheral nerve block is planned for an oral or dental procedure, some considerations should be made to limiting the potential morbidity associated with the procedure.

Clinical Considerations for Local Anesthesia and Peripheral Nerve Blocks

Preoperative assessment should always include gathering a complete history, as MS may predispose a patient to peripheral neuropathy or TN. Such neuropathy may increase vulnerability to local anesthetic toxicity or direct needle trauma during the injection. Careful documentation of existing neurologic dysfunction should be recorded by history and clinical examination. Risk benefit ratio should be weighed and consideration should be given to choosing local infiltrations over peripheral nerve blocks or using injection techniques to avoid direct nerve trauma whenever feasible before dental or oral surgery procedures. Concentrations of local anesthesia and the duration of exposure of the drug to the peripheral nerve correlate with histologic fiber damage.[31] It may be prudent to avoid local anesthetics with higher neurotoxic and ischemic potential for inferior alveolar and mental nerve block anesthesia such as 4% articaine 1:100,000 ratio epinephrine.[27] Epinephrine reduces the blood flow in the peripheral nerve.[32] This may be poorly tolerated in those who suffer from peripheral neuropathy. Epinephrine decreases the migration of the local anesthetic, which prolongs the duration of local anesthetic exposure and may potentiate toxicity to the compromised peripheral nerve. However, if the duration of action of the nerve blockade is inadequate, the provider may feel the need to give an additional nerve blockade. The planned duration of the procedure and risk/benefit analysis of the potential adverse effects of epinephrine versus the possibility for need in a second nerve blockage must be weighed.

Immunosuppressive Treatment in Multiple Sclerosis

Treatment and management of MS is targeted at relieving the symptoms, treating acute exacerbations, and preventing disease progression. Immunomodulation therapy, immunosuppressive therapy, and corticosteroids are widely used to treat MS because MS is thought to be a T-cell–mediated autoimmune disease. There are many perioperative oral surgical considerations, which must be addressed when treating patients who are taking immunosuppressants or chronic exogenous glucocorticoids. Patients with compromised immunity due to chronic steroid use or immunosuppressive drug therapy may be predisposed to surgical site infections following invasive oral surgical procedures or complications from bacteremia such as infective endocarditis. Additionally, patients with a history of chronic glucocorticoid therapy have a high risk of developing adrenal insufficiency during stressful surgical procedures. This section will review common guidelines for treating MS patients who may be taking immunomodulation therapy, immunosuppressive therapy, or corticosteroids.

Preoperative Assessment

A review of recent lab work may be warranted prior to invasive oral surgical procedures. Immunosuppressants can suppress the leukocyte count, which will predispose a patient to develop an infection whether it be local (surgical site infection) or distant (infective endocarditis). Absolute neutrophil count (ANC) which is part of the complete blood count with differential

(CBC with diff) will give a general indication of how well the immune system is functioning. An ANC of less than 1000/μL suggests that the immune system is compromised. As neutrophils make up the majority of the white blood cell (WBC) count, the WBC count is usually low when the neutrophil count is low.

Guidelines on Antibiotic Prophylaxis Before Dental or Oral Surgical Procedures in the Setting of Immunosuppression

Antibiotic prophylaxis refers to the administration of antimicrobials in situations where the risk of infection is substantial. Oral procedures such as dental extractions, root canal treatment, and oral prophylaxis which involve manipulation of the oral tissues in a contaminated site are known to cause bacteremia. A compromised immune system can predispose the patient to systemic odontogenic infection complications. Mortality in the perioperative setting is highest in these groups. Patients with MS who are immunosuppressed may benefit from antibiotic prophylaxis.

The Canadian Dental Association Position Paper on Antibiotic Prophylaxis for Dental Patients at risk recommends patients with a variety of immunocompromising conditions to receive antibiotic prophylaxis. It is recommended for those with a suppressed leukocyte count where the WBC count is less than 3500 cells/mm^3 (3.5 K/mm^3) or the ANC is less than 500 cells/mm^3 (0.5 K/mm^3) to receive antibiotic prophylaxis according to the guidelines of the American Heart Association (see Box 21.1). Consideration for antibiotic prophylaxis should be given for other patients with an impaired immune systems or those with delayed healing, such as those with ANC less than 1000 cells/mm^3 (1.0 K/mm^3). Consideration should be given for longer antibiotic prophylaxis schedules (7-10 d or longer) for those patients who may experience delayed healing following invasive procedures. This delayed healing would further expose them to ongoing surgical site infections or bacteremia.[33]

Glucocorticoid Therapy and Adrenal Sufficiency

Exogenous glucocorticoid therapy is often used for mild to moderate exacerbations of MS. Patients currently receiving steroid therapy have a high risk of developing adrenal insufficiency when placed in a stressful situation such as surgery or invasive dental procedures. Steroid usage for MS patients is generally for patients experiencing significant relapse symptoms, which vary from patient to patient. Most physicians will not prescribe the high-dose steroids for an acute episode more than three times a year. Typically a short course of prednisone (1250 mg dose) is used

Box 21.1 2007 AHA Guidelines for Infective Endocarditis Prevention

Patient Type	Drug[a]	Regimen: Single Dose 30-60 min Before Procedure	
		Adults	**Children**
Not allergic to penicillin	Amoxicillin	2 g	50 mg/kg
Not allergic to penicillin and unable to take oral meds	Ampicillin or	2 g IM or IV	50 mg/kg IM or IV
	cefazolin or ceftriaxone	1 g IM or IV	50 mg/kg IM or IV
Allergic to penicillins or ampicillin	Cephalexin[b]	2 g	50 mg/kg
	or clindamycin	600 mg	20 mg/kg
	or azithromycin or clarithromycin	500 mg	15 mg/kg
Allergic to penicillins or ampicillin and unable to take oral meds	cefazolin or ceftriaxone	1 g IM or IV	50 mg/kg IM or IV
	or clindamycin	600 mg IM or IV	20 mg/kg IM or IV

[a]Cephalosporins should not be used in an individual with a history of anaphylaxis, angioedema, or urticaria with penicillins or ampicillin.

[b]Or other first- or second-generation oral cephalosporins in equivalent adult or pediatric dosage.

orally for 3 to 5 days, or for more severe symptoms, IV methylprednisolone of 1 g/d for 3 to 5 days is given; this IV dosage has been used in acute optic neuritis, which has set a foundation for the treatment of MS exacerbations.[34] This can also be followed by an oral prednisone taper. Other options are 5 days of IV solumedrol for acute relapse or high-dose oral prednisone for 2 weeks with a tapering dose.[35,36]

Before initiating steroid therapy, infections need to be ruled out. Elective dental or oral surgical procedures theoretically could be done during short-term high-dose steroid treatment, but one recommendation would be to delay dental treatment for as many days as the treatment was given. However, if someone needs emergency dental care due to infection, pain or trauma, the short-term high-dose steroid therapy must continue so as not to exacerbate the underlying disease state and treatment of the emergency must occur along with appropriate antibiotics if indicated and pain management.

Chronic long-term steroid therapy is not commonly used in MS patients. However, if a patient has been on corticosteroids and that is equal to 5 mg of prednisone or 20 mg hydrocortisone per day or higher, for over 3 weeks, they should be considered at risk of hypothalamic-pituitary-adrenal (HPA) axis suppression.[37] If they require dental treatment, coordination with the patient's physician must ensue. Routine dental procedures with or without local anesthesia do not require additional steroid top off doses with gluco-corticoids. With complex invasive treatment or if a patient is anxious and emotionally stressed about the upcoming treatment, supplementation with additional morning dosing might be recommended. There is no standard mechanism for steroid modification, as this depends on the underlying disease that is being treated. Patients respond differently owing to their general health status and comorbidities, but collaboration with the patients care team is vital.

When treating patients with a history of glucocorticoid therapy, one must obtain a history of the duration and dosage of glucocorticoids therapy. The degree of adrenal suppression depends on the dose and duration of steroid treatment. The normal rise in plasma adrenocorticotrophic hormone (ACTH) and hence cortisol is in response to stress and severity of surgery. Intake of exogenous glucocorticoid by a patient can cause adrenal gland suppression, which causes a decrease glucocorticoid response to stress and may precipitate an adrenal crisis. The body releases about 30 mg of cortisol a day (equivalent to 7.5 mg prednisolone). Under stress, this may increase to 300 mg (60 mg prednisolone equivalent). Long-term steroid treatment of doses equivalent to 10 mg prednisolone or greater is most likely to cause HPA suppression. Additionally, patients taking doses above 50 mg prednisolone are close to the maximum cortisol level seen in patients during times of stress, therefore maintenance of current doses rather than supplementary doses are needed.[38]

The level of invasiveness of the procedure should be taken into consideration when considering glucocorticoid supplementation or "steroid cover." Patients undergoing minor surgical procedure under local anesthesia are very low risk for developing adrenal crisis. Supplementation is unnecessary for local anesthesia procedures. No cases of adrenal insufficiency have been reported in patients undergoing procedures under local anesthesia. In a study by Bunch et al, patients having third molar extractions under local anesthesia did not show significant increases of cortisol levels.[39]

For surgical procedures under general anesthesia, the need for perioperative glucocorticoid supplementation for patients on exogenous steroid should be determined by the severity of the surgery and the pre-existing glucocorticoid dose. There is no evidence to support glucocorticoid supplementation exceeding physiologic level of cortisol induced by stress. For patients undergoing general anesthesia for minor oral surgery, 100 mg hydrocortisone intramuscularly should be considered and the usual dose of glucocorticoid medications maintained.[40]

Clinical Considerations to Bisphosphonate Therapy and Oral Health

Patients that have been diagnosed with MS have decreased motility due to muscle weakness, loss of balance, and difficulty in coordination of bodily movements. Because of the progressive inactivity, they are more susceptible to osteoporosis. In addition, many patients with MS have taken corticosteroids multiple times throughout their disease state to treat relapses. This too can lead to decreased bone density and osteoporosis. Some patients in the later stages of MS are prescribed antiresorptive medications with bisphosphonates to treat and prevent osteoporosis, most commonly: alendronate (Fosamax®), risedronate (Actonel®), and ibandronate (Boniva®). As with all of the bisphosphonate medications as well as the RANK ligand inhibitor and antiangiogenic medications, there are potential risks for developing medication-related osteonecrosis of the jaw (MRONJ). While the risk is extremely low with the oral and IV medication in the treatment of osteoporosis, the true incidence of MRONJ is unknown and the pathophysiology is undefined. Therefore, it is still a risk and patients must be educated and informed. It is believed that the risk of MRONJ development increases with increasing doses and with exposure to more than one ONJ-related medication. Bisphosphonates have a long half-life; therefore, the risk of MRONJ is likely to remain even after therapy is discontinued. There is no known and established treatment for MRONJ, and management is focused on symptom palliation and prevention of superinfection.[41]

In general, before initiation of any antiresorptive therapy, dental health should be optimized. Any teeth with questionable prognosis should be extracted, and all necessary dental treatment should be done before initiation of the medication. Maintaining a healthy dentition and practicing excellent oral hygiene including the use of fluoride dentifrice and electric toothbrush is crucial. Patients along with their families should discuss with the dentist ways to minimize the risk of needing invasive procedures during drug therapy such as extractions, bone grafting, or any type of oral surgical intervention. Professional cleanings at least 2x/y, excellent home care with assistance, and attentive monitoring of any changes in the patient's mouth are extremely important. Preservation of teeth through restorations and endodontic therapy rather than extractions is ideal. Preventive treatment where dental work is planned and executed before therapy with bisphosphonates is key.

Treatment Recommendations for the Advanced MS Patient

As dentists, treating any patient with debilitating degenerative diseases of the CNS are a challenge especially when the disease has progressed. The majority of MS patients seen in dental practices are stable enough for treatment. Many individuals are taking newer disease-modifying therapies, which are mainly immunosuppressants, such as IV treatment with Tysabri®, Ocrevus®, Lemtrada®, and oral agents, such as Gilenya® and Tecfidera®. Lymphopenia is one of the side effects of these medications which can increase the patient's risk of infection so careful review of the patients blood cell count is often necessary before treatment. Patients may also be taking muscle relaxants to combat muscle spasticity and corticosteroids during relapse periods (see Table 21.3). Most MS patients can be treated routinely in a normal dental setting, but an understanding of their symptoms as well as their medication effects is important.

Shorter dental appointments, preferably in the mornings are best since fatigue tends to get worse in the later part of the day, but if longer appointments are needed, frequent breaks should be incorporated into the appointment. MS patients should not be fully reclined but semireclined to avoid airway compromise due to potential respiratory and swallowing difficulties. In the later stages of the disease, patients develop dysphagia and utilizing a rubber dam for some procedures might be indicated to prevent respiratory concerns. Mouth props may also be useful as it is difficult for many patients to keep their mouths open for extended periods of time (see Table 21.2).

More progressive dental disease with severe caries, gingival and periodontal inflammation, pulpal disease, and infection are more often seen at the advanced stages of MS where patients are wheelchair bound. Treatment for these patients is difficult in a regular dental office setting due to compromises with the patients' swallowing and breathing. These patients then require treatment in a hospital setting in an operating room under general anesthesia via nasotracheal intubation where the airway is secure. Often times, these patients are older with other comorbidities; risks and benefits need to be discussed with the family and medical team in deciding appropriate care of the patient.

If the patient is cared for in the operating room setting, a full set of X-rays are taken, and a comprehensive clinical evaluation is done after induction. The procedures that are done in this type of setting are meant to stabilize the patient's oral health. Generally complex multistep treatments such as root canals, crowns, and implants are not options, as these typically require consecutive appointments, which are not feasible for patients with advanced MS. The goal of treatment is to remove infection and active dental disease and restore comfort and function in these patients.

The Association of State and Territorial Dental Directors comprises a list of dental departments and contact information in each state if help referring patients to the appropriate center for care is needed (www. astdd.org). The National Foundation of Dentistry for the Handicapped is an option for care as this organization provides free comprehensive dental treatment in each state (http://dentallifeline.org). There are a number of dental residency programs and dental schools in each state that are more often equipped for treatment of patients with special needs (www.ada.org/ed/coda/find-a-program). Additionally, these programs provide excellent comprehensive care and often have more affordable treatment options for individuals that may have limited or no insurance coverage.

Conclusion

The progression of MS can pose significant challenges that affect the oral health of these individuals. With proper understanding and early management, the dental clinician will positively impact the patient's dental health and overall health. Although the goal of this section is to create a foundation for an approach to treatment, care for any patient with or without a chronic illness needs to be individualized and bidirectional.

References

1. Danesh-Sani RA, Soltani M, Rahimdoost A, et al. Clinical assessment of orofacial manifestations in 500 patients with multiple sclerosis. *J Oral Maxillofac Surg.* 2013;71(2):290-294.
2. Kovac Z, Uhac I, Buković D, et al. Oral health status and temporomandibular disorders in multiple sclerosis patients. *Coll Antropol.* 2005;29(2):441-444.
3. Fischer D, Epstein J, Klasser G. Multiple Sclerosis: an update for oral health care providers. *Oral Surg Oral Med Oral Pathol Oral Radiol Endod.* 2009;108(3):318-327.
4. Fragoso Y, Carvalho Alves H, Carvalho Alves L. Dental Care in multiple sclerosis: an overlooked and under-assessed condition. *J Disabil Oral Health.* 2010;11(2) 53-56.
5. McGrother CW, Dugmore C, Phillips M. Multiple sclerosis, dental caries and fillings: a case-control study. *Br Dent J.* 1999;187(5):261-264.
6. Baird W, Mcgrother C, Abrams KR. Factors that influence the dental attendance pattern and maintenance of oral health for people with multiple sclerosis. *Br Dent J.* 2007;202(4):1-5.
7. De Mattos M, Pinelli L, Ribeiro R, et al. Fabrication of an acrylic resin device used to increase the size of toothbrush handles. *J Prosthet Dent.* 1998;79(3):361-362.
8. Dickinson C, Millwood J. Toothbrush handle adaptation using silicone impression putty. *Dent Update.* 1999;26:288-289.
9. Buljevac D, Flach H, Hop W, et al. Prospective study on the relationship between infections and multiple sclerosis exacerbations. *Brain.* 2002;125(5):952-960.
10. Edwards S, Zvartau M, Clarke H, et al. Clinical relapses and disease activity on magnetic resonance imaging associated with viral upper respiratory tract infections in multiple sclerosis. *J Neurol Neurosurg Psychiatry.* 1998;64:736-741.
11. Correale J, Farez M. Monocyte-derived dendritic cells in multiple sclerosis: the effect of bacterial infection. *J Neuroimmunol.* 2007;190(1–2):177-189.
12. Correale J, Fiol M, Gilmore W. The risk of relapses in multiple sclerosis during systemic infections. *Neurology.* 2006;67:653-659.

13. Mulvey MR, Doupe M, Prout M, et al. *Staphylococcus aureus* harbouring enterotoxin A as a possible risk factor for multiple sclerosis exacerbations. *Mult Scler.* 2011;17(4):397-403.

14. Kriesel JD, White A, Hayden FG, et al. Multiple sclerosis attacks are associated with picornavirus infections. *Mult Scler.* 2004;10(2):145-148.

15. National Multiple Sclerosis Society. Medications. National Multiple Sclerosis Society. Available at nationalmssociety.org/Treating-MS/Medications. Accessed May 31, 2018.

16. Drugs, Herbs, and Supplements. *MedlinePlus.* U.S. National Library of Medicine; May 21, 2018. Available at medlineplus.gov/druginformation.html. Accessed May 31, 2018.

17. Fox PC, Cummins MJ, Cummins JM. Use of orally administered anhydrous crystalline maltose for relief of dry mouth. *J Altern Complement Med.* 2001;7(1):33-43.

18. Pedersen AM, Bardow A, Jensen SB, Nauntofte B. Saliva and gastrointestinal functions of taste, mastication, swallowing and digestion. *Oral Dis.* 2002;8(3):117-129.

19. Villa A, Connell CL, Abati S. Diagnosis and management of xerostomia and hyposalivation. *Ther Clin Risk Manag.* 2015;11:45-51.

20. Headache Classification Committee of the International Headache Society. The international classification of headache disorders. *Cephalalgia.* 2013;38:629-808.

21. Hooge JP, Redekop WK. Trigeminal neuralgia in multiple sclerosis. *Neurology.* 1995;45(7):1294-1996.

22. Fallata A, Salter AM, Cutter GR, Marie RA. Trigeminal neuralgia commonly precedes the diagnosis of multiple sclerosis. *Int J MS Care.* 2017;19(5):240-246.

23. Nurmikko TJ, Elrdige PR. Trigmeninal neuralgia-pathophysiology, diagnosis and current treatment. *Br J Anaesth.* 2001;87:117-132.

24. Scrivani S. *Trigeminal neuralgia.* In: *Oral Surgery, Oral Medicine, Oral Pathology, Oral Radiology and Endodontics*; 2005:527-538.

25. Klasser G, Gremillion HA. Dental treatment for patients with neuropathic orofacial pain. *J Am Dent Assoc.* 2013;144(9):1006-1008.

26. Foreman PA. Preemptive analgesia: the prevention of neurogenous orofacial pain. *Anesth Prog.* 1995;42(2):36-40.

27. Hillerup S, Jensen RH, Ersbøll BK. Trigeminal nerve injury associated with injection of local anesthetics. *J Am Dent Assoc.* 2011;142(5):532-539.

28. Markis A. Multiple sclerosis: basic knowledge and new insights in perioperative management. *J Anesth.* 2014;28(2):267-278.

29. Lirk P. Regional anesthesia in patients with pre-existing neuropathy. *Int Anesthesiol Clin.* 2011;49(4):144-145.

30. Pollack M, Calder C, Allpress S. Peripheral nerve abnormality in multiple sclerosis. *Ann Neurol.* 1997;2(1):41-48.

31. Kroin JS, Buvanendran A, Williams DK, et al. Local anesthesitic sciatic nerve block and nerve fiber damage in diabetic rats. *Reg Anesth Pain Med.* 2010;35(4):343-350.

32. Neal JM. Effects of epinephrine in local anesthetics on the central and peropheral nervous systems: neurotoxicty and neural blood flow. *Reg Anesth Pain Med.* 2003;28(2):124-134.

33. Directors, CDA Board of. CLL Canada Dental Antibiotic. CLL Canada; 2010. Retrieved from http://cllcanada.ca/2010/pages/dental_antibiotic.pdf.

34. Beck RW, Cleary PA, Anderson MM Jr, et al. A randomized, controlled trial of corticosteroids in the treatment of acute optic neuritis. The Optic Neuritis Study Group. *N Engl J Med.* 1992;326(9):581-588.

35. Morrow SA, Stoian CA, Dmitrovic J, Chan SC, Metz LM. The bioavailability of IV methylprednisolone and oral prednisone in multiple sclerosis. *Neurology.* 2004;63(6):1079-1080.

36. Thrower BW. Relapse management in multiple sclerosis. *Neurologist.* 2009;15(1):1-5.

37. Furst DE, Saag KG. *Glucocorticoid Withdrawal.* Uptodate; 2016.

38. Salem M, Tainsh RE Jr, Bromberg J, Loriaux DL, Chewnow B. Perioperative glucocorticoid coverage. A reassessment 42 years after emergence of a problem. *Ann Surg.* 1994;19(4):416-425.

39. Bunch FL, Allen GD, Jorgensen NB. Analysis of blood cortisol levels in oral surgery patients given various levels of intravenous medications. *J Dent Res.* 1975;53(6):965-967.

40. Gibson N, Ferguson JW. Steroid cover for dental patients on long-term steroid medication: proposed clinical guidelines based upon a critical review of the literature. *Br Dent J.* 2004;97(11):681-685.

41. Ruggiero SL, Dodson TB, Fantasia J, et al. American Association of Oral and Maxillofacial Surgeons position paper on medication-related osteonecrosis of the jaw – 2014 update. *J Oral Maxillofac Surg.* 2014;72:1938-1956.

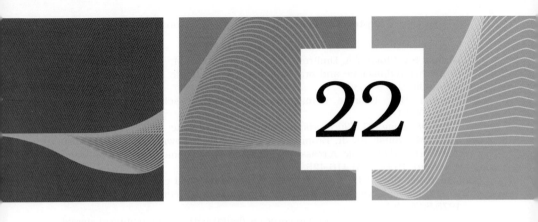

Otolaryngologic Manifestations of Multiple Sclerosis

■ ▨ ▨ Alisha N. Dua, Tiffany Peng, George Alexiades

Introduction

In the historical study of multiple sclerosis (MS), dysarthria takes on a prominent role as one of the three characterizing symptoms of MS described in Charcot triad from 1877. Although no longer considered pathognomonic for MS, dysarthria and other otolaryngologic manifestations are frequent components of the MS disease course. Up to 5% of patients with MS report a ear, nose, and throat (ENT) symptoms as the initial presenting symptom of their disease, whereas anywhere from 6% to 63% report experiencing an otolaryngologic symptom once diagnosed.[1,2] Thus, it is important for the otolaryngologist and other nonneurologists to be able to recognize and decipher the otolaryngologic presentations that warrant consideration of MS in the differential diagnosis. This chapter provides an overview of the clinical presentation, pathophysiology, and management options for each of the most common ENT symptoms observed in MS.

Hearing Loss

Clinical Presentation

Although hearing loss is considered a rare manifestation of MS, it is reported to occur at least once during the course of disease in 3.5% to 17% of patients with MS.[1-4] Rare reports of hearing loss as the initial symptom are also present in the literature.[1,5-7] A review of the case literature indicates a significant heterogeneity in the presentation of auditory abnormalities in MS, with cases describing patients presenting with different degrees of hearing loss, both unilateral and bilateral deficits, and temporal variation from sudden onset to progressive loss. Thus, no characteristic pattern of auditory abnormalities has been defined for MS. Still, certain more common features of MS-associated hearing loss can be extracted from the small cohort studies and cases in the literature.

Both vertigo and tinnitus are frequently associated with symptoms of hearing loss, although certain cases report hearing loss as a clinically isolated syndrome.[7-11] Presentations of progressive hearing loss in MS are likely a result of lesions in the auditory brainstem pathways, and symptoms are driven by the specific location of the patient's lesions. Notably, one study identified a greater than 4.5 times increased annual incidence of sudden sensorineural hearing loss (SSNHL) in people diagnosed with MS compared with the normal population.[5] Findings from other studies of SSNHL and acute deafness suggest that hearing loss associated with MS will have spontaneous recovery, often with no permanent audiological deficits.[3,7,8,12]

Diagnostic Evaluation

The workup and management of hearing loss in the setting of MS mirrors that of hearing loss in the typical patient without MS. These patients should undergo an otoscopic evaluation. If the hearing loss is persistent despite management of cerumen impaction, acute otitis media, tympanic membrane perforation, or other immediately apparent causes of hearing loss, the patient should be referred for complete audiometric evaluation. Brainstem auditory evoked responses are not routinely assessed but have been reported as frequently abnormal in patients with MS, even when hearing loss is not a reported symptom.[10,13,14] If hearing loss has been established with audiometric evaluation, magnetic resonance imaging (MRI) is the imaging modality of choice to identify lesions in the auditory brainstem[7,9] and should be performed whether the hearing loss recovers or not.

When a patient presents with acute, unilateral sensorineural hearing loss associated with tinnitus and/or vertigo, and no prior history of audiological symptoms, as with all cases of sudden sensorineural hearing loss, this constellation of symptoms is considered an otologic urgency and should be evaluated and treated. However, the differential for this constellation of symptoms remains broad, including diabetes mellitus, medication ototoxicity, Meniere disease, Susac syndrome, Wolfram syndrome, and autoimmune disease of the ear, among others.[15]

In the presence of concurrent facial nerve and vestibular deficits with audiogram-proven sensorineural hearing loss, MRI of the brain and internal auditory canals with gadolinium contrast should be pursued to rule out mass lesion. Although it requires a high index of suspicion, MS remains a consideration in the presence of multiple acute cranial neuropathies, and brainstem involvement has previously been reported as the presenting feature of MS in up to 15% of cases.[8,16]

Management in Patients With Known Multiple Sclerosis

The management of hearing loss in patients with known MS mirrors that of patients without MS. A complete audiometric evaluation will determine the patient's candidacy and likelihood of benefitting from amplification with a hearing aide. Deafness is an uncommon symptom in MS, reported to be less than 3% in large series of this patient population.[13] However, if profound sensorineural hearing loss is present, the patient may require cochlear implantation.

As previously mentioned, it is important to note that sudden sensorineural hearing loss is an otologic urgency. As such, a patient who has sudden-onset unilateral hearing loss with or without concurrent vertigo or tinnitus requires urgent evaluation with audiogram and treatment as warranted based on those results. For patients with known MS and a new-onset sudden unilateral sensorineural hearing loss, the limited data available on sudden sensorineural hearing loss in MS portend a relatively good prognosis. In one series of 11 patients with sudden sensorineural hearing loss, 5 of the subjects had spontaneous recovery before complete audiometric evaluation.[5] Thus, any patient with sudden unilateral hearing loss should undergo an urgent complete audiometric evaluation, and if medically able, consideration should be given to treatment with 1 week of high-dose oral steroids followed by a steroid taper.[17] If the patient cannot receive oral steroids, intratympanic steroid injection by an otolaryngologist should be considered.

Tinnitus

Clinical Presentation

Tinnitus has not been evaluated in large-scale series in the population with MS but has nonetheless been reported in the literature as a component of MS.

In light of the prevalence of hearing loss as a symptom of MS and the close clinical association between tinnitus and all causes of hearing loss, this does not come as a surprise. In a report of 12 patients with unilateral hearing loss and MS, 9 had tinnitus.[13] However, it is notable that there have been isolated case reports in which tinnitus was a primary symptom at the time of initial presentation. One such case was in an 11-year-old who was found to have persistent unilateral nonpulsatile tinnitus and remitting hearing loss.[18] Thus, a high index of suspicion should be maintained for any patient with persistent unilateral otologic symptoms.

Diagnostic Evaluation

The initial workup of both persistent bilateral and unilateral tinnitus in any patient should include complete audiometric evaluation. For persistent unilateral tinnitus, as in the case of any unilateral or elusive audiovestibular disorder, we further advocate for workup with an MRI of the internal auditory canals to rule out mass lesions or alternate diagnoses, even in the presence of a normal audiogram.[19] In the case report referenced previously in this section, a complete audiometric evaluation demonstrated unilateral high-frequency sensorineural hearing loss and subsequent MRI was initially unremarkable owing to artifact from concurrent dental hardware. However, repeat imaging following removal of the hardware demonstrated multiple demyelinating lesions consistent with a diagnosis of MS.[18]

Of note, tinnitus is also a reported side effect of interferon-beta, which may be used in the treatment of MS. It has been reported in isolation or in conjunction with sensorineural hearing loss at cumulative doses greater than 100 MIU of interferon-beta.[20]

Management in Patients With Known Multiple Sclerosis

In patients with known MS, new-onset tinnitus should prompt a complete audiometric evaluation to assess whether the tinnitus is occurring in isolation or in conjunction with hearing loss. If the patient is taking any ototoxic medications, consideration should be given to cessation of this medication if clinically able, particularly if the tinnitus is accompanied by true hearing loss, as this may be progressive and lead to permanent damage of the outer hair cells of the cochlea.

There is otherwise no special consideration in the management of tinnitus for the patient with MS. Management options parallel those that are available to patients without MS. When hearing loss is present, amplification with hearing aids may be beneficial in reducing the patient symptoms. Additionally, lifestyle and behavioral changes are helpful in the management of tinnitus, including optimization of sleep hygiene, limitation of caffeine intake, and white noise. However, it is important for any clinician to note that tinnitus can be extremely disturbing for patients and has previously been associated with both depression and suicidality.[21] For patients with severe, debilitating tinnitus, cognitive behavioral therapy has been shown to be efficacious in a systematic review of over 1000 patients.[22]

Vertigo and Dysequilibrium

Clinical Presentation

Imbalance is a common presentation in MS that can result from either central or peripheral causes: affecting proprioceptive, visual, and/or vestibular pathways. The differential for vertigo is broad and includes benign paroxysmal positional vertigo (BPPV), vestibular migraine, labyrinthitis, or vestibular neuronitis. A thorough history regarding the frequency and duration of symptoms is critical, as well as the quality of symptoms themselves, to differentiate between symptoms that may be characterized as "dizziness" by a given patient. Frank vertigo (self or room spinning sensation) and disequilibrium may result from central lesions such as those seen in MS, masses of the internal auditory canal, or a vascular event of the posterior cerebral circulation, as well as peripheral vestibular issues such as vestibular neuronitis, labyrinthitis, Meniere disease, or BPPV. Syncope, or presyncopal symptoms, are more suggestive of neurocardiac etiologies, as a peripheral vestibular issue never causes these symptoms. Concurrent auditory symptoms, facial nerve symptoms, or other cranial neuropathies may be helpful in localizing symptoms and identifying the underlying etiology.[23]

Vertigo is one of the more common otolaryngologic symptoms in MS with anywhere from 4% to 15% and 33% to 50% of patients experiencing vertigo at onset or after diagnosis, respectively.[1,15,24] However, a study by Pula et al of a cohort of patients presenting with acute vestibular syndrome (AVS) found that only 4% of the subjects studied had AVS resulting from demyelinating disease.[25] Furthermore, multiple studies have suggested that vertiginous episodes in patients diagnosed with MS can often be attributed to peripheral causes of imbalance, such as BPPV.[26] If the vertiginous episode is provoked by head movement and is short in duration lasting seconds to minutes, it is likely to be of BPPV etiology. However, a more chronic presentation of vertigo lasting at least 24 hours that is associated with other brainstem findings is more suggestive of a brainstem lesion resulting from MS.[27,28]

Diagnostic Evaluation

Patients reporting vertigo should undergo a thorough clinical examination, including assessment of the extraocular movements for nystagmus, a full cranial nerve examination to screen for concurrent cranial neuropathies, gait assessment, and Dix-Hallpike testing. The head thrust test is an additional bedside maneuver useful in assessing the vestibulo-ocular reflex. If the history of vertigo is unclear, consideration should be given to orthostatic blood pressure measurement.

For patients with vertigo, a complete audiometric evaluation is useful in the evaluation of subtle hearing deficits. There are a variety of options for thorough vestibular testing, including electronystagmography, vestibular evoked myogenic potential, and posturography, among others. Electronystagmography tests can be useful in differentiating and characterizing peripheral and central vestibular abnormalities and are thus potentially useful tests for guiding the diagnosis of patients presenting with vertigo.[29] Abnormal posturography scores have been identified in patients with MS with both high and low functional status.[30]

The imaging modality of choice for the evaluation of vertigo and for the diagnosis of MS in this setting is MRI. Special attention to the internal auditory canal (IAC) is warranted to rule out a mass lesion of the IAC as causative of the patient's symptoms. Vertigo in the patient with MS likely results from demyelinating lesions affecting the central vestibular pathways or associated fiber tracts in the lower pons and upper medulla.[24] In the study by Pula et al, of those patients whose AVS was determined to be caused by demyelinating disease, all but one patient was found to have at least one potentially causative posterior fossa lesion on MRI.[25]

Management in the Patient With Known Multiple Sclerosis

MS-associated vertigo often resolves spontaneously or responds to treatment with corticosteroids.[1] For patients with persistent vertigo or disequilibrium of all causes, vestibular therapy or vestibular rehabilitation is the standard of care for improving functional status and symptom management. In patients specifically with MS, vestibular rehabilitation has been demonstrated to improve symptoms of fatigue, balance, and disability[31] and to decrease fall rate.[32]

Sinusitis

Multiple Sclerosis and Sinusitis

Prior studies have reported on the increased incidence of sinus disease among patients with MS,[33] and this has been corroborated on objective review of MRI scans of patients with MS.[34] Patients with MS had a higher recorded rate of chronic and relapsing sinusitis, and MS attacks were more frequent during bouts of sinusitis, with similar results identified across 10 different clinical sites of evaluation.[33]

The exact reason for this association has yet to be clearly demonstrated, but authors postulate that chronic sinusitis in this population may be linked to a common environmental factor underlying both entities. Sibley et al postulated that respiratory infections may be triggers to MS exacerbations, but Gay et al argue that these entities share a causal link, citing their similarities in age-specific attack curves occurring at a mean close to 30 years of age and worldwide geographic distribution including rare incidence in tropical countries.[33,35] Thus, unlike the other entities described in this chapter, sinusitis is postulated to have a linked underlying cause, possibly immunologic, rather than a causative relationship with MS secondary to demyelinating lesions.

Clinical Presentation and Diagnostic Evaluation

Patients with chronic sinusitis should undergo a thorough clinical examination, including history. The diagnosis of chronic sinusitis requires two of the four primary symptoms (nasal discharge/postnasal drip, nasal obstruction, facial pain or headache, and hyposmia) for at least 12 weeks. Symptoms may be unilateral or bilateral. The differential for unilateral nasal congestion also includes neoplasm, septal deviation, allergy, or immunologic disorders, and physicians require a high index of suspicion for mass lesion in the presence of facial swelling, orbital symptoms, anosmia, or epistaxis. Imaging may be warranted with a noncontrast computed tomography scan of the sinuses to further evaluate disease extent and obtain objective confirmation.

Management in the Patient With Known Multiple Sclerosis

Patients with MS typically have chronic rhinosinusitis without nasal polyposis, for which the first-line management is medical. Initial treatment of this entity involves nasal irrigations, nasal steroids, and a sustained course of antibiotics lasting 3 weeks with an accompanied oral steroid taper. For patients who fail medical management, endoscopic sinus surgery by an otolaryngologist may be warranted.

Voice: Dysarthria and Dysphonia

Clinical Presentation

Dysarthria is defined as problems in the articulation, speed, intelligibility, and cadence of speech and results from alteration in the motor control of the muscles in the oral cavity, larynx, and diaphragm that contribute to speech production.[36] In MS, dysarthria is frequently accompanied by dysphonia—disordered sound production—that can result in changes in the pitch, loudness, voice quality, nasality, and emphasis of speech.[36] Historically, dysarthria and more specifically the presentation of "scanning speech" patterns were considered highly characteristic of MS. Earlier diagnosis and a deeper knowledge of the disease has now made it evident that speech and vocal deficits in MS are relatively infrequent in its early course. Studies suggest that the prevalence of dysarthria varies between 37% and 51% in patients with MS, with the wide range likely attributable to variability in disease severity of the cohorts studied and whether episodic and/or permanent vocal impairment was included.[1,37,38] In one text, the presence of dysarthria as a symptom at onset was found to have an incidence of just 0.6%.[1] Dysarthric speech is more frequent in patients with higher disability scores and in patients with more progressive forms of MS, supporting a classification of dysarthria as a late symptom of MS.[37]

MS-associated dysarthria most commonly presents as a mixed ataxic-spastic dysarthria, characterized by a combination of spastic-type presentations, such as decreased loudness, hypernasality, imprecise articulation, pitch breaks, reduced breath support/control, reduced stress, or slowed rate, and ataxic-type presentations, such as ataxic movement of the mouth, increased and varying loudness, irregular articulation, prolonged intervals, prolonged phonemes, scanning speech, or vocal tremor.[36] The most prominent deficits identified in a selection of studies included harsh quality, defective articulation, impaired loudness control, delayed onset, and prosodic difficulties such as elongated intervals.[37,38] Episodic presentations of dysarthria in the form of paroxysmal dysarthria-ataxia syndrome (PDA) are frequently reported in the MS literature. Such cases of paroxysmal dysarthria in the literature describe a characteristic presentation of rapid-onset vocal/speech impairment of short duration with subsequent full recovery. Episodes are accompanied by paroxysmal ataxia and are often repetitive in nature.[39-42] As PDA is also associated with stroke, Behçet disease, and inherited episodic ataxia, other characteristic findings of MS are necessary for diagnostic certainty.[39,42,43]

Dysphonia, characterized by disordered sound production, in MS has also been observed, occurring in one study among 70% of patients with MS compared with 33% of controls on objective acoustic voice analysis.[44] Dogan et al demonstrated on evaluation with videostrobolaryngoscopy, acoustic analysis, and subjective questionnaire that patients with MS have weakness of voice, with worsening acoustic parameters, including fundamental frequency, soft phonation index, and "jitter values," a measurement of vocal stability.[45]

Diagnostic Evaluation

As previously discussed, dysarthria in MS may be a paroxysmal symptom or a late symptom, and diagnosis is made based on a combination of clinical assessment at the time of symptomatology and patient report. Examination should include speech assessment, as well as a complete cranial nerve examination, including assessment of tongue deviation and fasciculations. Identification of this symptom with or without concurrent cranial neuropathies should prompt a thorough workup, including imaging, for MS. However, there is no current mechanism by which to objectively quantify dysarthria in this patient population. Patients with sustained dysphonia or frank hoarseness should be evaluated by an otolaryngologist with flexible laryngoscopy to rule out mass lesion or alternate voice disorder.

Management in Patients With Known Multiple Sclerosis

The management of dysarthria and dysphonia in MS is linked closely to the treatment of the underlying illness. However, referral to speech and language pathology is appropriate, as the patient may benefit from formal analysis and initiation of voice therapy or speech therapy as warranted. Intensive phonatory-respiratory treatment has been demonstrated to improve speech tasks, sustained vowel phonation, and voice loudness.[46] Although these therapies have no impact on disease progression, symptom-directed treatment improves quality of life among patients with MS by decreasing disability and handicap.[47]

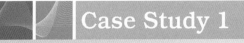

Case Study 1

Acute Vertigo and New-onset Dysarthria With No Prior Established MS Diagnosis

The patient is a 56-year-old woman with a history of positional vertigo 10 years ago, which resolved spontaneously and now returned with recurrent positional vertigo lasting a few seconds at a time. She was diagnosed with BPPV, and an Epley maneuver was performed in the office. There was no complaint of hearing loss or tinnitus. Two days after the office visit, the patient reported having difficulty with her handwriting and noted some difficulty initiating speech as well. An MRI of the internal auditory canals and brain with gadolinium contrast was ordered and revealed multiple T2-hyperintensities in the cerebellum, which were highly suspicious for a demyelinating disease (Figure 22.1).

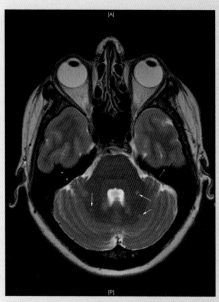

Figure 22.1. T2-weighted axial MRI image showing multiple hyperintensities consistent with demyelination (arrows).

A diagnosis of MS was made and intravenous corticosteroids were initiated, and her symptoms resolved. She was switched to Tysabri with no recurrence of her vertigo, dysarthria, or hand motor issues.

Commentary: Our patient initially fit the classic presentation for BPPV. With balance disorders there can often be neurocognitive issues such as tiredness, mental fog, memory issues, and difficulty concentrating. All these resolve as the balance issues resolve. This patient reported having difficulty with her speech and signing her name, which are not neurocognitive issues associated with dizziness and triggered the imaging study. In addition, this patient was older than the typical patient for newly diagnosed MS.

had a history of transient dysphagic symptoms. The incidence of permanent dysphagia was correlated with disease severity, as 65% of patients with severe disability presented with permanent dysphagia compared with 15.5% of mildly impaired patients.[48] As such, it is unlikely that symptoms of dysphagia due to MS will present in a previously undiagnosed patient.

Early stages of dysphagia in MS are associated with difficulty swallowing fluids. Difficulty with thin liquids is especially common in MS because of delays in initiating the pharyngeal phase of swallowing. Dysphagia in MS often progresses to include difficulty with solids in more disabled patients.[1,36,48] In a survey of patients with MS, a history of coughing or choking during meals and history of pneumonia were the most commonly reported signs indicative of impaired swallowing.[48] In comparison with other neurologic disorders, the dysphagia of MS is often episodic and follows the relapse-remitting course of the disease in earlier presentations.[36] Different texts suggest that MS-associated dysphagia is due to a variety of abnormalities in mostly the oral and pharyngeal phases of swallowing. More specifically, oral bolus formations, the previously mentioned delay in the swallowing reflex, and reduction in pharyngeal wall contraction are all common in MS.[36,48]

Diagnostic Evaluation

Patients with new-onset oropharyngeal dysphagia should be evaluated with a thorough history and physical examination. The differential is broad and includes oropharyngeal neoplasm, Zenker diverticulum, esophageal motility disorder, and neurologic disorder. Because oropharyngeal dysphagia may be caused by a mass lesion, referral to an otolaryngologist for flexible laryngoscopy should be considered in patients with concurrent symptoms of oropharyngeal or oral pain, voice changes such as hoarseness or muffled voice, or any symptoms of stridor or other changes to work of breathing. A modified barium swallow is indicated in patients with signs or symptoms of aspiration.

Management in Patients With Known Multiple Sclerosis

Patients with dysphagia in this population should be referred to speech and language pathology for formal swallow evaluation. This is recommended even in the absence of frank signs or symptoms of aspiration, as up to 40% of patients with MS have demonstrated silent aspiration.[50] Patients may require certain diet consistency restrictions to prevent aspiration pneumonia, and in severe cases in which swallow function is critically impaired, may require referral for an enteric feeding tube.

Special Senses: Gustatory and Olfactory Function

Clinical Presentation

Although gustatory and olfactory deficits are considered rare symptoms of MS, a review of the literature suggests that hypogeusia and hyposmia may be more common than expected. Reports of the incidence of hypogeusia and hyposmia in MS vary significantly, with studies reporting 5% to 32% and 11% to 44% of patients experiencing each symptom, respectively.[51-56]

In many cases, patients were aware of their olfactory deficits.[52,56] A study of 153 patients with MS found a correlation between later disease stages and the frequency of hyposmic symptoms, with 68.8% of patients with secondary progressive MS having significant deficits on a brief smell identification test (B-SIT). In the same study, only ~3% of patients with relapse remitting disease had deficits on the B-SIT, which was not significantly different from the results of the test for the healthy controls.[55] In a second study, patients with active disease, defined as a relapse in the last 12 months by Lutteroti et al, were interestingly found to have higher odor perception thresholds than those patients with MS with prolonged latent disease.[57] Together, these studies suggest that olfactory testing may be useful for discriminating the disease state and/or stage of a patient with MS. However, olfactory deficit is a hallmark presentation in other neurodegenerative disorders, such as Parkinson disease, and so it should be recognized that MS is an unlikely diagnosis if a patient is presenting with new-onset olfactory dysfunction.

As gustatory and olfactory sensation are closely tied functions, discriminating true taste dysfunction from taste dysfunction resulting from olfactory deficits can be difficult. Furthermore, the literature on taste deficits in MS is limited. Cases of dysgeusia as the presenting symptom of MS have been reported.[58-60] Hypoaguesia, when reported, is commonly tied to other trigeminal pathology.[1] The most comprehensive study to date on taste function in MS found that patients with MS had a significantly reduced ability to identify all four classic tastants—caffeine, citric acid, sucrose, and NaCl—compared with healthy controls. No difference in taste discrimination was found between the anterior (CN VII) and posterior (CN IX) regions of the tongue.[61]

Diagnostic Evaluation

Evaluation of gustatory and olfactory dysfunction may be challenging, as patients reporting these symptoms may not have an immediately apparent clinical correlate on examination. A high index of suspicion must be maintained to rule out a mass lesion affecting the cranial nerves. Those who have additional cranial neuropathies or specific examination findings may undergo further workup based on diagnostic suspicion.

Patients with olfactory dysfunction should undergo a thorough history, including risk factors of nasopharyngeal or sinonasal neoplasms such as smoking or exposure to Epstein Barr virus, epistaxis, unilateral nasal obstruction, chronicity of symptoms, and any associated orbital symptoms. Olfactory dysfunction may include decreased or absent olfaction (hyposmia, anosmia) or changes in perception to existing or nonexistent olfactory stimuli (parosmias or phantosmias). Examination should include a full cranial nerve examination and an anterior rhinoscopy. If cranial neuropathies or alarm symptoms are present, consideration should be given for a referral to otolaryngology for nasal endoscopy. Of note, objective evaluation of the olfactory sense may be performed with smell identification tests. One such test is the University of Pennsylvania Smell Identification Test (UPSIT), which can also screen for malingering. Importantly, hyposmia may be an early sign of Alzheimer disease by way of a neurologically mediated phenomenon.[62] Recent investigations further suggest a similar relationship with Parkinson dementia.[63,64] Thus, in patient populations at risk for dementia, consideration should be given for a mini-mental status examination, assessment of activities of daily living, and formal dementia screening.

Patients presenting with gustatory dysfunction (dysgeusia) should undergo a complete history with special consideration given to screening questions for dementia, history of cancer, and any medications, particularly chemotherapeutics. Gustatory dysfunction may include decreased taste sense (hypogeusia) or an altered perception of taste, usually noxious, without otherwise apparent stimulus or etiology (taste phantoms). Examination should include close attention to lesions of the tongue, the seventh and ninth cranial nerves including facial motor function and soft palate elevation, and an otoscopic examination. Chorda tympani provides taste sensation to the anterior two-thirds of the tongue, with a takeoff from cranial nerve VII arising in the middle ear. Importantly, patients with dysgeusia or hypogeusia may have difficulty describing their symptoms, and a close relationship exists between taste and olfaction. Thus, patients with dysgeusia should be screened for hyposmia or anosmia.

Olfactory and gustatory dysfunction is a symptom that can be quite distressing to the patient without an obvious clinical correlate for the clinician. The great American composer, George Gershwin, famously suffered from phantosmias manifesting as the smell of burnt rubber, before ultimately succumbing to an undiagnosed glioblastoma multiforme that had been causing olfactory seizures.[65] This symptom may be a sequela of MS, but a very high index of suspicion and thorough consideration should be maintained to rule out mass lesion or other organic neurologic disease.

Management in Patients With Known Multiple Sclerosis

In patients whose symptoms can be confidently attributed to MS, management of dysgeusia and dysosmia is limited to management of MS. In one large-scale study and literature review performed in the United Kingdom, diagnosis and management of olfactory disorders of all causes was focused on the underlying pathology, although corticosteroids are thought to be potentially helpful in improving the prognosis of new-onset hyposmia.[66] Damm et al reported in a 2014 *Laryngoscope* article that olfactory retraining with regular and timed exposure to specific scented oils led to improvement in olfactory function after postinfectious olfactory loss.[67] At this time, however, no studies have been performed on therapeutic interventions to improve alterations to taste or smell in MS, and the mechanisms leading to this association with MS are unclear.[68]

Conclusion

The hallmark demyelination and inflammation of the central nervous system (CNS) that characterizes MS is often indiscriminate in its localization in CNS tissues. As such, there is potential for lesion formation in brain regions associated with auditory, vestibular, sinonasal, and laryngeal function, as well as alteration to the special senses of taste and smell. Even though MS is not a common diagnosis in the ENT office, it is important for all clinicians to be able to recognize and decipher the ENT symptoms that warrant consideration of MS in the differential diagnosis.

References

1. Compston A, McDonald I, Noseworthy J, et al. *McAlpine's Multiple Sclerosis.* 4th ed. Edinburgh: Churchill Livingstone Elsevier; 2006.
2. Peyvandi A, Naghibzadeh B, Roozbahany NA. Neuro-otologic manifestations of multiple sclerosis. *Arch Iran Med.* 2010;13(3):188-192.
3. de Seze J, Assouad R, Stojkovic T, Desaulty A, Dubus B, Vermersch P. Hearing loss in multiple sclerosis: clinical, electrophysiologic and radiological study. *Rev Neurol (Paris).* 2001;157(11):1403-1409.
4. Oh YM, Oh DH, Jeong SH, Koo JW, Kim JS. Sequential bilateral hearing loss in multiple sclerosis. *Ann Otol Rhinol Laryngol.* 2008;117(3):186-191.
5. Atula S, Sinkkonen S, Saat R, Sairanen T, Atula T. Association of multiple sclerosis and sudden sensorineural hearing loss. *Mult Scler J Exp Transl Clin.* 2016;2. doi:10.1177/2055217316652155.
6. Franklin DJ, Coker NJ, Jenkins HA. Sudden sensorineural hearing loss as a presentation of multiple sclerosis. *Arch Otolarngol Head Neck Surg.* 1989;115(1):41-45.
7. Hellmann MA, Steiner I, Mosberg-Galili R. Sudden sensorineural hearing loss in multiple sclerosis: clinical course and possible pathogenesis. *Acta Neurol Scand.* 2011;124:245-249.
8. Daugherty WT, Lederman RJ, Nodar RH, Conomy JP. Hearing loss in multiple sclerosis. *Arch Neurol.* 1983;40:33-35.
9. Drulovic B, Ribaric-Jankes K, Kostic VS, Sternic N. Sudden hearing loss as the initial monosymptom of multiple sclerosis. *Neurology.* 1993;43(12):2703-2705.
10. Fernández-Menéndez S, Redondo-Robles L, García-Santiago R, García-González MA, Arés-Luque A. Isolated deafness in multiple sclerosis patients. *Am J Otolaryngol.* 2014;35:810-813.

11. Shea JJ 3rd, Brackmann DE. Multiple sclerosis manifesting as sudden hearing loss. *Otolarngol Head Neck Surg.* 1987;97(3):335-338.

12. Tekin M, Acar GO, Cam OH, Hanege FM. Sudden sensorineural hearing loss in a multiple sclerosis case. *North Clin Istanbul.* 2014;1(2):109-113.

13. Fischer C, Mauguière F, Ibanez V, Confavreux C, Chazot G. The acute deafness of definite multiple sclerosis: BAEP patterns. *Electroencephalogr Clin Neurophysiol.* 1985;61(1):7-15.

14. Chiappa KH. Brainstem auditory evoked potentials in multiple sclerosis. In: Poser CM, Paty DW, Scheinberg L, eds. *The Diagnosis of Multiple Sclerosis.* New York: Thieme-Stratton; 1984:120-130.

15. Zafarroni M, Baldini SM, Ghezzi A. Cranial nerve, brainstem and cerebellar syndromes in the differential diagnosis of multiple sclerosis. *Neurol Sci.* 2001;22:S74-S78.

16. Commins DJ, Chen JM. Multiple sclerosis: a consideration in acute cranial nerve palsies. *Am J Otol.* 1997;18:590.

17. Schreiber BE, Agrup C, Haskard DO, Luxon LM. Sudden sensorineural hearing loss. *Lancet.* 2010;375(9721):1203-1211.

18. Rodriguez-Casero MV, Mandelstam S, Kornberg AJ, Berkowitz RG. Acute tinnitus and hearing loss as the initial symptom of multiple sclerosis in a child. *Int J Pediatr Otorhinolaryngol.* 2005;69(1):123-126.

19. Schick B, Brors D, Koch O, Schäfers M, Kahle G. Magnetic resonance imaging in patients with sudden hearing loss, tinnitus and vertigo. *Otol Neurotol.* 2001;22(6):808-812.

20. Walther EU, Hohlfeld R. Multiple sclerosis. *Neurology.* 1999;53(8):1622, LP-1622.

21. Pridmore S, Walter G, Friedland P. Tinnitus and suicide: recent cases on the public record give cause for reconsideration. *Otolaryngol Neck Surg.* 2012;147(2):193-195.

22. Hesser H, Weise C, Westin VZ, Andersson G. A systematic review and meta-analysis of randomized controlled trials of cognitive-behavioral therapy for tinnitus distress. *Clin Psychol Rev* 2011;31(4):545-553.

23. Herndon RM, Horak F. Vertigo, imbalance, and incoordination. In: Burks JS, Johnson KP, eds. *Multiple Sclerosis: Diagnosis, Medical Management, and Rehabilitation.* New York: Demos Medical; 2000:333-339.

24. Schumacher GA. Demyelinating diseases as a cause for vertigo. *Arch Otolaryngol.* 1967;85(5):537-538.

25. Pula JH, Newman-Toker DE, Kattah JC. Multiple sclerosis as a cause of the acute vestibular syndrome. *J Neurol.* 2013;260:1649-1654.

26. Frohman EM, Zhang H, Dewey RB, Hawker KS, Racke MK, Frohman TC. Vertigo in MS: utility of positional and particle repositioning maneuvers. *Neurology.* 2000;55(10):1566-1569.

27. Frohman EM, Kramer PD, Dewey RB, Kramer L, Frohman TC. Benign paroxysmal positioning vertigo in multiple sclerosis: diagnosis, pathophysiology and therapeutic techniques. *Mult Scler* 2003;9:250-255.

28. El-Moslimany H, Lublin FD. Clinical features in multiple sclerosis. In: Raine CS, McFarland HF, Hohlfeld R, eds. *Multiple Sclerosis: A Comprehensive Text.* Philadelphia: Saunders Elsevier; 2008:10-23.

29. Degirmenci E, Bir LS, Ardic FN. Clinical and electronystagmographical evaluation of vestibular symptoms in relapsing remitting multiple sclerosis. *Neurol Res.* 2010;32(9):986-991.

30. Nelson SR, Di Fabio RP, Anderson JH. Vestibular and sensory interaction deficits assessed by dynamic platform posturography in patients with multiple sclerosis. *Ann Otol Rhinol Laryngol.* 1995;104(1):62-68.

31. Hebert JR, Corboy JR, Manago MM, Schenkman M. Effects of vestibular reha- bilitation on multiple sclerosis-related fatigue and upright postural control: a randomized controlled trial. *Phys Ther.* 2011;91(8):1166-1183.
32. Cattaneo D, Jonsdottir J, Zocchi M, Regola A. Effects of balance exercises on people with multiple sclerosis: a pilot study. *Clin Rehabil.* 2007;21(9):771-781.
33. Gay D, Dick G, Upton G. Multiple sclerosis associated with sinusitis: case-con- trolled study in general practice. *Lancet.* 1986;327(8485):815-819.
34. Jones RL, Crowe P, Chavda SV, Pahor AL. The incidence of sinusitis in patients with multiple sclerosis. *Rhinology.* 1997;35(3):118-119.
35. Sibley WA, Foley JM. Infection and immunization in multiple sclerosis. *Ann N Y Acad Sci* 2018;122(1):457-468.
36. Sorenson PM. Dysarthria. In: Burks JS, Johnson KP, eds. *Multiple Sclerosis: Diagnosis, Medical Management, and Rehabilitation.* New York: Demos Medical; 2000:385-404.
37. Hartelius L, Svensson P. Speech and swallowing symptoms associated with Parkinson's disease and multiple sclerosis: a survey. *Folia Phoniatr Logop.* 1994;46:9-17.
38. Hartelius L, Runmarker B, Andersen O. Prevalence and characteristics of dys- arthria in a multiple-sclerosis incidence cohort: relation to neurological data. *Folia Phoniatr Logop.* 2000;52:160-177.
39. Blanco Y, Compta Y, Graus F, Saiz A. Midbrain lesions and paroxysmal dysar- thria in multiple sclerosis. *Mult Scler.* 2008;14:694-697.
40. Gorard DA, Gibberd FB. Paroxysmal dysarthria and ataxia: associated MRI abnormality. *J Neurol Neurosurg Psychiatry.* 1989;52(12):1444-1445.
41. Iorio R, Capone F, Plantone D, Batocchi AP. Paroxysmal ataxia and dysarthria in multiple sclerosis. *J Clin Neurosci.* 2014;21(1):174-175.
42. Marcel C, Anheim M, Flamand-Rouvière C, et al. Symptomatic paroxysmal dys- arthria-ataxia in demyelinating diseases. *J Neurol.* 2010;257:1369.
43. Matsui M, Tomimoto H, Sano K, Hashikawa K, Fukuyama H, Shibasaki H. Paroxysmal dysarthria and ataxia after midbrain infarction. *Neurology.* 2004;63(2):345-347.
44. Feijó AV, Parente MA, Behlau M, Haussen S, De Veccino MC, de Faria Martignago BC. Acoustic analysis of voice in multiple sclerosis patients. *J Voice.* 2004;18(3):341-347.
45. Dogan M, Midi I, Yazıcı MA, Kocak I, Günal D, Sehitoglu MA. Objective and subjective evaluation of voice quality in multiple sclerosis. *J Voice.* 2007;21(6):735-740.
46. Sapir S, Pawlas AA, Ramig LO, Seeley E, Fox C, Corboy J. Effects of intensive phonatory-respiratory treatment (LSVT) on voice in individuals with multiple sclerosis. *J Med Speech Lang Pathol.* 2001;9(2):35-45.
47. Kesselring J, Beer S. Symptomatic therapy and neurorehabilitation in multiple sclerosis. *Lancet Neurol.* 2005;4(10):643-652.
48. De Pauw A, Dejaeger E, D'hooghe B, Carton H. Dysphagia in multiple sclerosis. *Clin Neurol Neurosurg.* 2002;104(4);345-351.
49. Danesh-Sani SA, Rahimdoost A, Soltani M, Ghiyasi M, Haghdoost N, Sabzali- Zanjankhah S. Clinical assessment of orofacial manifestations in 500 patients with multiple sclerosis. *J Oral Maxillofac Surg.* 2013;71(2):290-294.
50. Terré-Boliart R, Orient-López F, Guevara-Espinosa D, Ramón-Rona S, Bernabeu-Guitart M, Clavé-Civit P. Oropharyngeal dysphagia in patients with multiple sclerosis. *Rev Neurol.* 2004;39(8):707-710.
51. Doty RL, Li C, Mannon LJ. Olfactory dysfunction in multiple sclerosis. Relation to plaque load in inferior frontal and temporal lobes. *Ann N Y Acad Sci* 1998;855:781-786.

52. Fleiner F, Dahlslett SB, Schmidt F, Harms L, Goektas O. Olfactory and gustatory function in patients with multiple sclerosis. *Am J Rhinol Allergy.* 2010;24(5):e93-e97.

53. Goektas O, Schmidt F, Bohner G, et al. Olfactory bulb volume and olfactory function in patients with multiple sclerosis. *Rhinology.* 2011;49:221-226.

54. Rolet A, Magnin E, Millot JL, et al. Olfactory dysfunction in multiple sclerosis: evidence of a decrease in different aspects of olfactory function. *Eur Neurol.* 2013;69(3):166-170.

55. Silva AM, Santos E, Moreira I, et al. Olfactory dysfunction in multiple sclerosis: association with secondary progression. *Mult Scler J.* 2011;18(5):616-621.

56. Uecker FC, Olze H, Kunte H, et al. Longitudinal testing of olfactory and gustatory function in patients with multiple sclerosis. *PLoS One.* 2017;12(1):e0170492.

57. Lutterotti A, Vedovello M, Reindl M, et al. Olfactory threshold is impaired in early, active multiple sclerosis. *Mult Scler J.* 2011;17(8):964-969.

58. Benatru I, Terraux P, Cherasse A, Couvreur G, Girond M, Moreau T. Gustatory disorders during multiple sclerosis relapse. *Rev Neurol (Paris).* 2003; 159(3):287-292.

59. Nocentini U, Giordano A, Castriota-Scanderbeg A, Caltagirone C, Parageusia: an unusual presentation of multiple sclerosis. *Eur Neurol.* 2004;51:123-124.

60. Pascual-Leone A, Altafullah I, Dhuna A. Hemiageusia: an unusual presentation of multiple sclerosis. *J Neurol Neurosurg Psychiatry.* 1991;54:657.

61. Doty RL, Tourbier IA, Pham DL, et al. Taste dysfunction in multiple sclerosis. *J Neurol.* 2016;263(4):677-688.

62. Feldman JI, Murphy C, Davidson TM, et al. The rhinologic evaluation of Alzheimer's disease. *Laryngoscope.* 1991;101(11):1198-1202.

63. Baba T, Kikuchi A, Hirayama K, et al. Severe olfactory dysfunction is a prodromal symptom of dementia associated with Parkinson's disease: a 3 year longitudinal study. *Brain.* 2012;135(1):161-169.

64. Takeda A, Baba T, Kikuchi A, et al. Olfactory dysfunction and dementia in Parkinson's disease. *J Parkinson's Dis.* 2014;4(2):181-1871

65. Silverstein A. Neurologic history of George Gershwin. *Mt Sinai J Med.* 1995;62(3):239-242.

66. McNeill E, Ramakrishnan Y, Carrie S. Diagnosis and management of olfactory disorders: a survey of UK-based consultants and literature review. *J Laryngol Otol.* 2007;121(8):713-720.

67. Damm M, Pikart LK, Reimann H. Olfactory training is helpful in postinfectious olfactory loss: a randomized, controlled, multicenter study. *Laryngoscope.* 2014;124(4):826-831.

68. Lucassen EB, Turel A, Knehans A, et al. Olfactory dysfunction in multiple sclerosis: a scoping review of the literature. *Mult Scler Relat Disord.* 2016;6:1-9.

23

Orthopedic Issues in the Multiple Sclerosis Patient

■ ■ ■ Brandon J. Erickson, Joshua S. Dines

Introduction

Multiple sclerosis (MS) is an autoimmune, inflammatory disorder resulting in demyelination of the central nervous system axons with a wide array of symptoms that encompass everything from subtle numbness and tingling to profound muscle weakness. The pattern of symptoms is often undulating, and as such can present at varying stages. There are roughly 400,000 people in the United States who are affected by MS, with women more commonly affected than men.[1] Although the orthopedic surgeon is not commonly managing the majority of symptoms from MS, there are several issues that are relevant to orthopedists when evaluating a patient with MS who presents with a musculoskeletal complaint. Some of these issues include increased risk of fractures, osteoporosis, increased complications following total joint arthroplasty, difficulty in distinguishing neuropathy from MS symptoms, and lack of improvement following surgical intervention for cervical myelopathy.

Osteoporosis and Fractures

Some of the many symptoms patients with MS can have include dizziness, lightheadedness, loss of balance, numbness, and blurred vision, all of

427

which can lead to a propensity for falls.[2] Unfortunately, the actual disease process of MS, the immobility associated with MS, low vitamin D levels, as well as some of the treatments for MS (glucocorticoids) can lead to severe osteoporosis.[2] Although use of glucocorticoids is common in patients with MS, either the use of glucocorticoids or the disease process itself may predispose patients to a higher risk of osteonecrosis.[3] Delanois et al reviewed 34 patients who were treated for osteonecrosis of the talus and noted MS as one of the causes. Furthermore, 83% of patients in their study had a history of corticosteroid use, making the combination of MS and steroid use a high risk for osteonecrosis. Patients with MS who present with hip, ankle, shoulder, and other joint pain should be carefully evaluated for osteonecrosis. This evaluation includes radiographs of the involved joint(s) followed by magnetic resonance imaging if the radiographs are negative. This allows early diagnosis of the osteonecrosis, hopefully before the collapse stage, thereby greatly increasing the treatment options for the patient. Once osteonecrosis progresses to the collapse stage, the treatment options become much more limited, so catching this process in the early stages is extremely important.

The combination of increased risk of falls and osteoporosis puts patients with MS at increased risk of fractures, specifically those about the hip.[4] Bazelier et al used the Danish national registry to compare 11,157 patients with a diagnosis to MS with 57,273 controls without a diagnosis of MS.[4] The purpose of the study was to report the incidence rates of fracture in patients with MS and stratify these fractures by location, sex, and age. The authors also compared the fracture rates of patients with MS with those of controls to see if a difference existed. The average age of patients with MS was 46.4 years (45.9 for controls), and females made up 65.9% of the MS cohort. Of note, when reviewing the medication lists, patients with MS used significantly more antidepressants, anxiolytics, and anticonvulsants than controls. This is something to keep in mind when prescribing medications to patients with MS to avoid an unwanted medication interaction. Obtaining a thorough medication history can avoid any unnecessary complications. The fracture incidence in patients with MS was 22.84 per 1000 person-years compared with 16.53 per 1000 person-years in controls. This gave an incidence rate ratio for any fracture between patients with MS and controls of 1.40. However, when the fractures were broken down by location, the incidence rate ratio for patients with MS compared with controls was 3.36 for tibia fractures, 6.66 for femur fractures, and 3.20 for hip fractures. Hence, although patients with MS had an increased overall risk for fracture compared with controls, this risk was significantly higher in hip, femur, and tibia fractures. Although fractures about the lower extremity are common, the pelvis can also be fractured in patients with MS. There has been a report of spontaneous bilateral periacetabular fractures in patients with MS necessitating open reduction internal fixation.[5] The cause was thought to be a combination of osteoporosis and spasticity. This highlights the fragility of some patients with MS. When a patient with MS complains of bone pain, it is important to investigate that complaint and ensure it is not a fracture.

The increased risk of fracture and osteoporosis associated with MS is concerns not only for patients sustaining fractures in general but also for patients sustaining falls and fractures in the acute postoperative period. Many of the orthopedic surgeries performed require a period of limited weight bearing and use of an assist device. When patients are unsteady on their feet, using an assistive device can be challenging. An inability to adequately progress with therapy may require a longer in-patient hospital stay or a short stay in a rehabilitation center following discharge to make sure the patient is safe. Similarly, osteoporosis is a concern in many orthopedic procedures, as fixation of implants becomes a problem when the patient's bone is diseased.[6] This can become particularly relevant when treating ankle fractures, obtaining a good press fit in a total hip arthroplasty, and others.[6,7] In a patient with MS who is undergoing an elective orthopedic procedure, it is prudent to obtain a bone mineral density test to evaluate the degree of osteoporosis in the preoperative period. Furthermore, there may be a role for treating the osteoporosis in these patients before offering them an elective surgery to help increase their chances of a successful outcome.[8] This may not always be possible, especially in patients who present with a long bone fracture, but should be considered in patients who necessitate elective procedures. Interestingly, there is limited evidence regarding treatment of long bone fractures in patients with MS. One study did show excellent results when treating a patient with MS with a femur fracture using a retrograde nail.[9] The fracture fixation implant should be tailored to the individual patient and fracture pattern, taking into account bone stock.

Total Joint Arthroplasty

Studies have shown that patients with MS have roughly the same risk of developing arthritis as the general population.[2] Patients with MS may also suffer from spasticity, specifically spasticity of the adductors, which can lead to gait dysfunction, skin irritation, and difficulties with perineal hygiene.[10] This spasticity can be treated using injections of intramuscular botulinum toxin, which has been shown to be effective in increasing passive hip abduction and the space between the knees in patients with MS with adductor spasticity.[10] Aside from the abductor spasticity, patients with MS in need of a total hip arthroplasty (THA) provide a challenge to orthopedic surgeons in regards to operative technique as well as rehabilitation.[3] Newman et al performed a review of the National Inpatient Sample (the largest US all-payer database of inpatient admissions) to evaluate the short-term outcomes following THA in patients with MS. The authors wanted to specifically study patient factors that differed in patients with MS and patients without MS, as well as report patient outcomes (complications, length of hospital stay, etc.) in those who had MS and underwent THA compared with all non-MS patients who underwent THA. They matched the patients with MS who underwent THA to controls without MS who underwent THA in a 1:3 ratio to control for confounding variables.

The authors found that the annual prevalence of MS in patients who underwent THA increased from 1.36 to 2.54 per 1000 THA from 2002 to 2013. Patients with MS were younger and had a higher percentage of females, but there was no difference in race. As predicted, patients with MS were more likely to have gait abnormalities preoperatively and were more likely to have osteonecrosis of the hip (likely secondary to the fact that more patients with MS were on corticosteroids than controls). Patients with MS stayed in the hospital longer than controls and were more likely to go to a rehabilitation center than controls. In regards to complications, patients with MS were more likely to have perioperative complications (both medical and surgical) compared with controls. The specific postoperative complications that were higher in the MS group were hemorrhagic anemia, fever, genitourinary issues, and transfusion of blood. This study illustrates that patients with MS undergoing THA represent a different patient cohort and must be treated slightly differently when preparing for and recovering from a THA. These patients may necessitate a botulinum toxin injection or adductor tenotomy before THA to help prevent a postoperative gait abnormality and help with hygiene. Unfortunately, this study did not address potential complications with implant loosening (either early or late), ongrowth/ingrowth surfaces, and when to use cementation techniques in patients with MS undergoing THA.

To answer the questions surrounding survivorship, reasons for failure, and functional outcomes in patients with MS undergoing total hip or knee arthroplasty, Rondon et al performed a retrospective review of 108 total joint arthroplasties (TJAs) (46 total knee arthroplasties [TKA] and 62 THA) performed from 2000 to 2016 at a single institution.[11] The authors matched these patients to a group of controls who underwent TJA without a history of MS based on age, body mass index, joint undergoing replacement, and comorbidities. The authors achieved an average follow-up of 6.2 years and found that 19.4% of patients with MS who underwent a TJA required revision surgery within that time frame. The MS cohort compared with the controls demonstrated an odds ratio of 3.5 ($p = 0.0011$) for requiring a revision arthroplasty (odds ratio was 3.8 for THA and 3.2 for TKA). For the MS cohort, the overall survivorship of TJA at 2, 5, and 7 years was 96.5%, 86.3%, and 75.3%, respectively, all of which were significantly worse than the controls. The reasons for revision in the 19.4% of the MS cohort that required revision included periprosthetic fracture (19%), instability (5.6%), aseptic loosening (3.7%), periprosthetic joint infection (4.6%), patellar clunk syndrome (1.9%), extensor mechanism failure (1%), and wear/corrosion (1%). Similar to the previous study, the authors found an increased length of stay in the MS cohort (3.15 vs. 2.82 d).

There was no difference in preoperative knee deformity in the MS cohort compared with controls, but the functional outcome scores following TJA were significantly better in the controls than in patients with MS. Finally, patients in the MS cohort had higher rates of instability and periprosthetic joint infection than controls. The higher infection rate was likely secondary to the fact that the patients with MS were more often taking immunomodulators than the control group. This study clearly outlines the issues that can arise when patients with MS undergo a TJA. Unfortunately, survivorship of a TJA in a patient with MS is significantly less than in the general population, despite the same rate of arthritis as in the general population. Fortunately, no patient in this study who underwent a TKA experienced a severe contracture postoperatively. However, there has been a report of a severe knee contracture following TKA in a patient with MS. Hughes et al reported a case of a patient with MS who underwent an uncomplicated TKA without nerve block anesthesia and developed severe pain and a knee flexion contracture in the immediate postoperative period.[12] Despite pain medication and eventually botulinum toxin injections, the spasticity did not significantly improve. This is a rare but important point to bring up with patients with MS when having a preoperative discussion. Similarly, if a patient with MS does begin to develop any sort of contracture following TJA, it may be prudent to swiftly intervene with a botulinum toxin injection to prevent progression of the contracture. Further work must be done in this area to better understand why the failure rate is so high and develop techniques and implants that will bring the revision risk following TJA in a patient with MS down to that of the general population, especially as it relates to implant loosening.

Although there are several studies in the hip and knee literature evaluating patients with MS, there are far fewer in the shoulder arthroplasty literature. One study reported on a patient with MS who underwent total shudder arthroplasty, although the case report was not actually written to describe the results following shoulder arthroplasty. Koff et al described a severe brachial plexopathy following an ultrasound-guided single injection interscalene nerve block in a patient with MS who was undergoing a total shoulder arthroplasty.[13] This patient had persistent motor and sensory deficits in the operative extremity more than 8 months following the interscalene block that had not resolved at the time the case report was published. Although this complication appears to be uncommon, it is devastating. Therefore, it may be prudent to avoid nerve block anesthesia in patients with MS undergoing orthopedic procedures to prevent this debilitating complication.

Neuropathy

Neuropathic complaints are one of the most common complaints seen by orthopedic surgeons. These issues can range from carpal or cubital tunnel syndrome in the upper extremity to lower extremity compressive neuropathies.[14,15] Patients with carpal or cubital tunnel syndrome commonly complain of paresthesias in a specific area (pinky and ulnar half of the ring finger for cubital tunnel versus thumb, index, middle, and radial half of the ring finger in carpal tunnel). Unfortunately, although MS commonly involves the central nervous system, there are patients who develop peripheral neuropathic symptoms.[15] It is for this reason that, anytime a patient with MS presents with peripheral nerve symptoms, the orthopedist must obtain a detailed history and perform a thorough physical examination to determine if the neuropathy is secondary to the patient's MS or if the patient has a separate cause of the neuropathy. However, the reverse is also true. There will be some patients who present with symptoms of carpal or cubital tunnel syndrome (as these are the two most common neuropathies of the upper extremity) who should be evaluated for MS before undergoing cubital or carpal tunnel release.[14,16,17] Witt et al reported 12 cases of failed carpal tunnel release secondary to inability to recognize neurologic disorders preoperatively. Of these 12 patients, 2 had MS. One of these patients had a normal electromyography (EMG), whereas one had an EMG inconsistent with carpal tunnel syndrome. This is not to say that patients who have MS cannot also suffer from carpal or cubital tunnel syndrome. Rather, the treating orthopedist must be aware that other neurologic disorders such as MS can masquerade as compressive neuropathies and these patients should be carefully evaluated. Proper initial evaluation and diagnostic testing can prevent unnecessary surgeries in these patients with MS and can lead to a new diagnosis.

Radiculopathy

As previously mentioned, MS can coexist with, or mimic, peripheral neuropathy. In a similar manner, patients with MS can suffer from myelopathy and/or cervical radiculopathy secondary to cervical stenosis.[18] Lubelski performed a retrospective review of 77 patients with concomitant MS and myelopathy secondary to cervical stenosis to determine the benefits of cervical decompression in this patient cohort. The MS cohort was also matched to a cohort of patients with cervical myelopathy secondary to cervical stenosis but without MS to assess the difference in outcomes following surgery between the two groups. Interestingly, patients with MS were less likely to have neck pain or radiculopathy preoperatively than controls. Following cervical decompression in both the short and long term, patients with MS had a significantly lower rate of resolution of their myelopathic symptoms than the controls. The patients with MS did improve/stabilize, but to a much lesser extent than the non-MS patients. This study clearly demonstrates that, although patients with MS who undergo cervical decompression for cervical myelopathy do improve following surgery, their improvements are much less than those of patients with similar pathology who undergo decompression but who do not have MS. It is important to educate patients on this finding preoperatively to set proper expectations for the postoperative course.

Although myelopathy can be a difficult problem to treat in patients with coexistent MS, cervical radiculopathy is a different type of pathology and one that may be amenable to better outcomes following surgical intervention.[19] Myelopathy involves compression of the spinal cord, whereas radiculopathy involves compression of nerve roots as they exit the spinal canal. Tan et al performed a retrospective review of 18 patients with coexistent MS and cervical stenosis causing cervical radiculopathy and myelopathy who underwent cervical decompression and fusion. The authors found that radiculopathy symptoms improved in 80% of patients, whereas neck pain improved in 100% of patients. However, similar to the Lubelski study, myelopathy improved only in 28.6% of patients. Of note, myelopathic symptoms did stabilize and did not progress in 64.3% of patients. One important point is that 0% of patients with urinary dysfunction preoperatively had any improvement in their symptoms following cervical decompression and fusion. These studies highlight the fact that patients with MS can expect to see improvements in symptoms of cervical radiculopathy (shooting pain down the arm, numbness/tingling, etc.) following cervical decompression and fusion but that improvements in myelopathic symptoms (waddling gait, clumsiness with hands, etc.) and urinary dysfunction are less predictable.

Conclusion

Patients with MS can present difficult problems for the orthopedic surgeons. Meticulous history and physical examination along with setting proper expectations in this patient population can lead to more satisfied patients following any type of surgical intervention.

References

1. Tullman MJ. Overview of the epidemiology, diagnosis, and disease progression associated with multiple sclerosis. *Am J Manag Care.* 2013;19(suppl 2):S15-S20.
2. Marrie RA, Hanwell H. General health issues in multiple sclerosis: comorbidities, secondary conditions, and health behaviors. *Continuum (Minneap Minn).* 2013;19(4 Multiple Sclerosis):1046-1057.

3. Newman JM, Naziri Q, Chughtai M, et al. Does multiple sclerosis affect the inpatient perioperative outcomes after total hip arthroplasty? *J Arthroplasty.* 2017;32(12):3669-3674.

4. Bazelier MT, de Vries F, Bentzen J, et al. Incidence of fractures in patients with multiple sclerosis: the Danish National Health Registers. *Mult Scler.* 2012;18(5):622-627.

5. Aggarwal A, Parvizi J, Ganz R. Bilateral spontaneous periacetabular fracture: an unusual complication of multiple sclerosis. *J Orthop Trauma.* 2004;18(3):182-185.

6. Finnila S, Moritz N, Svedstro ME, Alm JJ, Aro HT. Increased migration of uncemented acetabular cups in female total hip arthroplasty patients with low systemic bone mineral density. A 2-year RSA and 8-year radiographic follow-up study of 34 patients. *Acta Orthop.* 2016;87(1):48-54.

7. Pidgeon TS, Johnson JP, Deren ME, Evans AR, Hayda RA. Analysis of mortality and fixation failure in geriatric fractures using quantitative computed tomography. *Injury.* 2018;49(2):249-255.

8. Kim SY, Zhang M, Bockman R. Bone mineral density response from teriparatide in patients with osteoporosis. *HSS J.* 2017;13(2):171-177.

9. Chin KR, Altman DT, Altman GT, Mitchell TM, Tomford WW, Lhowe DW. Retrograde nailing of femur fractures in patients with myelopathy and who are nonambulatory. *Clin Orthop Relat Res.* 2000(373):218-226.

10. Hyman N, Barnes M, Bhakta B, et al. Botulinum toxin (Dysport) treatment of hip adductor spasticity in multiple sclerosis: a prospective, randomised, double blind, placebo controlled, dose ranging study. *J Neurol Neurosurg Psychiatry.* 2000;68(6):707-712.

11. Rondon AJ, Schlitt PK, Tan TL, Phillips JL, Greenky MR, Purtill JJ. Survivorship and outcomes in patients with multiple sclerosis undergoing total joint arthroplasty. *J Arthroplasty.* 2018;33(4):1024-1027.

12. Hughes KE, Nickel D, Gurney-Dunlop T, Knox KB. Total knee arthroplasty in multiple sclerosis. *Arthroplast Today.* 2016;2(3):117-122.

13. Koff MD, Cohen JA, McIntyre JJ, Carr CF, Sites BD. Severe brachial plexopathy after an ultrasound-guided single-injection nerve block for total shoulder arthroplasty in a patient with multiple sclerosis. *Anesthesiology.* 2008;108(2):325-328.

14. Jarrett CD, Papatheodorou LK, Sotereanos DG. Cubital tunnel syndrome. *Instr Course Lect.* 2017;66:91-101.

15. Bales JG, Meals R. Peripheral neuropathy of the upper extremity: medical comorbidity that confounds common orthopedic pathology. *Orthopedics.* 2009;32(10). doi:10.3928/01477447-20090818-19.

16. Cutts S. Cubital tunnel syndrome. *Postgrad Med J.* 2007;83(975):28-31.

17. Witt JC, Stevens JC. Neurologic disorders masquerading as carpal tunnel syndrome: 12 cases of failed carpal tunnel release. *Mayo Clin Proc.* 2000;75(4):409-413.

18. Lubelski D, Abdullah KG, Alvin MD, et al. Clinical outcomes following surgical management of coexistent cervical stenosis and multiple sclerosis: a cohort-controlled analysis. *Spine J.* 2014;14(2):331-337.

19. Tan LA, Kasliwal MK, Muth CC, Stefoski D, Traynelis VC. Is cervical decompression beneficial in patients with coexistent cervical stenosis and multiple sclerosis? *J Clin Neurosci.* 2014;21(12):2189-2193.

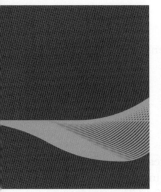
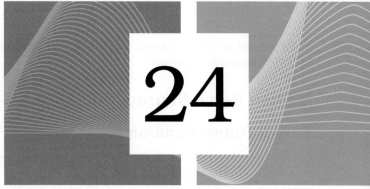

24

Upper Extremity Evaluation in Patients with Multiple Sclerosis

■ ▓ ▒ Kyle W. Morse, Michelle G. Carlson

Introduction

Multiple sclerosis (MS) can manifest with disabling symptoms of the upper extremities, including reduced grip strength, reduced pinch strength, tremor, decreased dexterity, and impaired sensation.[1-6] Patients with MS may also report worsening hand function as their disease progresses, and nearly 60% to 79% of patients with MS may have decreased dexterity or experience upper extremity symptoms.[1,2] Disabling upper extremity symptoms can cause significant functional impairment and lead to a decreased quality of life, unemployment, and use of an assistive device.[5] Compression neuropathies are commonly encountered in the general population as the median, ulnar, and radial nerves encounter multiple sites of potential constriction as they course distally from the brachial plexus. For patients with MS, the diagnosis of compressive neuropathies may be challenging, as patients may present with weakness, paresthesia, and numbness in the upper extremity that may mimic compression neuropathy.[4] The ability to differentiate peripheral compression from a central nervous system insult is critical in managing these pathologies. Peripheral nerve neuropathy can be explored through nerve anatomy,

435

pathophysiology, presentation, diagnosis, and treatment to aid clinicians in their diagnostic approach.

Median Nerve Neuropathies

Carpal Tunnel Syndrome

Carpal tunnel syndrome is the most common compression neuropathy that occurs in the upper extremity with an estimated incidence of 1 to 3 cases per 1000 and a prevalence of 50 cases per 1000.[7-9] The syndrome presents with paresthesia and numbness along the median nerve distribution to the radial three and a half digits. These symptoms typically begin at night, which may be the most sensitive predictor.[10] The symptoms can occur during the day as the syndrome progresses and becomes more severe. Shaking of the hand, often referred to as the "flick sign," may relieve symptoms. This sign is reported to have a sensitivity of 37% and specificity of 74%.[8] Weakness of thumb palmar abduction and thenar eminence atrophy may appear later in the clinical course as the syndrome progresses.[8]

The median nerve takes origin from the C5 to T1 nerve roots and arises from the medial and lateral cords of the brachial plexus.[11] After traversing the upper extremity, the nerve ultimately passes into the wrist through the carpal tunnel, which begins at the volar wrist crease. The scaphoid tubercle and trapezium create the radial border, whereas the triquetrum, pisiform, and hook of hamate form the ulnar border. The dorsal floor is formed by the scaphoid, capitate, hamate, and triquetrum. Soft tissue structures create the volar border, consisting of the flexor retinaculum or transverse carpal ligament.[9,11] The median nerve is accompanied by the four tendons of the flexor digitorum superficialis, the four tendons of the flexor digitorum profundus, and the tendon of the flexor pollicis longus through the carpal tunnel.[9,11]

Carpal tunnel syndrome occurs as a result of decreased space and increased pressure within the confined space of the cubital tunnel, which may result from tendon inflammation, edema, hormonal changes, or manual activity.[12] As a result, several risk factors have been associated with carpal tunnel syndrome, which include hypothyroidism, menopause, diabetes mellitus, obesity, arthritis, and pregnancy.[12] The increase in compartment pressure leads to decreased perfusion to the median nerve's epineurium, leading to local tissue edema, decreased myelination, and ultimately reduced signal transmission due to axonal transport dysfunction.[9,13] Venous return may also be compromised, leading to venous stasis and extraneural edema, whereas intraneural edema may occur chronically owing to the development of nerve fibrosis and scarring.[13] Symptoms may occur during positions that reduce the size of the carpal tunnel, such as wrist flexion or extension, which is why a wrist brace often helps. Carpal tunnel syndrome may also occur acutely, typically described following a distal radius fracture, carpal fracture/dislocation, and metacarpal fractures.[9] Acute fractures resulting in carpal tunnel syndrome are especially important to consider in patients with MS, as these patients have a 25% overall lower prevalence of bone mineral density and their risk of fracture may be increased because of corticosteroid therapy.[4]

The clinical history and examination are critical in the diagnosis of carpal tunnel syndrome. History focuses on acuity, aggravating factors, associated activities, and relevant past medical history, as patients with MS may adjust their activities to compensate for their upper extremity disabilities.[2] Several physical examination maneuvers are used to aid in the diagnosis of carpal tunnel syndrome. The first is Phalen sign, which is performed by holding the wrist in prolonged flexion. This position causes compression of the carpal tunnel, and the sign is positive after several minutes if the patient's symptoms are replicated. Phalen sign has a reported sensitivity between 42% and 85% and specificity of 54% to 98%.[12] Tinel sign, with a sensitivity of 38% to 100% and specificity of 55% to 100%, involves the replication of symptoms when the examiner repeatedly taps the patient's carpal tunnel.[8] Conducting a thorough sensory examination of the entire median nerve distribution with a comparison with the contralateral side is vital in patients with MS. Bertoni et al[1] reported decreased unilateral thumb sensation in 22% of patients with MS examined, and 68% of patients had decreased sensation bilaterally as measured by the Semmes-Weinstein monofilament test. Therefore, a patient with a unilateral sensory deficit affecting the index, long, and radial half of the ring finger may be due to carpal tunnel syndrome.[14] In addition, other etiologies such as cervical radiculopathy or cervical myelopathy should be considered. Cervical radiculopathy results from compression of a spinal nerve root that typically results in unilateral pain and paresthesias that follow a dermatomal distribution as illustrated in Figure 24.1.[15,16] In contrast, cervical myelopathy results from central spinal cord compression and the presentation may mimic that of MS with upper motor neuron symptoms, such as nondermatomal sensory disturbances, loss of balance, loss of coordination and difficulty with performing fine motor tasks, hyperreflexia, and weakness.[16] A patient with cervical radiculopathy may reveal decreased neck range of motion, and symptoms may be replicated or relieved with a variety of examination maneuvers. The Spurling test is performed by axially loading the neck and then rotating and extending it toward the affected side. This maneuver was found to be the most sensitive and specific physical examination test for cervical radiculopathy with a sensitivity between 30% and 100% and a specificity of 75% to 100%.[15,16] The shoulder abduction test, with a reported sensitivity between 17% and

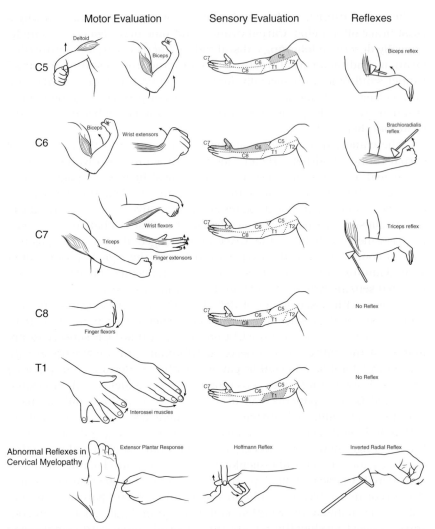

Figure 24.1. Neurologic evaluation of cervical radiculopathy and myelopathy. (Reprinted with permission from Micev AJ, Ivy AD, Aggarwal SK, Hsu WK, Kalainov DM. Cervical radiculopathy and myelopathy: presentations in the hand. *J Hand Surg Am.* 2013;38(12):2478-2481.)

78% and specificity of 75% to 92%, is another examination maneuver used, in which the patient's symptoms are relieved when the shoulder is abducted and externally rotated.[15] Lastly, the Valsalva maneuver may also elicit symptoms of cervical radiculopathy with a reported sensitivity of 22% and specificity of 94%.[15,16] If cervical radiculopathy or myelopathy is suspected, computed tomography (CT) and magnetic resonance imaging are used to evaluate for cervical spondylosis or spinal cord compression with appropriate referral to a spine surgeon.

In addition to the above-mentioned physical examination findings or in cases of an uncertain diagnosis or equivocal examination findings, further testing may be required, such as nerve conduction studies, electromyography, or ultrasonography. Nerve conduction studies are advantageous because they can measure the severity of nerve degeneration, such as the amount of demyelination and axonal loss, which is important for future outcome.[12] Changes in conduction velocity are often detected first in sensory fibers before motor fibers.[12] Recently, ultrasound has been used and compared with electrophysiological assessments for the diagnosis of carpal tunnel syndrome to identify compression of the median nerve by assessing the cross-sectional area of the nerve before and after it is compressed. Ultrasonography has been reported to have a sensitivity of 77.6% and specificity of 86.8% compared with clinical diagnosis.[12]

Management of carpal tunnel syndrome includes both nonoperative and operative approaches. The goal of management is to reduce compression within the carpal tunnel. A trial of nonoperative management is warranted before opting for surgery. The patient should be counseled on avoiding provocative wrist motions and reducing heavy lifting.[12] Options include nonsteroidal anti-inflammatory drugs (NSAIDs), corticosteroid injections, and nighttime bracing. When bracing the patient with MS, careful follow-up is needed for repeat skin examinations, as these patients are prone to developing pressure sores.[4] If symptoms do not resolve following initial nonsurgical treatment, a second nonsurgical modality can be trialed.[17] If nonoperative management fails to address symptoms, surgical management is indicated and involves transection of the entire flexor retinaculum above the carpal tunnel, which may be performed using open, minimally invasive, or endoscopic techniques, all with high degrees of success. There is no difference in long-term outcome between each technique.[12] Potential complications that may result from carpal tunnel release include the injury to surrounding neurovascular structures and tendons, development of complex regional pain syndrome, scar tenderness, neuropraxia, and revision surgery. Patients with MS-attributed weakness, spasms, and sensory loss not associated with carpal tunnel may have worsening of their symptoms following surgery.[4]

Other Median Nerve Neuropathies

Although carpal tunnel syndrome may be the most common compressive neuropathy associated with the median nerve, the nerve can become compressed along other sites as it traverses distally. Proximally, pronator syndrome can occur as the nerve can be compressed at the elbow, which results in pain in the proximal portion of the volar forearm along with weakness and numbness of the radial digits and the palm.[11,18] The anterior interosseous nerve (AIN), a purely motor branch of the median nerve, may also be compressed at the elbow. Compression of the AIN does not produce sensory findings, but weakness of the flexor pollicis longus and flexor digitorum profundus to the index finger typically occurs.[11,18] Patients with proximal median nerve or AIN involvement will be unable to bring the tips of their thumb and index finger together to make the Kiloh-Nevin sign or "OK sign."[18]

Ulnar Nerve Neuropathy

Cubital Tunnel Syndrome

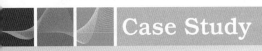

Case Study

Cubital tunnel syndrome with prior diagnosis of MS

A 35-year-old right-hand-dominant woman with a history of relapsing-remitting MS presents to the clinic with unilateral right-hand numbness. She has been treated with glucocorticoids in the past, which has resulted in good control of her symptoms acutely. Today, she notes numbness and tingling along her right small and ring fingers that is worse after the workday ends and is relieved when she stretches her arm. She works as a project manager and spends most of her day working on a computer at her desk. She denies radiating pain, weakness, imbalance, neck pain, or loss of grip strength. Her past episodes of MS have not yielded hand weakness, and she is concerned that this may be an acute MS flare. On examination, she is noted to be thin. Tapping of the medial elbow reproduces her symptoms as well as when her arm is flexed with the wrist extended. Two-point discrimination of the little and ulnar border of the ring finger is found to be 10 mm compared with 4 mm in the remaining digits. She does not have loss of sensation over the ulnar side of the forearm. Spurling maneuver was negative. The patient was referred for electrodiagnostic testing and found to have nerve conduction velocity of 40 m/s. She underwent uncomplicated surgical ulnar nerve decompression and had resolution of symptoms.

Commentary   The patient presented with signs and symptoms of cubital tunnel syndrome, which is ulnar nerve entrapment at the level of the cubital tunnel as will be discussed later. A differential diagnosis of cervical radiculopathy was also considered, but the patient had a negative Spurling test and no loss of ulnar sided forearm sensation, which would be seen in cervical radiculopathy. She displayed a positive Tinel sign at the elbow and a positive flexion test, both of which reproduced her symptoms. The diagnosis was confirmed with a nerve conduction velocity study.

Cubital tunnel syndrome is the second most common compressive neuropathy affecting the upper extremity with an incidence of 25 cases per 100,000 person-years in men and 19 cases per 100,000 person-years in women.[14,19] Patients present with numbness and paresthesia along the ulnar nerve distribution, especially the ring and little finger. Pain may also occur along the medial forearm. Symptoms are worsened by elbow flexion as the space in the tunnel decreases during this movement.[11,14]

The ulnar nerve arises from the C8 and T1 nerve roots and is the terminal branch of the medial cord of the brachial plexus. The nerve courses on the medial head of the triceps as it descends through the upper arm and encounters its first point of constriction proximal to the elbow as it pierces the intermuscular septum. It then passes through the arcade of Struthers, a fascial band between the medial head of the triceps and the intermuscular septum.[11,14] Continuing distally, the ulnar nerve passes posteriorly over the medial epicondyle and enters the cubital tunnel. The tunnel is formed primarily by fibrous attachments of Osborne ligament between the medial epicondyle, the humeral and ulnar heads of the flexor carpi ulnaris, and the olecranon, with the nerve exiting into the forearm between the two heads of the flexor carpi ulnaris.[11,14]

Similarly to other compression neuropathies, cubital tunnel syndrome results from decreased space and increased pressure within the cubital tunnel and commonly occurs during elbow flexion as pressure on the nerve increases past 90° of elbow flexion.[14] Thickening and fusion of the different layers of Osborne ligament are also attributed to causing decreased space in the tunnel.[14] Ulnar nerve neuropathy may also occur following traumatic elbow dislocation or distal humerus fracture, either acutely or following surgery as a result of scar tissue formation, deformity, or edema, so careful history taking remains important in understanding the etiology of the symptoms.[14]

The patient will often have decreased vibratory or two-point discrimination in the ring and little fingers. Hypothenar musculature atrophy due to innervation of the opponens digiti minimi and abductor digiti minimi can result. In addition, atrophy of the adductor pollicis may occur. Physical examination maneuvers are performed to recreate symptoms. The Froment sign occurs when the patient is asked to pinch a piece of paper between the thumb and radial side of the index finger as the examiner forcefully tries to remove it. The sign is positive if thumb interphalangeal joint flexion occurs. Owing to weakness of the ulnar nerve–innervated adductor pollicis, the flexor pollicis longus, which is not innervated by the ulnar nerve, is recruited to aid pinch strength, producing the unwanted flexion of the thumb interphalangeal joint. In patients with MS, the Froment sign may not be diagnostic, as these patients may have impaired pinch and grip strength.[1,3] The Wartenberg sign may also be produced as patients extend their fingers; the fifth finger "sticks out" because they are unable to adduct the digit due to weakness of the third palmar interosseous muscle.

Symptoms may also be reproduced with a Tinel sign over the cubital tunnel or when the elbow is positioned in full flexion and the wrist extended.[14] Electrodiagnostic testing may also be employed in the diagnostic assessment of the cubital tunnel syndrome, which will show a decrease in either ulnar nerve conduction velocity or conduction velocity about the elbow.[14]

Treatment of cubital tunnel syndrome is centered on nonoperative and operative approaches to relieve pressure on the ulnar nerve. Initially, conservative management is pursued, commonly in the form of splinting to restrict elbow flexion. In addition, patients should be counseled to avoid both direct pressure on the elbow and prolonged time in elbow flexion.[14] This treatment course may be most effective in patients presenting with mild or moderate disease. Patients who do not respond to conservative management may require surgical treatment to alleviate their symptoms. The goal of surgery is to decompress the ulnar nerve within the tunnel, and there are a variety of techniques that have been used, including decompression, medial epicondylectomy, and transposition. The choice of surgical procedure depends on the mobility of the ulnar nerve and the body habitus of the patient.[14]

Other Ulnar Nerve Neuropathies

When encountering ulnar-sided symptoms, it is essential to consider other points of possible compression distal to the cubital tunnel, although this is much less frequent. The ulnar nerve continues its course distally into the forearm alongside the ulnar artery between the flexor digitorum profundus and flexor carpi ulnaris and ultimately enters the wrist through Guyon canal. Similar to the carpal tunnel, Guyon canal is formed by fibro-osseous structures and begins just proximal to the distal wrist crease.[20] The radial border is made up of the hook of hamate and the ulnar border by the pisiform. Multiple soft tissue structures compose its roof and floor. The dorsal floor is formed primarily by the transverse carpal ligament with contributions from the flexor digitorum profundus, opponens digiti minimi, and pisohamate and pisometacarpal ligaments.[11] The roof is composed of contributions of the palmar carpal ligament, palmaris brevis, and fat and fibrous tissue from the hypothenar eminence.[11,20] The nerve subsequently divides into motor and sensory branches in varying zones of the canal as described by Gross and Gelberman[11,20,21] (Figures 24.2-24.4).

Multiple causative factors have been implicated in Guyon canal syndrome. The most common cause is reported to be ganglion cysts arising from the carpal joints.[18,20] Similar to other compression neuropathies, repetitive motions and provocative positions may lead to Guyon canal syndrome. Continuous pressure on the ulnar palm with the wrist in extension and persistent vibratory trauma are the second most common causes of Guyon canal syndrome and is observed in cyclists and ball/

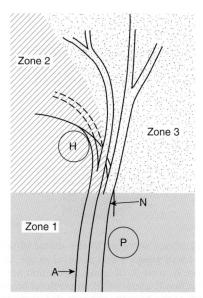

Figure 24.2. Schematic drawing of the distal ulnar tunnel showing the location of the three zones: zone 1 (coarse stippling), zone 2 (lines), and zone 3 (fine stippling). A, ulnar artery; H, hamulus; N, ulnar nerve; P, pisiform. (Reprinted with permission from Gross MS, Gelberman RH. The anatomy of the distal ulnar tunnel. *Clin Orthop Relat Res.* 1985;(196):238-247.)

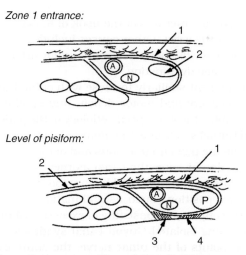

Figure 24.3. Schematic cross section of the distal ulnar tunnel in zone 1. Entrance to zone 1: 1, palmar carpal ligament; 2, tendon of flexor carpi ulnaris; A, ulnar artery; N, ulnar nerve. Level of the pisiform: 1, palmaris brevis; 2, transverse carpal ligament; 3, pisohamate ligament; 4, pisometacarpal ligament; A, ulnar artery; N, ulnar nerve; P, pisiform. (Reprinted with permission from Gross MS, Gelberman RH. The anatomy of the distal ulnar tunnel. *Clin Orthop Relat Res.* 1985;(196):238-247.)

Level of Bifurcation:

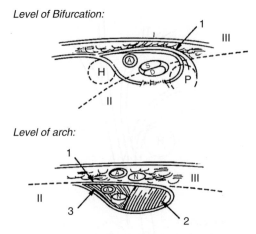

Level of arch:

Figure 24.4. Schematic cross sections of the distal ulnar tunnel at the proximal and distal boundaries of zones 2 and 3. Level of the bifurcation of the ulnar nerve: 1, palmaris brevis; II, zone 2; III, zone 3; A, ulnar artery; D, deep branch of the ulnar nerve; H, hamulus; P, pisiform; S, superficial branch of the ulnar nerve. Level of the fibrous arch of the hypothenar muscles: 2, abductor digiti minimi; 3, flexor digiti minimi. In zone II: A, deep branch of ulnar artery; N, deep branch of the ulnar nerve. In zone III: A, superficial branch of the ulnar artery forming the superficial arch; N, superficial branch of the ulnar nerve. (Reprinted with permission from Gross MS, Gelberman RH. The anatomy of the distal ulnar tunnel. *Clin Orthop Relat Res.* 1985;(196):238-247.)

stick athletes.[20] Acutely, fractures of the hook of hamate may cause ulnar nerve neuropathy at the wrist. Other causes include anomalous muscles, fibrous adhesions, arthritis, bony deformity, ulnar artery aneurysm, and edema due to metabolic dysfunction.[18,20]

Patients may present similarly to those with cubital tunnel syndrome with ulnar-sided sensory and motor deficit, and careful examination is warranted to determine the appropriate etiology of the patient's symptoms. Unlike in cubital tunnel syndrome, the ulnar palm and dorsum of the hand are not involved, as the palmar cutaneous and dorsal cutaneous branches of the ulnar nerve do not enter the canal as they branch from the ulnar nerve proximal to the canal.[18] A careful history that notes prolonged movement or provocative positions such as ambulation with a cane, cycling, weightlifting, and occupations consisting of excessive vibration are clinical clues when suspecting isolated Guyon canal syndrome. Given the multiple compression points of the ulnar nerve, the entire extremity should be inspected and compared with the contralateral side. In severe cases of ulnar nerve neuropathy, claw hand may occur with extension of the ring and little finger metacarpal phalangeal joints and flexion of the proximal interphalangeal joints owing to the absent intrinsic muscles but present flexor digitorum profundus with proximal innervation. Additionally, there is atrophy of the first dorsal interosseous muscle with hollowing of the appearance of the thumb web space.[18] Upper extremity contractures are not common in MS, and these findings warrant further exploration into their etiology.[4]

The remainder of the examination focuses on the innervation of the ulnar nerve's deep motor branch. Decreased pinch strength may occur because of weakness of the first dorsal interosseous muscles and adductor pollicis, and the Froment and Wartenberg signs may be present. The patient may have difficulty crossing the index and long fingers owing to weakness of the first palmar and second dorsal interosseous muscles. Similar to the diagnosis of other compression neuropathies, a detailed sensory examination is performed, noting deficits in light touch and two-point discrimination. Manual compression over Guyon canal may also replicate paresthesia and numbness along the ulnar nerve distribution, and a Tinel sign at the canal may also be present. If diagnostic uncertainty remains, further imaging and studies are warranted. If the neuropathy occurred acutely, x-ray and CT imaging are used to diagnose hook of the hamate fractures and other bony deformities. Nerve conduction and electromyography (EMG) are also employed to localize the lesion and would show decreased conduction along the wrist.[18] EMG can be used to evaluate the hypothenar muscles and first dorsal interosseous muscle.

Guyon canal syndrome is also managed nonoperatively and operatively. If it is caused by provocative movements, conservative management with braces and physical therapy can be used. Surgical management is indicated for persisting symptoms or those that continue to worsen, and tunnel decompression is performed. In cases that are caused by ganglion cysts, the cyst and its extensions are removed surgically.

Radial Nerve Injuries

Radial nerve compression presents less commonly than median and ulnar nerve compression neuropathies.[22] Two syndromes are commonly associated with radial nerve compression: radial tunnel syndrome and posterior interosseous nerve (PIN) syndrome. These syndromes are distinguished based on their presentation. The presentation of radial tunnel syndrome is pain without sensory deficit, whereas patients who present with PIN syndrome have weakness extending the digits.[18]

The radial nerve arises from the C5 to C8 nerve roots and is the termination of the posterior cord of the brachial plexus. The radial nerve divides into the superficial radial nerve and the PIN just distal to the lateral humeral epicondyle. The superficial radial nerve travels along the forearm on the lateral edge of the brachioradialis and ultimately becomes subcutaneous, providing sensory innervation to the skin on the radial aspect of the forearm and the dorsal aspects of the radial three and a half digits. The PIN passes through the supinator into the forearm, innervating the digital extensors as it descends toward the hand and terminates at the dorsal wrist capsule.[11]

The radial tunnel begins just after the radial nerve bifurcates into the superficial radial nerve and the PIN at the humeroradial joint and continues distally to the proximal edge of supinator, also referred to as the arcade of Frohse.[18,23] The tunnel's floor is composed of the radiocapitellar joint capsule proximally and the deep head of supinator distally, with the brachioradialis forming the roof.[18,23] Medially, it is enclosed by the biceps tendon and brachalis as the mobile wad consisting of the brachioradialis, extensor carpi radialis brevis and extensor carpi radialis longus compose the lateral border of the tunnel.[18,23]

Pain along the lateral forearm is a common presentation of radial tunnel syndrome.[18] The pain may worsen with forearm supination and pronation as pressure is increased in the tunnel as a result of stretching of the supinator.[23] Applying pressure over the supinator with the forearm in supination can reproduce pain.[18] Pain may also occur during resisted wrist and long finger extension.[18,23] It is critical to differentiate the potential diagnosis of radial tunnel syndrome from lateral epicondylitis, and this can be accomplished by localizing the pain's origin. Pain associated with lateral epicondylitis occurs at the lateral epicondyle, whereas pain associated with radial tunnel syndrome occurs 3 to 5 cm distally directly on the supinator muscle.[18,23] An anesthetic injection may also be used to differentiate the two pathologies.[18,23] Unlike the compression neuropathies of the median and ulnar nerves, electrodiagnostic studies are often normal in patients with radial tunnel syndrome[18,23]

The first-line treatment of patients with radial tunnel syndrome is nonsurgical and includes physical therapy, wrist splinting, NSAIDs, and activity modification, such as avoiding prolonged periods of elbow extension with the forearm pronated and wrist flexed.[18,23] Patients who fail conservative measures may progress to surgical treatment to decompress the radial tunnel.

Other Radial Nerve Neuropathies

Entrapment of the superficial branch of the radial nerve can also occur between the brachioradialis and the extensor carpi radialis longus. Compression of the superficial branch produces numbness and paresthesia over the dorsolateral aspect of the hand and may be provoked by wrist pronation.[11]

Conclusion

Patients with MS frequently present with upper extremity dysfunction. MS may cause sensory loss, weakness, and loss of grip strength, and the diagnosis of upper extremity neuropathy involving the median, ulnar, and radial nerves may become complicated in these patients. We can help clinicians dissociate MS versus peripheral nerve involvement by performing careful neurologic examination and often nerve conduction/EMG study. These tools can help in making a clear diagnosis between MS and peripheral nerve involvement.

References

1. Bertoni R, Lamers I, Chen CC, Feys P, Cattaneo D. Unilateral and bilateral upper limb dysfunction at body functions, activity and participation levels in people with multiple sclerosis. *Mult Scler.* 2015;21(12):1566-1574.
2. Kraft GH, Amtmann D, Bennett SE, et al. Assessment of upper extremity function in multiple sclerosis: review and opinion. *Postgrad Med.* 2014;126(5):102-108.
3. Chen CC, Kasven N, Karpatkin HI, Sylvester A. Hand strength and perceived manual ability among patients with multiple sclerosis. *Arch Phys Med Rehabil.* 2007;88(6):794-797.
4. Pidgeon TS, Borenstein T, Daniels AH, Murali J, Hayda RA. Understanding multiple sclerosis: essentials for the orthopaedic surgeon. *JBJS Rev.* 2014;2(7). doi:10.2106/JBJS.RVW.M.00120.
5. Marrie RA, Cutter GR, Tyry T, Cofield SS, Fox R, Salter A. Upper limb impairment is associated with use of assistive devices and unemployment in multiple sclerosis. *Mult Scler Relat Disord.* 2017;13:87-92.
6. Severijns D, Van Geel F, Feys P. Motor fatigability in persons with multiple sclerosis: relation between different upper limb muscles, and with fatigue and the perceived use of the arm in daily life. *Mult Scler Relat Disord.* 2018;19:90-95.
7. Fajardo M, Kim SH, Szabo RM. Incidence of carpal tunnel release: trends and implications within the United States ambulatory care setting. *J Hand Surg Am.* 2012;37(8):1599-1605.
8. Duckworth AD, Jenkins PJ, McEachan JE. Diagnosing carpal tunnel syndrome. *J Hand Surg Am.* 2014;39(7):1403-1407.
9. Gillig JD, White SD, Rachel JN. Acute carpal tunnel syndrome: a review of current literature. *Orthop Clin North Am.* 2016;47(3):599-607.
10. Szabo RM, Slater RR Jr, Farver TB, Stanton DB, Sharman WK. The value of diagnostic testing in carpal tunnel syndrome. *J Hand Surg Am.* 1999;24(4):704-714.
11. Mazurek MT, Shin AY. Upper extremity peripheral nerve anatomy: current concepts and applications. *Clin Orthop Relat Res.* 2001;(383):7-20.
12. Padua L, Coraci D, Erra C, et al. Carpal tunnel syndrome: clinical features, diagnosis, and management. *Lancet Neurol.* 2016;15(12):1273-1284.
13. Tapadia M, Mozaffar T, Gupta R. Compressive neuropathies of the upper extremity: update on pathophysiology, classification, and electrodiagnostic findings. *J Hand Surg Am.* 2010;35(4):668-677.

14. Staples JR, Calfee R. Cubital tunnel syndrome: current concepts. *J Am Acad Orthop Surg.* 2017;25(10):e215-e224.

15. Iyer S, Kim HJ. Cervical radiculopathy. *Curr Rev Musculoskelet Med.* 2016;9(3):272-280.

16. Micev AJ, Ivy AD, Aggarwal SK, Hsu WK, Kalainov DM. Cervical radiculopathy and myelopathy: presentations in the hand. *J Hand Surg Am.* 2013;38(12):2478-2481; quiz 2481.

17. Keith MW, Masear V, Amadio PC, et al. Treatment of carpal tunnel syndrome. *J Am Acad Orthop Surg.* 2009;17(6):397-405.

18. Strohl AB, Zelouf DS. Ulnar tunnel syndrome, radial tunnel syndrome, anterior interosseous nerve syndrome, and pronator syndrome. *Instr Course Lect.* 2017;66:153-162.

19. Soltani AM, Best MJ, Francis CS, Allan BJ, Panthaki ZJ. Trends in the surgical treatment of cubital tunnel syndrome: an analysis of the national survey of ambulatory surgery database. *J Hand Surg Am.* 2013;38(8):1551-1556.

20. Earp BE, Floyd WE, Louie D, Koris M, Protomastro P. Ulnar nerve entrapment at the wrist. *J Am Acad Orthop Surg.* 2014;22(11):699-706.

21. Gross MS, Gelberman RH. The anatomy of the distal ulnar tunnel. *Clin Orthop Relat Res.* 1985;(196):238-247.

22. Latinovic R, Gulliford MC, Hughes RA. Incidence of common compressive neuropathies in primary care. *J Neurol Neurosurg Psychiatry.* 2006;77(2):263-265.

23. Naam NH, Nemani S. Radial tunnel syndrome. *Orthop Clin North Am.* 2012;43(4):529-536.

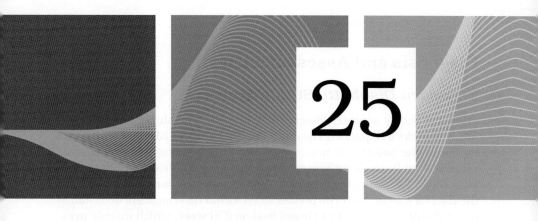

Foot and Ankle Manifestations of Multiple Sclerosis

■ ▓ ▓ Rock CJay Positano, Michael A. Ciaramella, Rock G. Positano, Molly Forlines

Introduction

The foot and ankle are often overlooked in the assessment of patients with multiple sclerosis (MS). Yet, much of our sense of balance and stability stems from the foundation provided by the foot and ankle. Given that mobility dysfunction consistently ranks among the most high-impact symptoms of MS, it is important to recognize the ways in which subtle alterations in the structure and function of the foot and ankle play an important role in symptom severity and disease progression in MS. It is also important to understand the ways in which common foot and ankle pathologies may interact with symptoms of MS in a way that either masks one or exacerbates both. The purpose of this chapter is to review the ways in which the foot and ankle contribute to the overall presentation of a patient with MS and to discuss treatments that involve the foot and ankle.

Diagnosis and Assessment Tests

Expanded Disability Status Scale

The most widely accepted diagnostic tool used to evaluate patients with MS is Kurtzke's Expanded Disability Status Scale, or EDSS.[1,2] The EDSS evaluates the severity of impairment due to MS using a 10-point scale ranging from 0, the least severe cases of MS, to 10, death resulting from MS.[2] Steps 1.0 through 4.5 refer to patients who are ambulatory without the use of a walking aid. The precise steps within this range are determined by a subscale called the Functional System (FS) score, which include pyramidal (motor function), cerebellar, brainstem, sensory, bowel and bladder, visual, cerebral or mental, and other functions. The FS subscale ranges from 0 to 5 or 6. An EDSS score between 1.0 and 4.5 should not change by 1.0 step unless there is also a change in the same direction in at least one FS.[3] A patient's ability to walk plays a critical role in determining the EDSS score because the difference between grades 4.0 through 6.0 are assigned based on how far a patient can walk without ambulatory assistance, with the differences between 4.0, 4.5, 5.0, and 5.5 being the ability to walk 500, 300, 200, or 100 m, respectively.[3,4] Patients with an EDSS score between 1.0 and 6.5 stand to gain the most from orthopedic interventions to improve balance and mobility.

Modified Ashworth Scale

About 84% of patients with MS are affected by spasticity, a disabling symptom of MS associated with reduced mobility, painful spasms, and sleep disturbances.[5] The Modified Ashworth Scale (MAS) measures muscle resistance during passive movement. Resistance is scored on a six-point scale (0, 1, 1+, 2, 3, 4), where 0 indicates no increased resistance and 4 indicates rigid flexion or extension.[6,7] The MAS is the preferred measure of spasticity because of its clinical interrater consistency. Knowledge of a patient's level of spasticity can help clinicians determine a treatment plan. The key to successful spasticity management is striking a balance between the beneficial and negative aspects of treatment, specifically with pharmacological interventions.[8]

The 25-Foot Walk

Another method of monitoring the disability status of patients with MS is the 25-Foot Walk (T25FW), a test of maximum walking speed on a short distance. When compared with other clinical measurements of ambulation, the results of the T25FW correlated strongly with those of the EDSS.[9] The T25FW is among the most commonly used standardized measurements of MS patient walking ability due to the ease of administration.

Foot and Ankle Involvement in Gait and Posture Dysfunction

Mobility dysfunction is one of the hallmark symptoms of MS and consistently ranks as the symptom with the largest impact on daily activities and quality of life.[10-13] Difficulty with walking affects more than 75% of individuals with the disease, and the degree of mobility dysfunction has been correlated with metrics of disease progression.[2,14,15] Additionally, it is estimated that between 50% and 63% of individuals with MS experience at least one fall over a 6- to 9-month period,[14,16,17] most commonly occurring while walking.[18,19] This places individuals with MS at risk for other traumatic musculoskeletal injuries resulting from falling[19,20] and cultivates a sense of fear of falling during ambulation, which can generate self-imposed limits on mobility.[16,21,22] Thus, a treatment plan targeting balance and mobility is important not only for reducing risk of injury due to falling but also for increasing overall quality of life and wellness.

Maintaining balance during standing and motion is a complex task involving several neurological mechanisms within the sensorimotor, vestibular, and visual systems.[23,24] In MS, each of these areas is affected to varying degrees. Owing to the heterogenous presentation of central nervous system lesions in MS, it was initially thought that impaired postural control and subsequent motor dysfunction in MS was multifactorial and inherently unpredictable from patient to patient.[25,26] This made the development of therapeutic strategies targeting mobility impairment very difficult. It has now been demonstrated that the origin of imbalance and mobility dysfunction in MS results primarily from a combination of slowed somatosensory conduction and impaired subsequent central integration,[27,28] impaired proprioceptive receptors in the lower extremity, and muscle weakness or spasticity.[27] A brief review of the ways in which these factors affect balance and movement is useful for understanding the compensatory movement strategies of individuals with MS and the overall burden of MS on the musculoskeletal system.

Neurological Origins of Gait and Posture Dysfunction

Spinal somatosensory conduction and central integration within the brain are closely related in coordinating balance and movement. Each of these is affected in individuals with MS.[25,29,30] Lesions in the dorsal column of the spinal cord are responsible for slowed somatosensory conduction. Regarding lower extremity motor control, slowed somatosensory conduction within the spinal cord results in the delayed transmission of proprioceptive information from the lower extremity to the brain. Consequently, the brain is given less time to integrate proprioceptive information and pro-duce an appropriate motor response. In a study assessing somatosensory conduction, individuals with MS exhibited delayed somatosensory evoked potentials within the cerebellum in response to an external stimulus per-turbing balance in comparison with healthy controls. This was shown to result in larger postural response latencies as well as exacerbated and asymmetric movement scaling during compensatory movements.[29] Slower postural response latencies have also been correlated with poorer mea-sures of balance, such as increased postural sway.[31] Additionally, the degree of MS lesions in the dorsal column has been correlated with poorer measures of sensation.[32]

Individuals with MS have been shown to recruit alternative neural circuitry in additional regions of the cerebellar and cerebral cortices for postural motor learning and rely more heavily on feed-forward control for balance involving other senses.[28,33] This is supported by the findings that individuals with MS may require higher cognitive demands during ambu-lation. This is evidenced by the observations that they perform poorly on dual tasks involving motion than healthy controls[34,35] and that individuals with MS rely more heavily on sight for balance than healthy controls.[36-39] It is hypothesized that this is an adaptation to allow more proactive main-tenance of balance to correct for impaired movement compensation ability stemming from corticocerebellar conduction impairment.[33] Owing to the reliance on proactive balance management, individuals with MS exhibit a more cautious gait pattern to avoid positions of instability and reduce the necessity of compensatory postural adjustments.

Impaired proprioception receptors within the foot and ankle of indi-viduals with MS contribute to a deficit in sensory information available to coordinate body position and maintain balance. Muscle spindles and other mechanoreceptors around the ankle joint are of particular impor-tance for reducing body sway while standing and for maintaining overall balance.[40] In MS, lack of dorsiflexion with a limited range of motion at the ankle joint from spasticity and muscle weakness reduces the amount of proprioceptive information provided from the ankle.[35,41-43] Individuals with MS therefore often compensate for reduced ankle mobility by increasing motion at the hip.[42,44] Additionally, mechanoreceptor sensitivity along the plantar surface of the foot, particularly beneath the heel and first meta-tarsal head, is often reduced in MS. Individuals with MS have been shown to score significantly worse on two-point discrimination tests along the plantar surface of the foot, indicating decreased light touch sensitivity, and degree of sensitivity has been correlated with balance performance and EDSS score.[45] It is unclear, however, if this lack of sensitivity is reflective of truly impaired peripheral sensation or impaired relay of sen-sory information via the spinal cord.[32] Regardless, because plantar sur-face mechanoreceptors provide important proprioceptive information, abnormal sensation also likely contributes to sensorimotor dysfunction via decreased proprioceptive information from the lower extremity. Thus, not only is proprioception information delayed via slowed somatosensory conduction, but it is also often incomplete owing to deficits in peripheral proprioceptive sensation.

Spasticity and Muscle Control

Impaired muscle control and spasticity in patients with MS stem from acquired imbalances between the intrinsic and extrinsic muscles of the foot due to the varying degrees of inflammatory involvement, progressive nerve demyelination, axonal disruption, interruption of efferent nerve conduction, and decreased inhibitory interneuron modulation. With disease progression, spasticity can lead to contractures, starting first with extensor spasms then later affecting flexor tone.[46,47] From these dynamic muscle imbalances comes the influence of equinus as a primary deforming force and its various compensations. Equinus is when the foot is in a more plantarflexed position (in relation to the lower leg) with limited ankle dorsiflexion and the subtalar joint in a neutral position.[48] Although contractures and deformities tend to occur later on in the disease progression, the most common site for contracture in patients with MS was noted to be at the ankle joint.[49] The ankle joint is a prime sagittal plane dominant joint (e.g., dorsiflexion/plantarflexion) of the distal extremity and is most capable of compensating for sagittal plane forces (e.g., equinus). When paired with an extended double support time as seen in MS,[50] equinus with spasticity and/or contracture affects the forefoot and medial aspects of the foot by increasing average ground reaction forces during mid to late stance and uncoupling the opposite "swing limb" during the swing phase of gait.[10,18,51] The degree of these imbalances is often determined by the level, extent, and areas of brain and spinal cord involvement. For example, lesions in the pyramidal tracts can cause varied weakness and spasticity, whereas lesions in the dorsal columns and cerebellar lesions can cause varied loss of coordination and proprioception (e.g., ataxia and postural sway).[1] Owing to the fact that the possible pedal deformities found in MS assume a more rigid or contracted attitude over time, stressing supination or mass flexion/adduction toward the midline of the body, the foot is never allowed to properly transition to an effective "mobile adaptor" during midstance to "accept" the ground and effectively. The combination of spasticity and/or contractures, equinus, postural balance/proprioceptive discoordination, and increased shearing ground reaction forces (especially vertical and horizontal/linear) creates an environment that is both destructive and kinesthetically inefficient to the maintenance of proper joint mechanics and bipedal ambulation in an already compromised individual.

Overall Movement Impairment and Compensation Strategies

Instability caused by the aforementioned factors results in overall movement impairment and a constant effort to remain balanced through compensatory movements. These strategies are generally aimed at better controlling the body's center of mass (COM) during gait, avoiding positions of instability imposed by motion, and allowing additional time for integration of sensory information and execution of compensatory movements. As the disease progresses, these compensatory strategies become increasingly noticeable clinically and contribute to decreased quality of life. However, even if there appears to be an absence of disability upon clinical presentation, motion analysis tools can be used to detect minute gait abnormalities in MS patients, leading to a more precise EDSS score.[2,52] Beyond disease progression, movement impairment has also been shown to correlate with increased incidence of falls and subsequent fear of falling in MS. Therefore, patients who have a history of falls in MS often exhibit more cautious movement strategies.[16,17,21,25]

There are several general alterations in gait that are commonly employed by patients with MS. These alterations are characterized by decreased walking velocity, shorter stride length, and wider step width. Additionally, individuals with MS exhibit a higher proportion of time in the double stance phase of gait, in which both feet are in contact with the ground. These alterations can be noticed clinically at later stages of disease progression and can also be detected in the absence of clinical disability through motion analysis tools. As the disease progresses, gait often becomes more variable owing to increasing difficulty controlling the body's COM within the region of stability.[53,54] The sum of these general alterations serves three purposes: (1) to allow increased time for somatosensory integration and planning of an appropriate response to maintain balance; (2) to control the COM within the margins of stability of the body and avoid unnecessary positions of imbalance; (3) to limit energy expenditure on compensation and therefore limit fatigue.

Impaired balance control also affects the anticipatory postural adjustments (APAs) individuals with MS employ before the initiation of gait. APAs are a form of feed-forward balance control in which muscle activation opposing the desired direction of movement occurs before motion to maintain balance during motion.[23] During gait, healthy individuals exhibit slight posterior and lateral COM displacement generated by APAs in anticipation of forthcoming anterior COM displacement during motion. Individuals with MS exhibit significantly less anticipatory posterior COM displacement. This reflects a combination of slower overall gait pattern and impaired ability to execute APAs owing to slowed sensorimotor conduction.[55,56] Additionally, individuals with MS show delayed onset of APAs both before gait and before an unanticipated balance perturbing stimulus.

Furthermore, these APAs show significantly less amplitude than in healthy controls regardless of the perturbing stimulus.[55] Finally, APA impairment is more significant before backward stepping than forward stepping, indicating that eye sight plays a role in APAs in individuals with MS.[57] The degree of APA impairment also correlates with the EDSS score.[57,58]

Owing to impaired feed-forward balance control, individuals with MS must employ greater compensatory movement strategies to maintain balance. However, the ability to execute these compensatory movements depends on the degree of disease progression in relation to the aforementioned factors of slowed somatosensory conduction, impaired proprioceptive sensation, and impaired muscle control or spasticity. Overall, one of the most common compensation strategies in patients with MS is to redistribute mechanical work of walking from the ankle joint to the hip.[56,59-61] This allows for reduced reliance on the ankle joint, which is most affected by spasticity or contracture.[43] Compensatory hip movement is often asymmetric, favoring less-impaired extremity. The hip increases the medial-lateral sway and plays a more significant role in anteroposterior control than in healthy controls. Although this compensatory strategy helps maintain balance, it has also been shown to require more energy and contribute to fatigue in patients with MS.[62,63]

Another result of increased hip motion is that it changes the COM movement pattern during gait and subsequently affects the average position of the ground reaction force. The culmination of this effect is a tendency for individuals with MS to avoid placing pressure near the lateral and posterior boarders of the foot. When the trunk moves in the lateral direction, the body aligns COM and COP closer within the base of support to maintain balance. Therefore, individuals with MS show a generally greater dynamic margin of stability, indicative of an avoidance of positions of instability.[64]

Local Alterations in Foot Structure and Function Affecting Movement

Each of the aforementioned mechanisms of balance impairment and compensation affect the function of the foot and ankle. Until recently, however, little attention has been spent on elucidating the specific alterations to foot structure and function in patients with MS. It is known that individuals with MS overpronate in an atypical way during gait.[65] Where typical pronation exhibits increased plantar pressure under the medial longitudinal arch and under metatarsal heads two and three, patients with MS show increased pressure under the first metatarsal head and the medial longitudinal arch. During gait, therefore, the trend is for patients with MS to exhibit more than usual pressure toward the midline and anteriorly. This appears to be consistent with previous work done on compensation strategies and sources of gait impairment in MS. For example, increased medial and anterior plantar pressure coincides well with the finding that individuals with MS avoid the lateral and posterior boarders of the feet, thereby shifting weight toward the midline and forward. This unique pressure distribution may reflect an attempt to compensate for balance and proprioception deficits and maintain a stable position. That said, more work needs to be done in this regard.

Interactions Between Foot and Ankle Musculoskeletal Pathologies and MS Symptoms

The Effect of MS Symptoms on Foot and Ankle Musculoskeletal Health

An important factor affecting musculoskeletal health in patients with MS is the effect of equinus due to impaired muscle coordination or spasticity. This equinus deforming force is found in the sagittal plane and increases the axial load stresses placed on the foot, specifically the forefoot and midfoot.[66,67] It is considered one of the most destructive forces on the foot and ankle.[68] Equinus is a congenital or acquired lack of ankle dorsiflexion or a plantarflexed attitude of the foot on the lower leg with the subtalar joint in a neutral position.[48] Plantar flexor muscles, such as the gastrocnemius and soleus, account for up to 54.5% of the force in the foot.[69] This makes it specifically difficult for the foot, even under nonpathological circumstances, to counterbalance this natural "equinus urge" of the body. What equinus does is displace the center of gravity more anteriorly, encouraging the body and foot to rock back more in an attempt to balance out forces to a limited extent. As a result, there is an increase or focus in axial loading forces on the forefoot and midfoot generally during mid to late stance around the second peak vertical force of gait when 2.7 to 9 times the body weight centers on the forefoot.[70] Owing to the added vestibular and proprioceptive challenges MS presents, the patient's ability to properly adjust for this anterior shift in the center of gravity becomes more difficult and subsequently increases forefoot shearing forces during stance and lateral postural "sway."[71] This deviation can further accelerate or magnify various forefoot/medial foot overuse injuries (e.g., bursitis, capsulitis, tendonitis) and fracture risk via abnormal joint reaction forces wherever and whenever the foot comes in contact with the ground and the muscles failed attempt to overpower the stronger ground reactive forces.[72] Also, as often with contractures, the lever arm of the specific muscles involved becomes shorter and less powerful and fatigues more easily owing to impaired excitation-contraction coupling and functional length.

Compensation for pedal deformities and derangements is generally based on where the next best or largest degree of available motion in that specific plane is found. The joints of the lower extremity affected the most by sagittal plane (equinus) forces include:

1. First ray/first metaphalangeal joint (MPJ) and/or MPJs 2 to 5
2. Oblique axis of the midtarsal joint and subtalar joint
3. Ankle
4. Knee
5. Hips/pelvis
6. Spine/lower back

Possible compensation mechanisms for an equinus deformity can include all or one of the following[27]:

1. Toe walking (e.g., toe-to-heel gait)
2. Early heel lift (e.g., pronation of the oblique midtarsal joint (MTJ) axis and subtalor joint (STJ) with an "abductory twist")
3. Abduction of the foot and leg/externally rotated "out toe"-type gait with possible leg circumduction (e.g., pronation of the MTJ and STJ or circumduction-type gait)
4. Shorter stride lengths (e.g., reduces demand placed on the first MPJ)
5. Knee extension (e.g., genu recurvatum—knee hyperextension or "back bend")
6. Lumbar lordosis (e.g., lumbar hyperextension or "swayback")

Any one or more of these components, although subtle especially to the untrained eye, may be part of a larger pathological process. Identification and/or prevention, if possible, of these manifestations would greatly improve the patient's quality of life by avoiding overuse injuries caused by unnecessary burden on the musculoskeletal system and by impeding progression of immobility.

The Interaction of Common Foot and Ankle Musculoskeletal Pathologies with MS Symptoms

Foot and/or ankle pain is highly common in the general population, affecting an estimated one in five adults and increasing with age and other factors such as obesity.[73,74] Given its high prevalence, foot and/or ankle pain of some type is likely to arise as a comorbidity at some point in the progression of a patient with MS, particularly when ambulation impairment is minimal. It is therefore important for MS specialists to understand the ways in which sources of foot and ankle pain may interact with MS symptoms.

Foot and ankle musculoskeletal pain can stem from several sources, including overuse, trauma, and structural alterations. A common source of foot and ankle pain stems from chronic overuse of tendon or ligament structures during ambulation causing either a degenerative or inflammatory process within the structure or surrounding soft tissues. This can be caused not only by an underlying biomechanical alteration in the function of the foot, placing excess pressure on a particular region, but can also arise idiopathically. This commonly manifests as Achilles tendinopathy, plantar fasciitis, posterior tibial tendon dysfunction, or capsulitis of one of the metatarsophalangeal joints (most commonly the first MTP joint). Overuse may also cause a Morton neuroma to become symptomatic. Additionally, sources of trauma such as an ankle inversion or eversion can contribute to or exacerbate tendon degeneration/inflammation, or even cause a tear. Ankle inversion injuries frequently cause damage to the lateral collateral ligaments (to a varying degree depending on the intensity of the inversion), as well as damage to the peroneal tendons and deltoid ligament. Significant ankle trauma may also result in a fracture. Finally, changes in the bony structures, such as midfoot, ankle joint, or forefoot arthritis, or deformities such as bunions or bunionettes (tailor's bunion) may also cause significant pain in the foot.

When patients with MS present with one of the aforementioned pathologies, the most significant interaction is between foot and ankle pain and gait dysfunction. Drawing upon the earlier discussion of compensation strategies observed in patients with MS, the following are a few examples of interactions in which a foot or ankle pathology negatively affects the ability of a patient with MS to ambulate with a compensation strategy:

- More frequent and shorter strides may exacerbate heel pain or Achilles tendinopathy by increasing the number of heel strikes and push-offs.[53,54]
- Increased pronation during gait may exacerbate first MTP capsulitis and generate increased inflammation of the capsule, causing pain. It may also generate increased inflammation and forefoot pain in the presence of a bunion deformity by creating a source of overuse in the region.[66]
- Avoidance of the lateral boarder of the foot may shift pressure medially, creating increasing medial longitudinal arch pressure and subsequently exacerbating posterior tibial tendinopathy.[65]

Although it is important to recognize these potential interactions, it is difficult to predict how foot and ankle pain would affect compensation more globally. It seems that the response to foot pain would be highly individual, likely including some method to reduce pressure on the injured region. However, in patients with MS with existing balance deficiencies, making these adjustments would likely be difficult. Given this uncertainty, it is all the more important to recognize, diagnose, and treat the accompanying foot and/or ankle pathology as to reduce pain and increase the ability to ambulate.

Other Foot and Ankle Pathologies Associated With Multiple Sclerosis

Foot Drop "Talipes Equinus"

Foot drop is commonly found in patients with MS.[31] It occurs from damage to or involvement of the common peroneal nerve (L4, L5, S1) creating a loss of function or weakness in the dorsiflexors of the foot and ankle (e.g., tibialis anterior, extensor digitorum longus muscle) and/or lateral compartments (e.g., peroneus longus and brevis). This deficit leads to an inability of the foot to clear the ground during the swing phase of gait, which can lead to an increased risk of trips and falls (e.g., steppage gait). The position of the foot is found in a plantarflexed and inverted attitude.

Erythromelalgia

Erythromelalgia is a rare acquired or inherited clinical syndrome that is characterized by erythematous, hot, and painful distal extremities, generally affecting the foot and ankle. Although this condition is associated secondarily to myeloproliferative disorders, diabetes, and spinal cord injury, it has also been linked to MS.[75]

Complex Regional Pain Syndrome

Complex regional pain syndrome is a painful disorder that involves changes to somatosensory, sympathetic, and sudomotor systems generally after a traumatic event with or without evidence of peripheral nerve injury. Although this condition is traditionally associated with trauma, it has also been linked to patients with MS.[76,77]

Onychomycosis

Onchomycosis is a fungal infection of the nail bed and nail plate most commonly by dermatophytes (*Trichophyton rubrum*). It can present in varied ways and locations on the nail depending on the infecting organism (e.g., fungus, mold, yeast) and comorbidities. MS is considered a neurological risk factor associated with developing onychomycosis, especially if the patient is taking an immune-modulating therapy.[78]

Nutritional Deficiencies

Either B12 or vitamin D deficiency has been seen in patients with MS. Both vitamins are essential components in maintaining nerve (e.g., myelin sheath) and bone health and structure. These deficiencies can lead to further muscle weakness and/or symptoms of distal peripheral neuropathy further complicating the decreased proprioceptive/balance abilities and increased risk of pathological fractures from osteoporosis in patients with MS.[79,80]

Treatment

Although there are many available options for treating the foot and ankle complications of MS and improving balance, the success of each therapy varies widely from one patient to the next. These options include exercise and balance-based therapies, functional electrical stimulation (FES), foot and ankle orthoses, and pharmaceutical therapies. The addition of one or more of these therapies to an MS treatment regimen can improve the quality of life for patients with MS by restoring confidence in their mobility, reducing the risk of falling, and potentially slowing down the deterioration of musculoskeletal function. An added benefit of these therapies is the prevention of secondary orthopedic complications, such as deterioration of the knees, hips, or lower back. However, because these complications originate in the central nervous system, the patient's neurologist should be consulted on any therapeutic intervention. A neurologist can also determine the source of a patient's impairment, which allows the musculoskeletal specialist to implement the therapy best suited for the patient.

Exercise-Based Therapy

For patients with MS who are still able to walk with minimum support (EDSS scores between 2.5 and 4.5), exercise-based therapies to improve balance and mobility should be considered as the primary treatment option for orthopedic complications of MS in the lower extremities.[81] Clinical trials have indicated that engaging in balance-training exercises 2 to 3 days a week for a duration of 10 to 40 minutes (depending on the severity of disability) can result in improved mobility, coinciding with an improvement in balance.[4,82] Balance exercises are those that target lower-limb strength and core muscle strength.

Exergaming, or a video game that incorporates physical exercise, has been proposed as a useful method of rehabilitating patients. The games used in trials for MS treatments require the patient to use a balance board while playing the game.[83] Unlike traditional exercise and balance-training routines, exergaming tends to be more enjoyable for patients. As a result, patients often demonstrate better adherence to training programs that incorporate exergaming in comparison with traditional methods. One study showed that exergaming enhanced balancing abilities not only during single-task walking but also during multitask walking. This is significant because the majority of patients with balance impairments report a higher incidence of falls while attempting to text, talk, read, or perform other activities while walking.[84,85]

In addition to rehabilitating balance and mobility, exercise training may also affect peripheral inflammatory markers and the physical structure of white and gray matter in the brain.[86,87] High aerobic capacity, achievable through exercises such as cycling, aquatic exercise, or walking, has been shown to correlate positively with gray matter volume, as well as white matter integrity in people with MS.[88] Because the loss of body functions in people with MS involves damage of white and gray matter in the brain, the discovery that exercise can retard that function could change the way MS is treated. However, a great deal more research is needed to prove the efficacy of exercise on neurological functioning in patients with MS.

The main limitation of exercise-based therapies is that the benefits seem to last only as long as the patient keeps up with the exercise routine.[81] Additionally, although balance-exercise routines have been shown to improve balance, more studies are needed to determine whether they have an effect on the number of falls that a patient with MS experiences. However, of the interventions available, exercise-rehabilitation therapy tends to be the most successful in restoring mobility.

Functional Electrical Stimulation

FES refers to an application of electrical stimulation to induce a muscle contraction that generates movement and is used to treat foot drop in patients with MS.[89] In the case of most clinical trials in which an FES device is used to stimulate dorsiflexion in people with MS, one electrode is placed over the common peroneal nerve where it passes the head of the fibula and the other electrode is placed over the motor point of the tibialis anterior.[90,91] Depending on the device, a built-in gait sensor or heel-switch worn on the heel synchronizes the stimulation with the patient's gait. The electrodes fire when the heel is lifted at the beginning of the swing phase and are turned off when the heel makes contact with the ground.[92] The FES activation helps to maintain dorsiflexion for the entire swing phase, reducing the energy cost and increasing the speed of walking.[89,93]

FES has been shown to increase walking speed both initially and for varying amounts of time after intervention.[94] Compared with custom orthoses, FES systems do not need to be custom made and are more readily available to a wider range of people. The electrical stimulation can also serve to stimulate blood circulation and contribute to improved overall cardiovascular health.[81,92] However, FES can only improve walking speed in individuals who are still able to walk with minimal assistance (EDSS: 1-4.5). FES surface stimulators are functional only if they are placed correctly. Because the surface stimulator devices are removed before a patient goes to sleep, they must be replaced each morning by the patient, so the margin of error for placement is high, especially in patients with impaired cognition.[11] Although implantable FES systems are available, they have the added complications associated with any internally placed device. Finally, there are little data to indicate that FES can stabilize balance issues in patients with MS.[89,93]

Orthotic

Custom foot and ankle orthoses have long been the stable of treatment for the orthopedic complications of MS, particularly in those who have a drop foot. As mentioned earlier, patients with MS tend to have decreased walking ability, caused by weakened plantar flexor muscles that reduce the patient's ability to push off with the ankle.[95] The classic construction of an ankle-foot orthotic (AFO) device consists of a dorsal leaf spring placed in the shoe and a right-angled carbon spring that extends vertically to the mid-calf.[96] Hinge-type devices with bilateral steel joints are also considered. The AFO is customized to each patient's ability and can help maintain the ankle's neutral position using the tension of the calf muscles, preserve some push-off, and, in some cases, provide push-off. One study showed that an AFO can reduce the energy cost of walking by up to 9.8%.[95]

There are some limitations to AFOs. Most significantly, they are only successful in increasing a patient's push-off ability while they are worn, whereas exercise and FES have been shown to have extended therapeutic effects on mobility. Additionally, the potential for muscle atrophy occurring in the calf should also be considered for treatment plans involving AFOs, because they reduce the muscular activity required. AFOs are also limited by the manufacturer and, if made incorrectly, could actually hinder a patient's ability to push off from the ankle.[97]

Medical

There are several pharmaceutical options available to reduce the musculoskeletal complications of MS. Clinical data suggest that cannabinoids, derived from the *Cannabis sativa* plant, could be useful in reducing spasticity and chronic pain associated with MS, as well as other inflammatory diseases.[98] Although our understanding of the neurobiological mechanisms has advanced significantly, there is still a need for more medicinal options for treating the physical symptoms of MS. Other treatments include isoniazid, an antibiotic used in the treatment of tuberculosis, which has been shown to reduce tremors in patients with MS, and benzodiazepines to control mild to moderate spasticity.[24,99] However, these medications should not be prescribed without consulting a neurologist, who can help determine what treatment would be the most effective for a patient with MS.

References

1. Kurtzke JF. On the origin of EDSS. *Mult Scler Relat Disord.* 2015;4(2):95-103.
2. Cao H, Peyrodie L, Boudet S, et al. Expanded Disability Status Scale (EDSS) estimation in multiple sclerosis from posturographic data. *Gait Posture.* 2013;37(2):242-245.
3. Kurtzke JF. Rating neurologic impairment in multiple sclerosis: an Expanded Disability Status Scale (EDSS). *Neurology.* 1983;33(11):1444-1452.
4. Dalla-Costa G, Radaelli M, Maida S, et al. Smart watch, smarter EDSS: improving disability assessment in multiple sclerosis clinical practice. *J Neurol Sci.* 2017;383:166-168.
5. Rizzo M, Hadjimichael O, Preiningerova J, Vollmer T. Prevalence and treatment of spasticity reported by multiple sclerosis patients. *Mult Scler.* 2004;10(5):589-595.
6. Charalambous CP. *Interrater Reliability of A Modified Ashworth Scale of Muscle Spasticity. Classic Papers in Orthopaedics.* Springer; 2014:415-417.
7. Waninge A, Rook R, Dijkhuizen A, Gielen E, Van Der Schans C. Feasibility, test–retest reliability, and interrater reliability of the Modified Ashworth Scale and Modified Tardieu Scale in persons with profound intellectual and multiple disabilities. *Res Dev Disabil.* 2011;32(2):613-620.
8. Ehling R, Edlinger M, Hermann K, et al. Successful long-term management of spasticity in patients with multiple sclerosis using a software application (APP): a pilot study. *Mult Scler Relat Disord.* 2017;17:15-21.
9. Bethoux FA, Palfy DM, Plow MA. Correlates of the timed 25 foot walk in a multiple sclerosis outpatient rehabilitation clinic. *Int J Rehabil Res.* 2016;39(2):134.
10. LaRocca NG. Impact of walking impairment in multiple sclerosis. *Patient.* 2011;4(3):189-201.
11. Zwibel HL. Contribution of impaired mobility and general symptoms to the burden of multiple sclerosis. *Adv Therapy.* 2009;26(12):1043-1057.
12. Sutliff MH. Contribution of impaired mobility to patient burden in multiple sclerosis. *Curr Med Res Opin.* 2010;26(1):109-119.
13. Heesen C, Böhm J, Reich C, Kasper J, Goebel M, Gold S. Patient perception of bodily functions in multiple sclerosis: gait and visual function are the most valuable. *Mult Scler.* 2008;14(7):988-991.
14. Nilsagård Y, Lundholm C, Denison E, Gunnarsson L-G. Predicting accidental falls in people with multiple sclerosis—a longitudinal study. *Clin Rehabil.* 2009;23(3):259-269.
15. Swingler R, Compston D. The morbidity of multiple sclerosis. *Q J Med.* 1992;83(1):325-337.
16. Peterson EW, Cho CC, Finlayson ML. Fear of falling and associated activity curtailment among middle aged and older adults with multiple sclerosis. *Mult Scler.* 2007;13(9):1168-1175.
17. Cattaneo D, De Nuzzo C, Fascia T, Macalli M, Pisoni I, Cardini R. Risks of falls in subjects with multiple sclerosis. *Arch Phys Med Rehabil.* 2002;83(6):864-867.
18. Peterson EW, Ari EB, Asano M, Finlayson ML. Fall attributions among middle-aged and older adults with multiple sclerosis. *Arch Phys Med Rehabil.* 2013;94(5):890-895.
19. Matsuda PN, Shumway-Cook A, Bamer AM, Johnson SL, Amtmann D, Kraft GH. Falls in multiple sclerosis. *PM R.* 2011;3(7):624-632.
20. Peterson EW, Cho CC, von Koch L, Finlayson ML. Injurious falls among middle aged and older adults with multiple sclerosis. *Arch Phys Med Rehabil.* 2008;89(6):1031-1037.

21. Peebles AT, Bruetsch AP, Lynch SG, Huisinga JM. Dynamic balance in persons with multiple sclerosis who have a falls history is altered compared to non-fallers and to healthy controls. *J Biomech.* 2017;63:158-163.

22. Matsuda PN, Shumway-Cook A, Ciol MA, Bombardier CH, Kartin DA. Understanding falls in multiple sclerosis: association of mobility status, concerns about falling, and accumulated impairments. *Phys Ther.* 2012;92(3):407-415.

23. Massion J. Movement, posture and equilibrium: interaction and coordination. *Prog Neurobiol.* 1992;38(1):35-56.

24. Winter DA. Human balance and posture control during standing and walking. *Gait Posture.* 1995;3(4):193-214.

25. Cameron MH, Lord S. Postural control in multiple sclerosis: implications for fall prevention. *Curr Neurol Neurosci Rep.* 2010;10(5):407-412.

26. Corradini ML, Fioretti S, Leo T, Piperno R. Early recognition of postural disorders in multiple sclerosis through movement analysis: a modeling study. *IEEE Trans Biomed Eng.* 1997;44(11):1029-1038.

27. Sosnoff JJ, Socie MJ, Boes MK, et al. Mobility, balance and falls in persons with multiple sclerosis. *PLoS One.* 2011;6(11):e28021.

28. Fling BW, Dutta GG, Schlueter H, Cameron MH, Horak FB. Associations between proprioceptive neural pathway structural connectivity and balance in people with multiple sclerosis. *Front Hum Neurosci.* 2014;8:814.

29. Cameron MH, Horak FB, Herndon RR, Bourdette D. Imbalance in multiple sclerosis: a result of slowed spinal somatosensory conduction. *Somatosens Mot Res.* 2008;25(2):113-122.

30. Cameron MH, Wagner JM. Gait abnormalities in multiple sclerosis: pathogenesis, evaluation, and advances in treatment. *Curr Neurol Neurosci Rep.* 2011;11(5):507.

31. Huisinga JM, St George RJ, Spain R, Overs S, Horak FB. Postural response latencies are related to balance control during standing and walking in patients with multiple sclerosis. *Arch Phys Med Rehabil.* 2014;95(7):1390-1397.

32. Zackowski KM, Smith SA, Reich DS, et al. Sensorimotor dysfunction in multiple sclerosis and column-specific magnetization transfer-imaging abnormalities in the spinal cord. *Brain.* 2009;132(5):1200-1209.

33. Fling BW, Dutta GG, Horak FB. Functional connectivity underlying postural motor adaptation in people with multiple sclerosis. *Neuroimage Clin.* 2015;8:281-289.

34. Hamilton F, Rochester L, Paul L, Rafferty D, O'Leary C, Evans J. Walking and talking: an investigation of cognitive—motor dual tasking in multiple sclerosis. *Mult Scler.* 2009;15(10):1215-1227. doi:10.1177/1352458509106712. PubMed PMID: 19667011.

35. Leone C, Patti F, Feys P. Measuring the cost of cognitive-motor dual tasking during walking in multiple sclerosis. *Mult Scler.* 2015;21(2):123-131.

36. Comber L, Sosnoff JJ, Galvin R, Coote S. Postural control deficits in people with multiple sclerosis: a systematic review and meta-analysis. *Gait Posture.* 2018;61:445-452.

37. Van Emmerik RE, Remelius JG, Johnson MB, Chung LH, Kent-Braun JA. Postural control in women with multiple sclerosis: effects of task, vision and symptomatic fatigue. *Gait Posture.* 2010;32(4):608-614. doi:10.1016/j.gaitpost.2010.09.002. Epub 2010/10/15. PubMed PMID: 20943393.

38. Huisinga JM, Yentes JM, Filipi ML, Stergiou N. Postural control strategy during standing is altered in patients with multiple sclerosis. *Neurosci Lett.* 2012;524(2):124-128. doi:10.1016/j.neulet.2012.07.020. Epub 2012/07/25. PubMed PMID: 22824302.

39. McLoughlin J, Barr C, Crotty M, Lord SR, Sturnieks DL. Association of postural sway with disability status and cerebellar dysfunction in people with multiple sclerosis: a preliminary study. *Int J MS Care.* 2015;17(3):146-151.
40. Fitzpatrick R, Rogers DK, McCloskey D. Stable human standing with lower-limb muscle afferents providing the only sensory input. *J Physiol.* 1994;480(2):395-403.
41. Lee Y, Chen K, Ren Y, et al. Robot-guided ankle sensorimotor rehabilitation of patients with multiple sclerosis. *Mult Scler Relat Disord.* 2017;11:65-70. doi:10.1016/j.msard.2016.12.006. Epub 2017/01/21. PubMed PMID: 28104260.
42. Chua MC, Hyngstrom AS, Ng AV, Schmit BD. Relative changes in ankle and hip control during bilateral joint movements in persons with multiple sclerosis. *Clin Neurophysiol.* 2014;125(6):1192-1201.
43. Psarakis M, Greene D, Moresi M, et al. Impaired heel to toe progression during gait is related to reduced ankle range of motion in people with multiple sclerosis. *Clin Biomech (Bristol, Avon).* 2017;49:96-100. doi:10.1016/j.clinbio-mech.2017.08.012. Epub 2017/09/13. PubMed PMID: 28898816.
44. Davies BL, Hoffman RM, Kurz MJ. Individuals with multiple sclerosis redistribute positive mechanical work from the ankle to the hip during walking. *Gait Posture.* 2016;49:329-333.
45. Citaker S, Gunduz AG, Guclu MB, Nazliel B, Irkec C, Kaya D. Relationship between foot sensation and standing balance in patients with multiple sclerosis. *Gait Posture.* 2011;34(2):275-278.
46. Perry J, Hoffer MM, Giovan P, Antonelli D, Greenberg R. Gait analysis of the triceps surae in cerebral palsy: a preoperative and postoperative clinical and electromyographic study. *J Bone Joint Surg Am.* 1974;56(3):511-520.
47. Perry J, Giovan P, Harris LJ, Montgomery J, Azaria M. The determinants of muscle action in the hemiparetic lower extremity:(and their effect on the examination procedure)The determinants of muscle action in the hemiparetic lower extremity:(and their effect on the examination procedure)The determinants of muscle action in the hemiparetic lower extremity:(and their effect on the examination procedure). *Clin Orthop Relat Res.* 1978;(131):71-89.
48. Chakravarty A, Mukherjee A. Spasticity mechanisms – for the clinician. *Front Neurol.* 2010;1:149.
49. Vachranukunkiet T, Esquenazi A. Pathophysiology of gait disturbance in neurologic disorders and clinical presentations. *Phys Med Rehabil Clin N Am.* 2013;24(2):233-246.
50. Dibble LE, Lopez-Lennon C, Lake W, Hoffmeister C, Gappmaier E. Utility of disease-specific measures and clinical balance tests in prediction of falls in persons with multiple sclerosis. *J Neurol Phys Ther.* 2013;37(3):99-104.
51. Cazeau C, Stiglitz Y. Effects of gastrocnemius tightness on forefoot during gait. *Foot Ankle Clin.* 2014;19(4):649-657.
52. Shanahan CJ, Boonstra F, Cofre Lizama E, et al. Technologies for advanced gait and balance assessments in people with multiple sclerosis. *Front Neurol.* 2017;8:708.
53. Sosnoff JJ, Sandroff BM, Motl RW. Quantifying gait abnormalities in persons with multiple sclerosis with minimal disability. *Gait Posture.* 2012;36(1):154-156.
54. Comber L, Galvin R, Coote S. Gait deficits in people with multiple sclerosis: a systematic review and meta-analysis. *Gait Posture.* 2017;51:25-35.
55. Krishnan V, Kanekar N, Aruin AS. Anticipatory postural adjustments in individuals with multiple sclerosis. *Neurosci Lett.* 2012;506(2):256-260.

56. Remelius JG, Hamill J, Kent-Braun J, Van Emmerik RE. Gait initiation in multiple sclerosis. *Motor Control.* 2008;12(2):93-108.

57. Peterson DS, Huisinga JM, Spain RI, Horak FB. Characterization of compensatory stepping in people with multiple sclerosis. *Arch Phys Med Rehabil.* 2016;97(4):513-521.

58. Galli M, Coghe G, Sanna P, Cocco E, Marrosu MG, Pau M. Relationship between gait initiation and disability in individuals affected by multiple sclerosis. *Mult Scler Relat Disord.* 2015;4(6):594-597.

59. Chua MC, Hyngstrom AS, Ng AV, Schmit BD. Movement strategies for maintaining standing balance during arm tracking in people with multiple sclerosis. *J Neurophysiol.* 2014;112(7):1656-1666.

60. Huisinga JM, Mancini M, George RJS, Horak FB. Accelerometry reveals differences in gait variability between patients with multiple sclerosis and healthy controls. *Ann Biomed Eng.* 2013;41(8):1670-1679.

61. Huisinga JM, Schmid KK, Filipi ML, Stergiou N. Gait mechanics are different between healthy controls and patients with multiple sclerosis. *J Appl Biomech.* 2013;29(3):303-311.

62. Motl RW, Sandroff BM, Suh Y, Sosnoff JJ. Energy cost of walking and its association with gait parameters, daily activity, and fatigue in persons with mild multiple sclerosis. *Neurorehabil Neural Repair.* 2012;26(8):1015-1021. doi:10.1177/1545968312437943. PubMed PMID: 22466791.

63. Motl RW, Suh Y, Dlugonski D, et al. Oxygen cost of treadmill and overground walking in mildly disabled persons with multiple sclerosis. *Neurol Sci.* 2011;32(2):255-262.

64. Peebles AT, Reinholdt A, Bruetsch AP, Lynch SG, Huisinga JM. Dynamic margin of stability during gait is altered in persons with multiple sclerosis. *J Biomech.* 2016;49(16):3949-3955.

65. Fields C, Abbot K, Positano RG, et al. Foot structure, function and flexibility in MS patents (abstract). International Foot and Ankle Biomechanics Meeting. April 8-11, 2018.

66. Lavery LA, Armstrong DG, Boulton AJ. Ankle equinus deformity and its relationship to high plantar pressure in a large population with diabetes mellitus. *J Am Podiatric Med Assoc.* 2002;92(9):479-482.

67. Hoang PD, Gandevia SC, Herbert RD. Prevalence of joint contractures and muscle weakness in people with multiple sclerosis. *Disabil Rehabil.* 2014;36(19):1588-1593.

68. Schmid S, Schweizer K, Romkes J, Lorenzetti S, Brunner R. Secondary gait deviations in patients with and without neurological involvement: a systematic review. *Gait Posture.* 2013;37(4):480-493.

69. Guthrie TC, Nelson DA. Influence of temperature changes on multiple sclerosis: critical review of mechanisms and research potential. *J Neurol Sci.* 1995;129(1):1-8.

70. Valmassy R. *Clinical Biomechanics of the Lower Extremities.* St. Louis, Missouri, USA: Ed Mosby; 1996. ISBN 0-8016-7986-9.

71. Ganesan M, Kanekar N, Aruin AS. Direction-specific impairments of limits of stability in individuals with multiple sclerosis. *Ann Phys Rehabil Med.* 2015;58(3):145-150.

72. Hearn AP, Silber E. Osteoporosis in multiple sclerosis. *Mult Scler.* 2010;16(9):1031-1043.

73. Hill CL, Gill TK, Menz HB, Taylor AW. Prevalence and correlates of foot pain in a population-based study: the North West Adelaide health study. *J Foot Ankle Res.* 2008;1:2. doi:10.1186/1757-1146-1-2. PubMed PMID: 18822153; PubMed Central PMCID: PMCPMC2547889.

74. Thomas MJ, Roddy E, Zhang W, Menz HB, Hannan MT, Peat GM. The population prevalence of foot and ankle pain in middle and old age: a systematic review. *Pain.* 2011;152(12):2870-2880.

75. Morgan UMS. *Hallux Varus.* StatPearls; March 20, 2017.

76. Mailis A, Wade T. Profile of Caucasian women with possible genetic predisposition to reflex sympathetic dystrophy: a pilot study. *Clin J Pain.* 1994;10(3):210-217.

77. Rogers JN, Valley MA. Reflex sympathetic dystrophy. *Clin Podiatr Med Surg.* 1994;11(1):73-83. Epub 1994/01/01. PubMed PMID: 8124658.

78. Walton L, Villani MF. Principles and biomechanical considerations of tendon transfers. *Clin Podiatr Med Surg.* 2016;33(1):1-13.

79. Schwarz S, Leweling H. Multiple sclerosis and nutrition. *Mult Scler.* 2005;11(1):24-32. doi: 10.1191/1352458505ms1119oa. PubMed PMID: 15732263.

80. Beard S, Hunn A, Wight J. Treatments for spasticity and pain in multiple sclerosis: a systematic review. 2003.

81. Sosnoff JJ, Sung J. Reducing falls and improving mobility in multiple sclerosis. *Expert Rev Neurother.* 2015;15(6):655-666.

82. Motl RW, Pilutti LA. The benefits of exercise training in multiple sclerosis. *Nat Rev Neurol.* 2012;8(9):487.

83. Kramer A, Dettmers C, Gruber M. Exergaming with additional postural demands improves balance and gait in patients with multiple sclerosis as much as conventional balance training and leads to high adherence to home-based balance training. *Arch Phys Med Rehabil.* 2014;95(10):1803-1809.

84. Nilsagard YE, von Koch LK, Nilsson M, Forsberg AS. Balance exercise program reduced falls in people with multiple sclerosis: a single-group, pretest-posttest trial. *Arch Phys Med Rehabil.* 2014;95(12):2428-2434. Epub 2014/07/09. doi: 10.1016/j.apmr.2014.06.016. PubMed PMID: 25004466.

85. Azadian E, Torbati HRT, Kakhki ARS, Farahpour N. The effect of dual task and executive training on pattern of gait in older adults with balance impairment: a randomized controlled trial. *Arch Gerontol Geriatr.* 2016;62:83-89.

86. Nicklas BJ, Brinkley TE. Exercise training as a treatment for chronic inflammation in the elderly. *Exerc Sport Sci Rev.* 2009;37(4):165.

87. Golzari Z, Shabkhiz F, Soudi S, Kordi MR, Hashemi SM. Combined exercise training reduces IFN-γ and IL-17 levels in the plasma and the supernatant of peripheral blood mononuclear cells in women with multiple sclerosis. *Int Immunopharmacol.* 2010;10(11):1415-1419.

88. Prakash RS, Snook EM, Motl RW, Kramer AF. Aerobic fitness is associated with gray matter volume and white matter integrity in multiple sclerosis. *Brain Res.* 2010;1341:41-51.

89. Springer S, Khamis S. Effects of functional electrical stimulation on gait in people with multiple sclerosis–a systematic review. *Mult Scler Relat Disord.* 2017;13:4-12.

90. Coote S, Hughes L, Rainsford G, Minogue C, Donnelly A. Pilot randomized trial of progressive resistance exercise augmented by neuromuscular electrical stimulation for people with multiple sclerosis who use walking aids. *Arch Phys Med Rehabil.* 2015;96(2):197-204.

91. van der Linden ML, Scott SM, Hooper JE, Cowan P, Mercer TH. Gait kinematics of people with multiple sclerosis and the acute application of functional electrical stimulation. *Gait Posture.* 2014;39(4):1092-1096.

92. Kottink AI, Oostendorp LJ, Buurke JH, Nene AV, Hermens HJ, IJzerman MJ. The orthotic effect of functional electrical stimulation on the improvement of walking in stroke patients with a dropped foot: a systematic review. *Artif Organs.* 2004;28(6):577-586.

93. Miller L, McFadyen A, Lord AC, et al. Functional electrical stimulation for foot drop in multiple sclerosis: a systematic review and meta-analysis of the effect on gait speed. *Arch Phys Med Rehabil.* 2017;98(7):1435-1452.

94. Street T, Taylor P, Swain I. Effectiveness of functional electrical stimulation on walking speed, functional walking category, and clinically meaningful changes for people with multiple sclerosis. *Arch Phys Med Rehabil.* 2015;96(4):667-672.

95. Bregman D, Harlaar J, Meskers C, De Groot V. Spring-like ankle foot orthoses reduce the energy cost of walking by taking over ankle work. *Gait Posture.* 2012;35(1):148-153.

96. Wolf SI, Alimusaj M, Rettig O, Döderlein L. Dynamic assist by carbon fiber spring AFOs for patients with myelomeningocele. *Gait Posture.* 2008;28(1):175-177.

97. Bregman D, Rozumalski A, Koops D, De Groot V, Schwartz M, Harlaar J. A new method for evaluating ankle foot orthosis characteristics: BRUCE. *Gait Posture.* 2009;30(2):144-149.

98. Chiurchiù V, van der Stelt M, Centonze D, Maccarrone M. The endocannabinoid system and its therapeutic exploitation in multiple sclerosis: clues for other neuroinflammatory diseases. *Prog Neurobiol.* 2018;160:82-100.

99. Samkoff LM, Goodman AD. Symptomatic management in multiple sclerosis. *Neurol Clin.* 2011;29(2):449-463.

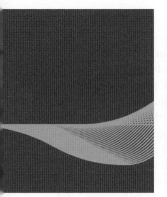
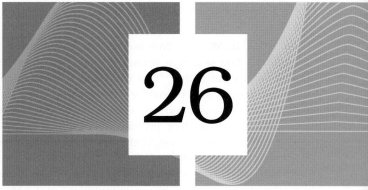

26

Common Foot and Ankle Conditions Associated With Multiple Sclerosis

■ ■ ■ Ronald Guberman, Waldemar Majdanski, Rock CJay Positano, Rock G. Positano

Introduction

Patients with multiple sclerosis (MS) are encouraged by their health care providers to remain active and exercise to maintain strength and agility of their musculoskeletal system. Foot and ankle conditions can interfere with mobility and affect balance. Presented below is a listing of some of the more common foot and ankle problems encountered in the general population.

Hallux Valgus

Hallux valgus, more commonly known as a bunion deformity, is a condition in which the first metatarsal abducts from the midline of the foot and the hallux adducts toward the midline of the foot.[1] It is often a combination of joint contracture and incongruity, combined with structural boney changes or adaptation that is present in this and many other developmental foot

469

deformities. In MS, one limb is often more supinatory and the other more pronatory.[2] The side that pronates more is also more likely to develop a hallux valgus deformity.[3] This condition is generally a progressive deformity, worsening and becoming more painful over time, as the adductor hallucis and extensor tendons gain a mechanical advantage. Conservative treatments such as foot orthoses, strappings, shoe gear modifications, anti-inflammatories, physical therapy, and ultrasound-guided corticosteroid injections are indicated. Surgical options are available to correct the deformity when conservative therapy fails. These include a wide variety of metatarsal osteotomies, musculotendinous and capsular balancing, and first metatarsophalangeal joint (MTPJ) or first metatarso-cuneiform fusions.

Hallux Varus

In hallux varus, the hallux abducts away from the midline of the foot at the first MTPJ. The first MTPJ and hallux may become painful owing to joint incongruity, positional deformity, and from direct shoe pressure on the hallux. The development of hallux varus in MS and other neurologic conditions is attributed to the neurologic deficits and biomechanical alterations associated with these conditions.[4] The neurologic deficits can cause an imbalance of the musculotendinous structures around the first MTPJ that lead to development of the deformity. As the adductor hallucis tendon gains a mechanical advantage, the condition continues to progress and increase in severity. Conservative treatments specific for this condition are categorically similar to those used for hallux valgus are indicated. In severe case, tendon transfers and capsulotendinous rebalancing, with or without osteotomy, are necessary to restore the integrity of the joint and eliminate pain. First MTPJ fusion is also an option, although should be considered a last resort until all conservative measures are exhausted.

Metatarsalgia/Plantar-Flexed First Ray/ Sesamoiditis/Hammered Hallux

A plantar-flexed first ray is a sagittal plane deformity. This condition is also a hallmark of neurogenic disorders such as MS. It is related to the progressive equinus or equinovarus attitude that the foot frequently assumes as the disease progresses.[5] Increase stress and strain on the peroneus longus tendon, one of the major invertors of the foot, may also contribute to the deformity. The musculotendinous imbalance caused by the neurologic deficit that leads to the plantar-flexed first ray is then exacerbated by the progressive deformity leading to increased mechanical advantage and eventually a rigidly plantar-flexed first ray.[6] A hammering of the hallux, with extension at MTPJ and flexion at the interphalangeal joint (IPJ), is often a sequela.

A plantar-flexed first ray is associated with sesamoiditis and submetatarsal bursitis/metatarsalgia.[7] In sesamoiditis of the first metatarsal, the tibial sesamoid is more commonly affected.[3] Stress fractures of this small bone are also known to occur. Nonunion or malunion of sesamoid fractures is not uncommon owing to their small size, location, and relatively poor blood supply. In addition, damage to the ligaments and tendons in this area is a common presentation that can best be visualized using magnetic resonance (MR) and diagnostic ultrasound.

Metatarsalgia is a general term that describes a number of conditions that cause pain underneath or around one or more of the metatarsal heads.[7] These conditions can be associated with the anterior cavus foot (anterior equinus) or global cavus foot associated with many central nervous system (CNS) conditions including MS. Hyperpronation in one foot, associated with MS, can also lead to imbalance and overloading of one or more MTPJs, causing metatarsalgia.[2] There may be an associated metatarsal bursitis or capsulitis and, in more extreme cases, degeneration and partial tearing of the plantar ligament. One or more of the lesser metatarsal phalangeal joints may also be involved in cases of global and/or forefoot equinus. Conservative care includes NSAIDs, orthoses, bracing, padding, corticosteroid injections, and physiotherapy. Surgery is indicated when conservative therapy fails and may involve metatarsal osteotomies to shorten or elevate the metatarsals and tendon balancing procedures. In the case of unresolved sesamoiditis, removal of the involved sesamoid may be indicated. Surgery for the hammered hallux includes fusion with or without tendon lengthening or transfer.[3]

Lesser Toe Deformities—Hammertoes/Clawtoes/Clinodactyly

A variety of lesser toe deformities can be related to or caused by MS. The specific causation and progressive nature of the deformities dictate the type of deformity observed. Hammertoes can be seen from hyperpronation and also in the earlier stages of supinatory conditions and equinovarus associated with MS.[8] With hammertoes, there is extension at the MTPJ and flexion at the proximal IPJ. Clawing of the toes is generally seen in both early or late stage supinatory conditions, the equinovarus foot, and conditions caused by CNS deficits such as MS.[6] In this condition, there is extension at the MTPJ and flexion at the proximal and distal IPJs. These deformities initially present as flexible deformities and may progress to semirigid or rigid deformities. Clinodactyly is a transverse plane deformity of the toes that may or may not coexist with hammertoes, clawtoes, and plantar plate tears. The presence of clinodactyly can be an indicator of neurologic deficit when not solely associated with a biomechanical cause or trauma. Shoe gear changes, strappings, paddings, orthoses, and debridement of associated hyperkeratotic lesions over a bony prominence are indicated as conservative treatments for all of these digital deformities. Surgical correction is often needed that includes arthroplasty, toe fusions and tendon balancing, lengthening, releases or transfers, and joint capsulotomy.

Plantar Fasciitis/Heel Spur Syndrome

The most common heel pathology is plantar fasciitis. Heel spur syndrome is a more broad term that describes a variety of symptoms and findings that are found with or without the presence of an actual spur and may include plantar fasciitis, bursitis, and neurogenic causes. Recent data suggest that the pathology results from degenerative nature of the fascia without the presence of inflammation.[9] This degenerative nature of the fascia stems from abnormal biomechanics of the foot particularly at the insertion of the plantar fascia into the calcaneus. Discomfort or pain in and around the plantar fascia can be caused by both over pronation and over supination as well as increased plantar pressure—all associated with MS.[2] The presence or absence of actual spurring and its location and quality should also be noted. The contribution of neurogenic factors, rheumatologic conditions, or neoplastic conditions must be evaluated. There is a wide array of conservative and surgical options available for the management of the condition. In addition to the other forms of treatment mentioned above for digital and metatarsal conditions, shock wave and EPAT (extracorporeal pulse activation technology) therapies are an option. The use of PRP and amniotic injections has also gained in popularity. Prescription orthoses are extremely useful in the management of heel pain. Surgical options include fasciotomy and fasciectomy, with or without resection of the heel spur.[7]

Neuroma/Neuritis/Neuropathy

Inflammation, pressure, and entrapment of neural structures can cause neurological symptoms to be observed. This can occur as a result of the proliferation of supportive tissues around the nerve and with lesions or damage to the nerve itself.[10] Morton neuroma and other intermetatarsal neuromas may be present as a consequence of biomechanical imbalances caused by MS. These conditions can be managed with biomechanical and pain therapies as listed above for other conditions, including prescription foot orthoses, but as in all conditions, specifically arranged for each condition and individual. Additional therapies for these neurologic symptoms in the lower extremity include neuroactive medications, sclerosing therapy, ultrasound-guided injections, EPAT, and surgery. Surgical options include neurectomy, ligament release, and radiofrequency ablation.

There are a number of other neuropathic conditions that occur as either a direct or indirect result of the CNS lesions associated with MS. The affects can be noted in both sensory and motor nerves. These conditions can cause pain or paresthesias and can also cause significant and progressive weakness, imbalance and loss of sensorimotor control leading to severe and complete dysfunction, and the inability to ambulate.[11] Providing appropriate conservative treatment including physiotherapy, bracing, protection, assistance, and support for the patient is very important. In the event that conservative therapy proves ineffective, there are surgical options to address weakness and contractors, including tendon lengthening transfers and tenotomies, release of joint contractures, and fusions.

Neuropathic and Pressure Wounds

Foot ulcers caused by pressure and the loss of protective sensation occur both in the plantar region of the foot and in other pressure areas from shoes and braces and while the patient is lying in bed or sitting in a chair. The ulcerations may be exacerbated by associated conditions such as diabetes and PVD and from the prevalence of higher than usual plantar pressures associated with MS during ambulation.[12] Areas of bony prominence in the foot, ankle, and heel may also predispose the patient to ulceration. Prevention through early and regular observation and intervention is an important and necessary function of the clinicians and caregivers. Once an ulcer has formed and even in the preulcerative stages, particular attention toward appropriate wound management is needed. This includes offloading, appropriate local wound care and antibiosis if needed, and the assessment of vascular status and intervention where indicated.[3] Surgical intervention for wound debridement and for boney prominences and deformities may be indicated to prevent further progression, deep infection, gangrene, and limb loss.

Hyperkeratotic Lesions

Hyperkeratotic skin lesions are a result of increased pressures over prominent areas in the foot and ankle. The flat broad lesions are called calluses, whereas the lesions with a defined central core are called corns.[3] When lesions with a defined core are present underneath the foot, they are often called porokeratomas or porokeratoses. Foot and ankle contractures, such as hammer toes, plantar-flexed metatarsals, equniovarus deformities, as well as excessive pronation or supination, may lead to minor or severe hyperkeratotic lesions. These lesions are commonly found in areas of boney prominence often present due to progressive deformities associated with conditions including MS.[6] These deformities create abnormal weight bearing on boney prominence thereby increasing the forces that lead to the development of hyperkeratotic lesions. These lesions can be painful and associated with or lead to skin ulceration. Routine evaluation and care are essential in the prevention of more serious sequelae that can arise from the condition. It should be noted that certain porokeratoses are not pressure related and come from a variety of unrelated developmental and inherited conditions. Debridement, as an initial treatment, is generally indicated for hyperkeratotic lesions. This may need to be repeated on a regular basis if the cause cannot be successfully eliminated by padding, the use of braces and orthoses, offloading, and surgical management. Surgery for deformity correction and elimination of boney prominences and stabilization of the foot and ankle is important in decreasing pain with ambulation.[7]

Ankle Contracture, Instability, and Weakness

Spastic or rigid equinovarus associated with MS can cause ankle instability.[13] The progression of muscular weakness in addition to equinovarus at the ankle, leads to an unstable structure and weakening of the ankle ligamentous support.[14] This can result in unstable gait, recurrent ankle sprains and falls, which can often lead to more debilitating fractures and dislocations of the foot, ankle and more proximal structures. Bracing with an AFO is often recommended, and in certain cases combined with functional electrical stimulation.[15] A knee orthosis (KO) or a knee ankle foot orthosis (KAFO) are other options when additional weakness, instability and/or deformity is present. Surgical options are also available including ankle stabilization, tendoachilles or tenotomy, gastrocnemius recession, ankle contracture releases, musculotendinous releases and transfers, ankle fusion, and pantalar fusions. Without assistive devices and the help of caregivers in addition to therapy and surgery where indicated, ankle instability and weakness can lead to a loss of the ability to ambulate safely and with progression can lead to a complete loss of ambulation.

Myopathies/Tendinopathies

The CNS lesions associated with MS may directly cause musculotendinous dysfunction, and secondarily, the biomechanical instability resulting from MS can lead to tendinopathy.[2] These conditions can involve the extrinsic and intrinsic muscles and tendons of the foot and ankle. Most commonly affected are the Achilles, peroneus longus and brevis, tibialis anterior, tibialis posterior, as well as the long extensors, and flexor tendons.

Treatment is aimed at providing stability, support, and balance through bracing, physical therapy, prescription foot orthoses, and surgical procedures as needed. Surgical intervention may involve tenotomy, tendon lengthening, and tendon transfers.

In summary, foot and ankle problems are not necessarily life-threatening but instead lifestyle threatening; however, recognizing the presence of these issues is imperative. The value of podiatric services cannot be underestimated, and podiatrists should be involved in the day-to-day care of these patients and included in the team approach when managing this patient population.

References

1. Ferrari J. Bunions. *BMJ Clin Evid.* 2009;2009:1112.
2. Rusu L, Neamtu MC, Rosulescu E, et al. Analysis of foot and ankle disorders and prediction of gait in multiple sclerosis rehabilitation. *Eur J Med Res.* 2014;19:73.
3. Southerland JT. *McGlamry's Comprehensive Textbook of Foot and Ankle Surgery.* 4th ed. Vols 1-2. New York, NY: Wolters Kluwer; 2001.
4. Ng AV, Miller RG, Gelinas D, Kent-Braun JA. Functional relationships of central and peripheral muscle alterations in multiple sclerosis. *Muscle Nerve.* 2004;29:843-852. doi:10.1002/mus.20038.
5. Picelli A, Valies G, Chemello E, et al. Is spasticity always the same? An observational study comparing the features of spastic equinusfoot in patients with chronic stroke and multiple sclerosis. *J Neurol Sci.* 2017;380:132-136.
6. Neamtu MC, Rusu L, Rusu PF, Marin M, Neamtu OM. Biomechanical disorders of foot in multiple sclerosis. *Rom J Morphol Embryol.* 2012;53(3 suppl):841-845.
7. Coughlin MJ, Mann RA, Salzman CL. *Surgery of the Foot and Ankle.* 8th ed. Vol 1. Philadelphia, PA: Mosby Elsevier; 2007.
8. Psarakis M, Greene D, Moresi M, et al. Impaired heel to toe progression during gait is related to reduced ankle range of motion in people with multiple sclerosis. *Clin Biomech.* 2017;49:96-100.
9. Lemont H, Ammirati KM, Usen N. Plantar fasciitis: a degenerative process (fasciosis) without inflammation. *J Am Podiatr Med Assoc.* 2003;93(3):234-237.
10. Thomson CE, Gibson JNA, Martin D. Interventions for the treatment of Mortons neuroma. *Cochrane Database Sys Rev.* 2004;(3):CD003118.
11. Pepping M, Ehde DM. Neuropsychological evaluation and treatment of multiple sclerosis: the importance of a neuro-rehabilitation focus. *Phys Med Rehabil Clin.* 2005;16(2):411-436.
12. Citaker S, Gunduz AG, Guclu MB, et al. Relationship between foot sensation and standing balance in patients with multiple sclerosis. *Gait Posture.* 2011;34(2):275-278.
13. Haselkorn JK, Loomis S. Multiple sclerosis and spasticity. *Phys Med Rehabil Clin.* 2005;16(2):467-481.
14. Hoang P, Saboisky JP, Gandevia SC, Herbert RD. Passive mechanical properties of gastrocnemius in people with multiple sclerosis. *Clin Biomech.* 2009;24(3):291-298.
15. Ogino M, Shiozawa A, Ota H, Okamoto S, Kawachi I. Treatment and comorbidities of multiple sclerosis in an employed population in Japan: analysis of health claims data. *Neurodegener Dis Manag.* 2018;8(2):97-103.

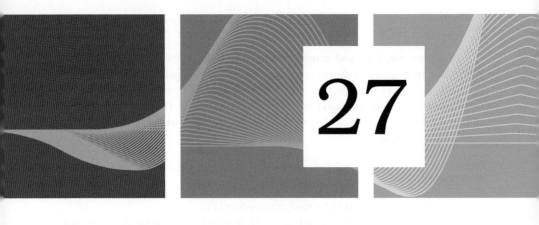

Perioperative Care of the Lower Extremity Orthopedic Patient With Multiple Sclerosis

■ ▥ ▦ W. Mark Richardson, Dale J. Lange, Karen Yanelli

Introduction

Multiple sclerosis (MS) is an immune-mediated disorder that causes a variably progressive neurological condition associated with demyelination throughout the central nervous system. We know much about the pathology of the disease, but there is uncertainty about the cause and the immunological determinants. Biomarker analysis and lesion classification may allow for diagnoses by pathological subtype in the near future.[1]

Individuals present with a clinically isolated syndrome (CIS) caused by a lesion of the optic nerve, cerebrum, cerebellum, brainstem, or spinal cord. Subsequent progression, if it occurs, is classified according to standardized McDonald diagnostic criteria.[2] It is estimated that approximately 70% to 80% of patients with both abnormal radiological findings and a CIS will convert to clinically definite multiple sclerosis (CDMS) over time.[3] According to the Multiple Sclerosis Society, there are three disease subtypes: relapsing remitting (RR), secondary progressive, and primary progressive.[2,4,5] These definitions are further refined by the frequency and magnitude of neuroinflammatory activity and remissions and progression through accumulation of neurological deficits over time.[6] Most patients are diagnosed with relapsing forms of the disease at an average age of 29 to 30 years, with a range 2 to 70 years. There is positive correlation between age at the time of diagnosis and progressive forms of the disease at its onset.[3,5] The majority of MS diagnoses are of the RR subtype, which has an estimated 80% likelihood of evolving into the progressive subtype within 25 years of diagnosis of CDMS.[3]

Patients with MS may require surgery for a variety of reasons. Given the age demographic, young patients often develop musculoskeletal injuries of the lower extremities such as torn menisci and lesions of the ligaments. Older patients with arthritic comorbidities and those with a history of long-term steroid use may require total hip arthroplasty (THA) or total knee arthroplasty (TKA).[7] Additionally, patients with progressive forms of the disease are at an increased risk of injury due to falls.

Owing to the pathogenic and clinical heterogeneity across patients, optimal management of the perioperative care of patients with MS requires careful planning and a multidisciplinary clinical effort. Any plan for lower extremity orthopedic procedures for patients with MS should account for the variables that, if managed properly, add the most value toward positive perioperative outcomes. These include preoperative neurological and medical evaluation, management of disease-related symptoms, steroid use, prophylactic use of antibiotics, anesthesiological technique, dosing and timing of disease-modifying therapies, and potential rehabilitation requirements. The purpose of this chapter is to organize the knowledge base around these aspects of care for patients with MS and their primary physicians and caregiver in preparation for lower extremity orthopedic surgery.

Preoperative Phase

Although there is uncertainty whether trauma, such as surgery, is able to cause a relapse,[8] anticipation of this potential is essential in the preoperative and perioperative evaluation of the patients with MS preparing for such procedures. Poor surgical outcomes may arise as a result of poor preoperative management, which may affect postoperative functionality, including risk of fracture in patients with a history of long-term steroid use, cardiovascular complications such as deep vein thrombosis in patients with impaired mobility, and cardiovascular comorbidities due to autonomic nervous system dysfunction.

It is imperative that the preoperative evaluation includes a thorough clinical examination and a review of the history of the patient's disease to account for the probability of relapse leading up to the procedure, to mitigate the risks of anesthesiological complications, and to predict the patients' capacity to effectively recover from the procedure, and to plan for rehabilitation.

The review of the history of the disease should include the date of the diagnosis, the disease subtype, symptoms, and their severity. The physical and neurological examinations should rule out an acute exacerbation and evaluate somatic and autonomic function as well as cognitive and psychological status.[7,9] Ambulatory function should be assessed for all patients. Those with a history of bladder dysfunction and urinary tract infections (UTIs) should be evaluated for infection.

Individuals with progressive forms of the disease may have accumulated neurological deficits that cause respiratory dysfunction and cardiovascular irregularities. The accumulated deficits would be associated with lesions in the medulla and spinal cord, which would be revealed on magnetic resonance imaging (MRI). Lesions in these regions may correlate with a respiratory condition, bulbar dysfunction, dysregulation of autonomic nervous system, and respiratory insufficiency.[10] Such patients should have pulmonary function tests administered preoperatively to determine the extent of respiratory dysfunction.[11,12]

Individuals with RRMS who have few residual neurological deficits may not require many resources beyond the standard of care for the general population.[5] However, it should be noted that onset of initial symptoms and date of a definitive diagnosis of RRMS is positively correlated with frequency of relapse; relapses have been shown to occur at a higher rate during the first years after a diagnosis of RRMS, slowing thereafter.[13] The preoperative examination should rule out an acute relapse.

Cognitive impairment can be assessed with a variety of tools, including the Symbol Digit Modalities Test and verbal fluency tests. Comorbid depression may affect cognition, prompting the need for tests that distinguish somatic symptoms and mood changes, such as the Depressive Mood Scale or a Beck Depression Inventory Fast Screen.[9,11]

A record of the patient's disease-modifying therapy program, concomitant medications, and history of steroid usage should be obtained.

Preoperative Symptom Management

Treatment of relapsing forms of MS generally includes immune-modulating therapies, whereas few treatments exist for progressive forms of the disease.[3] Of the most common deficits, those that require particular attention and management during the perioperative scope are spasticity, ambulatory dysfunction, fatigue, bladder dysfunction, and depression and cognitive impairment.[3]

Management of paroxsymal symptoms, such as spasticity, is especially important for optimal outcomes for hip and knee arthroplasty. Many patients with upper motor neuron involvement develop spasticity, which is usually managed with a combination of physical therapy and medications.[14] Common medications used to treat spasticity include baclofen, benzodiazepines, or tizanidine. If the patient can tolerate it, uptitration of antispasticity medication preoperatively may mitigate the risk of post-operative complications due to increased tone of the lower extremities.[7,15] However, as noted later, baclofen is contraindicated with some forms of anesthesia and therefore may not be administered intraoperatively.

A preoperative assessment of any surgical patient's airway is standard of care when preparing for endotracheal intubations. Patients with MS with surgical histories should have their notes reviewed for any incidence of difficulty with intubation. Given the possibility of paroxysmal symptoms throughout the perioperative period, head and neck range of motion assessment must be included in the preoperative neurological and physical examination. Less than 80° range of neck motion in flexion/extension is a risk factor for difficult intubation.[16,17]

Steroids

If acute exacerbation is encountered in the preoperative period, depending on its severity, treatment with high-dose intravenous glucocorticosteroids (GC) may be necessary. The typical dose given for acute flares is approximately 1000 mg of methyl prednisone daily for 3 to 5 days.[3] However, there is evidence that steroids may have a time- and dose-dependent impact on bone metabolism. It is well known that long-term use of glucocorticoids affects bone metabolism and leads to osteoporosis, more generally mediated by well-defined endocrinological mechanisms.[18,19] Studies show the association between steroids and osteonecrosis of the femoral head and increased risk of bone fracture. The latter may increase the likelihood of injury during positioning throughout the perioperative period.[13,20,21] Sahraian et al (2012) report from their case study analysis that symptoms of avascular necrosis of the femoral head may occur after 6 and 8 months of steroid therapy. Moreover, studies have also shown that short-term administration of high-dose GCs for young patients with RRMS with acute exacerbations may immediately increase bone resorption and decreased bone formation with high turnover after the steroids have been stopped.[22]

Randomized double-blind placebo-controlled trials of non-MS patients undergoing TKAs and THA show reduction in C-reactive protein with a preoperative dose of 125 mg intravenous methylprednisolone as well as favorable yet brief analgesic outcomes.[23] Prophylactic steroid use is required for patients who have recently used steroids for a relapse to prevent postoperative adrenal insufficiency.[12,13] However, steroid use within the perioperative period should be approached with caution given their potential hypothalamic-pituitary-axis suppressing effect. Rescheduling of the surgery should be considered if an acute relapse requiring high-dose corticosteroids reoccurs within the perioperative period for an elective surgery.

Antibiotic Prophylactics

Patients with a history of genitourinary symptoms who are prone to UTIs should be evaluated for infection throughout the perioperative period and provided with antibiotics to mitigate the risk of infection-induced pyrexia, which is associated with a higher risk of relapse. Urinalysis with culture should be performed in the preoperative period to rule out kidney dysfunction or an infection. Antibiotic prophylactics may be administered concurrently with glucocorticoids in the absence of systemic infection in the case in which UTI risk is high and catheters are used to prevent systemic infection.[24]

Anesthetic Implications of Multiple Sclerosis

An increase in temperature is thought to contribute to impaired conduction along demyelinated neuronal segments, rendering temperature management critical throughout the perioperative period. One study showed a high rate of lesions of the hypothalamus across a sample of patients with MS that affected the hypothalamic-pituitary-axis.[25] Furthermore, some cite evidence of lesions of the hypothalamus as possibly affecting thermoregulatory mechanisms, resulting in hyperthermia.[12,26] Pyrexia throughout the perioperative period can be managed through the use of cooling devices, antibiotics, and antipyretics.

Some advocate for the use of benzodiazepines during the preoperative and intraoperative phases as a way to manage stress, which may ultimately lower the risk of relapse. Caution should be applied in the case of patients with respiratory dysfunction.[12]

The prevalence of comorbid arthritis in the population with MS is between 16% and 26%.[27-29] There are also data that suggest a high prevalence of orthopedic injuries (lesions of the ligaments, cartilage, muscle, or bone) across the population with MS.[30] A wide variety of anesthetic algorithms that include one or a mix of general, regional, local, and intraoperative hypotension-inducing techniques exist for these procedures for the general population of orthopedic patients undergoing total joint replacement surgeries or partial arthroscopy.[31,32] In the context of the patient with MS, anesthesiologists must manage the risks and benefits between optimal application of anesthetic agents and techniques and the patient's disease-modifying therapy schedule, functional status, and the pathogenesis of MS lesions, more generally.

Some studies show the increased risk of relapse and disease activity upon discontinuation of disease-modifying therapies, so this should be done only after thorough examination of the patient and understanding treatment history.[12,33,34] Natalizumab (Tysabri), Fingolimod (Gilenya), Dimethylfumarate (Tecfidera) are associated with risk of diminished immune protection, resulting in one of the most severe complications, progressive multifocal leukoencephalopathy. Drug-induced immunosuppression also requires the intraoperative team to consider the possibility of opportunistic infections.[13]

Although there have been randomized controlled clinical trials for general versus regional anesthesia in the broader population of orthopedic patients, there have been no such studies for the MS community. There is conflicting evidence as to whether neuraxial anesthesia leads to exacerbations due to the possible toxic effect of the anesthesia on demyelinated nerves.[13,35] There is not enough evidence to conclude one way or the other, but general anesthesia leads to rates of exacerbation that fall closer to the rates of adverse events for the general populations.[35] There is evidence that neuraxial anesthesia reduces the risk of deep vein thrombosis, pneumonia, and respiratory depression.[36] Thus, the anesthesiologist must weigh the risks and benefits of neuraxial anesthesia depending on the extent of neurological deficits the patient presents with. Ultimately, use of neuraxial anesthesia may be warranted if the patient has a history of venous thromboembolisms and respiratory dysfunction.

The concern with spinal anesthesia in patients with MS versus epidural anesthesia rests on the notion that the former may increase the density of the anesthesia surrounding the nerves, which could be contraindicated for those with demyelination in those regions.[35] Obvious problems with this potential adverse mechanism would include hypotension, prolonged neural blockage, flaccid paralysis, urinary retention, and acute spinal syndrome.[35] Maintenance of general anesthesia with inhalational anesthetics, such as sevoflurane and desflurane, has been shown to be safe in patients with MS. McKay et al provide evidence that non-MS patients may show faster recovery of airway reflexes when desflurane is used.[37] Furthermore, Sahin et al present a case in which a male patient with MS with avascular necrosis of the femoral head due to long-term steroid intake was administered desflurane intraoperatively with no adverse events reported, noting more prompt return of respiratory airway functionality when compared with sevoflurane.[38] Beyond this evidence and case study, there are also evidence and cases that lend credence to the use of sevoflurane with regards to recovery and hemodynamic stability.[39,40]

Hypotensive anesthetic techniques should be avoided in patients with lesions to the thoracic spinal cord and a history of blood pressure instability, a symptom of autonomic involvement.[13,41] Symptoms of autonomic dysfunction include syncope, impotence, bladder and bowel dysfunction, vasomotor instability, or orthostatsis.[13] A preoperative MRI scan of the cervical and thoracic segments may be warranted even if there is no history of autonomic dysfunction given the risk of respiratory distress intraoperatively and postoperatively in patients with active lesion and plaques in the cervical spine. Dorotta et al note that there may also be lesions of medulla oblongata that compromise respiratory function, requiring adequate preoxygenation during the administration of the anesthesia.[13]

The upper motor neuron lesions from MS are associated with upregulation of nicotinic acetylcholine receptors (AChRs) beyond the neuromuscular junction and throughout the muscle tissue.[42] Succinylcholine, a common neuromuscular blocking drug (NMBD), is often used during general anesthesia to cause muscle paralysis. As an agonist of AChRs, it causes persistent depolarization of AChRs at the neuromuscular junction. However, in patients with MS, the efflux of potassium ions down their concentration gradient during this depolarization phase is not isolated to the area of the motor end plate, because the upregulation of AChRs extends past this area. Succinylcholine is nondiscriminatory in its effect on these AChRs, which may lead to an increase in plasma potassium levels (hyperkalemia) above the transient levels found in patients without disease.[43] Therefore, alternatives to succinylcholine may be considered for the patient with MS.[12,44] Management of spasticity with skeletal muscle relaxants, such as baclofen, may also increase the patient's sensitivity to NMBDs.[12] If NMBDs are required, these agents should be tapered slowly leading up to surgery.

Postoperative Considerations

Deep Vein Thrombosis

Managing the risk of postoperative venous thrombosis in patients undergoing THA and TKAs is imperative. Decreased mobility preoperatively put patients at an increased risk for developing a deep vein thrombus (DVT). Given that many patients undergoing TKA or THA are older with a more advanced form of the disease patients' thrombotic status should be monitored throughout the perioperative period. More generally, for both progressive and relapsing forms, regardless of age, if the preoperative evaluation indicates decreased ambulatory function or high levels of sedentarism, the patient may be at a higher risk of developing a DVT.[45] Moreover, the risk of bleeding due to anticoagulant prophylaxis needs to be measured against the risk of thrombosis. Mechanical treatments (e.g., pneumatics and leg compression) can be used as adjuncts. The use of COX-1 inhibitors and pharmacological interventions such as low-dose heparin and low-molecular-weight heparin analogues should be used as clinically indicated.

Rehabilitation

Patients with MS should prepare for longer rehabilitation than non-MS patients undergoing the same surgery. It is possible that the patient with more advanced disease will be exceptionally fatigued after surgery and symptoms may become worse as a result of a pseudorelapse. If a pseudorelapse occurs and the patient is experiencing sensory symptoms, depending on the extent of the sensory loss, they may lose the capacity to recognize anterior versus posterior weight-bearing sensation and thus will be considered at increased risk for falls due to decreased balance. If the patient was tapered off baclofen before surgery, he or she may retain spasticity. Patients who are nonambulatory and wheelchair bound will require additional resources. The hospital should be prepared with a lift if necessary and additional staff for transfers.

Acute rehabilitation is recommended for patients who may require a less protracted program to return them to their presurgical baseline. Patients who are expected to make a recovery to full independence in the household setting within 2 weeks go to acute rehabilitation centers. These patients should be able to handle 3 to 4 hours of physical and occupational therapy daily. The best candidates for this are patients with MS who, postoperatively, are ambulatory but would not yet be fully independent in the household owing to safety concerns or overall weakness and fatigue.

Subacute rehabilitation is recommended for patients who may require a more protracted rehabilitation program to return them to their presurgical baseline, for example, patients who are expected to make a recovery to full independence in their household setting within an estimated 3 to 12 weeks. These patients should be able to handle 2 hours of physical and occupational therapy daily. Candidates for subacute rehabilitation include patients who are nonambulatory postoperatively or patients who are able to ambulate short distances that are not functional in nature, more generally.

Conclusion

Given the variably progressive nature of MS, managing the perioperative care of the patient with MS undergoing lower extremity surgery requires careful planning with attention to the individual characteristics of each patient's condition. If an acute flare occurs within the preoperative window, rescheduling the surgery should be weighed against the risk of exacerbation of the condition. It is imperative to coordinate care between the neurologists and anesthesiologists, nurses, and physical therapists well before the day of the surgery.

Summary of Key Points

- For individuals with RRMS, rule out acute exacerbations preoperatively and assess the risk of an acute exacerbation occurring within the perioperative window.
- Spasticity must be managed aggressively for patients undergoing knee and hip arthroplasties. Increasing the dose of the antispasmodic may be beneficial but should be done under the guidance of the anesthesiologist given potential contraindications.

■ To mitigate the risk of infection-induced pyrexia, and possible relapse or increase in disease activity, rule out UTIs preoperatively and consider antibiotic prophylactics for patients with a history of frequent UTIs.

■ Some disease-modifying therapies, including Tysabri, Gilenya, and Tecfidera, are associated with an increased risk of progressive multifocal leukoencephalopathy and other immunosuppressant complications and need to be addressed preoperatively.

References

1. Reich DS, Lucchinetti CF, Calabresi PA. Multiple sclerosis. *N Engl J Med.* 2018;378:169-180.
2. Thompson AJ, Bandwell BL, Barkhof F, et al. Diagnosis of multiple sclerosis: 2017 revision of the McDonald criteria. *Neurology.* 2018;17(2):162-173.
3. Fabian MT, Krieger SC, Lublin FD. Multiple sclerosis and other inflammatory demyelinating diseases of the central nervous system. In: Daroff RB, Jankovic J, Mazziotta JC, Pomeroy SL, eds. *Neurology in Clinical Practice.* 7th ed. London: Elsevier Inc; 2016:1159-1186.
4. Miller D, Barkhof F, Montalban X, Thompson A, Filippi M. Clinically isolated syndromes suggestive of multiple sclerosis, part I: natural history, pathogenesis, diagnosis, and prognosis. *Neurology.* 2005;4(5):281-288.
5. Multiple Sclerosis FAQs [Internet]. Available at https://www.nationalmssociety.org/What-is-MS/MS-FAQ-s.
6. Lublin FD, Reingold SC, Cohen JA, et al. Defining the clinical course of multiple sclerosis. *Neurology.* 2014;83(3):206.
7. Hughes KE, Nickel D, Gurney-Dunlop T, Knox KB. Total knee arthroplasty in multiple sclerosis. *Arthroplast Today.* 2016;2:117-122.
8. Sibley WA, Bamford CR, Clark K, Smith MS, Laguna JF. A prospective study of physical trauma and multiple sclerosis. *J Neurol Neurosurg Psychiatry.* 1991;54:584-589.
9. Lange DJ, Shtilbans A, Reichler B, Leung D. Perioperative care of the orthopedic patient with neurological disease. In: MacKenzie CR, Memrsoudis SG, Cornell CN, eds. *Perioperative Care of the Orthopedic Patient.* New York: Springer; 2014:185-195.
10. Tzelepis GE, McCool FD. Respiratory dysfunction in multiple sclerosis. *Respir Med.* 2015;109(6):671-679.
11. Mutluay FK, Gurses HN, Saip S. Effects of multiple sclerosis on respiratory functions. *Clin Rehabil.* 2005;19(4):426-432.
12. Makris A, Piperopoulos A, Karmaniolou I. Multiple sclerosis: basic knowledge and new insights in perioperative management. *J Anesth.* 2014;28:267-278.
13. Dorotta IR, Schubert A. Multiple sclerosis and anesthetic implications. *Curr Opin Anaesthesiol.* 2002;15:365-370.
14. Pidgeon TS, Ramirez JM, Schiller JR. Orthopaedic management of spasticity. *R I Med J.* 2015;7:485-493.
15. Newman JM, Naziri Q, Chughtai M, et al. Does multiple sclerosis affect the inpatient perioperative outcomes after total hip arthroplasty? *J Arthroplasty.* 2017;32:3669-3674.
16. El-Ganzouri AR, McCarthy RJ, Tuman KJ, Tanck EN, Ivankovich AD. Preoperative airway assessment: predictive value of a multivariate risk index. *Anesth Analg.* 1996;82(6):1197-1204.

17. Karkouti K, Rose DK, Wigglesworth D, Cohen MM. Predicting difficult intubation: a multivariable analysis. *Can J Anesth.* 2000;47(8):730-739.
18. O'Brien CA, Jia D, Plotkin LI, et al. Glucocorticoids act directly on osteoblasts and osteocytes to induce their apoptosis and reduce bone formation and strength. *Endocrinology.* 2004;145(4):1835-1841.
19. Canalis E, Mazziotti G, Guistina A, Bilezikian JP. Glucocorticoid-induced osteoporosis: pathophysiology and therapy. *Osteoporos Int.* 2007;18(10):1319-1328.
20. Koo KH, Kim R, Kim YS, et al. Risk period for developing osteonecrosis of the femoral head in patients on steroid treatment. *Clin Rheumatol.* 2002;21:299-303.
21. Sahraian MA, Yadegari S, Azarpajou R, Forughipour M. Avascular necrosis of the femoral head in multiple sclerosis: report of five patients. *Neurol Sci.* 2012;33:1443-1446.
22. Dovio A, Perazzolo L, Osella G, et al. Immediate fall of bone formation and transient increase of bone resorption in the course of high-dose, short-term glucocorticoid therapy in young patients with multiple sclerosis. *J Clin Endocrinol Metab.* 2004;89(10):4923-4928.
23. Lunn TH, Andersen LO, Kristensen BB, et al. Effect of high-dose preoperative methylprednisolone on recovery after total hip arthroplasty: a randomized, double-blind, placebo-controlled trial. *Br J Anaesth.* 2013;110(1):66-73.
24. Mahadeva A, Tanasescu R, Gran B. Urinary tract infections in multiple sclerosis: under-diagnosed and under-treated? A clinical audit at a large University Hospital. *Am J Clin Exp Immunol.* 2014;3(1):57-67.
25. Huitinga I, Erkut ZA, van Beurden D, Swaap DF. The hypothalamo-pituitary-adrenal axis in multiple sclerosis. *Ann N Y Acad Sci.* 2003;992:118-128.
26. Martinez-Rodriguez JE, Munteis E, Roquer J. Periodic hyperthermia and abnormal circadian temperature rhythm in a patient with multiple sclerosis. *Mult Scler.* 2006;12(4):515-517.
27. Marrie RA, Horwitz R, Cutter G, Tyry T. Cumulative impact of comorbidity on quality of life in MS. *Acta Neurol Scand.* 2012;125(3):180-186.
28. Marrie RA. Comorbidity in multiple sclerosis: implications for patient care. *Nat Rev Neurol.* 2017;13(6):375-382.
29. Warren SA, Turpin KVL, Pohar SL, Jones CA, Warren KG. Comorbidity and health-related quality of life in people with sclerosis. *Int J MS Care.* 2009;11:6-16.
30. Mandell D, Tosches W. Orthopedic injuries in multiple sclerosis patients: incidence and patterns of injury types in this vulnerable population. *Neurol Bull.* 2012;4:12-23.
31. Turnbull ZA, Sastow D, Giambrone GP, Tedore T. Anesthesia for the patient undergoing total knee replacement: current status and future prospects. *Local Reg Anesth.* 2017;10:1-7.
32. Sharrock NE. Anesthesia for total hip arthroplasty. *Curr Opin Orthop.* 1992;3:455-560.
33. Havla JB, Pellkofer HL, Meinl I, Gerdes LA, Hohlfeld R, Kumpfel T. Rebound of disease activity after withdrawal of fingolimod (FTY720) treatment. *Arch Neurol.* 2012;69(2):262-264.
34. O'Connor PW, Goodman A, Kappos L, et al. No disease activity return during natalizumab treatment interruption in patients with multiple sclerosis. *Neurology.* 2011;76(22):1858-1865.
35. Hebl JR, Horlocker TT, Schroeder DR. Neuraxial anesthesia and analgesia in patients with preexisting central nervous system disorders. *Anesth Analg.* 2006;103(1):223-228.

36. Rodgers A, Walker N, Schug S, et al. Reduction of postoperative mortality and morbidity with epidural or spinal anaesthesia: results from overview of randomised trials. *BMJ.* 2000;321:1-12.

37. McKay RE, Hall KT, Hills N. The effect of anesthetic choice (sevoflurane versus desflurane) and neuromuscular management on speed of airway reflex recovery. *Anesth Analg.* 2016;122(2):393-401.

38. Sahin L, Korkmaz HF, Sahin M, Aydin T, Toker S, Gulcan E. Desflurane anaesthesia in a patient with multiple sclerosis in total hip replacement. *Arch Med Sci.* 2010;6(6):984-986.

39. Lee KH, Park JS, Lee S, et al. Anesthetic management of the emergency laparotomy for a patient with multiple sclerosis – a case report. *Korean J Anesthesiol.* 2010;59(5):359-362.

40. Shan J, Sun L, Wang D, Li X. Comparison of the neuroprotective effects and recovery profiles of isoflurane, sevoflurane and desflurane as neurosurgical pre-conditioning on ischemia/reperfusion cerebral injury. *Int J Clin Exp Pathol.* 2015;8(2):2001-2009.

41. Kytta J, Rosenberg PH. Anaesthesia for patients with multiple sclerosis. *Ann Chir Gynaecol.* 1984;73(5):299-303.

42. Martyn JAJ, White DA, Gronert GA, Jaffe RS, Ward JM. Up- and down-regulation of skeletal muscle acetylcholine receptors. *Anesthesiology.* 1992;76(5):822-843.

43. Martyn JAJ, Richtsfeld M. Succinylcholine-induced hyperkalemia in acquired pathological states. *Anesthesiology.* 2006;104(1):158-169.

44. Brett RS, Schmidt JH, Gage JS, Schartel SA, Poppers PJ. Measurement of acetylcholine receptor concentration in skeletal muscle from a patient with multiple sclerosis and resistance to atracurium. *Anesthesiology.* 1987;66:837-839.

45. Arpaia G, Bavera PM, Caputo D, et al. Risk of deep venous thrombosis (DVT) in bedridden or wheelchair-bound multiple sclerosis patients: a prospective study. *Thromb Res.* 2010;125(4):315-317.

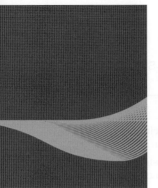
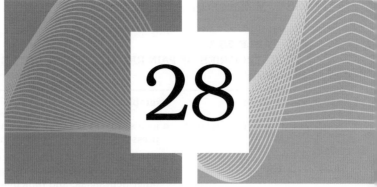

Pain Management in Multiple Sclerosis

■■■ Andrui Nazarian

Introduction

Multiple sclerosis (MS) is an inflammatory demyelinating disease with a high prevalence of pain.[1] Although one may not typically think of pain itself as a symptom of MS, many MS patients will develop pain syndromes throughout their disease state.[1,2] The reported range of prevalence of pain in MS patients ranges widely from near 50% up to 86%.[1-4] The pain can be classified into four main categories as listed in Table 28.1.

Some types of pain such as muscle spasms and low-back pain may fit into more than one category depending on their cause. O'Connor et al further proposed a separate classification for MS-related pain: neuropathic pain, musculoskeletal, and nociceptive (i.e., pain secondary to tonic spasms, spasticity, and headaches).[2] There are not many research studies on the assessment and treatment of MS-related pain, and most therapies recommended today are based on studies conducted in patients with similar symptoms from other disorders. Risk factors for pain in MS patients are included in Table 28.2.

Furthermore, individuals with neuropathic or chronic pain are more likely to experience sleep disturbances, anxiety disorders, and depression, therefore making it even more critical that pain is appropriately evaluated and managed.[3] Pain management is essential in improving

487

TABLE 28.1
CATEGORIES OF PAIN RELATED TO MULTIPLE SCLEROSIS (MS)[4,8]

Pain Category	Examples
■ Pain indirectly related to MS	■ as a sequel of MS symptoms including spasticity, pressure sores, abnormal posture
■ Pain directly related to MS	■ acute optic neuritis, Lhermitte sign, dysesthesias, paroxysmal syndromes such as trigeminal and other neuralgias, and radicular pain
■ Pain that is MS independent	■ low-back pain, primary headaches
■ Pain secondary to MS treatment	■ following drug therapy

the functionality and quality of life for MS patients. In this chapter, we will discuss some of the most common pain syndromes that MS patients may experience.

Spasticity and Muscle Spasm–Associated Pain

Spasticity and painful muscle spasms affect many individuals with MS including interfering with ambulation, performing activities of daily living, decreased functionality, and increased pain and suffering.[5] Spasticity can affect 60% to 80% of individuals with MS.[6] Treatment for spasticity aims to decrease muscle tone and spasms with the goal to improve function and decrease pain, without compromising all muscle tone. Although there are no conclusive studies on MS patients at this time, it is generally accepted that physiotherapy, with a focus on both active and passive treatment, can be helpful at all stages of management.[4,7-9] Physiotherapy can include training for appropriate posture and positioning, while avoiding triggers

TABLE 28.2
RISK FACTORS FOR PAIN IN MULTIPLE SCLEROSIS (MS) PATIENTS[2]

Increased age
Duration of disease
Depression
Degree of functional impairment
Fatigue

which worsen spasticity.[4] First-line oral therapy for spasticity includes the use of baclofen (10-120 mg/d oral) and tizanidine (2-24 mg/d oral), while diazepam and gabapentin are generally secondary agents.[4,5,7-9] Baclofen, diazepam, and gabapentin work via activating the inhibitory γ-amino butyric acid (GABA) receptors.[7] Tizanidine, on the other hand, functions on the presynaptic alpha 2 receptors to decrease excitatory output from these neurons.[7] Overall, there is limited evidence for the efficacy for these oral therapies at this time, particularly when it comes to functionality; however, they are commonly used for spasticity in clinical practice.[5,7] Additionally, there are side effects from these medications, particularly dry mouth, drowsiness, and weakness, which may not be well tolerated by patients.[4,7] When patients cannot tolerate oral medications or require higher doses of medications, an intrathecal baclofen delivery system is a good alternative. This system is an implanted intrathecal pump, which is more invasive and expensive, and as such, it is generally used as a last resort. The pump itself is positioned subcutaneously in the abdomen attached to a catheter, which is placed into the lumbar intrathecal space allowing for medication to be delivered into the spinal fluid. As there are high levels of GABA receptors in the lumbar spinal cord, much smaller doses of baclofen are needed for treatment.[7,8] There is good evidence for intrathecal baclofen therapy to reduce muscle tone and spasm frequency; however, this therapy comes with its own set of side effects including pump infections, catheter dislocations, muscle weakness, drowsiness, and headaches.[8]

Botulinum toxin muscle injections are an alternative treatment, particularly for focal spasticity.[4,7,8] Injections are especially helpful when initiated with physiotherapy.[4,8] Botulinum toxin is a neurotoxin which causes prolonged muscle relaxation by inhibiting the release of acetylcholine (ACH) at the neuromuscular junction, therefore blocking nerve conduction.[7,10,11] The effects of the injections are seen after 10 to 14 days and last a few months, after which the injections will need to be repeated.[7] In this case, the involved muscle groups need to be identified and the injections should be made into those specific muscles. Studies have shown that botulinum toxin injections can reduce muscle tone and improve passive function such as ease of dressing.[7]

Recently, there has been greater interest in cannabinoids for the management of spasticity. Studies looking at tetrahydrocannabinol (THC) or cannabis extract did not find a significant decrease in spasticity, although they may still have a role in pain management given that they did have an effect on the patient's overall mobility and subjective reduction of pain. Based on the available evidence and potential side effects; however, it is generally not recommended as a treatment for spasticity in MS patients except in specific refractory cases.[4,9]

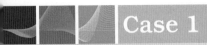

Case 1

MS Patient with Spasticity

A 45-year-old male with history of MS comes into your pain management clinic for evaluation and treatment for spasticity. The patient is particularly interested in improvement in his mobility and decreased pain from the spasticity and muscle spasms, and he is looking forward to an improvement in his quality of life. The patient has not undergone any treatment options in the past but states that he has heard of Botox injections for spasticity. He is highly interested in receiving these injections because his friend at church had the injections and said they were very helpful. Physical examination reveals a score of 2 on the Modified Ashworth Scale in both upper and lower extremities, and the patient also endorses pain and tightness of his muscles in the lower back. How would you approach the care for this patient? What would be your initial treatment plan and would you offer him botulinum toxin injections?

As this is a new patient to the clinic, a thorough assessment of the level and location of spasticity is warranted. The Ashworth Scale and Modified Ashworth Scale are common tools used in the assessment of spasticity (Table 28.3). These scales are determined during passive tissue stretching. The Ashworth Scale was particularly developed for spasticity in MS patients, and the Modified Ashworth Scale added a sixth point to the scale to differentiate between the lower levels of spasticity.[12]

In the case of our patient, based on history and physical examination, it appears as though the patient has back, lower extremity, and upper extremity spasticity and muscle spasms. Initial therapy for him should begin with physiotherapy, possible hydrotherapy, followed by initiation of oral antispasticity medications. Particularly given that his spasticity is global, the patient would benefit from systemic oral medications. Medications such as baclofen or tizanidine may be started at a low dose. As there is no one focal area of spasticity, botulinum injections would be less appropriate given there are many muscle groups involved, although a combination of oral therapy and specific muscle group botulinum injections would not be unreasonable. The patient's oral medication dose may be escalated until an appropriate dosage is reached where the patient has enough muscle relaxation, without excessive weakness or loss of muscle tone. Alternatively, the patient may be switched to second-line spasticity oral medications such as gabapentin or diazepam if the initially started

TABLE 28.3
THE ASHWORTH SCALE AND MODIFIED ASHWORTH SCALE

Score	Ashworth	Modified Ashworth
0	No increase in muscle tone	No increase in muscle tone
1	Slight increase in tone giving a catch when the limb is moved in flexion/extension	Slight increase in muscle tone manifested by a catch and release or by minimal resistance at the end of the range of motion (ROM) when the affected limb is moved in flexion or extension.
1+		Slight increase in muscle tone, manifested by a catch, followed by minimal resistance throughout the remainder (less than half) of the ROM
2	More marked increase in tone, but the limb is easily moved through its full ROM	More marked increase in muscle tone through most of the ROM, but affected part(s) easily moved
3	Considerable increase in muscle tone, passive movement difficult	Considerable increase in muscle tone, passive movement difficult
4	Affected part(s) rigid in flexion or extension	Affected part(s) rigid in flexion or extension

medication is not effective or poses undesired side effects. However, if the patient does well on baclofen, but cannot tolerate its side effects, and no other treatment options appear to be helpful, an intrathecal baclofen pump can be an excellent option as a last resort to provide long-term, low-concentration intrathecal baclofen with less chance for side effects.

Neuropathic Pain

Dysesthesias

Benzon's *Essentials of Pain Management* describes dysesthesia as "an unpleasant abnormal evoked sensation, whether spontaneous or evoked.[13]" In MS patients, dysesthesias are often burning, tingling, or aching sensations which can be located in the arms, legs, or trunk.[4,14] These can be uncomfortable, as well as painful, and decrease the activity level as well as quality of life for patients. Dysesthesias can be treated with tricyclic antidepressants (TCAs) or antiepileptic agents. Amitriptyline (25-150 mg/d), carbamazepine (200-1600 mg/d), gabapentin (300-2400 mg/d), and lamotrigine (200-400 mg/d) are first-line options for therapy while alternative options include topiramate, pregabalin, selective serotonin reuptake inhibitors (SSRIs), and, less desirably, opioids given their side effect profile.[4,8,9] Often times, combination therapy may be needed, particularly to avoid medication side effects from higher doses of one type of medication. Additionally, physiotherapy and carbonated baths may be helpful.[4] More invasive procedures including intrathecal baclofen pump and spinal cord stimulation may also be helpful in painful dysesthesias; however, further research is needed particularly in MS patients.[4]

Paroxysmal Syndromes

Paroxysmal syndromes include trigeminal neuralgia, other neuralgias including radicular pain syndromes, paroxysmal paresthesias, and Lhermitte sign.[9,14] MS-related disability and depression are commonly seen in MS induced neuropathic pain.[14] Classic trigeminal neuralgia is characterized by severe, sharp, stabbing, shock-like facial pain generally on one side of the face. The pain is intermittent, lasting for short periods of time, with pain-free intervals in between. The pain is generally triggered by activity such as speaking or chewing.[3,8,14] Trigeminal neuralgia is seen in 1% to 6.3% of MS patients.[13,14] Trigeminal neuralgia in MS patients is generally caused by inflammatory lesions, often with bilateral symptoms, and often with pain felt even between attacks.[4] In young individuals who present with bilateral facial pain, MS should be suspected.[13]

Generally, MS patients with trigeminal neuralgia are treated the same as trigeminal neuralgias of other origin. First-line treatment includes carbamazepine, while other options include oxcarbazepine, gabapentin, lamotrigine, topiramate, and baclofen.[3,4,8,9,13,14] While carbamazepine is the most effective initial drug of choice, it may be poorly tolerated as well as have side effects which mimic MS relapse such as dizziness and micturition problems. As such, second-line medications should be trialed to establish the best therapy for each individual patient.[14] Trigeminal nerve and gasserian ganglion blocks with local anesthetic and steroids can also provide temporary and less invasive pain relief, although their effects specifically in MS patients needs further evaluation.[15-18] Other invasive therapies include percutaneous techniques such as Gamma Knife radiation therapy, radiofrequency thermoablation, and pulsed radiofrequency ablation, as well as surgical microvascular decompression.[4,13] Gasserian ganglion neurostimulation is yet another form of therapy which may also provide pain relief.[13,19]

Lhermitte sign is an abrupt, transient electrical sensation which migrates from the neck, down into the spine, and can even progress to the lower extremities.[14,20,21] These paroxysmal symptoms are generally triggered by movement of the neck with lesions present within the cervical cord. According to a recent prospective study involving 694 patients with MS, 16% of patients experienced Lhermitte sign during their disease duration.[21] While there is no specific therapy for these symptoms, gabapentin, pregabalin, topical lidocaine, and antidepressants including TCAs, SSRIs and selective norepinephrine reuptake inhibitors can be helpful.[3,14,22] Second-line agents include medications such as carbamazepine, lamotrigine, topiramate, mexiletine, and oxcarbazepine.[14]

Patients with MS can also develop other neuralgias such as radicular pain and painful paroxysmal dystonias with muscle spasms.[8] Management for this type of pain is the same as for chronic neuropathic pain, with medications including those which were previously described above.[4,8,14] Often times a combination of drugs with different mechanism of action may be necessary. While medication management may be helpful for some patients, it may not be sufficient for others. In such cases, alternative therapies may include spinal cord stimulation, sympathetic nerve blocks, deep brain stimulation (DBS), transcutaneous electrical nerve stimulation (TENS), or repetitive transcranial magnetic stimulation (rTMS).[3,13]

Chronic Low-Back Pain With or Without Radiculopathy

Many MS patients will experience low-back pain at some point in their disease state. Low-back pain is present in 40% of patients with MS.[8] Patients may develop chronic low-back pain secondary to multiple causes including, but not limited to, degenerative disc disease, muscle tension, paralysis, immobility, truncal muscle spasticity, spinal stenosis, lumbar spondylosis, sacroiliac joint disease, or osteoporosis.[8,13] A more extensive list of causes of low-back pain can be found in Table 28.4.

It is particularly important to evaluate for any "red flags" in the medical history such as unexplained weight loss, history of neoplasm, loss of bowel or bladder control, constitutional symptoms such as fever/chills, history of recent trauma, or worsened pain to rule out serious causes of back pain.[3,13] It is key to differentiate the cause of the back pain (i.e., myofascial, discogenic, degenerative disease, herniated disc, etc.) so that appropriate therapies can then be sought. Pharmacological therapies for low-back pain include nonsteroidal anti-inflammatory drugs (NSAIDS) and muscle relaxants. Muscle relaxants are particularly helpful in pain secondary to immobility and muscle tension.[3,13] Oral corticosteroids can be prescribed in acute disc herniation, while a short very limited course of opioids may be initiated in acute low-back pain or exacerbations of chronic low-back pain.[13] Back pain with associated radiculopathy can be treated with neuropathic agents such as gabapentin.[8] While the evidence is not overwhelming, nonpharmaceutical therapies which can be incorporated into the management of back pain include physical therapy and rehabilitation interventions including posture awareness, ergonomics, activities of daily living (ADL) training, TENS unit, biofeedback, yoga, tai chi, hypnosis, and acupuncture.[3,8,13] A meta-analysis also demonstrated that massage therapy can be effective in low-back pain and that acupuncture massage may be more effective than conventional massage.[23]

TABLE 28.4
ETIOLOGY OF SPINE PAIN

Mechanical Spine Pain

- Lumbar spondylosis
- Sacroiliac joint pain
- Degenerative disc disease
- Myofascial pain syndrome
- Myofascial or ligament sprain/strain
- Kyphosis
- Scoliosis
- Spinal stenosis
- Osteoporosis
- Pars interarticularis defect
- Herniated discs
- Discogenic pain
- Transforaminal stenosis
- Neurogenic claudication

Nonmechanical Spine Pain

- Paget disease
- Vertebral body fractures
- Noninfectious inflammatory spine disorders (ankylosing spondylitis, psoriatic spondylitis, Reiter syndrome)
- Neoplasms of spine (primary or secondary)
- Osteomyelitis

Referred or Visceral Spinal Pain

- Renal disease (pyelonephritis, nephrolithiasis)
- Pancreatitis, cholecystitis, perforated bowel
- Pelvic visceral disorders (endometriosis, prostatitis)

While controlled studies have not consistently demonstrated the efficacy of spinal injections, particularly in the long term, minimally invasive therapies such as epidural steroid injections, facet joint injections, sacroiliac joint injections, and trigger point injections may be helpful in some types of back pain, particularly in the acute phase.[13] Alternatively, risk versus benefit analysis would be necessary to consider the next step of surgical intervention which may be particularly helpful or necessary in spinal stenosis, severe disc herniation, or cord compression. Emergent cases with red flag symptoms would necessitate emergent surgery to prevent further injury and potentially devastating outcomes such as paralysis. Additionally, surgical consideration should be made in cases where other modes of therapy have not been successful, where quality of life is severely affected, and where risks of surgery do not outweigh the benefits of pain relief and improvement in quality of life.

Pain Following Drug Treatment

Local pain at the site of the injection of beta-interferon or glatiramer acetate (GLAT) may be prevented or reduced by optimizing injection technique as well as placing ice packs on the skin before and after the injection. Ice packs should not be kept on for greater than 10 minutes as to avoid skin necrosis. Flulike symptoms may be reduced by administration of paracetamol, acetaminophen, ibuprofen, naproxen, or low-dose corticosteroids.[3,24,25] An increase in the frequency of headaches from B-interferon therapy may require prophylactic therapy, or optimization of headache medications.[3,8]

Effects of Cannabis on Neuropathic Patient

The role of cannabis and cannabinoid products for pain management is not well understood. Much research is still needed, particularly in regard to pain management specifically in the MS patient. The endocannabinoid system is involved in pain sensation and can be inhibited by the use of cannabinoids.[13,26] With regard to neuropathic pain, Rice found efficacy in cannabinoids relieving neuropathic pain, particularly in MS patients.[26] According to Liang et al, cannabis and cannabinoids may be potentially helpful in trigeminal neuralgia via modulation of pain pathways.[27] While there is little evidence for improvement in clinician-measured MS-related spasticity with oral cannabinoids, there is conclusive evidence for improvement in patient reported pain and overall mobility in MS patients.[8,28] A report published by The National Academies of Science, Engineering and Medicine which looked at over 10,000 scientific abstracts concluded that there is substantial evidence for improvement in pain in chronic pain patients, while there is moderate evidence showing cannabis or cannabinoids can improve short-term sleep outcomes in MS patients.[28] While further research is needed for stronger evidence for the role of cannabis and cannabinoids in pain management, some evidence does suggest that it may be helpful for MS patients. However, the benefits need to be outweighed by the side effects which patients may develop including dry mouth, dizziness, headache, and tiredness.[26]

Other Modalities for Pain Management

In any of the MS pain syndromes, the most effective treatment is one with a multimodal approach, involving different modalities of pain management. Previously, we discussed different pain syndromes with their therapies and now we will discuss in more detail a few other modes of therapies which can be helpful in pain management in MS patient. Physical therapy, including posture awareness, strengthening exercises, massage therapy, and TENS unit can be used in chronic low-back pain, neuropathic pain, and pain secondary to spasticity in MS patients.[3,7-9,13] Negahban et al found that in MS patients, massage therapy may be more effective in pain reduction, dynamic balance, and speed walking compared with exercise therapy, while the combination of the two therapies showed significantly greater reduction in pain.[29] Additionally, acupuncture therapy may be helpful in chronic low-back pain.[3,8,13] Some studies have also found that hydrotherapy can help reduce spasticity, baclofen need, pain, spasm, fatigue, disability, and autonomy.[30,31] Other complimentary therapies including biofeedback, cognitive behavioral therapy, and mindful meditation are not only helpful in decreasing self-reported pain, but they can also help with pain-associated comorbidities such as anxiety, depression, and disability.[3,8,13,32] As depression, anxiety disorders and sleep disturbances are more common in chronic pain patients versus the general population, consultation to psychologists, psychiatrists, and addition medicine specialists are also very important to address comorbidities that come with chronic pain.[3]

Conclusion

Many patients with MS develop symptoms of pain throughout their disease state. Pain can lead to increased depression and disability and subsequently a decrease in quality of life. A thorough examination and understanding of the patient's pain will allow for the appropriate mode of management. A multimodal approach specific for the patient's particular pain will be most beneficial in pain management in MS patients.

High-yield points:

- Regular physiotherapy is an important antispastic treatment at all stages of management.
- The goal of spasticity therapy is to decrease muscle tone to improve functionality and pain without causing excessive weakness or complete loss of muscle tone.
- Baclofen and tizanidine are first-line oral therapies for spasticity, while diazepam and gabapentin are second-line therapies which can be used. Medications should be titrated up slowly as needed.
- In focal spasticity, botulinum toxin injections can be helpful.
- In global spasticity, and when other options have failed, intrathecal baclofen delivery systems can be considered.
- Cannabinoids can be of benefit in helping with spasms and patient's subjective impression of their pain, and as such, their use should be in particular cases and under a physician's care.
- First-line therapy for trigeminal neuralgia is carbamazepine, followed by second-line therapies including oxcarbazepine, gabapentin, lamotrigine, topiramate, and baclofen.

- Interventional therapies for trigeminal neuralgia include trigeminal nerve and gasserian ganglion blocks, Gamma Knife radiation therapy, radiofrequency thermoablation, balloon microcompression, pulsed radiofrequency ablation, microvascular decompression, and gasserian ganglion neurostimulation.
- Other neuropathic pain including dysesthesias, Lhermitte sign, and radicular pain may be alleviated with the use of anticonvulsants, antidepressants, and opioids.
- Identifying the cause of low-back pain in MS patients is key in appropriately treating their pain.
- Physiotherapy with proper ergonomics and posture, TENS unit, acupuncture, massage therapy, and biofeedback may be incorporated into the treatment of back pain.
- While multiple strong research studies are lacking at this time, cannabis and cannabinoids may have a role in pain management in MS patients.
- The best approach to pain management in MS patients is using a multimodal approach.

References

1. Drulovic J, Basic-Kes V, Grigic S, et al. The prevalence of pain in adults with multiple sclerosis: a multicenter cross-sectional survey. *Pain Med.* 2015;16:1597-1602.
2. O'Connor AB, Schwid SR, Herrman DM, et al. Pain associated with multiple sclerosis: systematic review and proposed classification. *Pain.* 2008;137:96-111.
3. Vadivelu N, Urman RD, Hines RL, eds. *Essentials of Pain Management.* New York: Springer; 2011.
4. Pollmann W, Feneberg W. Current management of pain associated with multiple sclerosis. *CNS Drugs.* 2008;22(4):291-324.
5. Beard S, Hunn A, Wight J. Treatments for spasticity and pain in multiple sclerosis: a systematic review. *Health Technol Assess.* 2003;7:40 [executive summary].
6. Rizzo MA, Hadjimichael OC, Preiningerova J, et al. Prevalence and treatment of spasticity reported by multiple sclerosis patients. *Mult Scler.* 2004;10:589-595.
7. Thompson AJ, Jarrett L, Lockley L, et al. Clinical management of spasticity. *J Neurol Neurosurg Psychiatry.* 2005;76:459-463.
8. Henze T, Rieckmann P, Toyka KV. Symptomatic treatment of multiple sclerosis. *Eur Neurol.* 2006;56:78-105.
9. Pollman W, Feneberg W, Steinbrecher A, et al. Therapy of pain syndromes in multiple sclerosis—an overview with evidence based recommendations. *Fortschr Neurol Psychiatr.* 2005;73(5):268-285.
10. Odderson IR. *Botulinum Toxin Injection Guide.* New York: Demos Medical Publishing, LLC; 2008.
11. Frampton JE. Onabotulinum toxin A (BOTOX(R)): a review of its use in the prophylaxis of headaches in adults with chronic migraine. *Drugs.* 2012;72:825-845.
12. Ansari NN, Naghdi S, Arab TK, et al. The interrater and intrarater reliability of the Modified Ashworth Scale in the assessment of muscle spasticity: limb and muscle group effect. *Neuro Rehabil.* 2008;23(3):231-237.

13. Benzon H, Raja SN, Liu SS, et al, eds. *Essentials of Pain Medicine.* 3rd ed. Philadelphia, PA: Elsevier Saunders; 2011.

14. Zagon US, McLaughlin PJ, eds. *Multiple Sclerosis: Perspectives in Treatment and Pathogenesis [Internet].* Brisbane (AU): Codon publications; 2017.

15. Nader A, Kendall MC, De Oliveria GS, et al. Ultrasound-guided trigeminal nerve block via the pterygopalatine fossa: an effective treatment for trigeminal neuralgia and atypical facial pain. *Pain Physician.* 2013;16(5):E537-E545.

16. Nader A, Schittek H, Kendall M. Lateral pterygoid muscle and maxillary artery are key anatomical landmarks for ultrasound-guided trigeminal nerve blocks. *Anesthesiology.* 2013;118:957.

17. Adler P. The use of bupivacaine for blocking the Gasserian ganglion in major trigeminal neuralgia. *Int J Oral Surg.* 1975;4(60):251-257.

18. Greenberg C, Papper EM. The indications for gasserian ganglion block for trigeminal neuralgia. *Anesthesiology.* 1969;31(6):566-573.

19. Slavin KV, ed. *Stimulation of the Peripheral Nervous System. The Neuromodulation Frontier.* Prog Neurol Surg. Vol. 29. Basel: Karger; 2016:76-82.

20. Kanchandani R, Howe JG. Lhermitte's sign in multiple sclerosis: a clinical survey and review of the literature. *J Neurol Neurosurg Psychiatry.* 1982;45:308.

21. Beckman Y, Ozakbas S, Bulbur NG. Reassessment of Lhermitte's sign in multiple sclerosis. *Acta Neurol Belgica.* 2015;115(4):605-608.

22. Sakurai M, Kanazawa I. Positive symptoms in multiple sclerosis: their treatment with sodium channel blockers, lidocaine and mexiletine. *J Neurol Sci.* 1999;162(2):162-168.

23. Furlan AD, Imamura M, Dryden T, et al. Massage for low-back pain. *Cochrane Database Syst Rev.* 2008;8(4):CD001929.

24. Reess J, Haas J, Babriel K, et al. Both paracetamol and ibuprofen are equally effective in managing flu-like symptoms in relapsing-remitting multiple sclerosis patients during interferon-B1a (AVON-EX) therapy. *Mult Scler.* 2002;8:15-18.

25. Rio J, Nos C, Bonaventura I, et al. Corticosteroids, ibuprofen, and acetaminophen for IFN-B1a flu symptoms in MS. A randomized trial. *Neurology.* 2004;63:525-528.

26. Rice AS. Should cannabinoids be used as analgesics for neuropathic pain? *Nat Clin Pract Neurol.* 2008;4(12):654-655.

27. Liang YC, Huang CC, Hsu KS. Therapeutic potential of cannabindoids in trigeminal neuralgia. *Curr Drug Targets CNS Neurol Disord.* 2004;3(6):507-514.

28. National Academies of Sciences, Engineering, and Medicine. *The Health Effects of Cannabis and Cannabinoids: The Current State of Evidence and Recommendations for Research.* Washington, DC: The National Academies Press; 2017. doi:10.17226/24625.

29. Negahban H, Rezaie S, Goharpey S. Massage therapy and exercise therapy in patients with multiple sclerosis: a randomized controlled pilot study. *Clin Rehabil.* 2013;27(12):1126-1136.

30. Kesiktas N, Paker N, Erdogan N, et al. The use of hydrotherapy for the management of spasticity. *Neurorehabil Neural Repair.* 2004;18:268-273.

31. Castro-Sanchez AM, Mataran-Penarrocha GA, Lara-Palomo I, et al. Hydrotherapy for the treatment of pain in people with multiple sclerosis: a randomized controlled trial. *Evid Based Complement Alternat Med.* 2012;2012:1-8.

32. Senders A, Borgatti A, Hanes D, et al. Association between pain and mindfulness in multiple sclerosis: a cross-sectional survey. *Int J MS Care.* 2018;20:28-34.

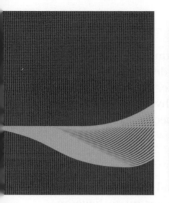
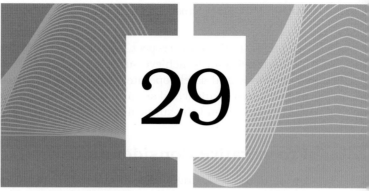

29

Multiple Sclerosis and General Anesthetic Considerations

■■■ Christopher Der, Guy Tran, Sydney Yee

Introduction

Although medical management is the mainstay of treatment of multiple sclerosis (MS), people with MS undergo operations and procedures on a daily basis. Things we now consider common procedures were impossible hundreds of years ago—until humans developed the ability to induce a state of anesthesia. The study of Anesthesiology has been around for centuries, but only recently in the early 1800s was it first described in Western medicine.[1] There are still a myriad of questions surrounding the pharmacokinetics and pharmacodynamics of anesthetics that patients ask commonly in clinical practice: Is it safe? What about in pregnancy? How does it affect MS and how does MS affect the type of anesthetic I receive?

In general, patients receive either general anesthesia, in which they are rendered unconscious, or a nerve block, either neuraxial or peripheral. No single type of anesthetic can be applied to all patients because each patient is complex and each procedure has its own surgical requirements. A pregnant mother may wish to receive a neuraxial anesthetic so that she can witness the birth of her newborn during her nonelective cesarean delivery, while realizing that there is an elevated risk of exacerbating

499

symptoms. In the same respect, a patient with debilitating MS may receive a muscle relaxant to achieve surgical conditions in order for the surgeon to effectively and safely operate. To plan an anesthetic, knowledge of the patient's past medical and surgical history, the pathophysiology of MS and its treatments, and the surgical requirements are all necessary.

Preoperative Considerations

Owing to the relapsing and remitting nature of MS and the ability of the perioperative period to provoke an MS flare, it is important to have an understanding and documentation of a patient's baseline function and deficits if present. The additional goals of anesthesia in patients with MS should encompass prevention of relapse, prevention of further neurological damage, and avoidance of drug interactions.

In patients with MS, neurological involvement can exist throughout the central nervous system, leading to various presentations and pathologies to be aware of before providing anesthetic. A thorough understanding of the preoperative neurological deficits is important. For example, cranial nerve involvement may increase the risk of aspiration due to deficits in laryngeal and pharyngeal function. Cervical spinal cord lesions may lead to respiratory abnormalities. Patients should be queried on their ability to clear secretions and strength of cough. If there is respiratory compromise, the severity, treatment, and episodes of mechanical ventilation should be noted and discussed.[2,3] Pulmonary function tests may show unchanged lung volumes and capacities, but diffusion capacity may be reduced.[2] An arterial blood gas may help establish baseline ventilatory physiology. Sleep disorders have been described in patients with MS. The combination of obesity and obstructive sleep apnea may increase postoperative respiratory failure. Because of the lifelong degenerative nature of the disease, optimization for surgery is relative to a patient's baseline function. Optimization with sleep studies and noninvasive continuous positive pressure may offer benefit in the perioperative period, as well as encouraging smoking cessation when applicable.[2] If a patient has any new neurological symptoms, it is prudent to delay elective surgery to consult with the patient's neurologist. Patients with cranial nerve or respiratory involvement should be counseled on the possibility of remaining intubated postoperatively, and the appropriate arrangements should be made with an institution's intensive care unit (ICU).

Involvement of the thoracic spinal cord may lead to autonomic dysfunction. Should autonomic dysfunction be present in this population it may manifest as episodes of syncope or arrhythmias. The severity of this should be noted as intraoperative fluctuations in blood pressure that may occur, and invasive monitoring may be considered. Invasive monitoring may include an arterial line, which would measure beat to beat blood pressure variations. In addition, a central venous catheter can be considered for central venous pressure measurements, which may assist with volume resuscitation.

Current treatment regimens should be explored and documented. Chronic use of steroids in patients with MS may require intraoperative administration of steroids, also known as stress dosing, or its osteoporotic sequelae may place the patient at risk for nerve injury. Additionally, certain anticonvulsants, which the patient may be taking, may increase resistance to muscle relaxant administration within the operating room. A list of medications should be provided to the anesthesiologist for consideration in the anesthetic plan.[4]

Numerous factors have been known to contribute to MS relapses including infection, emotional stress, physical trauma, and the perioperative and peripartum periods. Unfortunately for anesthesiologists, at least one of these conditions is met for a majority of the patients they care for on a routine basis. Also, because of the nature of the disease, it can often be impossible to distinguish if a relapse is secondary to anesthetic or is merely coincidental. Because we cannot completely alleviate any single one of these factors and the complicated clinical scenario, it is important to approach patients with MS with care and to involve them as much as possible in their anesthetic care plan, which should be documented in detail.

General Considerations for General Anesthesia and MS

The anesthetic care of any patient involves three phases of care: induction, maintenance, and extubation.

At induction, an anesthetic is generally given via an inhalational route or an intravenous route. Although cases have been reported of worsening of symptoms with general anesthesia, both routes of anesthetic administration have been safely used in this population and one route is not superior to the other. Another drug given during this phase is a muscle relaxant to obtain optimal intubating conditions, assuming an endotracheal tube is to be placed. Succinylcholine is a depolarizing muscular blocker that causes a well-known increase of extracellular potassium. Patients who are otherwise healthy have a mild increase in potassium, which is usually clinically insignificant, but patients with neuromuscular disease can have an upregulation of extrajunctional acetylcholine receptors, which can cause a life-threatening efflux of potassium from the cell. In patients with severe disease or in an active exacerbation, there have been reports of succinylcholine-induced hyperkalemic cardiac arrest.[2,3,5] Thus, this drug should be used with caution in patients with MS and usage should depend on the patient's current clinical status. In an emergency setting, if there is an alternative available, it would be prudent to avoid succinylcholine for intubation, particularly in patients with obvious neuromuscular involvement (contractures, muscle wasting, wheelchair usage). Alternatively, nondepolarizing muscular blockers, such as rocuronium or vecuronium, can be used. Patients with MS are particularly sensitive to these muscle relaxants. A nerve stimulator should be used to judiciously administer a muscle relaxant, and the anesthesiologist should monitor for return of muscle tone. Quantitative monitors may be more beneficial at centers with a high volume of MS patient population, as they may provide more reliable indicators of return of muscle function.[6]

The maintenance phase is the ongoing delivery of an anesthetic. No one particular anesthetic appears safer than another. In this phase, succinylcholine typically is not given. Nondepolarizing muscle relaxants are generally given during this phase, and as described earlier, a nondepolarizing muscle relaxant should be closely monitored, quantitatively or qualitatively, by an anesthesiologist. During any surgical procedure, the patient's temperature should be closely monitored as well. Hyperthermia is a well-described trigger of MS, and aggressive temperature control is important.[7] Special care should be taken when using warmers in the operative room. However, hypothermia is not advisable either and the goal should be to maintain normothermia. Care should also be taken with patient positioning, as further in the disease process, patients may have contractures and positioning may be difficult.

In the extubation phase, the anesthesiologist prepares for extubating the patient in a safe manner. As previously discussed, patients with MS may present with pharyngeal and laryngeal dysfunction, which may lead to aspiration.[2,3] As these patients wake up from anesthesia, they may be asked to perform certain functions, such as hand squeezing or head lifting. These clinical signs may provide the anesthesiologist indicators of strength, especially if a muscle relaxant was given. If a patient shows worsening signs of muscle function, even in the absence of muscle relaxant use, then further investigation may be necessary. This patient may remain intubated, sedated, and transferred to the ICU for further monitoring.

As discussed later, the use of neuraxial anesthesia has been shown to be safe in this population; however, there is controversy surrounding the use of neuraxial anesthesia in patients with ongoing symptoms. The concern arises from the idea of exposing demyelinated plaques to local anesthetic, which is potentially neurotoxic. Ultimately, it is believed that lower concentrations of local anesthetics may prove to be safer than higher concentrations and that epidural anesthesia may be safer than intrathecal anesthesia.[8-11]

Alternatively, some procedures may not require a general or regional anesthetic. This is considered monitored anesthesia care. An example of this may include obtaining a mass biopsy. Infiltration of a local anesthetic may be all that is needed. By injecting a local anesthetic into the skin and surrounding subcutaneous tissue, pain will be minimized during surgical incision. Intravenous benzodiazepines and opioids may be used additionally to provide more comfort and anxiolysis.

Pregnancy

Pregnancy is a time filled with excitement and joy, but it is also filled with fear and anxiety, which are known triggers of MS exacerbation. In the past, labor and delivery predominantly took place in one's home with the assistance of midwifery. Today, we have medicalized the labor and delivery process, with multiple teams, frequent vital measurements, and certain uncomfortable procedures, such as intravenous and urinary catheterizations. It is no wonder some of these mothers feel anxious and a lack of control! Ultimately, some of this control can be relinquished back to these mothers, and verbal anxiolysis may be the best initial approach to any patient, and especially those with known MS.

Mothers with MS can have a natural delivery. Even with MS symptoms affecting the pelvic floor, vaginal delivery is still possible. This may require instrumentation with forceps and/or vacuum for fetal delivery, and consultation with the obstetrician is important. Instrumented delivery can cause anxiety and pain, and in these cases, neuraxial anesthesia is beneficial. Neuraxial anesthesia can be delivered via two general methods. A catheter can be inserted into the epidural space via a large-bore needle. Once the catheter is positioned, the needle is removed and only the catheter remains. This catheter is used to infuse local anesthetic medication through and effectively blocking the transmission of neural signals. The other method is spinal anesthesia. Typically, this involves inserting a small-bore needle into the intrathecal sac, the space where cerebral spinal fluid resides. A small amount of local anesthetic is injected, effectively blocking the transmission of neural signals.

There is no contraindication to neuraxial analgesia and anesthesia for vaginal delivery via a labor epidural or cesarean delivery via an epidural or spinal. Because of a lack of studies and evidence being limited to case reports and observation, in the past, many anesthesiologists have been hesitant to provide neuraxial anesthesia for fear of triggering or worsening a patient's MS. There remains a long-standing concern of local anesthetics and direct neurotoxicity in the setting of demyelinated nerves. Thus, some anesthesiologists may only offer a general anesthetic if a cesarean delivery is indicated. However, causality is difficult to prove in patients with an unpredictable disease such as MS, particularly in the setting of temporarily induced motor and sensory blockade.

In general, pregnancy and its hypoimmunogenic state offers protection against MS.[7] However, because parturients are more likely to experience relapse in the postpartum period, distinguishing neurological sequelae from relapse versus neuraxial anesthesia is difficult. Good control of symptoms in the prepregnant state may offer some protection from relapse, so consultation with neurology may offer additional patient education and reassurance.[12,13] Despite this, some anesthesiologists may still reserve the right to withhold intrathecal administration of local anesthetics in this population, especially those with ongoing symptoms.[2,8,9,14]

Many anesthesiologists feel that it is important to give lower-dose local anesthetic and to combine with opioids when providing labor analgesia. This is because opioids both epidurally and intrathecally have not been shown to exacerbate MS symptoms.

Given this lack of consensus, the risks and benefits must be extensively discussed and documented with both the patient and obstetric team. A survey done in the United Kingdom revealed that a majority of obstetric anesthesiologists were comfortable with performing a neuraxial anesthetic for a patient with MS, as long as informed consent was obtained.[15] At this author's institution, patients with MS who are stable in their disease are eligible candidates for neuraxial anesthesia.

Regional blocks are considered generally safe because the majority of the disease process is limited to the central nervous system. However, it has been shown in autopsy studies that disease may spread along peripheral nerves. Cases of peripheral neuritis have been described, so it is recommended that ultrasound and the lowest possible dose of local anesthetic without epinephrine be used to achieve adequate results.[16]

As discussed previously, monitored anesthesia care can be provided with local infiltration for small procedures in our pregnant patients. Unlike above, the use of intravenous benzodiazepines may be avoided in this population.

General anesthesia may be required in some instances of failed neuraxial anesthesia. Failed neuraxial blocks are either ineffective or inadequate and can occur in the untimely instances of urgent and emergent cesarean delivery. When undergoing general anesthesia, muscle relaxants may be given. There have been reports of hyperkalemia in this population with succinylcholine use, but nondepolarizing muscle relaxants should also be cautiously used and monitored.[2,3,5] Although muscle relaxants may be avoided altogether, the use of volatile anesthetics not only may help with muscle relaxation but also induce uterine relaxation, which may worsen uterine atony and hemorrhage if it were to occur.

In the unfortunate event that a patient has a post-dural puncture headache, there are additional concerns. A post-dural puncture headache is a headache that typically arises approximately 24 hours post epidural placement. This occurs when the epidural needle traverses the dura, causing a loss of cerebrospinal fluid. A result of this decrease in fluid is a tugging of the central nervous system, causing what is commonly described as a headache that occurs in the upright position. A blood patch can be done to treat a post-dural puncture headache. A blood patch involves another epidural procedure, but rather than injecting a local anesthetic, blood is injected. However, there is concern that a blood patch may increase epidural pressure, affecting at-risk neural tissue. However, blood patches have been safely performed in this population. Slow and small-aliquot injection of blood into the epidural space may allow the practitioner to better recognize symptoms from increasing epidural pressure.[2]

Postoperative Considerations

Close monitoring is also important in the postoperative period. Vital signs should be monitored frequently, especially those with autonomic involvement. Signs of hyperthermia should be aggressively treated.[7] Patients already on continuous positive airway pressure (CPAP) should have their home use CPAP initiated in the recovery area, to assist with any hypoventilation and obstruction, especially when a general anesthetic or other substances that may affect one's respiratory physiology are given. Pharyngeal and laryngeal weakness may also lead to aspiration. In addition, the use of neuromuscular blockers should be clearly documented so physicians may quickly administer reversal drugs. Recently, sugammadex was available in the United States. Sugammadex provides quick-onset reversal of rocuronium and to a smaller degree with vecuronium, as compared with neostigmine. One small study comparing normal subjects with subjects with MS revealed no differences in onset time with sugammadex reversal.[17]

Although pregnancy overall is associated with a decreased rate of MS exacerbations, regardless of anesthetic choice or even without anesthetic exposure, the postpartum period is associated with an increased risk of relapse for patients with MS. This risk may be related to a patient's prepartum diseases status, and the obstetrician and neurologist should decide when to restart MS therapy after delivery.

Conclusion

MS is a disease with variable manifestations. These patients will undergo procedures that may not be MS specific. Although all types of anesthesia have been considered to exacerbate symptoms, anesthesia is considered safe for these patients, whether it is administered neuraxially, peripherally, or as a general anesthetic. It is ultimately important for the patients to have a thorough discussion with their neurologist, anesthesiologist, and proceduralist regarding the risks and benefits of their proposed care. A well-considered plan can provide the patient with knowledge, power, and comfort proceeding with their care. This author primarily cares for the obstetric population, and experience suggests that pregnant mothers appreciate the thorough discussion of epidural risk and safety in MS, whether they choose to use one or not.

References

1. Caton D. *The history of obstetric anesthesia.* In: *Chestnut's Obstetric Anesthesia Principles and Practice.* 5th ed. Elsevier Inc; 2014:3-11.
2. Makris A, Piperopoulos A, Karmaniolou I. Multiple sclerosis: basic knowledge and new insights in perioperative management. *J Anesth.* 2014;28(2):267-278.
3. Dorotta IR, Schubert A. Multiple sclerosis and anesthetic implications. *Curr Opin Anesthesiol.* 2002;15(3):365.
4. Houtchens MK, Kolb CM. Multiple sclerosis and pregnancy: therapeutic considerations. *J Neurol.* 2013;260(5):1202-1214.
5. Cooperman LH. Succinylcholine induced hyperkalemia in neuromuscular disease. *JAMA.* 1970;213:1867-1871.
6. Naguib M, Brull SJ, Kopman AF, et al. Consensus statement on perioperative use of neuromuscular monitoring. *Anesth Analg.* 2018;127(1):71-80. doi:10.1213/ANE.0000000000002670.
7. Pozzilli C, Pugliatti M. An overview of pregnancy-related issues in patients with multiple sclerosis. *Eur J Neurol.* 2015;22(S2):34-39.
8. Pastò L, Portaccio E, Ghezzi A, et al. Epidural analgesia and cesarean delivery in multiple sclerosis post-partum relapses: the Italian cohort study. *BMC Neurol.* 2012;12(1):165.
9. Lu E, Zhao Y, Dahlgren L, et al. Obstetrical epidural and spinal anesthesia in multiple sclerosis. *J Neurol.* 2013;260(10):2620-2628.
10. Bader AM, Hunt CO, Datta S, Naulty JS, Ostheimer GW. Anesthesia for the obstetric patient with multiple sclerosis. *J Clin Anesth.* 1988;1(1):21-24.
11. Vukusic S, Marignier R. Multiple sclerosis and pregnancy in the "treatment era". *Nat Rev.* 2015;11(5):280-289.
12. Coyle PK. Management of women with multiple sclerosis through pregnancy and after childbirth. *Ther Adv Neurol Dis.* 2016;9(3):198-210.
13. Hughes SE, Spelman T, Grammond P, et al. Predictors and dynamics of postpartum relapses in women with multiple sclerosis. *Mult Scler J.* 2014;20(6):739-746.
14. Perlas A, Chan V. Neuraxial anesthesia and multiple sclerosis. *Can J Anesth.* 2005;52(5):454-458.
15. Drake E, Drake M, Bird J, Russell R. Obstetric regional blocks for women with multiple sclerosis: a survey of UK experience. *Int J Obstet Anesth.* 2006;15(2):115-123. doi:10.1016/j.ijoa.2005.10.010.
16. Jangra K, Grover VK, Bhagat H. *Neurologic patients for non-neurosurgeries.* In: *Essentials of Neuroanesthesia.* 2017:783-803:chap 47.
17. Altunbay RA, Sinikoglu N, Bagci M. Train-of-four guard-controlled sugammadex reversal in patients with multiple sclerosis. *Niger J Clin Pract.* 2018;21(7):870-874. doi:10.4103/njcp.njcp_321_17.
18. Tantucci C, Massucci M, Piperno R. Control of breathing and respiratory muscle strength in patients with multiple sclerosis. *Chest.* 1994;105:1163-1170.

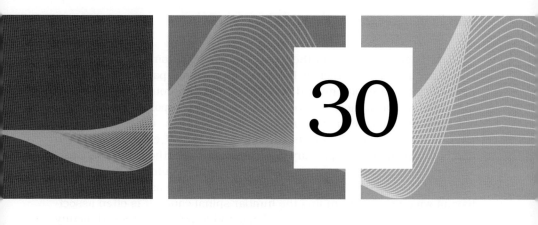

30

Neurosurgery

■■■ Mostafa El Khashab, Constantine J. Pella

Introduction

Neurologists are usually the principal providers for patients with multiple sclerosis (MS). However, there are many reasons when referral to neurosurgery is indicated. Conditions such as surgical removal of benign or malignant brain tumors and repair of aneurysms or arteriovenous malformations require neurosurgical consultation. This chapter will focus on problems seen in the MS patient such as back pain that often prompts referral to neurosurgery.

Low-Back Pain

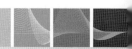

A 43-year-old female presented to the emergency department complaining of severe acute low-back pain and left-sided sciatic pain. The pain in the left lower extremity corresponded to the distribution of the L5 nerve root. The patient did have sensory impairment in the L5 dermatome and had pain on straight leg raising at 30°. Magnetic resonance imaging (MRI) scans revealed foraminal stenosis at L4/5 with disc bulge at this level. Patient has history of MS. Patient underwent pain management consult and was treated with epidural injections as well as nonsteroidal anti-inflammatory medications and physical therapy for 6 weeks. She continued to be followed up. Conservative treatment was not successful, and the patient elected to have microdiscectomy and laminectomy.

Low-back pain is one of the most common symptoms neurosurgeons encounter in everyday practice. Patients with low-back pain are referred for neurosurgical care for a myriad of reasons, and a thorough clinical examination as well as a thorough workup is needed to pinpoint the diagnosis.

Lumbar spine stenosis is one of the most common causes of low-back pain. It most commonly affects the middle-aged and elderly population and is primarily seen by primary care physicians or orthopedic surgeons.[1] The pathogenesis is due to entrapment of the cauda equine roots by hypertrophy of the osseous and soft tissue structures such as the ligamentum flavum which are surrounding the lumbar spinal canal. It is often associated with incapacitating pain in the back and lower extremities, difficulty ambulating, sensory impairment of lower extremities, and weakness and, if severe, may lead to a partial or a full-blown cauda equina syndrome with bowel or bladder disturbances.[2]

The characteristic syndrome associated with lumbar stenosis is termed neurogenic intermittent claudication, which must be differentiated from true intermittent vascular claudication, which is caused by atherosclerosis of the pelvic and femoral vessels. Although many conditions may be associated with lumbar canal stenosis, most cases are idiopathic and the symptoms are very vague on presentation. Imaging of the lumbar spine performed with computed tomography or MRI often demonstrates narrowing of the lumbar canal with compression of the cauda equina nerve roots by thickened posterior vertebral elements, facet joints, marginal osteophytes, or soft tissue structures such as the ligamentum flavum or herniated discs. Typically, treatment for symptomatic lumbar stenosis is usually surgical decompression with decompressive laminectomies at the level of stenosis with or without instrumented fusion. Surgical treatment would be considered after conservative treatment with medication and physical therapy as well as injections.[3-5] Examples of injection treatment used by pain management include epidural injections as well as paravertebral blocks. Medical treatment alternatives, such as bed rest, pain management, and physical therapy, should be reserved for use in debilitated patients or patients whose surgical risk is prohibitive as a result of concomitant medical conditions.

Lumbosacral radiculopathy follows a dermatomal distribution and is usually well circumscribed.[3] Sensory paresthesias are usually present in the involved root distribution, and MRI often reveals a disc herniation or bulge compromising the exiting nerve root within the spinal canal or at the foramen. Electromyography/nerve conduction testing can be helpful to demonstrate nerve root compression. Patients with lumbar disc disease are usually treated conservatively with medication, physical therapy, and injections. If conservative treatment fails, surgical microdiscetomy with or without foraminotomy is indicated.

Musculoskeletal disorders and back pain can occur as a result of irregular, asymmetric movement patterns and postures. This is typically what is referred to as mechanically induced low-back pain, and as this can be due to muscular weakness, spasticity, or imbalance, the diagnosis of MS must be strongly entertained. Typically, we will order an MRI scan as part of the workup and refer the patient to an MS center or to a neurologist. The aim is to investigate musculoskeletal disorders and risk factors of low-back pain in MS patients.

In the general population, **osteoarthritis** is a common cause of low-back pain. The prevalence of back pain is in the range of 5% to 22% and significantly limits work and daily activity.[6] Osteoarthritis is one of the most common diseases in adults and affects 22.7% of population. Of the patients with osteoarthritis, 25% are restricted in major activities of daily living.

Greater understanding is needed as to what causes musculoskeletal disorders in MS. The most common cause is low-back pain, with a prevalence of 21.4%.[6] Asymmetric posture, walking impairment, muscle weakness, sensory dysfunction, and spasticity could cause pain and musculoskeletal disorders. Lumbar disc degeneration as well as herniation is again one of the most common causes of low-back pain and sciatica due to nerve root irritation. Last but not least, vascular malformation of the spine with or without bleeding must be put in the differential diagnosis of low-back pain. It is not uncommon to miss this diagnosis without a thorough workup. MRI as well as CT imaging in addition to neurophysiological examination are important tools for the diagnostic workup.

Spasticity

Spasticity is a common symptom of MS, reported by 80% of patients.[7] This symptom could induce abnormal pattern of ambulation, gait impairment, or pain, with a prevalence ranging from 29% to 86%.[7] Spasticity is a term that defines a state of continuous increase in muscle tone. This immediately results in stiffness of muscles leading to interference in normal movement, speech, and gait.[7] It is expressed in neurosurgical literature as a state of increased resistance to passive muscle stretch. There are other conditions that may be clinically mistaken for spasticity, and it is paramount to differentiate those conditions from spasticity. Common hypertonic movement disorders grouped under the term dystonia are markedly differentiated by the quantification of the amount of abnormal movement.

Spasticity is defined as an **iso**kinetic disorder in which the movement is abnormal, but it is in fact not increased whereby dystonia is a **hyper**kinetic disorder in which the movement disorder is both increased and abnormal.[7,8]

Spasticity is clinically manifested by apparent tightness of muscles as well as a sensation of cramping associated with pain. As a result of those feelings, fatigue occurs even from attempted movement. There are variations in the degree and severity of spasticity ranging from mild to extremely disabling. The major components of spasticity are classified into whether they are of spinal origin or cerebral origin and denote damage to the portion of the brain or spinal cord that controls voluntary movement. The consequence of this damage is a disturbance of equilibrium between the central nervous system (CNS) and the muscular system represented in the muscles. This imbalance as we will show at a later stage is both mechanical as well as chemical and involves the release of chemical transmitters. The ultimate result of this imbalance is an increase in muscle activity.

Prevalence and Incidence

Spasticity is not only a common symptom of MS patients but also is condition that affects approximately 12 million people worldwide. Around 320,000 patients with MS have some degree of spasticity in the United States alone.[7] However, spasticity can have a high prevalence in people with other disorders, such as traumatic brain injury (TBI) or other neurological diseases. Statistics on precise prevalence rates of spasticity are difficult to obtain due to the varying causes of spasticity (Table 30.1).

It is noteworthy as we explore the incidence of spasticity in MS patients to point out that treating spasticity has a very profound effect on the quality of life in those affected.[9] In progressive types of MS, we know that there are neurological deficits that may not be very responsive to medical treatment. The inability to transfer combined with pain on movement and rest does cause great discomfort to the patient and can be an inconvenience to caregivers. In this context, the management of spasticity has proven to be of tremendous benefit in improving patient lives.

 TABLE 30.1
THE MOST COMMON CAUSES OF SPASTICITY

Causes of Spasticity
Traumatic brain injury (TBI)
Spinal cord injury (SCI)
Anoxic brain insults of traumatic or hypoxic origin
Central nervous system infections (i.e., encephalitis, meningitis, meningoencephalitis)
Endocrinopathies
Neurologic entities (amyotrophic lateral sclerosis)
Multiple sclerosis (MS)

Adapted from Spasticity. American Association of Neurological Surgeon. Available at https://www.aans.org/Patients/Neurosurgical-Conditions-and-Treatments/Spasticity. Accessed October 9, 2018.

Certain factors can worsen symptoms of spasticity in MS patients. Some of those factors are extremes of temperature, infection, humidity, or even tight-fitting clothes.

Spasticity in Multiple Sclerosis (MS)

As MS is being increasingly recognized in patients at an earlier stage, more referrals are being made to neurosurgeons from MS neurologists for evaluation of patients with severe spasticity, particularly those patients who fail oral medical treatment regimens. Spasticity in MS is divided into two types of MS-related spasms: flexor and extensor. **Flexor spasticity** is an involuntary bending of the hips or knees (involving the hamstring muscles on the back of the upper leg). Typically for flexor spasticity, the hips and knees bend up toward the chest. **Extensor spasticity** is an involuntary straightening of the legs. It involves the quadriceps (muscles on the front of the upper leg) and the adductors (inner thigh muscles).[7] The hips and knees typically remain straight, but the legs will be kept very close or even cross. See Figure 30.1 for reference. Spasticity involving the upper extremities is less common but does exist.

Symptoms

Spasticity is a very diverse phenomenon and may have multiple presentations and symptoms. These symptoms may vary in severity and presentation based on disease progression or the specific disease at hand. There may also be other factors affecting the presentation of symptoms, such as gender or age. Listed below are the most common symptoms of

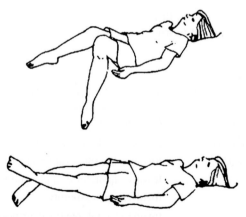

Figure 30.1. Diagram demonstrating the two types of spasticity commonly seen in multiple sclerosis (MS): flexor spasticity (above) and extensor spasticity (below). Reprinted with permission from Gibson B. Stretching for people with MS. National MS Society; 2016:1-26. Reprinted by permission of National Multiple Sclerosis Society.

spasticity. If left untreated, these factors can lead to decreased mobility and fatigue and ultimately can cause severe depressive symptoms and significant interference in family dynamics. Professional and social quality of life can deteriorate as well.[7-9]

- Hypertonicity (increased muscle tone), which often can cause muscle stiffness, rigid joints and bladder dysfunction.
- Spontaneous muscle activity in the form of uncontrollable muscle spasms that are either isolated in nature or present as a series of rapid muscle contractions in the form of clonus. These can be extremely painful in nature and cause significant discomfort to the patient. These spasms can also affect the bladder.
- Exaggerated tendon reflexes often associated with clonus.
- As spasticity worsens, it interferes with all forms of movements, including walking, transfers, and simple muscle movements.
- The tone changes associated with the inability of movement ultimately lead to change in posture, as the balance of flexor versus extensors of the trunk and limbs is disturbed.

Classification Criteria for Spasticity

Neurosurgeons tend to classify spasticity according to the anatomical categories, which were first described in cases of cerebral palsy (CP)[9] (Table 30.2). These classifications are the most important aspect of spasticity for the practicing neurosurgeon, as the anatomical location (as well as severity) influences treatment strategy.

Pathophysiology

Detailed knowledge is required to understand the neurophysiology of spasticity. It is important to know the mechanisms of the CNS that control

TABLE 30.2
THE MOST COMMON CAUSES OF SPASTICITY

Anatomical Categories	Description
Quadriparesis/tetraplegia	Involves all four extremities
Paraparesis/diplegia	Involves the bilateral lower extremities
Hemiparesis	Involves ipsilateral upper and lower extremities
Monoparesis	Involves one extremity
Truncal/cervical	Involving axial, postural, or neck muscles

Adapted from Levitt M, Browd S. *Spasticity: Classification, Diagnosis, and Management.* iKnowledge: Neurosurgery; 2015:chap 50. Available at https://clinicalgate.com/spasticity-classification-diagnosis-and-management.

and regulate movement and posture. In normal conditions, there is an equilibrium that exists between the alpha motor neurons being activated by pyramidal tracts and the alpha motor neurons being activated by basal ganglia, cerebellum and reticular activating system via contrary inhibition. This inhibitory influence is exercised by the reticulospinal tracts, which synapse on the motor neurons of the spinal cord. This is the fundamental cornerstone in understanding the baseline normal balance and which is the reason why those opposing influences create a normal muscle tone (Figure 30.2).[8,10]

Disturbance of this balance is how spasticity originates. The maintenance of posture and normal muscle tone is based on this concept. Spasticity results from any factor that can lead to decreased inhibition or facilitation of hypertonia.[8] Spasticity ultimately results in coactivation of agonistic and antagonistic muscle groups at the same time. This immediately leads to an imbalance of excitatory neurotransmitters in the spinal cord (in particular, a lack of the inhibitory substance γ-aminobutyric acid [GABA]). If left untreated, chronic spasticity may lead to denervation, super sensitivity, and ultimately permanent soft tissue contractures requiring some form of surgical release. This is particularly evident in the ankle joint and Achilles tendon.

Diagnosis

A careful history and physical examination is imperative for the precise and accurate diagnosis of both the cause and classification of spasticity. Steps need to be taken to exclude other causes of spasticity as listed in Table 30.1. For MS patients, spasticity is typically heterogeneous in presentation but largely depends on the areas of demyelination. It can often present with leg adductor and extensor imbalance. In physical examination, the hallmark of locating specific muscle groups affected by spasticity is the resistance to passive muscle stretching correlated to the speed of the stretch. This technique allows for better diagnosis of spasticity among the different spasticity-causing neurological diseases. Physicians often use clinical scales to determine the severity of symptoms of spasticity. Two scales that are often used are the Ashworth Scale and Modified Ashworth Scale, as seen in Table 30.3.

Treatment Philosophy of Spasticity

There are several types of treatment available that must be evaluated on a case-by-case basis. Owing to the diversity of causes, modes of presentation, and the age of patient besides other variables, treatment must be tailored to the individual patient. However, there are multiple guidelines for the treatment to achieve certain important goals. Those goals are summarized as follows.[7]

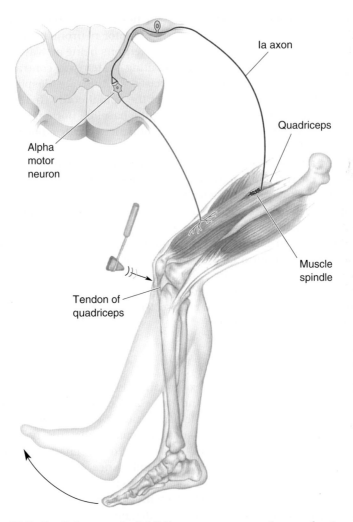

Figure 30.2. Excitatory and inhibitory processes of muscle tone and reflexes. Reprinted with permission from Bear MF, Connors BW, Paradiso MA. *Neuroscience: Exploring the Brain.* 4th ed. Wolters Kluwer Health: Philadelphia, PA. Figure 13-19.

1. Relieving the signs and symptoms of spasticity is the ultimate goal
2. Reducing the pain and frequency of muscle contractions that are a direct result of the spasticity syndrome
3. Improving gait, hygiene, activities of daily living, and ease of care
4. Reducing caregiver challenges such as dressing, feeding, transport, and bathing

TABLE 30.3
COMPARISON OF THE ASHWORTH SCALE AND MODIFIED ASHWORTH SCALE

Score	Ashworth	Modified Ashworth
0	No increase in muscle tone	No increase in muscle tone
1	Slight increase in tone giving a catch when the limb is moved in flexion/extension	Slight increase in muscle tone manifested by a catch and release or by minimal resistance at the end of the range of motion (ROM) when the affected limb is moved in flexion or extension.
1+		Slight increase in muscle tone, manifested by a catch, followed by minimal resistance throughout the remainder (less than half) of the ROM
2	More marked increase in tone, but the limb is easily moved through its full ROM	More marked increase in muscle tone through most of the ROM, but affected part(s) easily moved
3	Considerable increase in muscle tone, passive movement difficult	Considerable increase in muscle tone, passive movement difficult
4	Affected part(s) rigid in flexion or extension	Affected part(s) rigid in flexion or extension

Adapted from Spasticity. American Association of Neurological Surgeon. Available at https://www.aans.org/Patients/Neurosurgical-Conditions-and-Treatments/Spasticity. Accessed October 9, 2018.

5. Improving voluntary motor functions involving objects such as reaching for, grasping, moving, and releasing objects
6. Enabling more normal muscle growth in children

The treatment of spasticity is the best example of a multidisciplinary team effort. It involves multidimensional or multimodality therapy concept that includes physiotherapy, medical therapy (oral medications, percutaneous injections), neurosurgical therapy (surgical implantation of intrathecal infusion pumps, permanent selective denervation procedures such as selective dorsal rhizotomy), and orthopedic procedures.[6] This team effort allows for the best treatment of spasticity for patients.

Physical and Occupational Therapy

This is an integral component of the management of patients with spasticity; it is a long-term measure that continues with the patient from the time of diagnosis, and even with surgical treatment, physical treatment remains the cornerstone of long-term rehabilitation and treatment. Physical and occupational therapy for spasticity is designed to not only reduce muscle tone and maintain or improve range of motion and mobility but it also is aimed to increase strength and coordination and improve comfort.[7] Through those effects, together we can try to augment the effects of different treatments and have a synergistic effect on the patient. Therapy may include stretching and strengthening exercises, temporary braces or casts, limb positioning, application of cold packs, electrical stimulation, and biofeedback.

Medical Therapy

Baclofen, benzodiazepines, tizanidine, gabapentin, and pregabalin are the most commonly prescribed oral medications used to treat spasticity. Physicians today, owing to adverse effects and the availability of better treatments, do not commonly prescribe dantrolene. A summary of these medications is found in Table 30.4. The mechanism of action of each of these medicines involve one of two pathways: first is compensating for reduced GABA or other inhibitory neurotransmitter (NT) in the brain or spinal cord and secondly reducing the number of excitatory NTs through direct inhibition or activation of inhibitory interneurons. The common mechanism of action of these medications also results in a pattern of side effects comprising somnolence, ataxia, and muscle weakness.

Baclofen is the most widely used drug in treating spasticity.[11] Its mechanism of action is binding to $GABA_B$ receptors in the spinal cord. Activation of these receptors leads to increased cell permeability of K^+, causing cation efflux and resultant hyperpolarization of the cell membrane. This hyperpolarization leads to a reduction in the release of excitatory NTs, as well as substance P (polypeptide involved in synaptic transmissions). Important side effects of baclofen that should be noted include orthostatic hypotension and withdrawal symptoms (i.e., seizures, fever and hallucinations). It is important to titrate baclofen doses especially if a patient has been taking baclofen for extended periods as abrupt withdrawal can lead to seizure activity.

There is poor penetration of baclofen across the blood-brain barrier with cerebrospinal fluid (CSF) baclofen levels often 10-fold lower than serum concentrations. It is common that escalated dosage can lead to an increasing incidence of side effects before full therapeutic efficacy is reached. Intrathecal delivery of baclofen is highly effective and is considered when patients are unable to tolerate increased doses of oral baclofen.[6,12]

The mechanism of action of benzodiazepines is facilitation of the binding of existing GABA to the $GABA_A$ receptor, found in high concentrations in the reticular formation and polysynaptic spinal tracts. Unlike the $GABA_B$

TABLE 30.4
ORAL MEDICATIONS IN THE TREATMENT OF SPASTICITY

Drug	Mechanism of Action	Effect(s)	Additional Adverse Effects
Baclofen	Binds $GABA_B$ receptors, increasing K^+ efflux	Reduces release of excitatory NTs and substance P	Orthostatic hypotension; abrupt withdrawal may cause seizures, hallucinations, rebound spasticity, and fever
Benzodiazepines	Increase existing GABA affinity for $GABA_A$ receptors, increasing Cl^- influx	Increase presynaptic inhibition, reduce monosynaptic and polysynaptic reflexes	Hypotension, significant sedation. Withdrawal may cause seizures
Tizanidine	α_2-adrenergic agonist	Reduces excitatory NT release from spinal interneurons	Potential hepatotoxicity
Dantrolene[a]	Binds ryanodine receptor in skeletal muscle, decreasing intracellular calcium concentration by sequestering Ca^{2+} in sarcoplasmic reticulum	Excitation-concentration decoupler in skeletal muscle	Weakness may include respiratory muscles. Potential hepatotoxicity
Gabapentin Pregabalin	Binds to α_2-δ subunit of voltage-gated calcium channels	Reduces excitatory NTs in the brain and spinal cord	Well tolerated and less sedating. Isolated cases of myopathy

[a]Not commonly prescribed by physicians due to adverse effects.
Adapted from Spasticity. American Association of Neurological Surgeon. Available at https://www.aans.org/Patients/Neurosurgical-Conditions-and-Treatments/Spasticity. Accessed October 9, 2018.
GABA, γ-aminobutyric acid; NT, neurotransmitter.

receptor, the $GABA_A$ receptor is an ionotropic channel (changes orientation when a ligand binds to channel). Its activation results in the increase in cell permeability of Cl^-, causing anion influx and hyperpolarization. Different classes of benzodiazepines are available on the market with different speeds of action and duration of action, but they all share the same profile of side effects including sleepiness, sedation, and inability to maintain regular activities. Rapid reversal of benzodiazepine toxicity can be achieved with the administration of flumazenil. Additionally, habituation and tolerance may develop, and prolonged use is associated with addiction which is a very undesirable effect especially in children and young adults.

Tizanidine and related medications (such as clonidine) are classified as α_2-adrenergic agonists and act by decreasing the excitatory neurotransmitters in spinal interneurons. Tizanidine is particularly effective for treating spasticity in adults with MS or spinal diseases. Important adverse effects include nausea and vomiting, hypotension (clonidine), and sedation (tizanidine).

Dantrolene acts directly on skeletal muscles. Dantrolene binds to skeletal muscle ryanodine receptors, which prevents the release of calcium from the sarcoplasmic reticulum into the cytosol. Its action is defined as an "excitation-contraction decouple" in skeletal muscle. Its effect on skeletal muscle may result in significant weakness of both volitional and (in severe cases) respiratory muscles.

Surgical Intervention for Spasticity

Surgical intervention for the treatment of spasticity represents one of the different modalities of treatment and often is one component within the multidisciplinary pool of treatment options. Surgical treatment is not and should not be seen or regarded as a replacement of any of the other mentioned options which are mandatory for the treatment of spasticity depending on the type, cause, distribution, and age of patient. It should be considered in the context of optimal medical and rehabilitative management and rational goal setting provided by a multidisciplinary team of health care providers who specialize in spasticity. The surgical options currently considered for spasticity include selective dorsal rhizotomy (SDR), chronic administration of intrathecal baclofen (ITB), and orthopedic surgery.[13]

Selective Dorsal Rhizotomy

Understanding the physiologic substrate to normal muscle tone is the cornerstone to understanding the effects of SDR in the treatment of spasticity. Muscle tone is regulated by the output of the alpha motor neurons in the spinal cord.[10,13] The alpha motor neurons normally are regulated by interneurons in the spinal cord, which, through a balance of competing excitatory and inhibitory influences, exert a net inhibitory influence.

This is the main concept of the muscle tone physiology principle. Inhibitory impulses travel in descending corticospinal projections from the cerebellum and basal ganglia. Excitatory influences from the muscle spindles travel to the spinal cord in the sensory or dorsal roots where they mediate the local spinal reflex arc. In cases of spasticity due to CP, there is a reorganization of the corticospinal projection fibers which reduce the inhibitory influence on alpha motor neurons. The therapeutic goal of a rhizotomy procedure is to cause excitatory input from the dorsal roots to be attenuated by sectioning of individual rootlets. Theoretically, this selective sectioning results in restoration of the balance of the excitatory and inhibitory influences on the alpha motor neurons. The choice of those rootlets to be sectioned surgically relies on the skill of the surgical team and depends on very precise intraoperative neuromonitoring as well as a thorough understanding of the physiology of muscle tone.[10,11,13,14]

Techniques for SDR. Surgery is done under general anesthesia, and the patient is positioned in prone position to access the spine from a posterior approach. Anesthesia is performed without the use of any muscle relaxants to facilitate the neuromonitoring component of the operation which is very central to the success of the surgery. A midline incision over the lower lumbar region is marked under fluoroscopy, and the paravertebral muscles are retracted on both sides in a subfascial technique. In the old technique, exposure of the spinal cord and roots was achieved through a laminectomy from L1 to L5, but owing to the fear of creating spinal instability and the possible need for stabilization hardware fusion, we now mostly do the surgery through a one-segment laminectomy at L1. This approach can expose the cauda equine, thus allowing exposure of the dorsal and anterior roots. The segmental levels of the exposed roots are identified with electromyographic (EMG) recording electrodes placed in 4 to 10 target muscles with L1/L2–S2 innervation. The L1–S2 dorsal roots are separated from the anterior roots and lower sacral roots and divided into rootlets. This part of the surgical procedure is the most critical part of the whole surgery. The dorsal rootlets are stimulated, and their EMG responses are graded. The rootlets within each targeted root segment are selectively transected (Figure 30.3) based on their EMG responses.

The neurophysiologic methods used and the criteria applied to identify which rootlets are "abnormal"—that is, contributing most to spasticity—vary among centers performing SDR.[13,14] Discussion of these criteria at length is beyond the scope of this chapter.

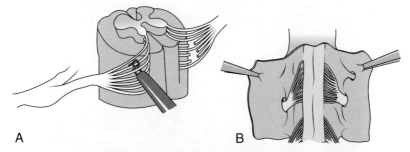

A   B

Figure 30.3. The technique used for selective dorsal rhizotomy (SDR). A. The stimulation of the dorsal roots. B. The transection of the dorsal roots. From Kolaski K, Frino J, Koman LA. Surgical Management of Spasticity in the Child With Cerebral Palsy. In: Brashear A, ed. *Spasticity Diagnosis and Managment.* 2nd ed. New York: Demos Medical. Reprinted with permission from L. Andrew Koman, MD.

Adverse Events of SDR. Serious adverse effects are rare. Strict pudendal nerve monitoring, both intraoperatively and perioperatively, is mandatory to lower side effects after SDR. Moreover, strict precautions and guidelines before sectioning of the rootlets is a standard of care that helps to minimize any side effects. In general, intraoperative and perioperative adverse events involving respiratory problems were more common (1.3%-6.9%),[13] as reported in earlier studies. Improvements in these rates reported in later series are attributed to refinements in surgical and anesthetic care.

Other studies have reported late-onset bowel and bladder dysfunction in 5.1% of patients in one series, and this was associated with the lack of pudendal nerve monitoring.[13] It also should be noted that SDR might increase the incidence of scoliosis, kyphosis, hyperlordosis, and lumbosacral spondylolisthesis.[13] Overall, lower rates of both early operative and late adverse events in the past 20 years are attributed to a variety of technical improvements and refinements.[13]

Intrathecal Baclofen

ITB treatment evolved due to the problems encountered with oral baclofen treatment: the low absorption of the drug through the blood-brain barrier resulted in low concentration of the drug in CSF, and consequently, the increased dose to achieve a satisfactory therapeutic effect can lead to an unacceptable level of side effects. Direct ITB delivery and continuous infusion via a device delivery system (Figures 30.4-30.6) evolved to compensate for the problems associated with the orally administered drug.[13,15-18]

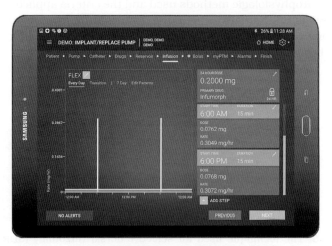

Figure 30.4. The SynchroMed II Clinician Programmer table with touch screen interface. (Image adapted from SynchroMed II Drug Infusion System. Medtronic; 2018. Available at http://www.medtronic.com/us-en/healthcare-professionals/products/neurological/drug-infusion-systems/synchromed-ii.html. Accessed October 16, 2018.) See eBook for color figure.

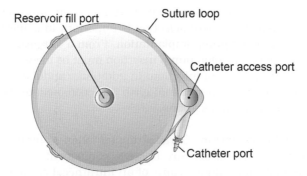

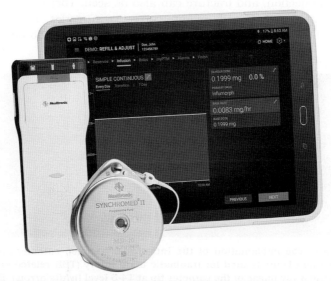

Figure 30.5. The SynchroMed II pump used for drug infusion. (Image adapted from SynchroMed II Drug Infusion System. Medtronic; 2018. Available at http://www.medtronic.com/us-en/healthcare-professionals/products/neurological/drug-infusion-systems/synchromed-ii.html. Accessed October 16, 2018.)

Spasticity patients who respond to oral baclofen but can not tolerate or do not respond to higher oral doses are candidates for ITB pump placement.[13,17,18] Patients who show satisfactory response after initial test ITB trial after injection of initial dose of 25 or 50 μg would be considered good candidates for pump placement. Following the test dose, patients are often evaluated by the neurologist involved in the care of the patient

Figure 30.6. The whole SynchroMed II Drug Infusion System. Includes the tablet, pump, and communicator. Image obtained from SynchroMed II Drug Infusion System. (Image adapted from SynchroMed II Drug Infusion System. Medtronic; 2018. Available at http://www.medtronic.com/us-en/healthcare-professionals/products/neurological/drug-infusion-systems/synchromed-ii.html. Accessed October 16, 2018.)

and physical therapist to ensure that there has been improvement from the baseline spasticity. Patient selection is important in achieving a good response after baclofen pump implantation. From a surgical perspective, patients chosen for a baclofen pump insertion must be medically and neurologically stable and free of infection; in addition, candidates must have adequate body mass and abdominal girth to accommodate the pump to avoid pump infection complications.

Technique of Implantation. Surgical implantation is performed under general anesthesia. The procedure has two components. The spine part involves insertion under fluoroscopy, of an intrathecal catheter at a level corresponding to the level of spasticity. Then the catheter is connected to the pump, which is implanted in the abdomen (Figure 30.7). Patient is positioned in lateral position to access the spinal part and the abdominal part, and the pump is inserted either subcutaneously or subfascial. Subfascial implantation is preferred in CP patients or in thin individuals to decrease the risk of infection.

Adverse Events of Intrathecal Baclofen. Adverse events of ITB are either related to the technical implantation or related to the dosing of ITB. Adverse effects amount to 25% of cases.[13] Infection is the most common complication. Catheter complications include kinking, migration, occlusion, disconnection, and fracture can also be seen. These occur at rates of 15% to 25% and typically require corrective surgeries. They often are considered when increases in the baclofen pump dosage do not seem to

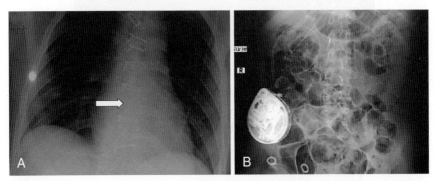

Figure 30.7. The implantation of the intrathecal baclofen catheter and pump inside a patient being treated for traumatic brain injury (TBI)–related spasticity. A. Shows the X-ray image of the catheter tip at T4-5 level (*white arrow*). B. Shows the X-ray image of baclofen pump located on the right abdominal wall. Image adapted with permission from Ungar L, Sharma M, Zibly Z. Intrathecal baclofen pump implantation in a patient 2 years following a traumatic brain injury resulted in regained oratory capabilities. *Neurol India.* 2015;63(4):618-619.

bring about any improvement in spasticity decrease. Primary problems with the pump itself occur at rates of less than 10%.[13] Baclofen over dosage or toxicity as well as withdrawal are potentially life-threatening problems. Long-term morbidity and mortality can be averted if symptoms are recognized and treated promptly. The acute ITB withdrawal syndrome is potentially fatal. Cases of serious over dosage of ITB are described more frequently than cases of withdrawal. Pump malfunction is also reported due to mechanical problems with the pump.

Signs of baclofen overdose are drowsiness, lightheadedness, difficulty breathing, seizures, loss of consciousness or coma, and low body temperature. Withdrawal symptoms may present as a return of spasticity, itchiness, low blood pressure, or tingling sensations.[19]

Radiosurgery for Trigeminal Neuralgia

Over the past two decades, significant change in the concept of treatment of trigeminal neuralgia (TN) has taken place in combination with traditional medical treatment. Stereotactic radiosurgery is now being considered as a first-line treatment of medically refractory trigeminal neuralgia.[20] Currently we have two modalities for radiosurgery, Gamma Knife radiosurgery (GKR) and CyberKnife radiosurgery(CKR). Gamma Knife uses an isocentric cobalt radiation unit. We currently have follow-up periods for almost 25 years post GKR for trigeminal neuralgia. There is ample literature as to the evaluation of the range of initial treatment radiation dosages, targets, and results with 1- to 10-year follow-ups as well as secondary effects, especially residual facial numbness.

The treatment of TN with GKR ranges from 70 to 90 Gy. It was found that more relief was reported with the higher range of 90 Gy but, at the same time, more risk of numbness. The area targeted is 4 to 6 mm along the trigeminal nerve or the root entry zone in the pons. The Barrow Neurological Institute (BNI) scale, which was introduced in the Barrow Neurological Institute, was based on assessment of the level of pain and medical treatment used. The BNI scale is used to assess and quantify the result after treatment. It is composed of stages from 0 to 5.[20]

Excellent result does correspond to BNI scale of 0 to 3 which would translate into no pain or mild to intermediate pain which responds to medical treatment. Long-term follow-up after an average of 1 year after GKR for TN shows excellent results with a BNI index 0 to 3 in approximately 72% to 86% of cases.[19] The improvement of pain can start within 2 to 3 days of treatment but more often it takes up to a month for the patient to report the beginning of improvement of the pain. This initial high percentage of pain relief after treatment does not last in most large long-term follow-up, and it is estimated that only 44% to 50% of cases continue to have excellent result of BNI 0 to 3.[20] There is a relationship between better long-term pain relief and development of mild postprocedure facial numbness, which is frequently related to extending the radiosurgical lesion 1 or 2 mm into the root entry zone. Oral medication can slowly be tapered as pain relief is obtained.

The nonisocentric robotic arm of CyberKnife represents the second method of radiosurgery for TN, and even though the GKR experience is much larger and older than the CKR, the CKR literature is now available with long-term follow-up results which are equivalent to those of GKR for TN. A recent report of 138 cases using the CyberKnife for initial treatment of trigeminal neuralgia with a mean dose of 75 Gy had an effective pain control rate (BNI class I-IIIa) at 6 months of 93.5%, 12 months 85.8%, 24 months 79.7%, and at 36 months 76%.[20]

As different nonisocentric and isocentric stereotactic radiosurgical systems have become available, the decision to initially treat trigeminal neuralgia with GK-, CK-, or even linear accelerator-based systems may be a result of machine proximity, insurance coverage, or physician training on the various systems rather than because there is any significant difference in results. Dosimetry comparisons have been made allowing conversion of dosing parameters based on the isodose lines from one system to another.

GKR has been show to be very effective in treating trigeminal neuralgia in patients with MS. GKR showed a significantly high rate of initial pain cessation (90.7%) and a low rate of numbness (16%) for a cohort of 43 different cases of trigeminal neuralgia caused by MS.[21]

Deep Brain Stimulation for Movement Disorders

Deep brain stimulation (DBS) as a concept of treatment is centered on a device that is implanted into the body, which sends electric signals to deep brain centers which control body movements. Electrodes are placed deep in the brain and are connected to a stimulator device. The stimulation regulates the activity of the brain and reduces symptoms of slowness, stiffness, and tremors. This ultimately contributes to improvement in quality of life and can lead to decrease in medication.

The DBS team consists of neurologists, neuropsychologists, and neurosurgeons who are the team assessing the condition of the patient and deciding as to whether the patient fulfills the criteria of being a surgical candidate. Cognitive functions as well as current medications and general health are evaluated. Multiple video images of the patient performing different movements (walking, finger tap, rising from a chair) while on and off medication are taken, monitored, and evaluated.

DBS surgery is performed by a neurosurgeon who has specialized training in functional neurosurgery. Electrodes are connected by long wires that travel under the skin and down the neck to a battery-powered stimulator under the skin of the chest. When turned on, the stimulator sends electrical pulses to block the faulty nerve signals causing tremors, rigidity, and other symptoms.

The stimulator settings can be adjusted as a patient's condition changes over time. Unlike other surgeries, such as pallidotomy or thalamotomy, DBS does not damage the brain tissue. Thus, if better treatments develop in the future, the DBS procedure can be reversed.

Electrodes can be placed in the following brain areas:

- Subthalamic nucleus (STN)—effective for tremor, slowness, rigidity, dystonia, and dyskinesia.
- Thalamus (vental intermediate nucleus)—effective for tremor. It is often used to treat essential tremor.
- Globus pallidus (GPi)—effective for tremor, slowness, rigidity, dystonia, and dyskinesia.

DBS is contraindicated in cases of severe depression, severe dementia, or atypical symptoms. DBS can help treat many of the symptoms caused by the following movement disorders[22]:

- Parkinson disease: tremor, rigidity, and slowness of movement caused by the decrease of dopamine-producing nerve cells responsible for relaying messages that control body movement.
- Essential tremor: involuntary rhythmic tremors of the hands and arms, occurring both at rest and during purposeful movement. Also, may affect the head in a "no-no" motion.
- Dystonia: involuntary movements and prolonged muscle contraction, resulting in twisting or writhing body motions, tremor, and abnormal posture. May involve the entire body or only an isolated area. Spasms can often be suppressed by "sensory tricks," such as touching the face, eyebrows, or hands.

Deep Brain Stimulation for Multiple Sclerosis

There is a growing interest in the use of DBS for treating patients with MS, owing to its success in treating Parkinson disease. Similar to Parkinson disease, tremors can be a debilitating symptom of MS. In cases where DBS was used to treat MS-related tremors, researchers found that most patients reported a reduction in tremor frequency and an overall improvement in functioning.[23,24] However, DBS has not proven to completely eliminate tremors due to MS. It is considered when patients have severe tremors resistant to oral medications, especially involving the upper extremities that interfere with activities of daily living such as eating.

Overall, DBS has been shown to be safe for treating tremors associated with MS. However, there are some adverse effects of DBS that should be noted by physicians that are considering using DBS as a treatment option. As the procedure involves invasive surgery, there is a possible risk of hemorrhage occurring during the implantation of the electrodes. However, hemorrhages are usually nonfatal and will often resolve months after surgery.[23] There is also the possibility of an infection occurring relating to DBS implantation procedure.[24] Safety of performing an MRI of the brain if a patient has DBS also has to be considered.

Conclusion

Neurosurgery is often considered for certain symptoms of MS that can be debilitating to the patient. In addition to trauma, brain tumors, and vascular issues, MS patients can be referred to neurosurgery for severe back pain, spasticity, tremors, and trigeminal neuralgia treatment. Neurosurgical evaluation is an important tool in the treatment armamentarium especially when medical therapy has been unsuccessful.

References

1. Genevay S, Atlas SJ. Lumbar spinal stenosis. *Best Pract Res Clin Rheumatol.* 2010;24(2):253-265.
2. Verbiest H. A radicular syndrome from developmental narrowing of the lumbar vertebral canal. *J Bone Joint Surg Br.* 1954;36-B(2):230-237.
3. Genevay S, Atlas SJ, Katz JN. Variation in eligibility criteria from studies of radiculopathy due to a herniated disc and of neurogenic claudication due to lumbar spinal stenosis: a structured literature review. *Spine (Phila Pa 1976).* 2010;35(7):803-811.
4. Rampersaud YR, Ravi B, Lewis SJ, et al. Assessment of health-related quality of life after surgical treatment of focal symptomatic spinal stenosis compared with osteoarthritis of the hip or knee. *Spine J.* 2008;8(2):296-304.
5. Ciol MA, Deyo RA, Howell E, Kreif S. An assessment of surgery for spinal stenosis: time trends, geographic variations, complications, and reoperations. *J Am Geriatr Soc.* 1996;44(3):285-290.
6. Massot C, Agnani O, Khenioui H, et al. Back pain and musculoskeletal disorders in multiple sclerosis. *J Spine.* 2016;5:285. doi:10.4172/2165-7939.1000285.
7. Spasticity. American Association of Neurological Surgeon. Available at https://www.aans.org/Patients/Neurosurgical-Conditions-and-Treatments/Spasticity. Accessed October 9, 2018.
8. Levitt M, Browd S. *Spasticity: Classification, Diagnosis, and Management.* iKnowledge: Neurosurgery; 2015:chap 50. Available at https://clinicalgate.com/spasticity-classification-diagnosis-and-management.
9. Arroyo R, Massana M, Vila C. Correlation between spasticity and quality of life in patients with multiple sclerosis: the CANDLE study. *Int J Neurosci.* 2013;123(12):850-858. doi:10.3109/00207454.2013.812084.

10. The spinal cord (Organization of the Central Nervous System) part 5. In: What-When-How: In Depth Tutorials and Information. Available at http://what-when-how.com/neuroscience/the-spinal-cord-organization-of-the-central-nervous-system-part-5/. Accessed October 16, 2018.

11. Pandey K. Spasticity Treatment & Management: Pharmological Therapy. MedScape. Available at https://emedicine.medscape.com/article/2207448-treatment#d8. Accessed October 16, 2018.

12. Gibson B. Stretching for people with MS. *Natl MS Soc.* 2016;1(5):1-26.

13. Kolaski K, Frino J, Koman A. Surgical management of spasticity in the Child with cerebral palsy. *Spasticity Diagn Manag.* 2010;29:450-465.

14. Abou Al-Shaar H, Imtiaz MT, Alhalabi H, Alsubaie SM, Sabbagh AJ. Selective dorsal rhizotomy: a multidisciplinary approach to treating spastic diplegia. *Asian J Neurosurg.* 2017;12(3):454-465.

15. SychroMed II Drug Infusion System. Medtronic; 2018. Available at http://www.medtronic.com/us-en/healthcare-professionals/products/neurological/drug-infusion-systems/synchromed-ii.html. Accessed October 16, 2018.

16. Ungar L, Sharma M, Zibly Z. Intrathecal baclofen pump implantation in a patient 2 years following a traumatic brain injury resulted in regained oratory capabilities. *Neurol India.* 2015;63:618-619.

17. Abou Al-Shaar H, Alkhani A. Intrathecal baclofen therapy for spasticity: a compliance-based study to indicate effectiveness. *Surg Neurol Int.* 2016;7(suppl 19):S539-S541. doi:10.4103/2152-7806.187529.

18. Anderson WS, Jallo GI. Intrathecal baclofen therapy and the treatment of spasticity. *Neurosurg Q.* 2007;17(3):185-192.

19. Awuor SO, Kitei PM, Nawaz Y, Ahnert AM. Intrathecal baclofen withdrawal: a rare cause of reversible cardiomyopathy. *Acute Card Care.* 2016;18(1):13-17.

20. Berti A, Ibars G, Wu X, et al. Evaluation of CyberKnife radiosurgery for recurrent trigeminal neuralgia. *Cureus.* 2018;10(5):e2598. doi:10.7759/cureus.2598.

21. Tuleasca C, Carron R, Resseguier N, et al. Multiple sclerosis-related trigeminal neuralgia: a prospective series of 43 patients treated with gamma knife surgery with more than one year of follow-up. *Stereotact Funct Neurosurg.* 2014;92:203-210. doi:10.1159/000362173.

22. *Deep Brain Stimulation (DBS).* Mayfield Brain and Spine; 2018. Available at https://mayfieldclinic.com/pe-dbs.htm. Accessed October 23, 2018.

23. Wishart HA, Roberts DW, Roth RM, et al. Chronic deep brain stimulation for the treatment of tremor in multiple sclerosis: review and case reports. *J Neurol Neurosurg Psychiatry.* 2003;74:1392-1397.

24. Oliveria S, Rodriguez R, Bowers D, et al. Safety and efficacy of dual-lead thalamic deep brain stimulation for patients with treatment-refractory multiple sclerosis tremor: a single-centre, randomised, single blind, pilot trial. *Lancet Neurol.* 2017;16(9):691-700.

31

Rehabilitation in Multiple Sclerosis

■ ■ ■ Francois Bethoux, Randy Karim, Robert W. Motl

Introduction

Multiple sclerosis (MS) is a disease that is commonly treated with disease-modifying drugs (DMDs), but there is increasing emphasis placed on rehabilitation as a core component of the comprehensive, multidisciplinary management of MS. For example, rehabilitation is integrated into the guidelines for management of MS symptoms such as fatigue[1] and spasticity.[2] The purpose of this chapter is to summarize key concepts, outcome measurement, and elements of evidence regarding the use of rehabilitation in individuals with MS.

Definition and Concepts

In an expert opinion paper published by the National Multiple Sclerosis Society, rehabilitation in MS was defined as "a process that helps a person achieve and maintain maximal physical, psychological, social and vocational potential, and quality of life consistent with physiologic impairment, environment, and life goals. Achievement and maintenance of optimal function are essential in a progressive disease such as MS."[3] This definition highlights one of the challenges of MS rehabilitation: in the context of a disease process generally resulting in worsening functional limitations over time, maintaining function is a valid goal, whereas the traditional model

528

of rehabilitation focuses on restoring or improving function. This does not mean that functional gains are not possible in MS, but often payors require periodic documentation of progress for continued coverage of rehabilitation services. This requirement in the context of Medicare coverage was challenged in a recent lawsuit (Jimmo v. Sebelius). In the settlement agreement, the Center for Medicare and Medicaid Services clarified that lack of improvement does not automatically lead to denial of coverage, as long as the need for skilled services can be demonstrated to "provide care that is reasonable and necessary to prevent or slow further deterioration."[4]

The application of rehabilitation requires a clear target and approach based on a conceptual framework in MS. The World Health Organization published the International Classification of Function, Disability, and Health (ICF), which proposes a conceptual framework and a classification system to describe and record the consequences of health conditions. These consequences are described in terms of impairment of body functions and structures, as well as limitations of activity and participation (defined as involvement in a life situation). Personal and environmental factors are taken into account in the model.[5] The ICF can be a useful tool for MS rehabilitation, particularly for the description of functional limitations and goal setting. Based on expert opinion, a brief and a comprehensive ICF core set was developed specifically for MS (Table 31.1).[6,7]

In addition to the ICF framework, the construct of health-related quality of life (HRQOL) is very relevant to rehabilitation. Several definitions of HRQOL have been proposed. It is generally accepted that quality of life (QOL) is a multidimensional construct encompassing judgments or evaluations of physical, mental, emotional, and social functioning. HRQOL focuses on the aspects of QOL related to general health and/or health conditions and their treatments.[8]

The term neurological rehabilitation (or neurorehabilitation) is commonly used when rehabilitation seeks to optimize function among people with disorders of the nervous system. For the sake of simplicity, we will continue to use the term "rehabilitation" in this chapter.

Strategies for Rehabilitation in MS

The strategies used in rehabilitation can be divided into two categories:

- Remediation, which directly aims at improving or restoring a body function or structure. This could involve muscle strengthening and gait training as remediation interventions for reversing walking impairment and gait disturbance.
- Compensation, which aims at developing compensatory strategies to "work around" the functional limitation. For example, the use of a scooter in a patient with severe gait and balance impairment can help preserve safe indoor and outdoor mobility.

TABLE 31.1
ICF BRIEF CORE SET FOR MULTIPLE SCLEROSIS

Body Functions	Body Structures	Activities and Participation	Environmental Factors
b130 Energy and drive functions b152 Emotional functions b164 Higher-level cognitive functions b210 Seeing functions b280 Sensation of pain b620 Urination functions b730 Muscle power functions b770 Gait pattern functions	s110 Structure of brain s120 Spinal cord and related structures	d175 Solving problems d230 Carrying out daily routine d450 Walking d760 Family relationships d850 Remunerative employment	e310 Immediate family e355 Health professionals e410 Individual attitudes of immediate family members e580 Health services, systems, and policies

ICF, International Classification of Function, Disability, and Health.

In practice, both strategies are combined to achieve desired functional goals.[9] Although the principles and effects of compensatory strategies are easily understood (albeit often insufficiently studied), one may question the potential for neurological restoration in the setting of multifocal central nervous system (CNS) damage from MS. However, rehabilitation targets several causes of functional limitations:

- Addressing secondary causes of functional limitations: although CNS damage is considered the primary cause of functional limitations from MS, secondary factors may be positively affected by rehabilitation. One common example is physiological deconditioning, which is thought to be related to decreased physical activity and was found to partially explain walking capacity.[10] Comorbidities (e.g., musculoskeletal, cardiovascular) are associated with worse disability in the context of MS, and some of them can be addressed or prevented in part through rehabilitation.[11]
- Promoting neuroplasticity: neuroplasticity can be defined as the ability of neurons within the CNS to adapt to new circumstances, including damage from disease or injury, through functional and structural changes.[12] Spontaneous cortical reorganization, representative of neuroplasticity, was demonstrated in MS and found to be associated with recovery of clinical function (adaptive plasticity).[13] Maladaptive plasticity may also occur and is thought to be related in part to disuse,

creating a negative reinforcement loop (e.g., motor impairment in one limb may lead to favoring the nonaffected limb in the performance of daily activities and in turn may lead to maladaptive cortical reorganization).[14] Therefore, rehabilitation aims at promoting adaptive plasticity while attempting to reverse maladaptive plasticity.

■ Neuroprotection and disease modification: animal studies and evidence from other CNS conditions suggest that a neuroprotective effect of physical exercise in MS is plausible, and limited clinical evidence seems to support this assumption.[15] Furthermore, possible effects of physical exercise on clinical and imaging markers of MS disease activity have been recently reported.[16,17] However, the evidence remains inconclusive. As pharmacological treatments promoting neural repair are being developed in MS, the effects of their combination with rehabilitation will hopefully be tested.

Evidence to Support and Guide the Use of Rehabilitation Services in MS

As in all other medical fields, there is a strong drive to develop a body of evidence to guide the prescription and delivery of rehabilitation services in MS, keeping in mind known challenges specific to this field and to the disease. Rehabilitation involves a variety of disciplines (e.g., physical therapy, occupational therapy, speech language pathology), and each discipline uses various techniques. Furthermore, rehabilitation interventions and techniques are often combined within a rehabilitation program and vary from patient to patient depending on needs, goals, and preferences. The resulting complexity and heterogeneity of the nature and contents of rehabilitation treatment, as well as the variability in outcome measures, complicate the comparison of study results and limit the ability to perform aggregate analyses. In addition, the design of a placebo intervention and participant blinding are difficult in the context of a rehabilitation randomized controlled trial (RCT). In a systematic review of published evidence from 1970 to 2013, the Guideline Development, Dissemination, and Implementation Subcommittee of the American Academy of Neurology pointed out a "paucity of well-designed studies," as did a more recently published "systematic review of systematic reviews."[18,19] Nevertheless, evidence on the efficacy of rehabilitation interventions in MS is accumulating, as we will illustrate in the section on rehabilitation interventions.

Outcome Measurement for MS Rehabilitation

A corollary to the drive for strong evidence is the need for consistent use of standardized, valid, and reliable measures of the outcomes of MS rehabilitation by clinicians and researchers. Increasingly, MS-specific measures are being developed, and generic measures are being validated in MS. In addition to psychometric properties, ease of use and relevance to the patients' characteristics and rehabilitation goals are important to consider when choosing a measure.

Providing an exhaustive list of outcome measures for MS rehabilitation is beyond the scope of this chapter. Compilations of relevant information are freely available online:

- The Rehabilitation Measures Database is maintained by the Shirley Ryan AbilityLab (formerly Rehabilitation Institute of Chicago) and provides detailed information on over 400 measures that can be used in rehabilitation (https://www.sralab.org/rehabilitation-measures). This database is not specific to MS.
- The Multiple Sclerosis Outcome Measures Task Force, appointed by the Academy of Neurologic Physical Therapy section of the American Physical Therapy Association, reviewed 63 outcome measures and issued recommendations for their use in clinical practice, education, and research in MS rehabilitation (http://neuropt.org/professional-resources/neurology-section-outcome-measures-recommendations/multiple-sclerosis).

We will briefly discuss tools that provide a global assessment but do not focus on a specific impairment or activity limitation (Table 31.2).

TABLE 31.2
OUTCOME MEASURES FOR MULTIPLE SCLEROSIS (MS) REHABILITATION

Category	Measures	Construct/ Domain	Comments
MS specific	Timed 25 Foot Walk (T25FW) Nine Hole Peg Test (NHPT) Low Contrast Letter Acuity (LCLA) Symbol Digit Modalities Test (SDMT)	Walking Upper extremity function Vision Cognition	Neuroperformance tests
	Expanded Disability Status Scale (EDSS)	Body functions Activity	Requires a neurological examination Score 0-10
	Incapacity Status Scale (ISS)	Body functions Activity	Interview/ observation 16 items Score 0-64

TABLE 31.2
OUTCOME MEASURES FOR MULTIPLE SCLEROSIS (MS)
REHABILITATION (CONTINUED)

Category	Measures	Construct/ Domain	Comments
	Patient-Determined Disease Steps (PDDS)	Body functions Activity	Self-report Score 0-8
	Multiple Sclerosis Impact Scale (MSIS-29)	Activity	Self-report 29 items: physical subscale 20 items, psychological sub-scale 9 items Score 0-100
	MS Quality of Life Inventory (MSQLI) Functional Assessment of MS (FAMS) Multiple Sclerosis International Quality of Life (MusiQol) MS Quality of Life-54 items (MSQOL-54)	Health-related quality of life	Self-report
Generic	Barthel Index (BI)	Activity (independence in daily activities)	Interview/ observation 10 items Score 0-100
	Functional Independence Measure (FIM)	Activity (independence in daily activities)	Observation 18 items: 13 motor, 5 cognitive Score 18-126
	Medical Outcomes Study 36-item Short Form Health Survey (SF-36) Quality of Life in Neurological Disorders (Neuro-QoL)	Health-related quality of life	Self-report SF-36: 36 items, physical and mental components Neuro-QoL: 13 sub-scales, short forms, and computer adap-tive testing available

MS-Specific Measures

■ The Multiple Sclerosis Outcome Assessments Consortium has issued evi-dence-based recommendations for outcome measures covering important domains of MS-related disability: the Timed 25 Foot Walk for walking, the Nine Hole Peg Test for manual dexterity, the Low Contrast Letter Acuity test for vision, and the Symbol Digit Modalities Test for cognition.[20]

- The Expanded Disability Status Scale (EDSS)[21] is widely used in clinical trials of DMDs for MS. Although it is called a measure of disability, the EDSS covers the ICF domains of body functions (reflected in the Functional Systems) and activities (particularly in relation to walking). Owing to its poor responsiveness to rehabilitation interventions, it is rarely a primary outcome measure in rehabilitation clinical trials but is often used to categorize or screen study participants based on the severity of the neurological "disability" from MS.[22]
- The Incapacity Status Scale (ISS) is a lesser known companion to the EDSS in the Minimal Record of Disabilities for MS, published by the National Multiple Sclerosis Society in 1985.[23] Most of the 16 items of the ISS are related to activities (e.g., climbing stairs, walking, bathing, dressing), whereas some are related to body functions (e.g., vision, speech, hearing). The scoring is based on difficulty performing activities (or the interference of impairments with activities and participation), the need for assistive equipment, and the need for human assistance. The ISS was recently shown to correlate with walking speed and with the EDSS in an outpatient rehabilitation population.[24]
- The Patient-Determined Disease Steps is a self-report outcome measure of MS-related disability, which is strongly correlated with the EDSS and with measures of walking.[25]
- The Multiple Sclerosis Impact Scale (MSIS-29) is a 29-item questionnaire that explores the consequences of MS on daily activities (2-week recall period). Most of the items inquire about the degree of bother relative to a variety of impairments, activity limitations, and participation restrictions.[26]
- MS-specific HRQOL measures include the MS Quality of Life Inventory, the Functional Assessment of MS (FAMS), the Multiple Sclerosis International Quality of Life (MusiQol) and the MS Quality of Life-54 items (MSQOL-54).[27]

Generic Measures

- Global measures of activity limitations: the Barthel Index (BI) and Functional Independence Measure (FIM) assess performance on activities of daily living based on the need for assistive devices or human assistance. The BI is a 10-item scale, whereas the (FIM) contains 18 items with defined motor and cognitive subscales. These instruments are most commonly used for inpatient rehabilitation and in that setting were found to be reliable and sensitive to change. A study focused solely on individuals with MS showed that FIM scores are correlated with care needs.[28] In a more recent study of the BI and FIM in a mixed inpatient neurological population of 149 patients (43% with MS), both scales exhibited satisfactory acceptability, reliability, convergent validity, and responsiveness to change.[29]

■ HRQOL scales: the Medical Outcomes Study 36-item Short Form Health Survey (SF-36) is arguably the most widely known generic HRQOL scale and has been used in studies of MS rehabilitation, although concerns have been raised regarding is psychometric properties in this population.[30] The Neuro-QoL (Quality of Life in Neurological Disorders) measurement tool, although not specific to MS, was validated in a sample of patients with MS during its initial development.[31] Neuro-QoL includes 13 scales to assess the various domains of HRQOL relevant to neurological disorders. Short versions of the scales (Short Forms) and computer-adaptive testing both decrease the responder burden.

Rehabilitation Interventions

Multidisciplinary Rehabilitation

Individuals with MS are not often admitted for inpatient multidisciplinary rehabilitation. One exception is severe functional loss from an MS relapse (or from an acute medical complication or surgery), wherein substantial functional recovery is expected and intensive skilled rehabilitation services are necessary. In one RCT, inpatient rehabilitation was found to be superior to standard outpatient care on measures of neurological disability and physical function.[32] Favorable results were also reported (vs. home exercise or wait list) after inpatient rehabilitation in patients with relapsing and progressive MS without acute worsening of disability. Although referrals for multidisciplinary outpatient rehabilitation are more common, this modality has not been more extensively studied. A Cochrane review of multidisciplinary inpatient or outpatient rehabilitation programs in adults with MS concluded that there was strong evidence of short-term gains on activity and participation but not on impairment.[33] Another review concluded that evidence supported the effectiveness of outpatient rehabilitation on disability but was otherwise inconclusive.[18]

Motor Rehabilitation

Motor rehabilitation generally involves multiple components: education and goal setting, exercise training (including stretching, aerobic, resistance, and task-specific training), and training to the use of assistive devices and orthotics. Increasingly, technology-assisted training is proposed as a means to enhance motor rehabilitation.

Mobility (Gait and Balance) Rehabilitation

A variety of interventions have been proposed to enhance mobility in individuals with MS, although not all of them have been extensively tested in

RCTs.[34] Although clinical trials of exercise and motor rehabilitation often focus on individuals with mild to moderate mobility disability, a few studies have specifically enrolled patients with progressive MS who have severe mobility disability.[35]

Exercise training

A meta-analysis of exercise training in MS showed significant improvement of walking.[36] The optimal frequency, duration, and type of training depending on individual goals and characteristics remain to be fully defined. The Canadian physical activity guidelines set minimum exercise requirements for people with mild to moderate disability from MS: 30 minutes of moderate intensity aerobic activity twice per week, and strength training for major muscle groups twice per week. The guidelines can be found at: http://www.csep.ca/CMFiles/Guidelines/specialpops/CSEP_MS_PAGuidelines_adults_en.pdf. Project GEMS (Guidelines for Exercise in Multiple Sclerosis) aims at testing the feasibility and efficacy of a 4-month home-based exercise training program based on physical activity guidelines and social cognitive theory. The feasibility and acceptability of this program was demonstrated in a recently published RCT.[37] Further discussion of exercise prescription for individuals with MS can be found in Chapter 35.

Physical Therapy

Ideally, physical therapy (PT) should be delivered by neurotrained therapists familiar with MS. The treatment plan may involve an array of interventions based on individual needs and goals, including stretching, combinations of exercise modalities (aerobic training, resistance training, and a common emphasis on task-specific training), as well as recommendations for and training to the use of orthotics and assistive devices. Overall, PT was found to produce a significant, albeit small, improvement of walking[38] and balance[39] in meta-analyses. In wheelchair-bound patients, optimization of trunk control and transfer ability constitutes an important rehabilitation goal. Wheelchair users also often exhibit impaired respiratory function, particularly restrictive dysfunction, a significant cause of morbidity and mortality in MS.[40] Unfortunately, respiratory function is rarely monitored in patients with MS, even though respiratory rehabilitation may be beneficial.[41]

The combination of symptomatic therapies affecting motor symptoms with PT for motor training is generally desired, particularly if improvement of active function is sought. This is often done in the management of spasticity, although the functional benefits of this combination have not been systematically studied to our knowledge. A small single-blind RCT of botulinum toxin A for treatment of spasticity with or without PT showed a greater improvement of spasticity as measured by the Modified Ashworth Scale in the physiotherapy group.[42] A recent chart review study showed that absence of ongoing rehabilitation was an independent predictor of discontinuation of botulinum toxin therapy for spasticity.[43] There is emerging evidence suggesting that the combination of motor training and treatment with extended-release dalfampridine results in further functional improvement.[44,45] Although these findings appear to agree with clinical intuition, they will need to be confirmed in large randomized clinical trials.

Technology-Enhanced Rehabilitation

Virtual reality (VR) is an enticing technology for gait and balance training, as it allows the manipulation of visual input, a greater variety of tasks (e.g., dual-task training) and training customization, and often adds a "fun" component to the training, which may enhance motivation and adherence. VR can be coupled with a balance platform, a treadmill, or an immersive environment such as the Computer Assisted Rehabilitation Environment (CAREN) system (Motekforce Link, Amsterdam, Netherlands). In addition, the availability of consumer VR products opens an opportunity for home use. Although current evidence suggests that VR-enhanced gait and balance rehabilitation is safe and leads to improvement compared with no intervention, superiority to traditional rehabilitation has not been demonstrated.[46,47]

Rhythmic auditory stimulation (RAS), in the form of a metronome or rhythmic music, has been shown to enhance gait training in patients with Parkinson disease and poststroke hemiparesis. The presumed mechanism of action of RAS is rhythmic entrainment within the CNS. A pilot RCT using rhythmic music in 10 patients with MS showed a greater improvement of double support time with an RAS-enhanced home-based walking program compared with no intervention.[48] A more recent RCT in 18 patients with MS using a metronome showed greater improvement of gait parameters after in-clinic gait training with RAS, compared with gait training without RAS.[49]

Technology-enhanced rehabilitation can be particularly useful in individuals with severe mobility disability. Body weight–supported treadmill training and robot-assisted gait training require significant time, equipment, and personnel involvement but have shown promising results, although they may not be superior to traditional gait training with a physical therapist.[50] Functional electrical stimulation (FES)-assisted cycling was shown to be safe in small uncontrolled trials, although RCTs are needed to determine its efficacy.[51]

Mobility Devices and Orthotics

A variety of assistive devices and orthotics are prescribed to enhance mobility.[52] Decision making is mainly based on clinical experience, patient preference, and individual results observed during rehabilitation visits after proper fitting and training. There is limited evidence showing improved gait parameters and walking capacity with use of a cane[53] or an ankle foot orthosis (AFO).[54,55] Empirically, the use of mobility devices is recommended when it is felt that the risk of falling is high in the context of gait and/or balance impairment. Use of an assistive device has been associated with a higher likelihood of "faller" status, but a recent study found that individuals with MS and mobility limitations who did not yet use an assistive device had a greater prevalence of multiple falls.[56] Although the use of a wheelchair as the primary mode of mobility may lead to a decreased frequency of falls, wheelchair users with MS remain at high risk of falling.[57]

The use of "active" devices providing assistance during walking has generated great interest, but functional results are variable. A small uncontrolled trial of the Hip Flexion Assist Device showed improvement on short and long walking tests.[58] There is a larger body of evidence on FES of the peroneal nerve delivered via surface electrodes to control foot drop, although mostly from case series.[59] A recent study comparing FES with an AFO on walking tests and oxygen cost of walking found a difference in performance on a long walking test at self-selected speed favoring FES but no difference on a short walking test or on oxygen cost.[60] An implanted FES device for foot drop is commercially available (ActiGait, OttoBock, Berlin, Germany) and improved walking capacity in a case series of six patients with MS.[61] Finally, exoskeleton technology, although commercially available, has been more extensively tested in spinal cord injury than in MS.[62] In practice, the use of technologically advanced mobility aids in MS has been limited by a lack of evidence to guide the selection of optimal candidates, and by the cost of the devices, which are often not covered by health insurance.

Upper Extremity Motor Rehabilitation

Evidence regarding upper extremity motor rehabilitation outcomes is more limited. A recent systematic review found only 30 studies meeting their search criteria, and only half of these studies specifically targeted the upper extremity.[63] In general, resistance and endurance training were effective on impairment, whereas multidisciplinary interventions and robot-assisted training were effective on activity.

Constraint-induced movement therapy (CIMT) is a well-known motor rehabilitation strategy in patients with poststroke hemiparesis, in which restoration of motor function, primarily in the upper extremity, is promoted through forced use of the paretic limb and restraint of the nonaffected limb.[64] A recently published phase 2 randomized clinical trial of CIMT in patients with MS with asymmetrical upper extremity motor impairment, compared with a holistic complementary and alternative medicine program, has shown a greater improvement with CIMT on the Motor Activity Log, a self-report measure of quality of movement of the more affected upper extremity (sustained at 1 year) but no between-group difference on the Wolf Motor Function Test.[65] Improvement on white matter integrity metrics derived from diffusion tensor imaging was noted immediately after CIMT, particularly in the contralateral thalamus and corticospinal tract, and in the ipsilateral superior temporal gyrus.[66]

Cognitive Rehabilitation

Considering the high prevalence of cognitive impairment in MS,[67] its impact on function, and the lack of pharmacologic treatments with demonstrated efficacy, cognitive rehabilitation (CR) appears as the only treatment modality that has shown promising effects on impairment and CNS plasticity.[9] Similar to motor rehabilitation, CR in practice often combines compensatory and restorative strategies. Most of the recent clinical trials of CR in MS have been primarily focused on restoration.

Computer-assisted programs are increasingly utilized for CR, owing to the fact that they ensure optimal standardization of contents, combined with a greater adaptability of exercise progression to an individual's abilities and progress during treatment. Computer-assisted programs also allow independent training, possibly from home, facilitating access to CR. In a recent systematic review of the literature, Goverover et al.[9] formulated evidence-based recommendations on currently available computer-assisted programs, including:

■ The modified Story Memory Technique, a 10-session program (two sessions per week for 5 weeks), which was shown to enhance learning and memory (at end of treatment and 6-month follow-up)[68] and changes in brain activation.[69]
■ The RehaCom program, which is composed of several modules covering multiple aspects of cognition and has been administered over periods varying from 5 weeks to 15 weeks in the literature. Benefits were noted after completion of RehaCom (and at follow-up) on attention, information processing, and memory, as well as brain activation.[70,71]
■ The Attention Process Training program, specifically focused on attention training and consisting of two sessions per week for 3 months. Improvement of performance on the Paced Auditory Serial Addition Test was noted at the end of treatment and maintained 3 months later.[72]

Many CR programs in MS involve individual or group sessions, sometimes combined with computer-based training. For example,

ReMind is a manualized program consisting of 10 group sessions supplemented with individual homework, which targets memory.[73] Group programs have also been developed to target metacognition (a person's ability to reflect on his or her own thought processes), and preliminary results, particularly on self-efficacy, are encouraging.[74,75] One intriguing study investigated the effects of music on learning and memory by asking participants to learn a 15-word list that was either read or sung 10 times; those in the music group exhibited significantly better word memory.[76]

Literature reviews on CR in MS emphasize the need for larger RCTs to better understand the effects of various techniques and programs. Furthermore, although evidence of efficacy on neuropsychological test performance is overall positive, results on self-reported cognitive limitations, mood, daily activities, and quality of life are more inconsistent.[77]

Interactions between cognitive and motor performance, and between the effects of motor rehabilitation and those of CR, remain insufficiently studied. Cognitive-motor coupling has been demonstrated in MS through associations between motor and cognitive impairment and through the dual task effect (i.e., altered performance on a motor task while performing a cognitive task). Recent evidence further suggests that physical exercise may enhance cognitive performance in individuals with MS.[78] Therefore, combining motor and CR may help enhance performance in both domains of function.[79]

Specialized Rehabilitation Services

In addition to general neurorehabilitation services, patients with MS may need help with important aspects of activity and participation, which is delivered by subspecialized professionals. When wheeled mobility is needed (manual or power wheelchair, power scooter), referral to a **wheelchair/seating clinic** is recommended to ensure that the most appropriate device is ordered[80] and to satisfy documentation requirements when reimbursement from health insurance is sought.

Driving is a high-level instrumental activity of daily living, which is generally very important for the outdoor mobility of individuals with MS, particularly in areas where public transportation is insufficient or not available.[81] At the same time, impairments from MS, side effects from medications, and other factors directly or indirectly related to the disease, may limit or render unsafe this activity. Indeed, visual, cognitive, and motor deficits were found to correlate with on-road performance in people with MS and various levels of disability or disease types.[82] When concerns arise, a referral to a **driver rehabilitation specialist** (often an occupational therapist [OT]) may be indicated. The initial step in driver rehabilitation is an extensive evaluation including in-office testing and performance testing on the road or in a driving simulator.[83] In addition to basic on-road or simulator training, driver rehabilitation specialists may recommend vehicle adaptations (such as hand controls, wheelchair ramp or lift) and train the individual to drive with these adaptations. Access to driver rehabilitation services is limited in some areas. The Association for Driver Rehabilitation Specialists website is a useful resource to locate driver rehabilitation professionals (https://www.aded.net/). One issue faced by clinicians involved in the care of patients with MS is when to refer them for driver rehabilitation, as patients are often reluctant to disclose issues with driving for fear of being told to stop driving altogether. On the other hand, impaired driving performance has been noted even in patients with mild to moderate MS symptoms compared with healthy controls, particularly on tasks of divided attention.[84] Screening tests may help predict on-road driving performance in MS[85,86] but do not replace clinical judgment.

Another important aspect of the life of patients with MS is work, because the disease most often affects them at the peak of their productive years. Unemployment in MS is higher than in the general population.[87] Body function impairments (motor, cognitive, fatigue) from MS were found to be associated with or predictive of unemployment,[88,89] and many other personal and environmental factors are involved in a given individual, requiring a personalized rehabilitation strategy. In addition to addressing impairments, work adaptations (reduced or adapted work schedule and work assignments, modifications to the work environment) may help preserve the ability to work. To help determine and document the need for accommodations, and to help facilitate the communication with employers, patients can be referred to government-funded or private **vocational rehabilitation services**. When the ability to work is fully compromised, the resulting loss of income can be partially compensated through disability benefits. Both government-funded and private disability insurance require that the individual satisfy a number of criteria to qualify for benefits, and this generally involves detailed documentation of the inability to work by clinicians. In the United States, the Social Security Administration has published specific criteria for MS.[90] A **functional capacity evaluation** (FCE) is a specialized rehabilitation evaluation that can help document functional limitations related to MS and help guide requests for accommodations or support an application for disability benefits. Owing to the specific challenges faced by patients with MS, an MS-specific FCE protocol has been proposed.[91]

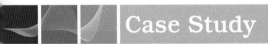

Case Study

The following case presentation illustrates the strategy for utilizing rehabilitation interventions to maximize function in a patient with MS over time, as her disability level, life circumstances, and priorities evolve.

STAGE 1

Jennifer is a 28-year-old Caucasian woman who was diagnosed with relapsing-remitting MS shortly after giving birth to her second child.

She lives with her husband and two children, ages 2 and 5 years, in a two-story single-family home. Jennifer played volleyball in college and currently enjoys running outdoors for 3 miles, twice per week. She has noticed that her running times are much faster in the mornings. She has attempted to run in the evening; however, she reports feeling much more fatigued. Six months ago, Jennifer sprained her right ankle during an evening run by stepping improperly on the sidewalk while mid-stride.

She works full-time as a mid-level accounts manager at a local accounting firm. Jennifer spends approximately 75% of her workday sitting at her desk and the remaining 25% walking around the office to different workstations to interact with her coworkers. Toward the end of her workday, she has been noticing her right foot feeling "stuck" to the carpet and occasionally catching her toes on the stairs, although she has never fallen to the ground. She stopped wearing high heels in the past year. Her supervisor recently had a meeting with her to discuss her productivity. He noticed that Jennifer has been forgetting to complete small errands and that it has been taking her much longer to type out her reports. On further examination, it was noted that her typing speed had decreased by 40% since she was first hired. She reports a slight "brain fog" by the end of her workday. Her coworkers noticed that Jennifer sometimes has difficulty finding the right word to say in the middle of conversations.

Lately, Jennifer reports feeling exhausted when returning home from work. She needs to nap for at least 1 hour before preparing meals for her family. Her husband is very supportive and frequently assists with cooking dinner and helps the children with their chores. Jennifer's husband voiced concerns when Jennifer burned her right hand twice in the past month while preparing a meal in the kitchen. She reports feeling tightness and occasional spasms in her right calf during the evening. Her husband reports that her legs would often "jump" or spasm during the middle of the night, frequently waking him up.

Jennifer was referred to physical, occupational, and speech therapy, with the goals of learning appropriate exercises to maintain her physical fitness and avoid tripping, and learning strategies for managing the housework, improving her typing skills, and improving her memory.

Motor examination showed overall mild right spastic hemiparesis, with distal right upper extremity weakness (wrist flexion 4/5 and finger flexion 3+/5), mild hip abduction/flexion and ankle dorsiflexion/eversion weakness, and mild spastic hypertonia in the finger flexors and ankle plantarflexors. Performance on motor and cognitive tests is presented in Table 31.3.

 TABLE 31.3
EVOLUTION OF OUTCOME MEASURES

Measure	First Presentation	6 y Later	21 y Later
Timed 25 Foot Walk Test	4.6 s	7.8 s	12.3 s
Timed Up and Go Test	9.5 s	14.2 s	21.1 s
Five Times Sit to Stand Test	12.8 s	15.3 s	19 s
Timed Up and Go Cognitive Test	11.2 s	17.7 s	28.4 s
Six-Minute Walk Test	1850 ft	1325 ft	975 ft
Berg Balance Scale	48 of 56	41 of 56	32 of 56
Nine Hole Peg Test Left Hand	18 s	22 s	26 s
Nine Hole Peg Test Right Hand	24 s	30 s	34 s
Montreal Cognitive Assessment	25 of 30	23 of 30	22 of 30

During the initial visit, the physical therapist taught Jennifer exercise guidelines that would promote strength and aerobic capacity, without causing any excess fatigue. The physical therapist educated her on a stretching program for her upper and lower extremities and recommended to perform stretching at least twice daily. During this visit, she was able to try a light-weight, carbon fiber AFO for her right lower extremity to prevent her toes from catching when she was fatigued. Although this orthosis supported a neutral position for her ankle, she declined to use this and opted to use a soft, elastic, external AFO called the Ossur Foot-Up instead.

The OT educated Jennifer on energy conservation tips while cooking in kitchen. He taught and reviewed coordination exercises for her right upper extremity.

The speech-language pathologist reviewed word finding and conversation strategies with Jennifer. She also taught her techniques for accomplishing her work tasks efficiently.

She followed up with PT, OT, and speech and language pathologist (SLP) for two additional visits to review her home exercise program.

STAGE 2

Jennifer is now 34 years old. She feels completely "wiped out" from trying to keep up with managing her household, her children's sporting events, and her work schedule. She stopped running long distances 4 years ago but still walks her dog for nearly a mile each day. She has difficulty with walking up and down steep slopes, noticing frequent toe-catching. Jennifer notices that her right calf muscle spasms in the evening. She started using a straight cane 6 months ago.

She switched jobs and now works 32 hours per week at a different firm. Owing to the increasing demands and high stress at her previous position, she opted to leave management and now works as a payroll specialist. She spends nearly 100% of her day seated at her workstation. She continues to feel fatigued, physically and cognitively, toward the end of her workday and still feels pressure to meet deadlines by her boss.

During a recent midday family outing to the zoo, she needed to have frequent seated rest breaks on the bench. Toward the end of their trip, while returning to their car in the parking lot, her right leg seemed to drag behind. She reports, "I really had to think about picking up my foot, otherwise I would have fallen." Her primary care physician had prescribed a prefabricated, plastic AFO; however, Jennifer found that it was bulky and made her leg too warm and that it really did not keep her leg from dragging.

Jennifer notices that her right hand is much clumsier recently. She recently dropped and broke her favorite coffee mug. Her fingers feel much stiffer, especially early in the morning and late at night.

Jennifer was referred to physical, occupational, and speech therapy, with the goals of improving her gait and balance, improving her fatigue with activities of daily living, and being able to hold meaningful conversations with her family and coworkers.

Motor examination revealed more diffuse right hemiparesis with weakness and spastic hypertonia at the shoulder, elbow, wrist, fingers, hip, and ankle. Spastic hypertonia was moderate in the finger flexors and ankle plantarflexors. There was a decline in performance on all outcome measures (Table 31.3).

The rehabilitation team recommended follow-up for six visits, over an 8-week period. During this time, the physical therapist reviewed safe ways to perform aerobic exercise for cardiovascular health, improving activity tolerance, and managing fatigue. He also recommended obtaining a cooling vest and a rollator walker with a seat so she can participate safely in family outings. Jennifer was fitted with a hip flexion assist device, as her right hip flexion weakness was the primary cause of her gait dysfunction. The PT also recommended consulting with a physiatrist for focal botulism toxin injection to her right ankle plantarflexors and continuing to perform stretching exercises using an incline board.

The OT created a home exercise program for upper extremity strengthening and coordination exercises. He also recommended home modifications to decrease the risk of falls. The OT also used a computer-based application to train Jennifer on how to improve her time management skills.

The SLP created a home program that included ways to incorporate word-finding strategies in everyday conversations. She educated and instructed Jennifer on compensatory strategies for complex auditory comprehension.

STAGE 3

Jennifer is now 49 years old. She has fallen twice in the past year but did not sustain any significant injuries. She uses her rollator walker regularly but is limited to walking only 100 ft before requiring a seated rest break. Jennifer expresses deep concern about her balance, especially at home and outdoors. She was unable to attend her son's baseball game because she was not confident with walking a long distance over uneven surfaces from the parking lot to the field. Although her family is supportive, her fatigue, balance, and mobility difficulties have put a strain on her marriage and family relationships.

Jennifer developed a small-amplitude tremor in her right hand, which interferes with her computer work and activities of daily living. She has been on short-term leave from her work for the past 4 months, because of not being able to keep up with the responsibilities. She reports feeling a brain fog by 2:00 PM every day. Her family notices that her voice is not as loud and articulate lately.

Jennifer was referred to physical, occupational, and speech therapy, with the goals of improving and maintaining her ability to walk, finding out ways to participate in community events safely, improving her right-hand coordination, and improving her voice volume.

Examination demonstrated further worsening of right-sided weakness, now affecting all of the muscle groups tested, and weakness in the left shoulder, hip, knee, and ankle. Spastic hypertonia was present in all but one of the muscle groups tested (overall moderate), as well as the left hip adductors and ankle plantarflexors. This was accompanied by markedly worse performance on all walking and balance tests but not on cognitive testing (Table 31.3).

The rehabilitation team recommended follow-up for 16 visits, over an 8-week period. The PT performed a neurological-based FCE to assess her ability to perform her duties at work. The PT recommended a more thorough stretching program for her lower extremities, including use of a stretching strap. After a thorough gait analysis was performed, the PT recommended a custom-fit, thermal plastic-molded AFO for her right foot to control for medial-lateral ankle stability. Gait training was performed on a treadmill with a harness to improve her gait quality and activity tolerance.

The OT evaluated the patient for a power wheelchair, so that she may perform her activities of daily living and community mobility safely.

The speech therapist taught Jennifer a home exercise program for improving her voice volume and articulation.

References

1. http://www.pva.org/media/pdf/fatigue1b772.pdf. Accessed July 20, 2018.
2. Gold R, Oreja-Guevara C. Advances in the management of multiple sclerosis spasticity: multiple sclerosis spasticity guidelines. *Expert Rev Neurother.* 2013;13(12 suppl):55-59.
3. Medical Advisory Board of the National Multiple Sclerosis Society. *Rehabilitation: Recommendations for Persons with Multiple Sclerosis.* National Multiple Sclerosis Society; 2005:10 pp. Avaialble at https://www.nationalmssociety.org/NationalMSSociety/media/MSNationalFiles/Brochures/Opinion-Paper-Rehabilitation-Recommendations-for-Persons-with-MS.pdf. Accessed July 20, 2018.
4. CMS.gov. Jimmo V. Sebelius Settlement Agreement Fact Sheet. Available at https://www.cms.gov/Medicare/Medicare-Fee-for-Service Payment/SNFPPS/Downloads/Jimmo-FactSheet.pdf. Accessed July 20, 2018.
5. *Towards a Common Language for Functioning, Disability and Health: ICF International Classification of Functioning, Disability and Health.* Geneva: World Health Organization; 2002:22 p. Available at http://www.who.int/classifications/icf/icfbeginnersguide.pdf. Accessed July 20, 2018.
6. Coenen M, Cieza A, Freeman J, et al. The development of ICF core sets for multiple sclerosis: results of the International consensus conference. *J Neurol.* 2011;258(8):1477-1488.
7. Conrad A, Coenen M, Schmalz H, et al. Validation of the comprehensive ICF core set for multiple sclerosis from the perspective of physical therapists. *Phys Ther.* 2012;92(6):799-820.
8. Karimi M, Brazier J. Health, health-related quality of life, and quality of life: what is the difference? *Pharmacoeconomics.* 2016;34(7):645-649.
9. Goverover Y, Chiaravalloti ND, O'Brien AR, DeLuca J. Evidenced-based cognitive rehabilitation for persons with multiple sclerosis: an updated review of the literature from 2007 to 2016. *Arch Phys Med Rehabil.* 2018;99(2):390-407.
10. Sandroff BM, Klaren RE, Motl RW. Relationships among physical inactivity, deconditioning, and walking impairment in persons with multiple sclerosis. *J Neurol Phys Ther.* 2015;39(2):103-110.

11. Marrie RA. Comorbidity in multiple sclerosis: implications for patient care. *Nat Rev Neurol.* 2017;13(6):375-382.
12. Sharma N, Classen J, Cohen LG. Neural plasticity and its contribution to functional recovery. *Handbook Clin Neurol.* 2013:110:3-12.
13. Tomassini V, Matthews PM, Thompson AJ, et al. Neuroplasticity and functional recovery in multiple sclerosis. *Nat Reviews Neurol.* 2012;8(11):635-646.
14. Reddy H, Narayanan S, Woolrich M, et al. Functional brain reorganization for hand movement in patients with multiple sclerosis: defining distinct effects of injury and disability. *Brain.* 2002;125(Pt 12):2646-2657.
15. Giesser BS. Exercise in the management of persons with multiple sclerosis. *Ther Adv Neurol Disord.* 2015;8(3):123-130.
16. Motl RW, Pilutti LA. Is physical exercise a multiple sclerosis disease modifying treatment? *Expert Rev Neurother.* 2016;16(8):951-960.
17. Kjolhede T, Siemonsen S, Wenzel D, et al. Can resistance training impact MRI outcomes in relapsing-remitting multiple sclerosis? *Mult Scler.* 2018;24(10):1356-1365. doi:10.1177/1352458517722645.
18. Haselkorn JK, Hughes C, Rae-Grant A, et al. Summary of comprehensive systematic review: rehabilitation in multiple sclerosis: report of the guideline development, dissemination, and implementation subcommittee of the American Academy of Neurology. *Neurology.* 2015;85(21):1896-1903.
19. Khan F, Amatya B. Rehabilitation in multiple sclerosis: a systematic review of systematic reviews. *Arch Phys Med Rehabil.* 2017;98(2):353-367.
20. LaRocca NG, Hudson LD, Rudick R, et al. The MSOAC approach to developing performance outcomes to measure and monitor multiple sclerosis disability. *Mult Scler.* 2018;24(11):1469-1484. doi:10.1177/1352458517723718.
21. Kurtzke JF. Rating neurologic impairment in multiple sclerosis: an expanded disability status scale (EDSS). *Neurology.* 1983;33(11):1444-1452.
22. Grasso MG, Pace L, Troisi E, Tonini A, Paolucci S. Prognostic factors in multiple sclerosis rehabilitation. *Eur J Phys Rehabil Med.* 2009;45(1):47-51.
23. National Multiple Sclerosis Society. *Minimal Record of Disability for Multiple Sclerosis.* New York: National Multiple Sclerosis Society; 1985.
24. Bethoux FA, Palfy DM, Plow MA. Correlates of the timed 25 foot walk in a multiple sclerosis outpatient rehabilitation clinic. *Int J Rehabil Res.* 2016;39(2):134-139.
25. Learmonth YC, Motl RW, Sandroff BM, Pula JH, Cadavid D. Validation of patient determined disease steps (PDDS) scale scores in persons with multiple sclerosis. *BMC Neurol.* 2013;13:37.
26. Hobart J, Lamping D, Fitzpatrick R, Riazi A, Thompson A. The Multiple Sclerosis Impact Scale (MSIS-29): a new patient-based outcome measure. *Brain.* 2001;124(Pt 5):962-973.
27. Miller DM, Allen R. Quality of life in multiple sclerosis: determinants, measurement, and use in clinical practice. *Curr Neurol Neurosci Rep.* 2010;10(5):397-406.
28. Granger C, Cotter A, Hamilton B, Fiedler R, Hens M, Functional assessment scales: a study of persons with multiple sclerosis, *Arch Phys Med Rehabil.* 1990;71:870-875.
29. Hobart J, Lamping D, Freeman J, et al, Evidence-based measurement: which disability scale for neurologic rehabilitation? *Neurology.* 2001;57:639-644.
30. Hobart J, Freeman J, Lamping D, Fitzpatrick R, Thompson A. The SF-36 in multiple sclerosis: why basic assumptions must be tested. *J Neurol Neurosurg Psychiatry.* 2001;71(3):363-370.

31. Miller DM, Bethoux F, Victorson D, et al. Validating Neuro-QoL short forms and targeted scales with people who have multiple sclerosis. *Mult Scler.* 2016;22(6):830-841.

32. Craig J, Young CA, Ennis M, et al. A randomised controlled trial comparing rehabilitation against standard therapy in multiple sclerosis patients receiving steroid treatment. *J Neurol Neurosurg Psychiatry.* 2003;74:1225-1230.

33. Khan F, Turner-Stokes L, Ng L, et al. Multidisciplinary rehabilitation for adults with multiple sclerosis. *Cochrane Database Syst Rev.* 2007;(2):CD006036.

34. Baird JF, Sandroff BM, Motl RW. Therapies for mobility disability in persons with multiple sclerosis. *Expert Rev Neurother.* 2018;18(6):493-502.

35. Pilutti LA, Edwards TA. Is exercise training beneficial in progressive multiple sclerosis? *Int J MS Care.* 2017;19:105-112.

36. Pearson M, Dieberg G, Smart N. Exercise as a therapy for improvement of walking ability in adults with multiple sclerosis: a meta-analysis. *Arch Phys Med Rehabil.* 2015;96(7):1339-1348.e7.

37. Learmonth YC, Adamson BC, Kinnett-Hopkins D, et al. Results of a feasibility randomized controlled study of the guidelines for exercise in multiple sclerosis project. *Contemp Clin Trials.* 2017;54:84-97.

38. Learmonth YC, Ensari I, Motl RW. Physiotherapy and walking outcomes in adults with multiple sclerosis: systematic review and meta-analysis. *Phys Ther Rev.* 2016;21(3–6):160-172.

39. Paltamaa J, Sjögren T, Peurala SH, et al. Effect of physiotherapy interventions on balance in multiple sclerosis: a systematic review and meta-analysis of randomized controlled trials. *J Rehabil Med.* 2012;44(10):811-823.

40. Levy J, Bensmail D, Brotier-Chomienne A, et al. Respiratory impairment in multiple sclerosis: a study of respiratory function in wheelchair-bound patients. *Eur J Neurol.* 2017;24(3):497-502.

41. Rietberg MB, Veerbeek JM, Gosselink R, et al. Respiratory muscle training for multiple sclerosis. *Cochrane Database Syst Rev.* 2017;12:CD009424.

42. Giovannelli M, Borriello G, Castri P, et al. Early physiotherapy after injection of botulinum toxin increases the beneficial effects on spasticity in patients with multiple sclerosis. *Clin Rehabil.* 2007;21(4):331-337.

43. Latino P, Castelli L, Prosperini L, et al. Determinants of botulinum toxin discontinuation in multiple sclerosis: a retrospective study. *Neurol Sci.* 2017;38(10):1841-1848.

44. Plummer P, Bohling CJ, Nickles LE. Combining dalfampridine with multicomponent exercise and gait training in a person with multiple sclerosis. *Int J MS Care.* 2018;20(5):238-243.

45. Jacques F, Schembri A, Nativ A. Prolonged-release fampridine as adjunct therapy to active motor training in MS patients: a pilot, double-blind, randomized, placebo-controlled study. *Mult Scler J Exp Transl Clin.* 2018;4(1). doi:10.1177/2055217318761168.

46. Casuso-Holgado MJ, Martín-Valero R, Carazo AF, et al. Effectiveness of virtual reality training for balance and gait rehabilitation in people with multiple sclerosis: a systematic review and meta-analysis. *Clin Rehabil.* 2018;32(9):1220-1234. doi:10.1177/0269215518768084.

47. Streicher MC, Alberts JL, Sutliff MH, et al. Effects of physical therapy training in an immersive virtual reality system or traditional physical therapy training in MS patients: a case series. *Int J Ther Rehabil.* In press.

48. Conklyn D, Stough D, Novak E, et al. A home-based walking program using rhythmic auditory stimulation improves gait performance in patients with multiple sclerosis: a pilot study. *Neurorehabil Neural Repair.* 2010;24(9):835-842.

49. Shahraki M, Sohrabi M, Taheri Torbati H, et al. Effect of rhythmic auditory stimulation on gait kinematic parameters of patients with multiple sclerosis. *J Med Life.* 2017;10(1):33-37.

50. Swinnen E, Beckwée D, Pinte D, et al. Treadmill training in multiple sclerosis: can body weight support or robot assistance provide added value? A systematic review. *Mult Scler Int.* 2012;2012:240274.

51. Pilutti LA, Motl RW, Edwards TA, et al. Rationale and design of a randomized controlled clinical trial of functional electrical stimulation cycling in persons with severe multiple sclerosis. *Contemp Clin Trials Commun.* 2016;3:147-152.

52. Souza A, Kelleher A, Cooper R, et al. Multiple sclerosis and mobility-related assistive technology: systematic review of literature. *J Rehabil Res Dev.* 2010;47(3):213-223.

53. Gianfrancesco MA, Triche EW, Fawcett JA, et al. Speed- and cane-related alterations in gait parameters in individuals with multiple sclerosis. *Gait Posture.* 2011;33(1):140-142.

54. Sheffler LR, Hennessey MT, Knutson JS, et al. Functional effect of an ankle foot orthosis on gait in multiple sclerosis: a pilot study. *Am J Phys Med Rehabil.* 2008;87(1):26-32.

55. Boes MK, Bollaert RE, Kesler RM, et al. Six-minute walk test performance in persons with multiple sclerosis while using passive or powered ankle-foot orthoses. *Arch Phys Med Rehabil.* 2018;99(3):484-490.

56. Coote S, Finlayson M, Sosnoff JJ. Level of mobility limitations and falls status in persons with multiple sclerosis. *Arch Phys Med Rehabil.* 2014;95(5):862-866.

57. Rice L, Kalron A, Berkowitz SH, et al. Fall prevalence in people with multiple sclerosis who use wheelchairs and scooters. *Medicine (Baltimore).* 2017;96(35):e7860.

58. Sutliff MH, Naft JM, Stough DK, et al. Efficacy and safety of a hip flexion assist orthosis in ambulatory multiple sclerosis patients. *Arch Phys Med Rehabil.* 2008;89(8):1611-1617.

59. Street T, Taylor P, Swain I. Effectiveness of functional electrical stimulation on walking speed, functional walking category, and clinically meaningful changes for people with multiple sclerosis. *Arch Phys Med Rehabil.* 2015;96(4):667-672.

60. Renfrew L, Lord AC, McFadyen AK. A comparison of the initial orthotic effects of functional electrical stimulation and ankle-foot orthoses on the speed and oxygen cost of gait in multiple sclerosis. *J Rehabil Assist Technol Eng.* 2018;5. doi:10.1177/2055668318755071.

61. Martin KD, Polanski WH, Schulz AK, et al. ActiGait implantable drop foot stimulator in multiple sclerosis: a new indication. *J Neurosurg.* 2017;126(5):1685-1690.

62. Kozlowski AJ, Fabian M, Lad D, et al. Feasibility and safety of a powered exoskeleton for assisted walking for persons with multiple sclerosis: a single-group preliminary study. *Arch Phys Med Rehabil.* 2017;98(7):1300-1307.

63. Lamers I, Maris A, Severijns D, et al. Upper limb rehabilitation in people with multiple sclerosis: a systematic review. *Neurorehabil Neural Repair.* 2016;30(8):773-793.

64. Corbetta D, Sirtori V, Castellini G. Constraint-induced movement therapy for upper extremities in people with stroke. *Cochrane Database Syst Rev.* 2015;(10):CD004433.

65. Mark VW, Taub E, Uswatte G. Phase II randomized controlled trial of constraint-induced movement therapy in multiple sclerosis. Part 1: effects on real-world function. *Neurorehabil Neural Repair.* 2018;32(3):223-232.

66. Barghi A, Allendorfer JB, Taub E. Phase II randomized controlled trial of constraint-induced movement therapy in multiple sclerosis. Part 2: effect on white matter integrity. *Neurorehabil Neural Repair.* 2018;32(3):233-241.

67. Chiaravalloti ND, DeLuca J. Cognitive impairment in multiple sclerosis. *Lancet Neurol.* 2008;7:1139-1151.
68. Chiaravalloti ND, Moore NB, Nikelshpur OM, et al. An RCT to treat learning impairment in multiple sclerosis: the MEMREHAB trial. *Neurology.* 2013;81:2066-2072.
69. Chiaravalloti ND, Wylie G, Leavitt V, et al. Increased cerebral activation after behavioral treatment for memory deficits in MS. *J Neurol.* 2012;259:1337-1346.
70. Cerasa A, Gioia MC, Valentino P, et al. Computer-assisted cognitive rehabilitation of attention deficits for multiple sclerosis: a randomized trial with fMRI correlates. *Neurorehabil Neural Repair.* 2013;27:284-295.
71. Mattioli F, Stampatori C, Zanotti D, et al. Efficacy and specificity of intensive cognitive rehabilitation of attention and executive functions in multiple sclerosis. *J Neurol Sci.* 2010;288:101-105.
72. Amato MP, Goretti B, Viterbo RG, et al. Computer-assisted rehabilitation of attention in patients with multiple sclerosis: results of a randomized, double-blind trial. *Mult Scler J.* 2014;20:91-98.
73. Carr SE, Nair R, Schwartz AF, et al. Group memory rehabilitation for people with multiple sclerosis: a feasibility randomized controlled trial. *Clin Rehabil.* 2014;28:552-561.
74. Shevil E, Finlayson M. Pilot study of a cognitive intervention program for persons with multiple sclerosis. *Health Educ Res.* 2010;25:41-53.
75. Pöttgen J, Lau S, Penner I, et al. Managing neuropsychological impairment in multiple sclerosis. *Int J MS Care.* 2015;17(3):130-137.
76. Thaut MH, Peterson DA, McIntosh GC, et al. Music mnemonics aid verbal memory and induce learning - related brain plasticity in multiple sclerosis. *Front Hum Neurosci.* 2014;8:395.
77. Mitolo M, Venneri A, Wilkinson ID, et al. Cognitive rehabilitation in multiple sclerosis: a systematic review. *J Neurol Sci.* 2015;354:1-9.
78. Briken S, Gold SM, Patra S, et al. Effects of exercise on fitness and cognition in progressive MS: a randomized, controlled pilot trial. *Mult Scler J.* 2013;20:382-390.
79. Motl R, Sandroff B, DeLuca J. Exercise training and cognitive rehabilitation: a symbiotic approach for rehabilitating walking and cognitive functions in multiple sclerosis. *Neurorehabil Neural Repair.* 2016;30:499-511.
80. De Souza LH, Frank AO. Problematic clinical features of powered wheelchair users with severely disabling multiple sclerosis. *Disabil Rehabil.* 2015;37(11):990-996.
81. Archer C, Morris L, George S. Assessment and rehabilitation of driver skills: subjective experiences of people with multiple sclerosis and health professionals. *Disabil Rehabil.* 2014;36(22):1875-1882.
82. Devos H, Ranchet M, Backus D, et al. Determinants of on-road driving in multiple sclerosis. *Arch Phys Med Rehabil.* 2017;98(7):1332.e2-1338.e2.
83. Kotterba S, Orth M, Eren E, Fangera T, Sindern E. Assessment of driving performance in patients with relapsing-remitting multiple sclerosis by a driving simulator. *Eur J Neurol.* 2003;50:160-164.
84. Devos H, Brijs T, Alders G, et al. Driving performance in persons with mild to moderate symptoms of multiple sclerosis. *Disabil Rehabil.* 2013;35(16):1387-1393.
85. Morrow SA, Classen S, Monahan M, et al. On-road assessment of fitness-to-drive in persons with MS with cognitive impairment: a prospective study. *Mult Scler.* 2018;24(11):1499-1506. doi:10.1177/1352458517723991.
86. Akinwuntan AE, O'Connor C, McGonegal E, et al. Prediction of driving ability in people with relapsing-remitting multiple sclerosis using the stroke driver screening assessment. *Int J MS Care.* 2012;14(2):65-70.

87. Bøe Lunde HM, Telstad W, Grytten N, et al. Employment among patients with multiple sclerosis-a population study. *PLoS One.* 2014;9(7):e103317.
88. Cadden M, Arnett P. Factors associated with employment status in individuals with multiple sclerosis. *Int J MS Care.* 2015;17(6):284-291.
89. Morrow SA, Drake A, Zivadinov R, et al. Predicting loss of employment over three years in multiple sclerosis: clinically meaningful cognitive decline. *Clin Neuropsychol.* 2010;24(7):1131-1145.
90. National Multiple Sclerosis Society. *Applying for Social Security Benefits. A Guide Book for People with MS and Their Healthcare Providers*; 2017. Available at http://www.nationalmssociety.org/nationalmssociety/media/msnational-files/brochures/guidebook-social-security-disability-for-people-with-ms.pdf. Accessed July 20, 2018.
91. Sutliff MH, Miller D, Forwell S. Developing a functional capacity evaluation specific to multiple sclerosis. *Int J MS Care.* 2012;14(suppl 3):17-28.

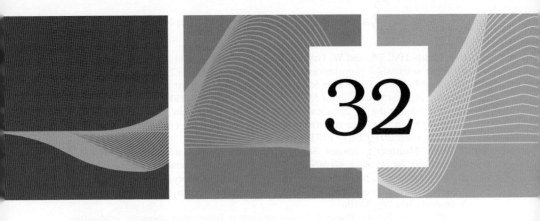

32

The Presence, Type, and Burden of Walking, Gait, and Balance Dysfunction in Multiple Sclerosis

■■■ Stephanie L. Silveira, Robert W. Motl, Francois Bethoux

Introduction

Multiple sclerosis (MS) is a chronic and nontraumatic, disabling disease of the central nervous system (CNS) characterized by axonal demyelination and transection as well as neurodegeneration involving loss of neurons and dendrites.[1] There are an estimated 1.1 million people currently living with MS in the United States, and the majority of cases are women of European descent between 20 and 50 years of age.[2] The CNS damage in MS is initially the result of immune-mediated demyelination and transection of axons that results in white-matter lesions and later the consequence of insufficient neurotrophic support for maintaining neurons and dendrites within the CNS that results in gray and white matter atrophy.[3] The CNS damage, depending on its location, can manifest as a range of symptoms including fatigue, depression, cognitive and visual impairment, muscle weakness, spasticity, and bowel and bladder problems. Another major consequence of MS is mobility disability, including difficulty with walking, dysfunction of gait, and compromised balance.[4] This chapter provides an overview of walking, gait, and balance dysfunction as prominent and life-altering consequences of MS that are important for disease management and rehabilitation by clinicians.

Definition of Mobility Disability in MS

We define mobility disability based on problems with walking, gait, and balance that may require the use of an assistive device and interfere with activities of daily living and community integration and participation (i.e., community ambulation). Walking is a form of locomotion (i.e., moving between places) that includes bipedal ambulation across different surfaces, short or long distances, and over or around obstacles.[5] Gait is an underlying feature of walking and involves describing the spatial and temporal parameters or characteristics of walking (i.e., the manner in which one walking). Gait is described in part based on step/stride length, cadence, base of support, double-support time, and side-to-side step variability or asymmetry.[6] Gait is one of the underlying factors for understanding walking speed, ambulatory endurance, and community ambulation. Balance, defined as maintaining upright stance or posture while standing or moving, can be described by the status or functioning of three sensory systems, namely, visual, somatosensory, and vestibular.[1] Balance is important for mobility and walking in MS, as its disruption could result in increased falls or near falls while walking and can certainly be associated with disturbance of gait (e.g., base of support) and walking. These three factors collectively represent major features in the description and understanding of mobility and its disability in MS.

Prevalence of Mobility Disability in MS

Mobility disability is a primary feature associated with the clinical manifestation of MS and its progression over time. This is commonly reported based on Expanded Disability Status Scale (EDSS) scores (i.e., a standardized clinical rating system for MS-related disability)[7] in natural history studies of MS, mostly based on the walking distance and the use of mobility aids. These natural history studies have examined the rate or time course and predictors of disability progression in persons with MS based on the time for reaching EDSS scores of 4.0 and 6.0 as benchmarks of irreversible mobility disability. For example, the median times from onset of MS until the assignment of benchmark EDSS scores of 4.0 (i.e., limited walking ability, but able to walk more than 500 m without aid or rest) and 6.0 (i.e., ability to walk with unilateral support no more than 100 m without rest) are approximately 10 and 20 years, respectively.[8-10] The median interval of time from the onset of MS until those benchmarks has been predicted by sex, age, symptoms and course at onset of disease, degree of recovery from the first relapse, time to a second neurological episode, and number of relapses in the first 5 years of the disease.[8-10]

Population-based studies further indicate that 75% of people with MS report problems with mobility, and difficulty with walking itself is reported by over 40% of people with MS.[4,11] Another study of patients with MS in Europe indicated that nearly 50% of people with MS reported experiencing mobility impairments within the first month of diagnosis, and more than 90% of people with MS reported experiencing mobility impairments within 10 years of diagnosis.[12] Nearly 70% of people with MS identified walking difficulty as the most challenging part of the disease, and common mobility problems reported by persons with MS included needing to concentrate on walking, difficulty standing, increased effort needed to walk, and needing support such as furniture, walls, or someone's arm when walking indoors.[13] Approximately one-third of people with MS report using at least one mobility device, such as a cane, walker, or wheelchair. Mobility aid use for ambulation is associated with age, worsening health, and secondary progressive MS.[13]

Balance problems are common among persons with MS and can increase the risk and prevalence of falls as well as decrease physical activity and quality of life (QOL).[14,15] Balance problems include increased postural sway during standing, abnormal patterns of movement in static and dynamic balance, and delayed postural reactions.[16-18] Balance problems typically manifest early in the disease course and worsen over time, with over 50% of persons with MS reporting a loss of balance two or more times weekly.[4,19,20] Falls represent a common marker of the presence of balance problems in MS. One prospective cohort study that included persons with MS between 21 and 74 years of age documented the occurrence, over a 6-month period, of three or more falls in 33% of the sample, and between one and two falls in 27%.[21] Another study reported a similar fall prevalence in persons with MS who used mobility aids, with 50% reporting 1 or more falls in last 3 months and a range between 1 and 18 falls overall.[22] Another study focused specifically on persons with moderate MS-related disability and reported that those who experienced frequent falls (i.e., classified as "fallers") had more gait dysfunction, including variability in step length and single support.[23] This suggests that mobility disability, including balance problems and gait disturbance, is related with falling among persons with MS and is prevalent in a large segment of this population.

Personal Value of Mobility in MS

Mobility is one of the most valued functions among people with MS, as it is critical for independence and its loss increases concern of dependence on caregivers or transition into a nursing home.[24] For example, one national survey of persons with MS reported that 41% of the sample had difficulty walking and 13% were unable to walk at least two times per week.[4] Among those who had difficulty walking, 70% reported that it was the most challenging aspect of living with MS.[4] The inability and difficulty with walking were rated as the most disruptive problems associated with the management of MS. Furthermore, most people reported at least some adverse impact on one or more everyday activity in the past 6 months because of difficulties maintaining balance (76%). Another study indicated that loss of lower extremity function was rated the highest concern among 13 domains of body function, followed by loss of vision, among persons with MS who had a more recent diagnosis (i.e., less than 5 y) and among those who had a longer time elapsed since diagnosis (i.e., 15 or more years).[25] One more recent study had persons with relapsing MS and physicians rate the value of 13 bodily functions from the most to least important using a standard questionnaire.[26] Persons with MS rated visual functioning as the primary concern, followed by thinking and memory and walking, whereas physicians rated mobility as the highest concern, followed by thinking and memory.[26] Overall, mobility dysfunction is rated as one of the primary concerns among people with MS, and its maintenance is a priority across the disease progression spectrum for both those affected by this disease and their health care providers. These findings are supported by evidence on the burden of mobility disability, as described in the next section.

Burden of Mobility Dysfunction in MS

Mobility disability portends considerable burden for people living with MS. The burden ranges from worsening of symptoms to reduced QOL. Furthermore, there are economic burdens associated with mobility disability as well as influences on participation and employment. The effect of mobility disability even extends into the lives of caregivers. This section provides an overview regarding the effect of mobility on a variety of outcomes in MS.

Fatigue and Depression

Fatigue and depression are two of the most common symptoms of MS, and these two symptoms have been associated with mobility disability in MS. In turn, fatigue and depression further affect community participation and activities. Upward of 95% of persons with MS report fatigue as a burden of the disease that can be severe.[27] Fatigue is further a significant predictor of physical functioning and QOL.[28,29] One study reported that self-reported fatigue was associated with self-report walking limitations, but it was only mildly associated with objective walking performance tests.[30] Additionally, gait abnormalities analyzed with a body sensor during the 6-minute walk test were associated with higher self-reported overall fatigue impact scores in persons with MS.[31] Another study of participants with MS reported that fatigue measured using the Fatigue Severity Scale was significantly associated with the 6-minute walk distance.[32] That study also measured self-report depression using the Hospital Anxiety Depression Scale (HADS-D) and reported that the 6-minute walk distance was associated with the HADS-D score.[32] Other studies have reported a significant relationship between depression and mobility disability (i.e., gait and balance problems) in MS.[33,34] One study demonstrated that persons scoring over 8 on the HADS-D (i.e., elevated depression symptom group) walked slower with a decreased cadence compared with those who had HADS-D scores of 8 or less; depression symptom scores were further correlated with self-perceptions of walking ability.[34] Another common measure of depression is the Beck Depression Inventory-II (BDI-II). Depression scores based on the BDI-II were significantly related to both objective and subjective balance scores in a study of ambulatory participants with MS.[33] Collectively, mobility disability may be associated with worse fatigue and depression in persons with MS.

Cognition

There is increasing evidence that mobility disability is associated with cognitive dysfunction in MS (i.e., cognitive-motor coupling). For example, one early study examined the association between motor impairments of the upper and lower extremities and cognitive functioning in MS. That study identified speed of processing and executive function as correlates of upper and lower extremity motor function based on the 9-Hole Peg Test and Timed 25-Foot Walk (T25FW) in persons with MS.[35] Another study reported that cognitive processing speed using the Symbol Digit Modalities Test was associated with self-reported and objective walking measures as well as EDSS scores in persons with MS.[36] One study of balance using the Six Spot Step Test and cognitive processing speed based on the Paced Auditory Serial Addition test reported an association between balance and cognition.[37] These data suggest that persons with MS who have more significant mobility disability have greater cognitive impairments.

There is further evidence of cognitive-motor coupling based on the dual-task paradigm. This paradigm involves examining changes in walking performance or balance (i.e., two metrics of mobility disability) when performing a concurrent cognitive task compared with not performing the cognitive task. One study examined the effect of performing alternate letter alphabet test while walking and reported that the concurrent performance of a cognitive task resulted in significantly slower velocity and cadence, shorter step length, increased step time, and increased double-support time in persons with MS.[38] Other research has demonstrated that balance can be significantly affected while concurrently performing a cognitive task in persons with MS. For example, one study of balance using the dual-task paradigm in persons with both mild and moderate MS reported that postural sway measured using posturography was significantly increased when completing a word generation task, and the change was significant across disease severity levels.[39] These data provide a direct link between cognitive functioning and walking and balance function in MS.

Quality of Life

QOL is defined as the subjective evaluation or judgment regarding satisfaction with life and can be directly influenced by mobility disability. One study of 103 patients with MS reported that QOL, rated using the Multiple Sclerosis Quality of Life-54, was significantly associated with disability level, depression, and fatigue.[40] Another study reported that persons with MS scored significantly lower than controls on the Quality of Life Index (QLI), and the degree of disability measured by EDSS scores was predictive of QLI score.[41] Health-related quality of life (HRQOL) has further been examined as a correlate of walking dysfunction in persons with MS. One retrospective study of three clinical trials of patients with MS reported that HRQOL measured using the SF-36 was significantly correlated with walking speed, with participants with faster speed reporting higher SF-36 physical component scores. That study further examined the association between longitudinal changes in SF-36 scores and walking speed over time and reported that participants with MS whose walking speed decreased had decreased SF-36 scores; these changes in both SF-36 scores and walking speed were in the clinically significant range, with a 20% to 25% decrease in walking speed being associated with a five-point decrease in SF-36 physical component score.[42] Other research has reported that impaired balance and coordination is among one of the common problems associated with diminished QOL of persons with MS.[43] This collectively suggests that disability severity and mobility disability are associated with worse QOL and HRQOL in persons with MS.

Economic Burden

The economic burden of MS can be understood, in part, based on the association between EDSS scores and costs of the disease. Costs associated with MS include medications and hospitalization as well as other direct costs, indirect costs, informal costs, and intangible costs.[44] Reviews of the literature report a stark increase in disease-related costs with increasing EDSS scores (i.e., overall mobility disability) in persons with MS.[44,45] In one study, those with mild MS (EDSS <3) incurred approximately $16,646 in annual disease-related costs, compared with $27,151 in those with moderate disease (EDSS 3-6), and even higher costs were presumed for those with severe disability (EDSS >6).[46] One study of health care–related costs for persons with MS reported that the average annual cost for medical care in persons with abnormal gait was $20,871.[47] Disease-modifying drugs (DMDs) are more often prescribed to those with abnormality in gait, and the average additional cost associated with DMDs in persons with MS is $7901 annually.[47] Overall, patients with walking impairment are more likely to need a variety of expert medical services outside of primary care and long-term DMD treatments that can contribute to the economic burden of MS disease management.[48]

Participation/Employment

Participation is defined as involvement in a life situation,[5] and employment is one of the primary determinants or indicators of participation. Mobility disability is associated with early retirement and work absences that significantly affect income in this population.[49] For example, an estimated $17,000 annually per patient is lost in relapse-related absences, reduced time spent at work, and early retirement.[49] North American Research Committee on Multiple Sclerosis (NARCOMS) patient registry data demonstrate that, on average, over 50% of patients with MS are not employed and those who are unemployed are more likely to have progressive disease, longer symptom duration, greater levels of disability, and greater functional limitations.[50] Furthermore, mobility performance subscale scores of the performance scales were predictive of work loss and work initiation longitudinally, with increased mobility problems predictive of loss and reduced mobility problems predictive of initiation.[50] Another study reported that only 34% of people who report walking difficulty were employed.[4] Objective measures of walking, including the T25FW, and self-report measures, such as the 12-item Multiple Sclerosis Walking Scale (MSWS-12), have been used to measure the association between mobility disability and employment.[51,52] For example, one study reported that longer T25FW times were associated with permanent disability (collecting Supplemental Security Income), government health care assistance (Medicaid/Medicare), and change in occupational status.[51] Issues with mobility and the subsequent impact on participation, particularly employment status, can affect feelings of independence in patients with MS.

Independence

Independence is defined as having choice and control over life and your environment and is directly associated with the presence and degree of mobility disability in MS. The need for assistance in activities of daily living further contributes to feelings of loss of independence and burden in persons with MS.[24] One study reported that approximately two-thirds of people with MS were dependent on a caregiver for assistance in activities of daily living, specifically mobility-related activities, such as walking outside, negotiating stairs, and navigating to social and lifestyle activities.[24] In studies using both objective and self-reported measures of walking disability, participants with greater disability severity reported a greater need for assistance with instrumental activities of daily living, such as preparing meals and managing medications.[51,52] In another study examining T25FW performance, participants who took longer than 8 s to complete the task had more difficulties in performing instrumental activities of daily living.[51] Balance problems associated with MS can further affect independence as suggested in one study reporting that persons with MS demonstrated significant postural challenges when performing movements involved in execution of activities of daily living, particularly during head, hand, and dynamic movements.[53] Overall, activities that seem to be most affected by MS are mobility related and include walking outside, cleaning indoors, negotiating stairs, dressing, outdoor transportation, and social and lifestyle activities.[54] Factors related to mobility disability and decreased independence are interrelated with employment and economic burden of MS, themselves closely related to dependence on caregivers.

Caregivers

The burden of disability extends beyond the person with MS and into the lives of others, notably caregivers. One study of unpaid assistance for patients with MS reported that those with moderate to severe disability require 1 to 8 hours per day of direct patient care (e.g., nursing and personal care) and 1 to 2 hours of indirect care (e.g., housekeeping and social activities).[55] Patients with mild disability require less hours of direct and indirect care but still need assistance from informal caregivers such as partners, parents, children, or other family members.[55] There is often a disconnect between the amount of time people perceive that caregivers spend helping them and caregiver perceptions of time spent that may affect the relationship between the patient and caregiver.[54,56] One study examining caregivers and persons with MS reported that the participants with MS with more walking impairment based on the MSWS-12 had lower QOL scores and caregivers of persons with higher MSWS-12 scores reported greater burden.[57] Need for caregiver support has been associated with objective measures of walking disability, with one study reporting that a longer T25FW time is associated with the need for additional hours of caregiver support.[48] The physical, emotional, psychological, social, and economic burdens that caregivers incur provide a critical area for future research and interventions providing resources for dyads.[54]

Descriptive Pattern of Walking Dysfunction in MS

There are many approaches for measuring walking dysfunction in MS. Some of the common measures include the T25FW, 6-minute walk (6MW), Timed Up and Go (TUG), Six Spot Step Test (SSST), oxygen (O_2) cost of walking, (i.e., milliliters of O_2 consumed per kilogram of body weight per meter traveled [mL/kg/m]), patient-reported outcomes, and free-living assessments (Table 32.1). We describe these measures and comparisons between MS and controls, across EDSS levels, and between MS clinical courses or phenotypes (i.e., relapsing remitting vs. progressive MS) as an approach for describing walking dysfunction as an index of mobility disability in MS.

TABLE 32.1

MEASUREMENTS OF MOBILITY DISABILITY IN PERSONS WITH MULTIPLE SCLEROSIS

Measure	Mobility-Related Outcome
Walking	
Timed 25-Foot Walk	Short distance walking speed
6-Minute Walk	Walking endurance
Timed Up and Go	Functional mobility and balance while walking
Six Spot Step Test	Short distance walking coordination, dynamic balance, lower limb strength
O_2 Cost of Walking	Energetic cost of walking
Patient-Reported Outcomes	Multiple Sclerosis Walking Scale-12
Free-Living Assessment	Ambulation in community: pedometer and accelerometer axis and step counts
Gait	
Pressure-Sensitive Walkways	Temporal (e.g., step time) and spatial (e.g., step length) parameters
Body-Worn Motion Sensors	Sway acceleration amplitude, sway velocity, sway frequency, and sway jerk
Balance	
Static Posturography Force Plates	Postural control, postural sway, and center of pressure path length
Computerized Dynamic Posturography	Postural control, postural sway, and center of pressure path length while manipulating stability and visual environment
Commercial Gaming Systems	Path length, weight distribution, vertical ground reaction forces

Timed 25-Foot Walk

The T25FW is a measure of walking speed over a short distance and involves having a person walk 25 feet as quickly and safely as possible. The time is recorded in seconds and averaged across two consecutive trials. The T25FW was recognized as the best characterized, objective measure of short distance walking disability in persons with MS across a wide range of walking impairment.[58] There are data indicating that performance on the T25FW is compromised in MS compared with controls who do not have MS or any other neurological disease.[59,60] For example, one study compared T25FW performance between persons with MS who had mild disability (EDSS 0-1.5) and normal controls and reported that those with MS performed worse on the T25FW (4.3 s) than controls (3.6 s).[59] The difference in T25FW performance across levels of disability status was reported in a recent paper validating T25FW benchmarks in MS.[51] That study reported distributions of participants who completed the T25FW in <6, 6 to 7.99, or ≥8 s, and this corresponded with groups of mild, moderate, and severe disability based on EDSS scores, respectively.[51] The T25FW further differs across relapsing-remitting and progressive MS disease courses, whereby participants with progressive MS on average took longer (9.2 s) than those with RRMS (5.1 s) to complete the T25FW.[17] Overall, this indicates that short-distance fast walking speed (i.e., velocity) is compromised in MS, particularly as a function of increasing disability severity or progressive clinical courses.

The 6-Minute Walk

The 6MW provides a measure of walking endurance and involves having a person walk as fast and as far as possible during a 6-minute period and recording the distance in feet or meters.[61] Some data demonstrate that people with MS across a wide range of EDSS scores consistently perform worse than healthy controls on the 6MW. For example, healthy controls on average walked 620 m, whereas those with mild, moderate, and severe MS walked 603, 507, and 389 m, respectively.[61] There are additional data indicating that the 6MW distance varies as a function of both EDSS and Patient-Determined Disease Steps (PDDS) scores.[62-64] For example, one study specifically comparing the 6MW performance between persons with mild and moderate MS demonstrated a significant difference between groups, with the mean distance walked for the mild and moderate groups of 482 and 259 m, respectively.[64] One study has reported a difference in 6MW performance for those with relapsing and progressive MS with means of 225 and 169 m, respectively.[65] Collectively, this indicates that compromised endurance walking capacity is another manifestation of MS that varies with disability severity and MS phenotype.

Timed Up and Go

The TUG provides a measure of functional mobility and balance within a walking performance test. The TUG requires that persons rise from a chair, walk 3 m, turn around, walk back, and sit down as quickly and safely as possible.[66] Validation studies of the TUG in people with MS demonstrated that higher EDSS scores were associated with longer times to complete the TUG.[67] One study reported that TUG scores were significantly higher in participants with relapsing MS (7.74 s) than controls (5.77 s).[68] Another study compared TUG scores across groups of persons with varying MS disease severity based on EDSS scores compared with control participants. The mean TUG score for controls was 7.3 s, whereas times were higher for mild, moderate, and severe MS groups: 7.4, 9.9, and 10.0 s respectively.[69] These data suggest that walking tests of functional mobility and balance are compromised in MS and become worse with increasing disability severity.

Six Spot Step Test

The SSST is an alternative measure of short-distance walking that engages coordination, dynamic balance, lower limb strength, vision, and cognition as it involves fast crisscross walking over a 5-m course and kicking cones/blocks off resting markers. The SSST further requires use of both the dominant and nondominant foot and provides additional information about patient mobility disability while exhibiting strong reliability and test-retest agreement in persons with MS.[70] One study of Brazilians with MS reported a significant difference between MS and controls on the SSST with a mean of 14.91 s in MS and 7.22 s in controls.[71] Furthermore, in a validation study of the SSST in persons with MS, disability severity based on EDSS was significantly associated with performance on SSST.[70] This study showed strong precision of the SSST by disability severity (EDSS scores), type of MS (relapsing remitting vs. progressive), and fall risk when compared with the T25FW and TUG.[37] Participants with relapsing MS performed the SSST task faster than those with progressive MS, and participants with a lower fall risk performed the SSST faster than those with a high fall risk.[37] Results from these studies show the SSST is a valid, reliable, multifaceted measure of walking dysfunction in persons with MS that is being more widely used in research and clinical practice.

O_2 Cost of Walking

Another way of describing walking dysfunction that occurs with MS involves measurement of physiological parameters during walking performance tests. The O_2 cost of walking is expressed in milliliters of O_2 consumed per kilogram of body weight per meter traveled (mL/kg/m) and is a physiological marker that reflects the degree of locomotor impairment in pathologic conditions based on the energetic cost of movement. The O_2 cost of walking can reflect an increase in the rate of O_2 consumption (VO_2) with normal walking speed (i.e., increased energy expenditure for doing the same movement) or a reduction in walking speed with a normal VO_2 (i.e., same energy expenditure for doing less movement). One study of persons with mild MS demonstrated that the O_2 cost of walking was higher for persons with MS in slow, moderate, and fast treadmill walking than for controls.[72] Disability severity is associated with the energetic cost of walking.[72,73] The previous study reported that, among persons with MS disability, severity was associated with O_2 cost of walking in over-ground walking at varying paces.[72] These data support that walking is more costly for persons with MS than for controls and is a function of disability severity.

Patient-Reported Outcomes

There is increasing interest in the documentation of walking dysfunction in MS based on the patient's perspective (i.e., patient-reported outcome or PRO). To that end, the Multiple Sclerosis Walking Scale-12 (MSWS-12) has been designed and validated as a common PRO of walking in MS.[11] The MSWS-12 has 12 items that are rated on a four-point scale with anchors of 1 and 4, and items scores are summed and then linearly transformed into a scale that ranges between 0 and 100. The MSWS-12 composite score reflects the patient's perspective regarding the impact of MS on walking such that higher scores reflect a larger degree of perceived walking impairment. There are consistent data indicating that MSWS-12 scores are strongly associated with disability severity in MS.[11,74,75] For example, the original development of the scale reported a strong association between MSWS-12 and EDSS scores in patients with MS undergoing steroid treatment ($r = 0.65$).[11] This association was later replicated in another study of community-dwelling persons with MS who had progressive and relapsing MS ($r = 0.80$). Collectively, this indicates that patient perception of walking dysfunction is another manifestation of MS that covaries with disability severity and is reliably reported in persons with different phenotypes of MS.

Free-Living Assessments

Walking dysfunction in MS has typically been documented based on assessments performed in a laboratory or clinical setting. These measurements are accurate, reliable, and valid but lack ecological validity for understanding ambulation that occurs in the context of daily life.[76] Another approach for measuring ambulation in free-living conditions in MS involves using accelerometers and pedometers. These devices are motion sensors that provide accurate counts of vertical displacement of the body, indicating times of activity and ambulation. Devices can be worn around the waist near the center of mass during all waking hours without disrupting normal activities. There is consistent evidence for reduced community ambulation based on motion sensor data in persons with MS and across the disability spectrum.[77-80] One recent meta-analysis demonstrated based on free-living assessments using accelerometry that persons with MS engage in less ambulatory physical activity than healthy controls.[81] For example, one study reported a large difference in effect size ($d = \sim 1.0$) in activity counts per day from a waist-worn ActiGraph accelerometer between persons with MS and a matched control sample such that the patients were engaging in less community-based ambulation.[81] We further note that lower step counts using accelerometers is directly associated with EDSS scores in persons with MS.[82,83] For example, one study reported a linear reduction in activity counts per day from a waist-worn ActiGraph accelerometer as a function of increasing disability severity (mild, moderate, and severe).[80] The effect of disability status has been confirmed in other research using the StepWatch Step Activity Monitor and metric of steps per day in persons with MS.[84] One recent paper reported a linear gradient between steps per day and disability status in 786 persons with MS, such that a one-point increase in disability was associated with a reduction of 900 steps per day.[85] Additionally, this study reported a significant difference by clinical course of MS with a difference of 2233 steps/day in participants with relapsing versus progressive MS phenotype.[85] Such data suggest that the association between disability severity and walking impairment extends beyond the laboratory or clinic and into the community thereby affecting one's ambulation as part of everyday life.

Descriptive Pattern of Gait Dysfunction in MS

There are many approaches for measuring gait (i.e., the spatial and temporal parameters or characteristics of walking) in MS presented in Table 32.1. Gait is a significant indicator of mobility disability in MS that provides a latent, descriptive basis for walking dysfunction. Gait is commonly measured using a gait mat and provides measures such as velocity, cadence, stride length, step length, double support duration, step width, stride time, and swing phase duration.[20] Body worn sensors further can capture measures of gait. Importantly, these measures of gait vary between MS and controls, across disability level in MS, and between MS clinical courses.[20]

Pressure-Sensitive Walkways

One common measure of gait dysfunction is pressure-sensitive walkways, such as the GAITRite mat (CIR Systems, Inc., Franklin, New Jersey, USA). The GAITRite system consists of a rubberized mat with embedded sensors for detecting footfalls during walking and provides measures of temporal and spatial parameters associated with gait (e.g., step time and step length). Participants typically walk across the mat at a normal, comfortable speed for capturing temporal and spatial measures of gait that are processed in real time, recorded, and stored. One study using the GAITRite compared persons with MS who had minimal gait impairment with healthy controls and reported that persons with MS took fewer, shorter, and wider steps; both feet were left on the ground for a greater percentage of the gait cycle; and walking velocity was slower.[86] Gait impairment further varies by disability severity as reported in a recent study.[87] EDSS was significantly correlated with walking velocity, step length, step time, and step width in a sample of persons with MS.[87] Additionally, persons who used assistive devices demonstrated greater step length variability and lower walking velocity and step length than those who did not use assistive devices.[87] Overall, studies demonstrate that pressure-sensitive walkways, such as the GAITRite system, are effective in quantifying subtle gait abnormalities in persons with minimal disability as well as more pronounced changes in persons with further progressed MS.

Body-Worn Motion Sensors

Body-worn sensors provide rich information through gyroscope and accelerometer measurement. Specific metrics include sway acceleration amplitude, sway velocity, sway frequency, and sway jerk that can be converted to both temporal and spatial gait parameters. One study comparing persons with MS and healthy controls demonstrated no significant difference in temporal measures (e.g., cadence, swing, and double support time) but significant differences in dynamic balance metrics.[18] Persons with moderate MS-related disability performed worse than those with mild MS, who performed worse than healthy controls on both body sensor and self-reported measures of walking and balance.[88] Current studies have not examined body-worn motion sensor results by clinical course of MS, leaving a gap in the literature on the efficacy of this gait measurement. Body worn sensor technology is now recommended as an option for clinicians to objectively quantify gait and balance abnormalities, providing more sensitive analysis of subtle changes over time, and this method is cost-effective and convenient.[89]

Descriptive Pattern of Balance Problems in MS

Balance problems are related but distinct from gait and walking dysfunction in persons with MS. Methods for measuring balance problems in MS include posturography force plate protocols, both static and dynamic, and more recently commercially available gaming systems (Table 32.1).

Balance problems in persons with MS are pervasive, and measurement of balance shows significant impairment in sensory systems associated with balance among persons with MS compared with healthy controls, by disease severity and MS clinical course.

Static Posturography Force Plates

Posturography is an objective measure of standing postural control and considered the gold standard for measuring balance problems in persons with MS. Persons with MS stand on a force plate in which data can be collected in multiple planes and sensitive detectors are used to measure oscillations. This method is effective for both quantifying and comparing postural sway in persons with MS versus healthy controls. One study comparing persons with MS with controls showed that the mean three-dimensional mean angular sway velocity of persons with MS was above the 95th percentile for controls.[90] Posturography is also effective in identifying changes in postural control related to disability severity. For example, one cross-sectional study of persons with varying disability severity demonstrated that posturography measures, specifically center of pressure path length, were significantly worse in individuals with moderate and severe MS (EDSS 3.0-5.5 and 6.0-6.5, respectively) compared with mild MS.[23] Further research is needed comparing persons with MS by clinical course; however, static posturography measurement in persons with MS indicates significant balance problems compared with healthy controls and by disability severity.

Computerized Dynamic Posturography

Another method for quantifying balance using posturography is computerized dynamic posturography. One example is the NeuroCom Balance Master (NeuroCom International, Inc., Clackamas, Oregon, USA), which provides objective measurement of postural balance using a support platform where stability and visual environment can be empirically manipulated. With this device, patients with loss of balance can be placed in a harness for safety, and measurements via force plates are taken in different dynamic and sensory conditions (e.g., dynamic phase with eyes closed vs. eyes open). One study of persons with MS with the relapsing remitting type and mild disability (i.e., EDSS ≤3.5) demonstrated significant differences between MS and healthy controls in postural sway when tested on a foam surface with eyes closed.[91] Specifically, this test allows participants to use their vestibular system but removes vision by closing eyes and compromises somatosensory system with a soft surface.[91] Unilateral stance was also tested with eyes closed and open, showing significantly different sway velocity between patients with MS and healthy controls.[91]

Another study compared persons with MS to healthy control norms using the Kistler 9281 force plate and demonstrated significant impairment in all postural sway variables; furthermore, participants with the relapsing MS type exhibited a better vibration sensation for the less and more sensitive toe than those with the progressive MS type.[92] Studies using varying protocols help identify and quantify the intricate systems involved in balance problems in persons with MS, and further research by disability severity is needed.

Commercial Gaming Systems

Commercially available gaming systems are of interest in current research to help improve balance, coordination, and aerobic capacity. These systems are typically more affordable than research-grade force plates and widely available. One example is the Nintendo Wii Balance Board, equipped with four force sensors in the corners of the board that are used to evaluate the distribution of weight on the board and vertical ground reaction forces. One recent validation study demonstrated that the Nintendo Wii Balance Board discriminated well between persons with MS and healthy controls in identifying path lengths, but not for absolute values compared with laboratory-grade force plates.[93] However, this provides an avenue for future research in using commercially available measurement tools to identify balance problems in persons with MS with varying disability severity and MS clinical course and to complement clinical assessments.

Importance of Focal Rehabilitation

The prevalence, scope, and burden of mobility disability in MS underscores the importance of focal medical management and rehabilitation for improving measures of walking, gait, and balance. One avenue of interest is DMDs that potentially slow the rate of atrophy of brain tissue in regions associated with mobility; however, there is minimal evidence supporting the efficacy of DMDs for improving mobility outcomes in persons with MS. To that end, one recent paper provided a review that outlines symptomatic pharmacologic and nonpharmacologic therapeutic approaches that target mobility disability with the goal of restoring and improving walking function in MS.[94] That review noted the efficacy of dalfampridine, currently the only symptomatic pharmacologic agent approved by the Food and Drug Administration that improves walking in persons with MS. However, dalfampridine seems to be effective only for a small portion (~30%) of persons with MS, often termed as "responders"[95]; therefore, there is a pressing need for alternate therapies. The review further outlines the efficacy of nonpharmacologic therapies for improving walking, included exercise training, physical therapy, and gait training. Exercise training is shown to be the most efficacious nonpharmacological treatment for walking function in persons with MS as evidenced in a meta-analysis of 22 studies.[96] Importantly, exercise interventions are efficacious in persons with varying disability severity and phenotype, demonstrating significant improvements in both objective measures of mobility and brain structures.[97,98] Physical therapy is the most widely prescribed method for managing mobility disability in persons with MS. These therapies often focus specifically on task-specific gait and balance training and vary greatly between therapists and approaches, which leads to heterogeneity in treatment effects.[99] Gait training via body-weight supported treadmill training and robot-assisted treadmill training are proposed as innovative strategies for reducing mobility disability in persons with MS. Efficacy of these protocols has been shown in improving walking endurance and ambulation[65,100]; however, the clinical meaningfulness of changes and lack of protocol standardization are significant concerns regarding the efficacy of these therapies.

Additionally, the review of therapies for mobility disability further noted the importance of future research on mobility in MS,[94] specifically the need for treatment plans that combine multiple intervention modalities in a comprehensive, multidisciplinary approach. Such an approach might involve standardized exercise interventions created in conjunction with physical therapists and further research on the characteristics of responders versus nonresponders to pharmacological therapies as they can have significant negative side effects. Overall, there has been an increased effort to develop impairment-specific treatments in MS that directly target mobility disability; however, more research is needed to determine the efficacy of these rehabilitative strategies alone and together for improving walking in persons with MS.

Summary

Mobility disability is a common consequence of MS that significantly affects independence in activities of daily living, navigation through the environment, and QOL. The burden of mobility disability further affects employment, mental health status, and relationships with others such as informal caregivers and is rated as one of the most significant concerns by persons with MS and their health care providers. Mobility disability includes dysfunction in walking, gait, and balance specifically, and valid measures of each component are outlined in this chapter Impairments in walking, gait, and balance between persons with MS and controls are apparent, as well as significant increase in dysfunction with increases in disability measured by clinician-rated (EDSS) or self-report (PDDS) measures. Further research is needed comparing mobility disability by MS phenotype (i.e., relapsing vs. progressive MS), but evidence currently available demonstrates significantly more impairment in persons with progressive MS. This research is important as persons with MS are living to older ages where mobility disability is common in all populations, while at the same time disability severity generally increases over time and the majority of people shift from a relapsing to a progressive course. Further focal rehabilitation is needed to aid in enhancing symptom-specific therapies created for this heterogeneous population that can have a significant positive impact on the lives of persons with MS.

References

1. National Multiple Sclerosis Society. *Multiple Sclerosis Information Sourcebook.* New York: Information Resource Center and Library of the National Multiple Sclerosis Society; 2005.
2. National Multiple Sclerosis Society. *Multiple Sclerosis Information Sourcebook.* New York: MS Prevalence; 2018
3. Lublin FD. Clinical features and diagnosis of multiple sclerosis. *Neurol Clin.* 2005;23(1):1-15, v.
4. LaRocca NG. Impact of walking impairment in multiple sclerosis. *Patient.* 2011;4(3):189-201.
5. WHO. *International Classification of Functioning, Disability and Health: ICF.* World Health Organization; 2001.
6. Givon U, Zeilig G, Achiron A. Gait analysis in multiple sclerosis: characterization of temporal-spatial parameters using GAITRite functional ambulation system. *Gait Posture.* 2009;29(1):138-142.
7. Kurtzke JF. Rating neurologic impairment in multiple sclerosis: an expanded disability status scale (EDSS). *Neurology.* 1983;33(11):1444-1452.
8. Confavreux C, Vukusic S. The natural history of multiple sclerosis. *La Revue du praticien.* 2006;56(12):1313-1320.
9. Confavreux C, Vukusic S, Adeleine P. Early clinical predictors and progression of irreversible disability in multiple sclerosis: an amnesic process. *Brain.* 2003;126(Pt 4):770-782.
10. Confavreux C, Vukusic S, Moreau T, Adeleine P. Relapses and progression of disability in multiple sclerosis. *N Engl J Med.* 2000;343(20):1430-1438.
11. Hobart J, Riazi A, Lamping D, Fitzpatrick R, Thompson A. Measuring the impact of MS on walking ability the 12-Item MS walking scale (MSWS-12). *Neurology.* 2003;60(1):31-36.
12. Van Asch P. Impact of mobility impairment in multiple sclerosis 2–patients' perspectives. *Eur Neurol Rev.* 2011;6(2):115-120.
13. Iezzoni LI, Rao SR, Kinkel RP. Patterns of mobility aid use among working-age persons with multiple sclerosis living in the community in the United States. *Disabil Health J.* 2009;2(2):67-76.
14. Klevan G, Jacobsen C, Aarseth J, et al. Health related quality of life in patients recently diagnosed with multiple sclerosis. *Acta Neurol Scand.* 2014;129(1):21-26.
15. Nilsagård Y, Lundholm C, Denison E, Gunnarsson LG. Predicting accidental falls in people with multiple sclerosis—a longitudinal study. *Clin Rehabil.* 2009;23(3):259-269.
16. Cameron MH, Lord S. Postural control in multiple sclerosis: implications for fall prevention. *Curr Neurol Neurosci Rep.* 2010;10(5):407-412.

17. Fritz NE, Newsome SD, Eloyan A, Marasigan RER, Calabresi PA, Zackowski KM. Longitudinal relationships among posturography and gait measures in multiple sclerosis. *Neurology*. 2015;84(20):2048-2056.

18. Spain RI, St George RJ, Salarian A, et al. Body-worn motion sensors detect balance and gait deficits in people with multiple sclerosis who have normal walking speed. *Gait Posture*. 2012;35(4):573-578.

19. Cavanaugh JT, Gappmaier VO, Dibble LE, Gappmaier E. Ambulatory activity in individuals with multiple sclerosis. *J Neurol Phys Ther*. 2011;35(1):26-33.

20. Comber L, Galvin R, Coote S. Gait deficits in people with multiple sclerosis: a systematic review and meta-analysis. *Gait Posture*. 2017;51:25-35.

21. Hoang PD, Cameron MH, Gandevia SC, Lord SR. Neuropsychological, balance, and mobility risk factors for falls in people with multiple sclerosis: a prospective cohort study. *Arch Phys Med Rehabil*. 2014;95(3):480-486.

22. Coote S, Hogan N, Franklin S. Falls in people with multiple sclerosis who use a walking aid: prevalence, factors, and effect of strength and balance interventions. *Arch Phys Med Rehabil*. 2013;94(4):616-621.

23. Kalron A, Nitzani D, Achiron A. Static posturography across the EDSS scale in people with multiple sclerosis: a cross sectional study. *BMC Neurol*. 2016;16(1):70.

24. Finlayson M, van Denend T. Experiencing the loss of mobility: perspectives of older adults with MS. *Disabil Rehabil*. 2003;25(20):1168-1180.

25. Heesen C, Bohm J, Reich C, Kasper J, Goebel M, Gold SM. Patient perception of bodily functions in multiple sclerosis: gait and visual function are the most valuable. *Mult Scler*. 2008;14(7):988-991.

26. Heesen C, Haase R, Melzig S, et al. Perceptions on the value of bodily functions in multiple sclerosis. *Acta Neurol Scand*. 2018;137(3):356-362.

27. Wynia K, Middel B, van Dijk JP, De Keyser JH, Reijneveld SA. The impact of disabilities on quality of life in people with multiple sclerosis. *Mult Scler*. 2008;14(7):972-980.

28. Chen K, Fan Y, Hu R, Yang T, Li K. Impact of depression, fatigue and disability on quality of life in Chinese patients with multiple sclerosis. *Stress Health*. 2013;29(2):108-112.

29. Fernandez-Munoz JJ, Moron-Verdasco A, Cigaran-Mendez M, Munoz-Hellin E, Perez-de-Heredia-Torres M, Fernandez-de-las-Penas C. Disability, quality of life, personality, cognitive and psychological variables associated with fatigue in patients with multiple sclerosis. *Acta Neurol Scand*. 2015;132(2):118-124.

30. Dalgas U, Langeskov-Christensen M, Skjerbæk A, et al. Is the impact of fatigue related to walking capacity and perceived ability in persons with multiple sclerosis? A multicenter study. *J Neurol Sci*. 2018;387:179-186.

31. Qureshi A, Brandt-Pearce M, Goldman MD. Relationship between gait variables and domains of neurologic dysfunction in multiple sclerosis using six-minute walk test. *Conf Proc IEEE Eng Med Biol Soc*. 2016;2016:4959-4962.

32. Motl RW, Balantrapu S, Pilutti L, et al. Symptomatic correlates of six-minute walk performance in persons with multiple sclerosis. *Eur J Phys Rehabil Med*. 2013;49(1):59-66.

33. Alghwiri AA, Khalil H, Al-Sharman A, El-Salem K. Depression is a predictor for balance in people with multiple sclerosis. *Mult Scler Relat Disord*. 2018;24:28-31.

34. Kalron A, Aloni R. Contrasting relationship between depression, quantitative gait characteristics and self-report walking difficulties in people with multiple sclerosis. *Mult Scler Relat Disord*. 2018;19:1-5.

35. Benedict RH, Holtzer R, Motl RW, et al. Upper and lower extremity motor function and cognitive impairment in multiple sclerosis. *J Int Neuropsychol Soc.* 2011;17(4):643-653.

36. Motl RW, Cadavid D, Sandroff BM, Pilutti LA, Pula JH, Benedict RHB. Cognitive processing speed has minimal influence on the construct validity of multiple sclerosis walking scale-12 scores. *J Neurol Sci.* 2013;335(1):169-173.

37. Sandroff BM, Motl RW, Sosnoff JJ, Pula JH. Further validation of the six-spot step test as a measure of ambulation in multiple sclerosis. *Gait Posture.* 2015;41(1):222-227.

38. Learmonth YC, Sandroff BM, Pilutti LA, et al. Cognitive motor interference during walking in multiple sclerosis using an alternate-letter alphabet task. *Arch Phys Med Rehabil.* 2014;95(8):1498-1503.

39. Boes MK, Sosnoff JJ, Socie MJ, Sandroff BM, Pula JH, Motl RW. Postural control in multiple sclerosis: effects of disability status and dual task. *J Neurol Sci.* 2012;315(1):44-48.

40. Amato M, Ponziani G, Rossi F, Liedl C, Stefanile C, Rossi L. Quality of life in multiple sclerosis: the impact of depression, fatigue and disability. *Mult Scler.* 2001;7(5):340-344.

41. Lobentanz IS, Asenbaum S, Vass K, et al. Factors influencing quality of life in multiple sclerosis patients: disability, depressive mood, fatigue and sleep quality. *Acta Neurol Scand.* 2004;110(1):6-13.

42. Cohen JA, Krishnan AV, Goodman AD, et al. The clinical meaning of walking speed as measured by the timed 25-foot walk in patients with multiple sclerosis. *JAMA Neurol.* 2014;71(11):1386-1393.

43. Zwibel HL, Smrtka J. Improving quality of life in multiple sclerosis: an unmet need. *Am J Manag Care.* 2011;17(5):S139.

44. Naci H, Fleurence R, Birt J, Duhig A. Economic burden of multiple sclerosis. *Pharmacoeconomics.* 2010;28(5):363-379.

45. Patwardhan M, Matchar D, Samsa G, McCrory D, Williams R, Li T. Cost of multiple sclerosis by level of disability: a review of literature. *Mult Scler.* 2005;11(2):232-239.

46. Grima DT, Torrance GW, Francis G, Rice G, Rosner AJ, Lafortune L. Cost and health related quality of life consequences of multiple sclerosis. *Mult Scler.* 2000;6(2):91-98.

47. Prescott JD, Factor S, Pill M, Levi GW. Descriptive analysis of the direct medical costs of multiple sclerosis in 2004 using administrative claims in a large nationwide database. *J Manag Care Pharm.* 2007;13(1):44-52.

48. Pike J, Jones E, Rajagopalan K, Piercy J, Anderson P. Social and economic burden of walking and mobility problems in multiple sclerosis. *BMC Neurol.* 2012;12:94. doi:10.1186/1471-2377-12-94.

49. Kobelt G, Berg J, Atherly D, Hadjimichael O. Costs and quality of life in multiple sclerosis: a cross-sectional study in the United States. *Neurology.* 2006;66(11):1696-1702.

50. Julian LJ, Vella L, Vollmer T, Hadjimichael O, Mohr DC. Employment in multiple sclerosis. *J Neurol.* 2008;255(9):1354-1360.

51. Goldman MD, Motl RW, Scagnelli J, Pula JH, Sosnoff JJ, Cadavid D. Clinically meaningful performance benchmarks in MS timed 25-foot walk and the real world. *Neurology.* 2013;81(21):1856-1863.

52. Goldman MD, Ward MD, Motl RW, Jones DE, Pula JH, Cadavid D. Identification and validation of clinically meaningful benchmarks in the 12-item multiple sclerosis walking scale. *Mult Scler.* 2017;23(10):1405-1414.

53. Lanzetta D, Cattaneo D, Pellegatta D, Cardini R. Trunk control in unstable sitting posture during functional activities in healthy subjects and patients with multiple sclerosis. *Arch Phys Med Rehabil.* 2004;85(2):279-283.

54. Dunn J. Impact of mobility impairment on the burden of caregiving in individuals with multiple sclerosis. *Expert Rev Pharmacoecon Outcomes Res.* 2010;10(4):433-440.

55. Carton H, Loos R, Pacolet J, Versieck K, Vlietinck R. A quantitative study of unpaid caregiving in multiple sclerosis. *Mult Scler.* 2000;6(4):274-279.

56. Aronson K, Cleghorn G, Goldenberg E. Assistance arrangements and use of services among persons with multiple sclerosis and their caregivers. *Disabil Rehabil.* 1996;18(7):354-361.

57. Ertekin O, Ozakbas S, Idiman E. Caregiver burden, quality of life and walking ability in different disability levels of multiple sclerosis. *NeuroRehabilitation.* 2014;34(2):313-321.

58. Kieseier BC, Pozzilli C. Assessing walking disability in multiple sclerosis. *Mult Scler.* 2012;18(7):914-924.

59. Novotna K, Sobisek L, Horakova D, Havrdova E, Preiningerova JL. Quantification of gait abnormalities in healthy-looking multiple sclerosis patients (with expanded disability status scale 0-1.5). *Eur Neurol.* 2016;76(3–4):99-104.

60. Phan-Ba R, Pace A, Calay P, et al. Comparison of the timed 25-foot and the 100-meter walk as performance measures in multiple sclerosis. *Neurorehabil Neural Repair.* 2011;25(7):672-679.

61. Goldman MD, Marrie RA, Cohen JA. Evaluation of the six-minute walk in multiple sclerosis subjects and healthy controls. *Mult Scler.* 2008;14(3):383-390.

62. Scalzitti DA, Harwood KJ, Maring JR, Leach SJ, Ruckert EA, Costello E. Validation of the 2-minute walk test with the 6-minute walk test and other functional measures in persons with multiple sclerosis. *Int J MS Care.* 2018;20(4):158-163.

63. Learmonth YC, Dlugonski DD, Pilutti LA, Sandroff BM, Motl RW. The reliability, precision and clinically meaningful change of walking assessments in multiple sclerosis. *Mult Scler.* 2013;19(13):1784-1791.

64. Langeskov-Christensen D, Feys P, Baert I, Riemenschneider M, Stenager E, Dalgas U. Performed and perceived walking ability in relation to the expanded disability status scale in persons with multiple sclerosis. *J Neurol Sci.* 2017;382:131-136.

65. Lo AC, Triche EW. Improving gait in multiple sclerosis using robot-assisted, body weight supported treadmill training. *Neurorehabil Neural Repair.* 2008;22(6):661-671.

66. Podsiadlo D, Richardson S. The timed "Up & Go": a test of basic functional mobility for frail elderly persons. *J Am Geriatr Soc.* 1991;39(2):142-148.

67. Sebastião E, Sandroff BM, Learmonth YC, Motl RW. Validity of the timed up and go test as a measure of functional mobility in persons with multiple sclerosis. *Arch Phys Med Rehabil.* 2016;97(7):1072-1077.

68. Fritz NE, Keller J, Calabresi PA, Zackowski KM. Quantitative measures of walking and strength provide insight into brain corticospinal tract pathology in multiple sclerosis. *Neuroimage Clin.* 2017;14:490-498.

69. Ciol MA, Matsuda PN, Khurana SR, Cline MJ, Sosnoff JJ, Kraft GH. Effect of cognitive demand on functional mobility in ambulatory individuals with multiple sclerosis. *Int J MS Care.* 2017;19(4):217-224.

70. Callesen J, Richter C, Kristensen C, et al. Test–retest agreement and reliability of the six spot step test in persons with multiple sclerosis. *Mult Scler.* 2018. doi:10.1177/1352458517745725.

71. Pavan K, Tilbery CP, Lianza S, Marangoni BE. Validation of the "six step spot test" for gait among patients with multiple sclerosis in Brazil. *Arq Neuropsiquiatr.* 2010;68(2):198-204.

72. Motl RW, Suh Y, Dlugonski D, et al. Oxygen cost of treadmill and overground walking in mildly disabled persons with multiple sclerosis. *Neurol Sci.* 2011;32(2):255-262.

73. Franceschini M, Rampello A, Bovolenta F, Aiello M, Tzani P, Chetta A. Cost of walking, exertional dyspnoea and fatigue in individuals with multiple sclerosis not requiring assistive devices. *J Rehabil Med.* 2010;42(8):719-723.

74. McGuigan C, Hutchinson M. Confirming the validity and responsiveness of the multiple sclerosis walking scale-12 (MSWS-12). *Neurology.* 2004;62(11):2103-2105.

75. Motl RW, Snook EM. Confirmation and extension of the validity of the multiple sclerosis walking scale-12 (MSWS-12). *J Neurol Sci.* 2008;268(1):69-73.

76. Motl RW, Sandroff BM, Sosnoff JJ. Commercially available accelerometry as an ecologically valid measure of ambulation in individuals with multiple sclerosis. *Expert Rev Neurother.* 2012;12(9):1079-1088.

77. Coulter EH, Miller L, McCorkell S, et al. Validity of the activPAL3 activity monitor in people moderately affected by multiple sclerosis. *Med Eng Phys.* 2017;45:78-82.

78. Ng AV, Kent-Braun JA. Quantitation of lower physical activity in persons with multiple sclerosis. *Med Sci Sports Exerc.* 1997;29(4):517-523.

79. Sandroff BM, Motl RW. Comparison of ActiGraph activity monitors in persons with multiple sclerosis and controls. *Disabil Rehabil.* 2013;35(9):725-731.

80. Sosnoff JJ, Goldman MD, Motl RW. Real-life walking impairment in multiple sclerosis: preliminary comparison of four methods for processing accelerometry data. *Mult Scler.* 2010;16(7):868-877.

81. Kinnett-Hopkins D, Adamson B, Rougeau K, Motl R. People with MS are less physically active than healthy controls but as active as those with other chronic diseases: an updated meta-analysis. *Mult Scler Relat Disord.* 2017;13:38-43.

82. Weikert M, Suh Y, Lane A, et al. Accelerometry is associated with walking mobility, not physical activity, in persons with multiple sclerosis. *Med Eng Phys.* 2012;34(5):590-597.

83. Snook EM, Motl RW, Gliottoni RC. The effect of walking mobility on the measurement of physical activity using accelerometry in multiple sclerosis. *Clin Rehabil.* 2009;23(3):248-258.

84. Sandroff BM, Motl RW, Pilutti LA, et al. Accuracy of StepWatch™ and ActiGraph accelerometers for measuring steps taken among persons with multiple sclerosis. *PLoS One.* 2014;9(4):e93511.

85. Motl RW, Pilutti LA, Learmonth YC, Goldman MD, Brown T. Clinical importance of steps taken per day among persons with multiple sclerosis. *PLoS One.* 2013;8(9):e73247.

86. Sosnoff JJ, Sandroff BM, Motl RW. Quantifying gait abnormalities in persons with multiple sclerosis with minimal disability. *Gait Posture.* 2012;36(1):154-156.

87. Socie MJ, Motl RW, Pula JH, Sandroff BM, Sosnoff JJ. Gait variability and disability in multiple sclerosis. *Gait Posture.* 2013;38(1):51-55.

88. Spain RI, Mancini M, Horak FB, Bourdette D. Body-worn sensors capture variability, but not decline, of gait and balance measures in multiple sclerosis over 18 months. *Gait Posture.* 2014;39(3):958-964.

89. Mancini M, King L, Salarian A, Holmstrom L, McNames J, Horak FB. Mobility lab to assess balance and gait with synchronized body-worn sensors. *J Bioeng Biomed Sci.* 2011(suppl 1):007.

90. Behrens JR, Mertens S, Krüger T, et al. Validity of visual perceptive computing for static posturography in patients with multiple sclerosis. *Mult Scler.* 2016;22(12):1596-1606.

91. Fjeldstad C, Pardo G, Bemben D, Bemben M. Decreased postural balance in multiple sclerosis patients with low disability. *Int J Rehabil Res.* 2011;34(1):53-58.

92. Fritz NE, Marasigan RE, Calabresi PA, Newsome SD, Zackowski KM. The impact of dynamic balance measures on walking performance in multiple sclerosis. *Neurorehabil Neural Repair.* 2015;29(1):62-69.

93. Severini G, Straudi S, Pavarelli C, et al. Use of Nintendo Wii Balance Board for posturographic analysis of multiple sclerosis patients with minimal balance impairment. *J Neuroeng Rehabil.* 2017;14(1):19.

94. Baird JF, Sandroff BM, Motl RW. Therapies for mobility disability in persons with multiple sclerosis. *Expert Rev Neurother.* 2018;18(6):493-502.

95. Yapundich R, Applebee A, Bethoux F, et al. Evaluation of dalfampridine extended release 5 and 10 mg in multiple sclerosis. *Int J MS Care.* 2014;17(3):138-145.

96. Snook EM, Motl RW. Effect of exercise training on walking mobility in multiple sclerosis: a meta-analysis. *Neurorehabil Neural Repair.* 2008;23(2):108-116.

97. Klaren RE, Hubbard EA, Motl RW, Pilutti LA, Wetter NC, Sutton BP. Objectively measured physical activity is associated with brain volumetric measurements in multiple sclerosis. *Behav Neurol.* 2015;2015:482536.

98. Edwards T, Pilutti LA. The effect of exercise training in adults with multiple sclerosis with severe mobility disability: a systematic review and future research directions. *Mult Scler Relat Disord.* 2017;16:31-39.

99. Learmonth YC, Ensari I, Motl RW. Physiotherapy and walking outcomes in adults with multiple sclerosis: systematic review and meta-analysis. *Phys Ther Rev.* 2016;21(3–6):160-172.

100. Pompa A, Morone G, Iosa M, et al. Does robot-assisted gait training improve ambulation in highly disabled multiple sclerosis people? A pilot randomized control trial. *Mult Scler.* 2017;23(5):696-703.

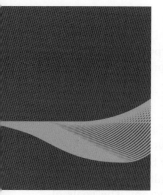
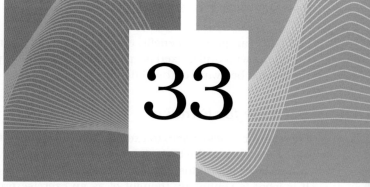

33

Exercise Prescription in Multiple Sclerosis

■■■ Herbert I. Karpatkin

Introduction

Multiple sclerosis (MS) is a disease of mobility. Although the underlying pathology of demyelination, inflammation, and axonal loss is the target of medical and pharmacologic interventions, the reason that persons with MS (pwMS) often seek medical attention is because they notice a decreased ability to perform mobility tasks such as gait and balance. Although medical management has shown effectiveness in decreasing the underlying pathology of MS, exercise as a means of addressing mobility loss is underutilized. This is somewhat puzzling, as decreased strength and flexibility can be remediated with the proper exercise regime. The limited usage of exercise as a means of treating MS mobility loss suggests that many pwMS are not receiving optimal treatment. Physicians who treat pwMS could potentially achieve better outcomes for their patients if they include as part of their intervention referral to a physical therapist with expertise in MS.

Exercise for Fitness Versus Exercise for Function

To understand the manner in which exercise programs can be effective in pwMS, it is necessary to divide exercise into two basic purposes: exercise for fitness and exercise for function. Although both are types of exercise,

575

and both can provide benefit, each has a distinct purpose and outcome. Clinicians who utilize exercise programs for pwMS or provide referrals for them must be aware of this difference.

Exercise for Fitness

Exercise for fitness refers to exercise that is intended to result in a generalized response to the body. It has been defined as "any bodily activity that enhances or maintains physical fitness and overall health and wellness."[1] It is what is commonly thought of as an exercise program. The goals of such a program tend to be more generalized as well, that is, exercise for weight loss, general conditioning, and aerobic fitness. Although exercises such as these are clearly beneficial for all persons, it is important to understand their limitations in MS. Specifically, improving overall fitness may not remediate specific impairments that are re-experienced by pwMS. For example, an impairment such as a foot drop, which can lead to gait and balance difficulties, would be unlikely to be remediated by a biking or swimming program. Although the biking and swimming program may be helpful for achieving general fitness, they would do little, if anything, to remediate the foot drop.

Exercise for Function

In contrast with exercise for fitness, exercise for function is highly specific. It has been defined by O'Sullivan as "interventions designed to incorporate task and context specific practice in areas meaningful to each patient, with an overall goal of functional independence."[2] The overarching idea behind this type of exercise is that each exercise is specifically prescribed to achieve a specific functional goal. In this manner, prescribing exercise for function is similar to how a physician prescribes medication; each exercise is intended to address a specific issue affecting the mobility of the patient with MS. Each exercise is prescribed for a specific indication, with a specific dosage. Exercise for function is prescribed following a physical therapy evaluation that has identified specific impairments and functional limitations that restricts the patient's mobility. The exercises that are prescribed are done so with the specific intention of remediating or ameliorating the diagnosed deficits in movement. The success of the exercises is determined by improvements seen on reevaluation.

The difference between these two types of exercises is important. Like medication, exercise can have both specific and general effects. Like medication, the incorrect exercise for a specific condition can be ineffective and potentially dangerous. Clinicians who provide exercise programs for pwMS or who refer to physical therapists who do should be aware of the distinction. The following are theoretical examples of (1) an exercise prescription for general fitness and (2) an exercise prescription for specific function.

1. Exercise prescription for general function
   1-Stationary bike, 15 minutes a day
   2-Sit-ups, 20 repetitions, every day
   3-Leg raises, 10 on each leg, every day

   Analysis: Even without knowing anything about the patient for whom this exercise program was prescribed, it is obvious that the program is unlikely to address specific deficits. Although stationary bike may have a cardiopulmonary and weight loss effect, it is unlikely to address a walking deficit, which is common in MS. The sit-ups and leg raises would strengthen abdominal and lower extremity muscles, but it is unclear as to how this may relate to specific tasks and activities of daily living that are limited to a patient with MS. Although leg and abdominal weakness may certainly occur in pwMS, these exercises do not appear to be related to a functional activity

1. Exercise prescription for specific function
   1-Slow sit to stand exercises, 5 every day
   2-Calf stretch on the right calf only, 30 s
   3-Toe raises in standing on the right, 5 repetitions, perform right after each calf stretch

   Analysis: Again, even without knowing anything about the patient for whom this is prescribed, much can be inferred from the exercises themselves. Sit to stand is an exercise that not only is extremely limited in multiple diagnostic entities[3,4] but has also been shown to be an excellent means of testing and strengthening lower extremity strength and function.[5]

The Impact of Fatigue on Exercise in Persons With MS

Fatigue is one of the most common findings in MS.[6] Although it is common in most neurologic conditions,[7] its prevalence is the highest in MS. Fatigue in MS is multifactorial with both subjective and objective components, central and peripheral components, and primary and secondary components. Each of these components has a unique pathophysiologic substrate and as a result requires different tools for evaluation and intervention.[8]

One of the most important effects of fatigue on pwMS is that it may limit the ability of the patients to exercise at a high-enough volume to achieve optimal benefit. Physical activity is generally lower in pwMS[9]; therefore, asking them to engage in an exercise program when they are already more sedentary than persons without MS is problematic.

For exercise to be of the greatest effect, it needs to be delivered at an appropriate dosage. A certain amount of practice of a task or a certain number of repetitions of an action is needed for exercise training to achieve its goals. However, because of fatigue, many pwMS are unable to achieve this volume. This presents a distinct problem for exercise prescription for patients with MS; exercise is needed to remediate the impairments and functional limitations seen in MS; however, because of one of the primary signs and symptoms of MS, patients are unable to exercise effectively.

Part of the issue with MS fatigue and exercise is due to thermosensitivity. The decreased ability of demyelinated nerves to transmit impulses when temperature is increased is a well-observed phenomenon in MS. During sustained exercise, core temperature increases occur, which decrease conduction through demyelinated nerves, a phenomenon known as activity-dependent conduction block (ADCB).[10] The effect of this is that the very act of exercising in MS decreases the ability to exercise in MS.

Two specific interventions have been utilized to address the limitations in exercise due to fatigue in pwMS. These are intermittent training and cooling.

Intermittent training, also known as interval training and fractionated training, refers to interspersing periods of exercise with periods of rest. Most exercise programs for persons with disabilities are continuous in nature, with patients often urged to push themselves harder when they encounter fatigue. Although this technique may be effective in nondisabled populations, it may be contraindicated in pwMS because of presence of fatigue. Studies showing that pwMS experience less subjective[11] and objective[12] fatigue when walking intermittently as opposed to continuously have been conducted. A pilot study by Karpatkin et al suggested that intermittent walking results in greater improvements in gait endurance than continuous walking.[13] Improved performance with intermittent as opposed to continuous training in pwMS during a straight leg raise training task suggests that intermittent training can be used for resistance training as well as for walking.[14]

Multiple modalities for cooling have been suggested, including cooling garments,[15] cold-water immersion,[16] and reflex cooling,[17] with none showing any clear advantage over the other. Multiple studies have supported the effectiveness of cooling in improving physical performance in pwMS. White et al[13] reported improvements in 25-foot walk test performance following cooling via whole body immersion. Schwid et al[18] found improvements in motor performance and vision following a high-dose cooling regime. Neither of these authors noted sustained improvements in motor function following cooling, and the question of whether a greater volume of exercise resulting in better rehabilitation outcomes would occur with cooling has not been addressed.

Loss of Function due to Inactivity

Although it is presumed that mobility impairments in MS are due predominantly to the primary aspects of the disease (e.g., demyelination of motor tracts, spasticity, sensory loss, diminished motor control), consideration must be paid to the possibility that a great deal of the impairments seen is due to secondary aspects of the disease such as inactivity. Owing to the multiple physical and cognitive impairments that are experienced by pwMS, they are generally less active than those without the disease.[9,19] Therefore, much of the mobility loss may not be due to the primary aspects of the disease such as demyelination and inflammation but due to secondary aspects of the disease such as disuse atrophy and learned helplessness. More simply, pwMS may have impaired mobility not just because of the damage to their central nervous system (CNS) but also because they move less. Tasks that are practiced less become more difficult to accomplish. This may in fact underlie a great deal of the weakness and fatigue seen in pwMS.[20] This may in fact be positive news for patients with MS, as it suggests that the mobility impairment that they are experiencing is not entirely due to central nervous system damage but at least in part to learned adaptations. Because mobility limitations due to inactivity would be more remediable than those due to CNS damage, improvement in mobility might be more achievable than otherwise thought.

Although there is no known way of determining by evaluation whether mobility loss is due to primary or secondary causes, it is probably the case that mobility loss due to secondary causes would remediate more quickly than those due to primary, as improvements in the former would be due to reconditioning, whereas improvements in function due to remediation of primary impairments would be due to neuroplastic processes.

Dosage/Intensity

The idea that pwMS could benefit from exercise is a relatively recent one. Until recently, it was thought that pwMS should limit exercise, as it could lead to an exacerbation.[21] A landmark article by Petejean[22] et al showed this to not only not be the case but that pwMS responded to exercise in a manner similar to persons without MS, that is, they improved in response to the exercise. However, the question of not only what exercises to perform but also what the dosage and intensity of the exercises should be still remains.

Most of the reviews of the exercise in pwMS have examined the use of relatively mild protocols, presumably to avoid fatigue. Clinicians and patients may confuse postexercise fatigue, which may present as a temporary worsening of signs and symptoms, as an exacerbation. However, the worsening of symptoms following aggressive exercise is transient and probably related to ADCB.[7] They may therefore more accurately be referred to as pseudoexacerbations. Some studies have in fact examined the use of a more aggressive exercise program in pwMS and found not only no worsening of status but also an improvement in strength and function. Fimland et al[23] examined the use of a maximal strength training program in pwMS, where subjects performed lower extremity resistance training at 85% to 90% of their one repetition maximum. Electromyography analysis was used to determine that the training resulted in increased CNS activation, suggesting that strength training at this level may result in neuroplasticity. Functional outcomes were not measured, and no adverse effects were reported. Karpatkin et al[24] performed a similar study but used functional performance as a primary outcome measure and found significant improvements in gait and balance measures for all subjects. Again, no adverse effects were reported. Marks et al[25] utilized a form of constraint-induced therapy in patients with MS, where the patients underwent 3.5 hours of aggressive functional training daily for 2 weeks. All subjects experienced notable improvements in function that were sustained at follow-up 4 years later. No adverse events were reported. These studies suggest that pwMS may not only tolerate but also benefit from more aggressive exercise interventions than might have been previously thought.

Specific Examples of Exercises to Improve Strength, Range of Motion, Balance, and Gait

The following are examples of specific exercises to improve specific impairments and functional limitations found in MS. This list is obviously not intended to be exhaustive, because given the nature of MS, there is practically an infinite number of possible reasons that mobility could be limited. This list represents some of the more common limitations seen in MS and exercises meant to specifically address them. These examples also demonstrate the use of specific exercises to treat specific mobility limitations.

Foot Drop

Foot drop is defined as a combination of tightness of the ankle plantiflexors, usually accompanied by weakness of the ankle dorsiflexors. It causes decreased or absent toe clearance during gait resulting in a toe first initial contact, which can lead to tripping over the foot and resultant falls and fall-related injuries. Recent evidence suggests that diminished ankle push off is a common finding in MS gait,[26] and the diminished ankle range and strength may be a component of this. The decrease in walking and standing that occurs in pwMS due to inactivity and fatigue can lead to a decreased amount of time that the patient's ankle is in dorsiflexion, which can increase predisposition to foot drop. Patients may compensate for this by using techniques such as ipsilateral hip circumduction, contralateral vaulting, or increased swing phase hip flexion (i.e., steppage gait). An ankle foot orthosis (AFO) is often prescribed to address this; however, the AFO results in decreased movement of the ankle that can further decrease range of motion and strength.

Although foot drop is a common finding in many neurologic diseases, the progressive nature of MS suggests that it happens relatively slowly over time, as opposed to its relatively sudden appearance as might occur in stroke. This suggests that evaluation and intervention for foot drop should be performed relatively early in the disease. Goniometric measurements of ankle dorsiflexion less than 15° to 20°[27] and Manual Muscle Testing strength of less than 4/5 should lead to suspicion of a developing foot drop. Observation of a foot slap, especially toward the end of a walk when the patient is more fatigued, would also be a strong indication.

A program of ankle plantiflexor stretching and ankle dorsiflexor strengthening can help to restore diminished movement and strength. Plantiflexor stretching can be performed in sitting or standing. The relative volume of stretch should be high, e.g. 30 to 60 s several times a day,[28] whereas the relative intensity of the stretch should be rather mild. It should be remembered that the foot drop developed over an extended period of time and therefore the period of time that the stretching exercise is given may also need to be extended, that is, performed many times daily for several months. Alternatively, a passive stretching device such as a night splint can be used that places the patient's foot in mild dorsiflexion and holds it in place for as long as the device is worn. This gives the advantage of the patient not needing to be standing during the stretch, an advantage for patients with poor standing balance or endurance.[29]

Concomitantly with the stretching, exercises to increase ankle dorsiflexion strength should occur.[30] In order for the exercise to be performed in a manner similar to what would be experienced in actual walking activities, it is recommended that the exercise be performed with the heel of the foot in contact with the floor to simulate heel strike. Similarly, performing the exercise with the foot slightly in front of the other foot also simulates how active dorsiflexion is actually utilized during gait. As with stretching, a large volume of active dorsiflexion should be performed to achieve optimal exercise response; using intermittent training can assist with attaining these high volumes.

Once the patient has achieved an increase in flexibility and strength, training to have the patient utilize these improvements in actual gait is indicated. Having patients practice gait where they focus on heel strike under a variety of different conditions (e.g., indoors, outdoors, even vs. uneven terrain, uphill, downhill [Figures 33.1-33.4]) will not only connect the reasons for the three exercises in patients' mind but also train them to practice the task in the appropriate environmental context.

Decreased Gait Endurance

As MS pathology progresses, mobility issues worsen. Decreasing gait endurance over time is an example of this. As a result of the combination of primary deficits such as demyelination of CNS motor tracts and secondary deficits such as disuse atrophy due to increasing sedentary behavior, gait endurance in pwMS often worsens over time. Patients with MS state that gait endurance is one of their most common issues[31] and is experienced by pwMS as a decrease in the maximum distance walked. The reason for this progressive decrease in endurance is multifactorial and may include primary and secondary findings, diminished lower extremity strength and flexibility, fatigue, diminished motor control, and pain. Remediation of this can be complicated. Increasing endurance in other activities such as biking or swimming may increase overall fitness but may not generalize to walking. Training to increase walking distance will be limited by the

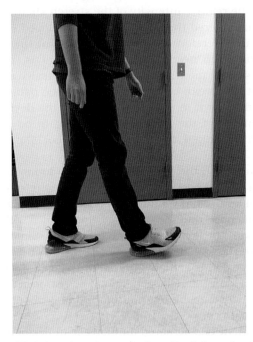

Figure 33.1. Level surface gait. See eBook for color figure.

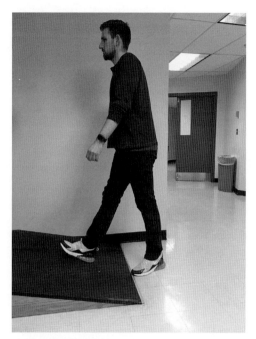

Figure 33.2. Uphill gait. See eBook for color figure.

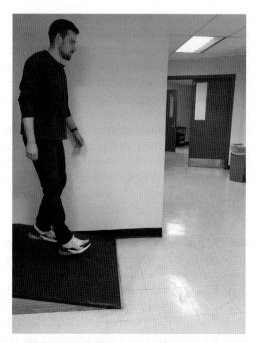

Figure 33.3. Downhill gait. See eBook for color figure.

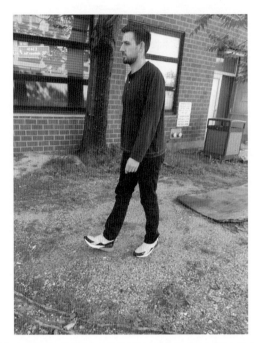

Figure 33.4. Outdoor gait. See eBook for color figure.

original complaint itself; it is hard to increase walking endurance by walking longer distances if the original complaint was decreased ability to walk longer distances. An intermittent walking program where walking multiple bouts of shorter distances and stopping to recover before the accrual of significant fatigue occurs can allow pwMS to achieve a greater total volume of walking than if the persons walked continuously. Karpatkin et al[24] found that pwMS achieved greater improvements in the 6-minute walk test (6MWT) when they trained intermittently than when they trained continuously. A program in which the patient walks until the onset of mild fatigue, then stops and recovers before resuming walking will be less affected by ADCB and allow for a greater volume of training to occur.

Balance Loss

As is the case with most mobility deficits in pwMS, balance loss is multifactorial. Impairments in strength, flexibility, sensation, motor control, attention, and vision can all result in balance loss and lead to falls. A patient with MS may be more likely to fall when fatigued than when unfatigued.[32] Balance loss can be very context specific, with loss of balance occurring in some tasks and not in others. Balance loss may also be secondary to inactivity and diminished task practice; as patients' balance becomes worse, they will try to avoid placing themselves in situations in which their balance is challenged. This sets up a cycle of inactivity, disuse, and decreasing practice of more difficult tasks. For this reason, pwMS who complain of loss of balance need to be evaluated at regular intervals with a task-specific evaluation, such as the Berg Balance Scale, the Dynamic Gait Index, or the MiniBESTest.[33,34] Each of tests examines a patient's ability to perform functional balance activities, such as balance while reaching, standing with narrow base of support, standing on an incline, and gait with head turns. The advantage of tests such as these is that they will reveal the type of task that a patient has trouble with. The treatment then becomes practice of that specific task. For example, an item in the Berg Balance Scale requires the person being tested to stand with his or her feet as close together as possible. Difficulty with this task may predispose the patient to loss of balance at times when a narrow base of support is needed. The exercise to improve this skill then becomes practice of standing with a progressively narrower base of support, using hand support as needed. Possible impairments that lead to difficulty with this task could include loss of ankle flexibility and/ or strength, diminished sensation, inability to utilize visual or vestibular cues, and fatigue. Exercises to remediate these impairments can be practiced as well.

Case Study

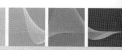

A case study has been used to illustrate the principles discussed earlier. The case is of an actual patient the author has worked with. Identifying characteristics have been changed.

The patient is a 44-year-old single white male diagnosed with relapsing-remitting MS 5 years ago. His Expanded Disability Status Scale score is 3.5. He has been taking Tysabri for the last year. He is employed full time in a position where he is mainly seated at a desk but must walk several blocks to get to and from work. He has noticed recently that it is getting harder and harder to walk to and from work without fatigue and loss of balance. He is particularly noticing that he is tripping over his toes while walking later in the day. He reports a recent fall occurring late at night when he got out of bed to use the bathroom.

Significant evaluation findings include 0° to 10° of right ankle passive dorsiflexion (normal = 0-20), right angle dorsiflexion manual muscle test 3-/5. There is mild to moderate sensory loss in both lower extremities. His Berg Balance Scale revealed particular difficulties in balance with eyes closed. His 6MWT was 1450 (441 m) feet, but his last 3 minutes was significantly slower than the first 3 minutes.

Based on these evaluative findings the following interventions were performed.

Right Plantiflexor Stretch

The subject was shown how to perform a standing plantiflexion stretch. He was advised to hold the stretch for a minimum of 30 s, 5 to 6 times a day. He was advised to stretch to the point where he "feels a pull" in his calf and not to the point of pain.

Rationale

The tripping he experiences while walking is due to insufficient plantiflexion, especially when fatigued, which leads to his toes becoming caught on elevations in the sidewalk. The lack of flexibility in his plantiflexors acts as a mechanical barrier to the lengthening needed for toe clearance. The prolonged stretching period is needed as tissues undergo lengthening as a response to stretching slowly. Some reports show that tissue lengthening does not occur unless the muscle is held in a lengthened position for at least 30 s.[25] He will need to perform these stretches everyday possibly for as long as he has the disease to prevent worsening of the condition. The stretch should be relatively mild rather than extreme to avoid the risk of tearing and inflammation of the stretched tissue.

Active Right Ankle Dorsiflexion in Standing

This should be done shortly after the plantiflexion stretch. The patient will be instructed to stand with his feet shoulder width apart, right foot a few inches forward of the left foot, then to raise the front of the right foot as high as he can, hold it in dorsiflexion for a few seconds, then slowly lower it down. He should perform as many of these as he can until he begins to experience fatigue. When fatigue occurs, he should stop and rest until he feels his fatigue decreasing, then repeat.

Rationale

The foot drop is due to a combination of plantiflexor tightness and dorsiflexor weakness. Therefore, the exercise program needs to address both issues. The dorsiflexor strengthening should be performed shortly after the plantiflexion stretch so that the increased range of motion from the stretch can be utilized. To regain strength a large number of repetitions must be performed, as part of the reason the dorsiflexors became weak was lack of use over many years. By taking frequent breaks as opposed to doing the exercise continuously, the patient will experience less fatigue and will perform a greater volume of repetitions. The exercise should be done with the foot on the floor to better simulate the manner in which the dorsiflexors would be used during the actual task of gait.

Practicing Walking With Emphasis on Heel Strike

After the impairments of decreased ankle dorsiflexion range and strength are addressed, practice of the specific task should be emphasized. Having the patient perform focusing on ankle dorsiflexion during the initial contact stage of swing phase will address this. The patient would first be asked to perform shorter walks with emphasis on heel strike and then progress to longer walks. Similarly, the walks can first be performed indoors, then outdoors on progressively more uneven surfaces to better simulate the types of conditions he is most likely to encounter.

Rationale

Specific practice of the task and task components are needed for the patient to learn to appropriately use the improvements in strength and range. Without practicing the specific task, the patient's range and strength may improve in isolated testing, but it may not carry over to the specific task that requires remediation.

Balance Training

To improve balance with eyes closed, it is necessary to practice that specific task. This will drive the patient's nervous system to adapt by "forcing" the use of other systems, in particular lower extremity position sense. The training can start with having the patient stand with eyes closed and use his hand to lightly touch on a stable surface for support. The patient can be asked to remove his hand for brief periods so that his primary sensory input will be from his feet. After he can maintain balance for 15 to 30 s with eyes closed and no hand support, he can be asked to perform movements that result in mild perturbations, such as head turns or arm movements. Retesting with the Berg Balance Scale will confirm improvements.

Rationale

The loss of balance at nighttime raises the suspicion that his balance is impaired when vision is limited. Evaluation with the Berg Balance Scale showed a specific loss of balance with eyes closed. The decreased sensation in both of his feet suggests that, when vision is limited, he cannot use proprioception to sufficiently compensate. However, it cannot be determined to what extent the decreased use of proprioception is due to demyelination of sensory tracts and to what extent it is due to a learned decrease in use of sensory modalities for balance and an overreliance on vision.

Gait Endurance Training

Gait endurance can be measured using the 6MWT. A normal value for the 6MWT is 571 ± 90 m,[35] which is well above the patient's value of 441 m. If the 6-minute walk is further analyzed to examine change in gait speed over time, it is noted that the patient's first 3 minutes are much faster than the last 3 minutes. It is also noted that there is increased incidence of foot slap and foot drag in the second 3 minutes, indicating the presence of motor fatigability.

To improve gait endurance, an intermittent walking program can be used. Asking the patient to perform walks that lead to minimal fatigue, and then to recover and then repeat, will allow him to achieve a greater total volume of walking practice. Based on the 6MWT performance, the patient can be asked to perform a 3-minute walk, rest, and perhaps stretch his calf muscles, then repeat.

Rationale

The patient will be able to perform a much greater total distance walked by taking breaks than if he tries to walk continuously. A higher volume of training can be achieved.

Summary Points for Exercise Prescription for Persons With MS

1. Treat the task—Exercise for pwMS should emphasize tasks that are specific to the lost function rather than generalized fitness activities.
2. Determine the underlying impairments—Specific mobility tasks are often limited in pwMS because of impairments in specific areas such as strength and flexibility. These need to be evaluated for so that the exercise program can correctly address them.
3. Function can be lost for primary and secondary reasons; mobility loss in MS can be due to both demyelination of CNS structures required for mobility and disuse atrophy. This suggests that much of the disability seen in MS may not be due to the disease itself but to lifestyle, which is more immediately remediable.
4. Fatigue is the most common finding in MS, and it limits the ability to engage in exercise programs in the same manner as persons without MS. The use of interventions such as intermittent training as well as the use of cooling modalities can reduce the effects of fatigue and allow pwMS to exercise at higher volumes.

References

1. Kylasov A, Gavrov S. *Diversity of Sport: Non-Destructive Evaluation.* Paris: UNESCO: Encyclopedia of Life Support Systems; 2011:462-491. ISBN:978-5-8931-7227-0.
2. O'Sullivan SB. *Physical Therapy.* 5th ed. Glossary: F.A. Davis Company; 2007:1335. ISBN:0-8036-1247-8.
3. Lord SR, Murray SM, Chapman K, Munro B, Tiedemann A. Sit-to-stand performance depends on sensation, speed, balance, and psychological status in addition to strength in older people. *J Gerontol A Biol Sci Med Sci.* 2002;57(8):M539-M543.
4. Cheng PT, Liaw MY, Wong MK, Tang FT, Lee MY, Lin PS. The sit-to-stand movement in stroke patients and its correlation with falling. *Arch Phys Med Rehabil.* 1988;79(9):1043-1046.
5. Bohannon RW. Sit-to-stand test for measuring performance of lower extremity muscles. *Percept Mot Skills.* 1995;80(1):163-166.
6. Krupp L. Fatigue is intrinsic to multiple sclerosis (MS) and is the most commonly reported symptom of the disease. *Mult Scler.* 2006;12:367-368. PMID: 16900749.
7. Chaudhuri A, Behan PO. Fatigue in neurological disorders. *Lancet.* 2004;363(9413):978-988.
8. Kluger BM, Krupp LB, Enoka RM. Fatigue and fatigability in neurologic illnesses proposal for a unified taxonomy. *Neurology.* 2013;80(4):409-416.
9. Ng AV, Kent-Braun JA. Quantification of lower physical activity in persons with multiple sclerosis. *Med Sci Sports Exerc.* 1997;29:517-523.
10. Vucic S, Burke D, Kiernan MC. Fatigue in multiple sclerosis: mechanisms and management. *Clin Neurophysiol.* 2010;121(6):809-817.
11. Karpatkin H, Rzetelny A. Effect of a single bout of intermittent versus continuous walking on perceptions of fatigue in people with multiple sclerosis. *Int J MS Care.* 2012;14(3):124-131.
12. Karpatkin H, Cohen ET, Rzetelny A, et al. Effects of intermittent versus continuous walking on distance walked and fatigue in persons with multiple sclerosis: a randomized crossover trial. *J Neurol Phys Ther.* 2015;39(3):172-178.
13. Karpatkin HI, Cohen ET, DiCarrado S, et al. The effect of intermittent versus continuous training on walking endurance and fatigue in people with multiple sclerosis: a randomized, crossover, trial. *Crit Rev Phys Rehabil Med.* 2016;28(1-2).
14. Karpatkin H, Evans D, Avolio M, Lang E, Ock S. Intermittent as opposed to continuous strengthening leads to improved straight leg raise performance in persons with multiple sclerosis [Abstract] (2013) Fifth Cooperative Meeting of CMSC and ACTRIMS. *Int J MS Care.* 2013;15(S3):1-151. doi:10.7224/1537-2073-15.S3.1.
15. Özkan Tuncay F, Mollaoğlu M. Effect of the cooling suit method applied to individuals with multiple sclerosis on fatigue and activities of daily living. *J Clin Nurs.* 2017;26(23–24):4527-4536.
16. White AT, Wilson TE, Davis SL, Petajan JH. Effect of precooling on physical performance in multiple sclerosis. *Mult Scler.* 2000;6(3):176-180.
17. Grahn DA, Murray JV, Heller HC. Cooling via one hand improves physical performance in heat-sensitive individuals with multiple sclerosis: a preliminary study. *BMC Neurol.* 2008;8(1):14.

18. Schwid SR, Petrie MD, Murray R, et al. A randomized controlled study of the acute and chronic effects of cooling therapy for MS. *Neurology.* 2003;60(12):1955-1960.

19. Motl RW, McAuley E, Snook EM. Physical activity and multiple sclerosis: a meta-analysis. *Mult Scler.* 2005;11:459-463.

20. Rudroff T, Kindred JH, Ketelhut NB. Fatigue in multiple sclerosis: misconceptions and future research directions. *Front Neurol.* 2016;7:122.

21. Rusk HA. *Rehabilitation Medicine.* CV Mosby; 1977.

22. Petajan JH, Gappmaier E, White AT, Spencer MK, Mino L, Hicks RW. Impact of aerobic training on fitness and quality of life in multiple sclerosis. *Ann Neurol.* 1996;39(4):432-441.

23. Fimland MS, Helgerud J, Gruber M, Leivseth G, Hoff J. Enhanced neural drive after maximal strength training in multiple sclerosis patients. *Eur J Appl Physiol.* 2010;110(2)435-443.

24. Karpatkin H, Cohen E, Klein S, et al. The effect of maximal strength training on strength, walking, and balance in people with multiple sclerosis: a pilot study. *Mult Scler Int.* 2016;2016:5235971. doi:10.1155/2016/5235971.

25. Mark VW, Taub E, Uswatte G, et al. Constraint-induced movement therapy for the lower extremities in multiple sclerosis: case series with 4-year follow-up. *Arch Phys Med Rehabil.* 2013;94(4):753-760.

26. Kempen JC, Doorenbosch CA, Knol DL, de Groot V, Beckerman H. Newly identified gait patterns in patients with multiple sclerosis may be related to push-off quality. *Phys Ther.* 2016;96(11):1744-1752.

27. Baggett BD, Young G. Ankle joint dorsiflexion. Establishment of a normal range. *J Am Podiatr Med Assoc.* 1993;83(5):251-254.

28. Bandy WD, Irion JM. The effect of time on static stretch on the flexibility of the hamstring muscles. *Phys Ther.* 1994;74(9):845-850.

29. Gao F, Ren Y, Roth EJ, Harvey R, Zhang LQ. Effects of repeated ankle stretching on calf muscle–tendon and ankle biomechanical properties in stroke survivors. *Clin Biomech.* 2011;26(5):516-522.

30. Mount J, Dacko S. Effects of dorsiflexor endurance exercises on foot drop secondary to multiple sclerosis: a pilot study. *NeuroRehabilitation.* 2006;21(1):43-50.

31. A Patient Survey of Mobility and Exercise Issues Among MS Patients [poll]. Poll commissioned by: Acorda Therapeutics®, Inc., and the Multiple Sclerosis Association of America; February 21, 2008.

32. Karpatkin H, Cohen E, Rzetelny A, et al. Performance on the berg balance scale in fatigued versus nonfatigued states in people with multiple sclerosis. *Crit Rev Phys Rehabil Med.* 2013;25(3–4):223-230.

33. Cattaneo D, Jonsdottir J, Repetti S. Reliability of four scales on balance disorders in persons with multiple sclerosis. *Disabil Rehabil.* 2007;29(24):1920-1925.

34. Ross E, Purtill H, Uszynski M, et al. Cohort study comparing the berg balance scale and the Mini-BESTest in people who have multiple sclerosis and are ambulatory. *Phys Ther.* 2016;96(9):1448-1455.

35. Casanova C, Celli BR, Barria P, et al. The 6-min walk distance in healthy subjects: reference standards from seven countries. *Eur Respir J.* 2011;37:150-156. doi:10.1183/09031936.00194909.

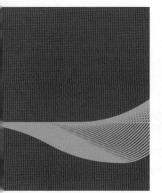
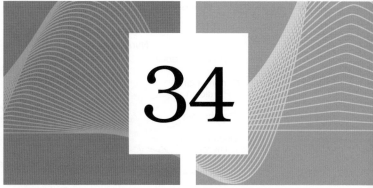

34

Comprehensive Care in Multiple Sclerosis: The Nursing Professional as a Linchpin

■■■ June Halper

Introduction

Multiple sclerosis (MS) is a complex, chronic, lifelong condition of adults that has a widespread impact on the patient, family, and society at large. Health care in MS requires the knowledge and skills of numerous medical and related professionals in a variety of health care settings: private practices, MS centers, rehabilitation settings, day treatment programs, and extended care facilities.

The nursing professional is often a key member of the MS health care team that includes physicians, rehabilitation specialists, mental health professionals, and patient advocates.[1] This model of comprehensive care may occur in MS centers or in centers without walls because care varies throughout the United States and throughout the world. However, in facilities where there is a nursing professional, patient contact usually places the nursing professional as a key player in this system.

The nurse is ideally prepared to make periodic assessments in person or via other means of contact (phone, email) and is in an ideal position

591

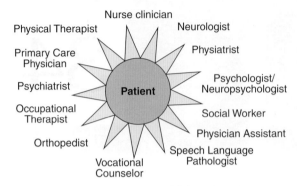

Figure 34.1. Comprehensive care in multiple sclerosis: a team approach.

to identify problems when subtle changes in MS symptoms may occur. Changes in bowel or bladder function, mobility, swallowing, or vision may portend overall problems with the patient's function or safety. Psychological and cognitive assessments are also within the nurse's scope of practice. It is well known that patients with MS are at an increased risk of depression and suicide, so screenings are essential. Cognitive changes, such as short-term memory loss or slowed information processing, may be misinterpreted by the family as stubbornness and irritability.[2] Because of the chronic and long-term nature of MS, it is crucial for the patient and family to be involved in the management of the disease and to consider themselves part of the health care team (see Figure 34.1). The nurse can explain and educate why changes occur and promote understanding and adjustment to these challenges.

The Nursing Role—The Diagnosis of MS

Although the diagnosis of MS is a clinical one, it involves the expertise of a neurologist who is familiar with MS and the newer diagnostic criteria, which were updated in 2017.[3] The patient must undergo a series of tests, including neuroimaging (magnetic resonance imaging) and laboratory testing (blood work and possible spinal fluid analysis), to rule out conditions that mimic the disease. This process may be prolonged owing to the need for third-party approval for the costs of the tests (prior authorization), scheduling, patient preparation, and other issues such as the need for transportation. The nurse functions as a facilitator, educator, and advocate during this process, ensuring that the tests ordered are completed, educating the patient and family as to why the tests are needed and what the results will tell the clinician, and advocating for insurance approval and reimbursement for the testing.[4]

Subsequently, once the testing is complete and the patient is given the results (should the patient be given the diagnosis of MS or another condition), the nurse's role is one of support and education. Please note that the importance of just "being there" cannot be underestimated. Reassurance and comfort are sometimes all that are required during the early phase of the diagnostic period. Once the realization has set in, patients and families need education about MS, particularly information relevant to the person with MS, not generalities. Sometimes, patients do not want in-depth information. Others want specifics. Tailoring education to the patient's needs, ethnocultural background, and specific for the time and place is a skill that nurses acquire over many years. Establishing a trusting relationship with open lines of communication is vital during the diagnostic phase and will carry over into subsequent interactions.

Treating Multiple Sclerosis—Nursing's Contributions

Management strategies for MS fall into three general categories: treatment of relapses caused by the underlying disease; prevention of progression or reduction of the frequency of relapses; and control of symptoms that affect the total patient, affect his or her quality of life, and influence the disease itself. Until the early 1990s, symptomatic care, rehabilitation services, and mental health interventions were the best that health care could offer those affected by MS. The entry of injectable therapies in the latter part of the 20th century, followed by infusible medications and subsequently by oral treatments, heralded a new era in the pharmacologic and nonpharmacologic approach to MS. Consequently, nursing responsibilities have expanded exponentially. Nursing care in MS falls into four general categories: relapse management, ongoing assessment and interventions, sustaining adherence, and contributing to the patient's and family's health-related quality of life.[5]

Relapse Management

A relapse or an exacerbation is unpredictable as to when it may occur and how it can manifest itself. It may involve a variety of symptoms, including abrupt changes in sensation, pain, cognition, coordination, bladder control, balance, strength, or vision. Treatment of a relapse is disruptive itself, and nursing support can ease a patient's anxiety. Education, reassurance, and coaching through the treatment process may ease the uncertainty and renewed concerns that reoccur during this period because, even in a clinically stable patient, a relapse is a powerful reminder of the presence of an "unwelcome guest," MS. Nursing professionals must help patients cope with a variety of challenges: dosing schedule, side effects, possible loss of income, costs of care, and additional health care needs such as rehabilitation, use of assistive devices, and the uncertainty about the extent of recovery. Like a pebble dropped in a pond, the effects of a relapse reverberate to affect the patient's family, friends, and vocational and social work, so the nurse's role may extend beyond the patient to educate others should the patient need that assistance.[6]

Ongoing Assessment and Interventions

MS has a widespread impact on a person's activities of daily living and his or her quality of life. The nursing professional has a complex role in addressing those issues in each interaction with the patient and family. In this author's experience, it is valuable to utilize the nursing process to ascertain the impact of MS on the patient's activities of daily living. By doing so, one can determine if the primary symptoms of MS (weakness, fatigue, tremor, pain, elimination dysfunction, speech and language problems, visual disturbance, and mood disorders) are affecting activities of daily living as well as a person's functional status. Then, in collaboration with the patient, the nurse can prioritize a plan of care to address those issues of greatest importance. For example, although elimination dysfunction may be a nursing concern, the patient's priority may be on changing roles and relationships with family and friends. Counseling, referrals to appropriate services, and education may be effective strategies in addressing issues related to these types of interpersonal challenges.

Comprehensive nursing management may include the following:

1. Improving elimination patterns and preventing infections and incontinence
2. Modifying sleep and rest patterns and reducing fatigue
3. Addressing and treating sensory symptoms such as dysesthesias and pain
4. Assessing for risks such as falls, contractures, and skin breakdown and instituting preventive measures
5. Working with rehabilitation specialists to maximize function and minimize risks
6. Counseling and educating patients and referrals to mental health care when indicated to improve coping skills and attain maximal quality of life
7. Referrals for and coordination to community care services such as home nursing care, social services, and other supportive programs (meals on wheels, food stamps, day care, to name a few)

8. Initiating and coordinating necessary testing required throughout the course of the disease (neuroimaging, laboratory studies, special tests for cognition, etc.)

9. Assessing and treating complications such as infected wounds and skin breakdown

10. Working with agencies and service organizations to obtain needed services and support for patients and families[7]

Sustaining Adherence to MS Treatments

Sustaining patient adherence to MS treatments, pharmacologic and non-pharmacologic, is an ongoing challenge to nursing professionals. Helping patients to maintain a realistic outlook and working on an individualized plan of care for each patient is one approach that helps improve adherence and optimize therapeutic outcomes. It is usually a nurse who has a partnership with the patient from the time of diagnosis throughout the journey with this lifelong disease. Adherence to therapy starts at this point and continues throughout the course of the disease with the adoption of new tasks such as self-injection, having regular blood work, scheduling infusion therapies, working with a rehabilitation team, undergoing diagnostic procedures, or facing changes in functioning. An open and honest relationship and free communication between the nurse and patient can promote adherence to new behaviors required for successful management of MS.[8]

Contributing to Health-Related Quality of Life

Because MS usually strikes during the most financially productive years of life, employment issues are usually of high importance to patients and families. Fatigue, increasing disability, and the unpredictable nature of the disease represent major obstacles to continued employment. Nevertheless, people with MS should be encouraged to work if possible, because the ability to remain productive is a strong deterrent to depression.

The very high frequency of depression should be a red flag for nursing professionals. It is important to assess patients at each encounter for signs and symptoms of mood change. Similarly, cognitive changes can invade every aspect of a person's life. MS nursing professionals need to ask the right questions to delve into the problems and, together with the patient, plan for the correct assessments and interventions. Psychological counseling, support groups, and advocacy by MS professionals are essential throughout a lifetime with MS.[9]

Partners in Wellness

Despite the medical, rehabilitative, and pharmacologic advances during the past 3 decades, people with MS must be vigilant to their ongoing health and wellness needs. In addition to seeking neurologic care, patients with MS should seek to maintain a desired and realistic level of activity and exercise, a well-balanced diet, routine health checks and vaccinations, and optimal weight. Recent evidence has revealed the impact of obesity, smoking, vitamin D, and inactivity on MS. The nursing professional plays an important role as a partner in wellness. In this ideal model, the nurse can provide education, support, guidance, and expert health management with the patient and family. As a caregiver, educator, advocate, and liaison for the MS patient, family, and the dedicated team of health care professionals, the MS nurse is a partner in wellness in MS.[10]

It is essential that MS nurses be aware that each individual affected by MS is unique. To provide optimal care, MS nursing must be a collaborative effort with patients, families, and other professional colleagues to address the dynamic condition that defines MS.

Nursing Care in Multiple Sclerosis— Comprehensive Management

With the advent of disease-modifying agents, the focus of care in MS has changed from one of monitoring and crisis intervention to a more positive and proactive approach. The nurse working in the field of MS has emerged as an important member of the health care team, playing a vital role in the ongoing care of and interaction with patients and their families. Nursing care in MS is a collaborative effort whose goal is self-awareness and self-responsibility; its activities involve supporting a growing array of self-care activities by patients, families, and care partners.

The Changing Face of Multiple Sclerosis

Common symptoms of MS include fatigue, cognitive changes, emotional problems (particularly depression), altered mobility, visual abnormalities, bladder and bowel dysfunction, and sensory problems. Emotional changes related to MS may encompass a wide variety of phenomena. They may include depression, grieving, reactions to stress, emotional lability, affective release (also known as pseudobulbar affect), euphoria, and anger. People who are diagnosed with MS are faced with a dynamic rather than a static illness. Problems confronted on one day may change on the next. The disease itself may wax and wane; symptoms may come and go; function can be altered by environmental factors and personal symptoms such as fatigue.[11]

Managing change in MS calls for creative solutions within a flexible and accepting environment. The element of chronicity implies the need for adaptation over time so that management becomes the goal rather than the cure. In acknowledging this, principles of care must change from those of the acute medical model to one that is individualized and ongoing throughout a person's lifetime. The aims of emotional support are to support the person in accordance with his or her life goals with the preservation of autonomy and maintenance of a role in the family and society at large. This requires maintenance of emotional stability and positive interpersonal relationships.[12]

Strategies to assist people manage change throughout the spectrum of the disease consist of education; individual, group, and family counseling; support groups; and networks of peers. The nature of MS challenges the people affected by the disease to seek appropriate support services with understanding professionals who can develop and implement individualized, culturally sensitive, and dynamic programs to meet the needs of all those affected by the disease throughout a lifetime.[12]

Acute Exacerbations and Nursing Care

Acute exacerbations or relapses are a hallmark of MS.

They are usually treated with oral or intravenous corticosteroids, which have been shown to shorten the duration of the attacks. Steroids have no long-term benefit on the disease course. Intravenous therapy may or may not be followed by an oral taper or dexamethasone or prednisone. Some physicians treat patients with a course of oral corticosteroids only. Long-term administration of corticosteroids is not recommended because of the significant toxic effect of these drugs. Side effects of long-term steroid use include susceptibility to opportunistic infections, hypertension, cataracts, muscle wasting, osteoporosis, and diabetes. Nurses play a role in the acute management of MS by educating patients about the proposed therapy, overseeing adherence to the prescribed regimen, monitoring patients for side effects, and encouraging patients during this difficult period.[13]

Symptom Management in MS

Primary symptoms in MS are those that are the direct result of demyelination in the central nervous system. Symptoms most commonly experienced include weakness, fatigue, tremor, pain, bladder and bowel dysfunction, paralysis, spasticity, visual changes, and diminished sexual function, including impotence in men.

Secondary symptoms are complications that are caused by the underlying impairment in MS. These include falls, injury, reduced activities of daily living, lack of sleep, urinary tract infections (UTIs), incontinence of bowel and bladder, skin breakdown, contractures, problems with the environment, and diminished opportunities for intimacy.

Tertiary symptoms are psychosocial or vocational problems that occur as a result of primary and secondary symptoms in MS, which are not treated and become an overwhelming part of the patient's life. These include loss of job; shift in roles; divorce; loss of financial, social, vocational, and environmental mobility; the stigma of disability; and reactive depression. The nurse and the MS team should take measures to alleviate primary symptoms, thereby dramatically reducing the incidence of secondary and tertiary symptoms. It is important to note, however, that the greatest impact on the patient's quality of life is taking measures to reduce social isolation and promoting participation and productivity despite the persistence of primary symptoms.[14]

Fatigue

Fatigue is a common symptom in MS that does not correlate well to the patient's physical status. Typically, a patient becomes tired after exercise or as the day progresses. Some may also complain of sudden episodes of fatigue. Regular rest periods or short naps, performing moderate exercises, and using assistive devices such as motorized scooters are effective energy-conserving techniques. It has been found that depression can be a cause of fatigue, and treatments such as counseling and a supportive social environment can be therapeutic in combating this problem. The role of nursing is to acknowledge the problem and to assist the patient and family to seek help either with their neurologist or through rehabilitation services. Individualizing care is important in addressing this problem, which can be unique to each individual. Underlying causes such as poor sleep patterns or medical issues such as anemia should be identified and treated.[15]

Spasticity

Spasticity is caused by involuntary muscle contractions and is characterized by stiffness. This symptom can also result in pain and limitation of motion. Sudden stretching of muscles, changes in position, and use of tight clothing or equipment may trigger and worsen spasticity. Treatment consists of slow stretching programs, appropriate physical activity such as swimming, mechanical aids, and medications. This class of medications may have sedative effects, and nurses can instruct patients about the potential effect on function as well as dosage and administration. A baclofen pump, in which medication is delivered continuously through intrathecal infusion, may be the next step should these interventions prove ineffective. Botulinum toxin can also promote relief in spasticity in small muscle groups. Here again, the MS nurse can provide valuable guidance and education to patients and their families about these treatments and expected outcomes.[16]

Bladder and Bowel Dysfunction

Many patients with MS experience some type of bladder problem during the course of the disease. Symptoms may include urinary urgency, frequency, incontinence, nocturia, and frequent UTIs. Bladder dysfunction is managed by obtaining a careful history, ruling out a UTI through a urine analysis and culture and sensitivity test, and obtaining a postvoid residual volume of urine. Nurses can be extremely important in ascertaining whether a patient is experiencing voiding problems, which many people do not recognize as related to MS, thus failing to disclose this information to the neurologist.

Bowel dysfunction can manifest itself as either constipation or diarrhea. With constipation, an adequate intake of fluids and fiber, a bowel program that consists of regular and adequate time for evacuation, and stool softeners usually are effective in the management of this problem. Patient and family education by a nursing professional can contribute to improving the patient's quality of life and self-management of this difficult problem.[17]

Sensory Symptoms

Sensory symptoms such as pain, numbness, burning, and tingling may be a great source of concern to the patient. Avoidance of noxious stimuli, investigation for underlying infections, and neurologic evaluation for exacerbations are recommended for these symptoms, especially if they occur acutely.

Secondary pain is usually musculoskeletal in nature and is the consequence of poor posture or balance. Patients who ambulate with inappropriate assistive devices, sit with poor posture, or fall frequently are subject to this symptom. Treatment consists of moist, moderate heat, massage, physical therapy, pain relievers, anti-inflammatory agents, and correction of the underlying problem. An important task for nurses regarding pain is to clarify the myth that MS is not a painful disease and help the patient seek appropriate interventions.[18]

Cognitive Implications of MS

Cognitive dysfunction is common in patients with MS. It is estimated that up to 65% of those with the disease experience some degree of cognitive loss—some so mild that it does not affect their lives. Others have such a great degree of loss that they are no longer able to function independently. Temporary lapses in cognitive function may also occur during exacerbations.

Although at the present time there is no pharmacological treatment for cognitive dysfunction in MS, nursing assessment of cognitive dysfunction can lead to referrals for services. Documentation of a severe cognitive disorder may qualify patients for disability benefits. Frequently, behaviors in the patient that are caused by diminished cognition—stubbornness, crankiness, mood swings, and inattentiveness—must be interpreted to family members and coworkers by the professional team. Nursing education, along with individual and family counseling, can help the patient and care partner cope with this problem.[19]

Preparing for Disease-Modifying Therapies

The wide variety of disease-modifying agents poses increasing challenges for MS nursing professionals. Injectable treatments require patient and family education about the injection technique itself, meticulous skin care, regular blood work (with interferons), and facilitation of sustained adherence to an injection schedule.

Oral medications, although more convenient for the patient, require vigilant monitoring, sustained contact with MS professionals, and side-effect management. Regular patient contact is essential to ensure maximal benefit from treatment and minimal potential complications.

Infusion therapies have almost become a standard of care in MS, from intravenous steroids to treatment with approved as well as off-label therapies. Appointments must be made, time must be allotted for treatment, and monitoring for complications is extremely important. Patient and family education are the bedrock of successful treatment along with ongoing monitoring for adverse events and side effects.[20]

Planning for the Patient's Future

Nurses who care for patients with MS should be aware of specific concerns that the patients have about their disease, such as: What will happen to me and my family? Can I continue working? How disabled will I become? Often, preexisting insecurities in the patient become exaggerated. Nurses must assist these patients to become educated about their disease and suggested treatments. Patients should be encouraged to seek counseling to overcome depression and possibly to affiliate with support groups for an ongoing supportive social environment.

Because MS usually strikes during the productive years of life, issues related to employment can be a prominent concern. It is estimated that 25% of patients with MS are working and that another 25% desire to return to the workforce. Fatigue and other symptoms experienced during relapses and in progressive disease and the unpredictability of future disease course in MS can impose major obstacles to employment. Nurses, social workers, and physicians can be supportive in encouraging a patient to continue to work, if possible. Working and productivity are important to a person's quality of life. Finding a job that does not require physically demanding work, staggering work hours, taking naps, and working from home are strategies used to assist patients to remain in the workforce. Those who are no longer able to work should be encouraged to find volunteer activities appropriate to their physical and mental function. Adaptive devices such as scooters, voice-activated computers, and visual aids can assist patients in these activities.[21]

Family Issues in MS

The patient and his or her partner must consider all aspects of parenting before deciding whether or not to start a family. Pregnancy has been shown to have a protective effect on MS, whereas the postpartum period results in a higher risk of relapses. It is very likely that many couples would welcome information about this choice. A nurse should encourage couples to be realistic about the problems associated with MS; to evaluate their emotional, financial, and family support; to assess their flexibility with parenting roles; and to think beyond the initial stages of infancy. Couples should also be made aware of the resources available to them, including educational materials, family therapists, and support groups.

A parent's diagnosis of MS can be difficult for a young child. A child's sense of security can be threatened by the disability of the parent. In addition, a child may have to shift roles and assume increased responsibility in the home. Although a parent with MS should avoid giving elaborate details of symptoms and disability, children become more anxious when they sense that the truth is being kept from them. Parents should give age-appropriate answers to questions and seek supportive material from sources of information. Family counseling can allow family members the opportunity to air their concerns and develop strategies for coping.[22]

Nursing Care in Advanced MS

The severely disabled patient with MS has a need for intensive nursing care. Patients with dysphagia must be given dietary modifications to prevent aspiration and nutritional deficits. Thick fluids, soft foods, and special feeding techniques must be initiated and taught to care partners and providers. In patients who are no longer able to swallow safely, adequate nutrition may be supported by modified diet or in extreme situations, via PEG feeding tube. Skin care is another concern for the severely disabled. Pressure sores often occur over bony prominences, such as on the sacrum, ankles, and elbows, and on pressure points, such as on the heel. Measures to prevent pressure sores include the use of wheelchair cushions, wheelchairs that are well fitted to the patient, assistive devices (e.g., side rails, trapezes) to promote repositioning, and good skin care to promote skin integrity.

A person with reduced mobility requires the following:

- Regular skin inspection for breakdown
- Meticulous personal hygiene
- Skin lubrication
- Frequent change of position
- Prompt treatment of pressure sores
- Adequate nutrition and hydration

With patients with advanced MS, the nurse is challenged to provide the patients and families with a realistic hope and a message of caring. This is particularly difficult today in light of the new disease-modifying medications, which are prescribed for patients with relapsing forms of MS but which are not appropriate for the severely disabled individual. Nursing care may consist of rehabilitation strategies, such as a program of stretching; linking patients to supportive services and networks; and intermittent appropriate psychosocial interventions as indicated by the needs of the patient and family. For the person with significant immobility, home care services are essential to sustain health, well-being, and connection to the health care community.[23]

Conclusion

The nurse working with patients with MS has many roles: care provider, facilitator, advocate, educator, counselor, and innovator. Additionally, the nurse often serves as a liaison between the patient, family, and health care providers and can be instrumental in the design, implementation, and coordination of a comprehensive treatment plan for the patient. A nurse's support, advice, education, and expertise as part of a therapeutic partnership can do much to advance MS from an overwhelming disease to a set of solvable problems in the lives of patients and their families.

References

1. Nygren K, Hartley G. Multiple sclerosis nursing. In: Giesser BS, ed. *Primer on Multiple Sclerosis*. New York: Oxford University Press; 2016:410-413.
2. LaRocca NG. Cognitive impairment and mood disturbances. In: Giesser BS, ed. *Primer on Multiple Sclerosis*. New York: Oxford University Press; 2016:283-309.
3. Thompson AJ, Banwell BL, Barkhof F, et al. Diagnosis of multiple sclerosis: 2017 revisions of the McDonald criteria. *Lancet Neurol*. 2018;17(2):162-173.

4. Nygren K, Hartley G. Multiple sclerosis nursing. In: Giesser BS, ed. *Primer on Multiple Sclerosis.* New York: Oxford University Press; 2016:410-413.
5. Schapiro RT. *Managing the Symptoms of Multiple Sclerosis.* New York: Demos Health; 2014:15.
6. Giesser B. Relapses, immunosuppressive and novel therapies. In: Giesser BS, ed. *Primer on Multiple Sclerosis.* New York: Oxford University Press; 2016:441-443.
7. Halper J, Holland NJ. *Comprehensive Nursing Care in Multiple Sclerosis.* New York: Demos Medical Publishing; 2010.
8. Harris C, Halper J, Kennedy P, et al. *Moving Forward: Adherence to Therapy and the Role of Nursing in Multiple Sclerosis.* Hackensack, NJ: IOMSN; 2013:17-29.
9. Murray TJ. *Coping With Multiple Sclerosis. Multiple Sclerosis A Guide for the Newly Diagnosed.* New York: Demos Health; 2017:115-132.
10. Harris C, Halper J, Kennedy P, et al. *Moving Forward: Adherence to Therapy and the Role of Nursing in Multiple Sclerosis.* Hackensack, NJ: IOMSN; 2013:13-15.
11. Harris C., Halper J. *Multiple Sclerosis: Best Practices in Nursing Care.* Teaneck, NJ: IOMSN; 2009. Available at www.iomsn.org.
12. LaRocca NR. Cognitive impairment and mood disturbances. In: Giesser BG, ed. *Primer on Multiple Sclerosis.* New York: Oxford University Press; 2016:283-310.
13. Harris C., Halper J. *Multiple Sclerosis: Best Practices in Nursing Care.* Teaneck, NJ. IOMSN; 2009:14-15. Available at www.iomsn.org.
14. Harris C., Halper J. *Multiple Sclerosis: Best Practices in Nursing Care.* Teaneck, NJ. IOMSN; 2009:15-18. Available at www.iomsn.org.
15. Bhise V, Charvet L, Krupp LB. Fatigue in multiple sclerosis. In: Geisser BG, ed. *Primer on Multiple Sclerosis.* New York: Oxford University Press; 2016:331-346.
16. Campea S, Haselkorn J. Disorders of mobility in multiple sclerosis. In: Geisser BG, ed. *Primer on Multiple Sclerosis.* New York: Oxford University Press; 2016:233-248.
17. Choi JM, Kim JH. Management of urinary and bowel dysfunction in multiple sclerosis. In: Geisser BG, ed. *Primer on Multiple Sclerosis.* New York: Oxford University Press; 2016.
18. Namerov NS. Multiple sclerosis and pain. In: Geisser BG, ed. *Primer on Multiple Sclerosis.* New York: Oxford University Press; 2016:311-330.
19. LaRocca NR. Psychosocial issues in multiple sclerosis. In: Halper J, ed. *Comprehensive Nursing Care in Multiple Sclerosis.* New York: Demos Medical Publishing; 2002:107-111.
20. Halper J. Pharmacotherapeutics in multiple sclerosis and nursing implications. In: Halper J, ed. *Comprehensive Nursing Care in Multiple Sclerosis.* New York: Demos Medical Publishing; 2002:175-182.
21. Kennedy PK. Interfacing with rehabilitation services. In: Halper J, ed. *Comprehensive Nursing Care in Multiple Sclerosis.* New York: Demos Medical Publishing; 2002:147-176.
22. Holland NJ. Patient and family education. In: Halper J, ed. *Comprehensive Nursing Care in Multiple Sclerosis.* New York: Demos Medical Publishing; 2002:191-204.
23. Harris CJ. Preventions of complications in the severely disabled. In: Halper J, ed. *Comprehensive Nursing Care in Multiple Sclerosis.* New York: Demos Medical Publishing; 2002:77-92.

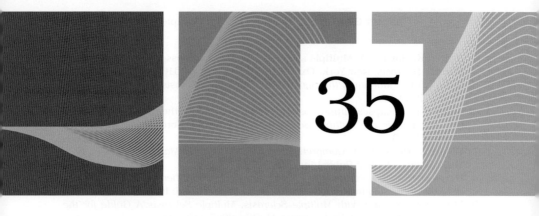

Palliative Medicine in Multiple Sclerosis

■ ■ ■ Misa Hyakutake, Mary Ann Picone

Introduction

Although significant strides have been made in treatment, multiple sclerosis (MS) is often a debilitating disease, and patients are susceptible to conditions such as pressure sores, intractable spasticity, and chronic pain. It is also true that MS is very difficult to prognosticate, as there is a wide range in the trajectory of the disease course; some patients may live a nearly normal life expectancy with death from cancer or heart disease, while other patients may lead a progressive disease course, with severe and debilitating symptoms. MS is an unpredictable disease even in the eye of the experts, which necessitates the providers to discuss about wishes and goals for each patient from early into the disease and continuously throughout the disease course. Additionally, providers should work together with the patient and the interdisciplinary team to ensure the most comfortable living environment. Palliative care is a multidisciplinary approach, encompassing the physical, emotional, social, and spiritual care for people with serious illnesses. Palliative care can be provided to patients regardless of the stages of their diseases and in numerous care settings, such as home, outpatient, in-hospital, or hospice. In contrast to traditional medical care that focuses on patient's disease or illness, asking "what is the matter?", palliative care focuses on patient's and family's needs, asking "what matters to you?"[1]

In this chapter, we will focus on ways to improve comfort and quality of life in MS patients.

When to Consider Getting Palliative Care Involved

Given complexity of MS and its incurable nature, it is never too early or too late to consider getting palliative care involved as the extra layer of support in the care of MS patients. Below are possible triggers for consulting palliative care.[2]

- When pain or other complex symptoms are not well controlled
- When high psychosocial or spiritual distress is suspected
- When family member or caregivers seem overburdened
- When patient or any of the members of the care team are concerned about the quality of life or the advance care planning
- When there is a concern for patient's decision-making capacity or identification of surrogate decision-maker

The Kurtzke disability status scale or DSS and the expanded version or EDSS are commonly used to assess the disability in MS.[3,4] The number ranges from 0 for normal examination and function up to 10 for death due to MS.

MS patients are generally considered to be in "advanced" stage when EDSS is 6.5 or greater, defined as requiring constant bilateral walking assistance (canes, crutches, or braces), or is mostly wheelchair-bound. At this stage, patients are at significantly higher risk of increase in symptoms that can cause life-threatening complications.

Increase in EDSS indices is an opportune timing to consider getting palliative care involved, if not done yet.

Starting the Conversation

When triggers as above are recognized, providers should further explore what the patients and families are experiencing. Open-ended questions and attentive listening are very useful in exploring the values and concerns and often can be therapeutic for the emotional distress. Studies have shown that people with disabilities have consistently stated that they want to be heard and to have their providers learn from them; it is important that providers let go of any preconceived ideas about what is important to the patients and make no assumptions about what they may want.[5]

We will introduce some of the communication skill tools and resources that any providers can use to facilitate palliative care conversation. However, if providers feel uncomfortable with the conversation, getting palliative care specialists involved early in the process is recommended.

1. SPIKES: Protocol for breaking bad news[6]

   Although SPIKES, the six-step protocol for disclosing unfavorable information, was originally developed for cancer patients, this can be applied to any providers who are discussing serious conditions with the patients.

   S = **"Setting up the interview."** Arrange for some privacy, involve significant others of the patient, arrange for most comfortable physical positioning (e.g., sitting down, level with patient), and manage time constraints and interruptions (e.g., inform the patient of any time constraints you may have).

   P = **"Perception."** Explore the patient's perception of the current situation by using open-ended questions (e.g., "What is your understanding of your medical situation right now?").

   I = **"Invitation."** While a majority of patients desire full information, some patients do not. Aim to get a clear invitation from the patient to share information, but accept the patient's right not to know (e.g., "How would you like me to give the information about...?" "Are you the sort of person who...?").

   K = **"Knowledge."** Start at a place compatible with patient's current comprehension when giving knowledge and information to the patient. Avoid medical jargon, and give information in small chunks. Check periodically as to the patient's understanding.

   E = **"Empathizing and Exploring."** Acknowledge patient's emotions and their origins. Explore, validate, and empathize their emotional responses.

   S = **"Strategy and Summary."** Make a plan via explanation and collaboration. Summarize main areas. Contract for next contact.

2. NURSE: Responding to patient emotions[7]

   NURSE is a useful mnemonic for ways to address emotions and articulate empathy.

   N = **"Naming."** Naming emotion shows you are attuned to what she is experiencing. (e.g., "It sounds like you are frustrated.")

   U = **"Understanding."** Empathize with and legitimize the emotion. (e.g., "This helps me understand what you are thinking," "I cannot imagine what it is like to...")

   R = **"Respecting."** Praise the patient for strength. (e.g., "I can see you have really been trying to..." "I am very impressed with how well you've care for your mother during this.")

   S = **"Supporting."** Providers can express concern, articulate their understanding of patient's situation, express willingness to help, make statements about partnership, and acknowledge the patient's efforts to cope. (e.g., "I will do my best to make sure you have what you need.")

   E = **"Exploring."** Ask the patient to elaborate on the emotion. (e.g., "Could you tell me more about what you mean when you say that...")

3. REMAP: Address goal of care[8]

REMAP is the mnemonic of the talking map designed to give guidance through a complex conversation regarding goals of care. The processes of REMAP encourage providers to remain flexible and adapt their recommendations to what they hear from the patient based on the shared decision-making.

R = "**Reframe.**" Provider can paint a big picture "headline" that lets the patient know things are in a different place. You may need to share serious or bad news first. (e.g., "We're in a different place," "Given this news, it seems like a good time to talk about what to do now.")

E = "**Expect emotion.**" Actively attend to the patient's emotional response and respond with empathy. Refer to the mnemonic **NURSE** as explained above. (e.g., "It's hard to deal with all this," "I can see you are really concerned about...")

M = "**Map out patient goals.**" Ask open-ended questions to help patients think about the values and what's important to them. (e.g., "Given this situation, what's most important to you?" "As you think toward the future, what concerns you?")

A = "**Align with goals.**" Align with the patient's values by explicitly reflecting them back to the patient. (e.g., "As I listen to you, it sounds like the most important things are...")

P = "**Propose a plan.**" If the patient gives permission, use those values to propose a medical plan that matches patient values. (e.g., "Here's what I can do now that will help you do those important things.")

Symptom Management

MS patients are susceptible to conditions such as pressure sores and intractable spasticity, which can lead to chronic and complex symptoms that are difficult to manage.

When patients are close to the end of life, most of the symptom management approaches become similar; using opioids for dyspnea, trying atropine, glycopyrrolate, or scopolamine for excessive secretions, treating constipation with stimulant laxatives, such as sennosides, to name a few.

However, there are a few major differences in palliative symptom management of MS patients compared with other diseases. One is management of spasticity and another is pain management.

We will highlight these two symptoms' management below.

Spasticity

Spasticity is a common and disabling symptom that often has significant impact to functionality. There are multiple management options for spasticity, including therapeutic exercise, physical modalities, complementary/alternative medicine intervention, oral medications, chemodenervation, and implantation of an intrathecal baclofen pump. Often, treatment should be a combination of above options, depending on the extent of symptoms, patient preference, and availability of services.

Below are the recommendations of oral agents by the National Institute for Health and Care Excellence (NICE) guideline.[9]

- Consider baclofen or gabapentin as a first-line drug to treat spasticity in MS
- Consider tizanidine or dantrolene as a second-line option
- Consider benzodiazepine as a third-line option and be aware of their potential benefit in treating nocturnal spasms

Also, in addition to above oral medications, according to the Clinical Practice Guidelines on Spasticity Management in Multiple Sclerosis by Multiple Sclerosis Council,[10] it is Level A recommendation to

- Perform neuromuscular block
- Apply skilled rehabilitation strategies
- Refer for intrathecal therapy for patients with Expanded Disability Status Scale (EDSS) of 7 or above (Level C recommendation for patients with EDSS 5.0-6.5)

Concurrently, it is important to assess for factors that may aggravate spasticity such as constipation, urinary tract or other infections, inappropriately fitted mobility aids, pressure ulcers, posture, and pain.

Spasticity can be just a mere annoyance, but it can also lead to significant disability and result in unnecessary morbidity and mortality. Managing and treating spasticity effectively and sufficiently will minimize impairments, disability, and reduced quality of life.

Pain Management

When discussing pain in MS patients, we often focus mainly on neuropathic pain. However, we must be aware that most of MS patients also suffer from nociceptive or musculoskeletal pain, largely due to problems with mobility and posture.

For neuropathic pain, below are the recommendations by the NICE guideline in nonspecialist settings.[11]

- Offer a choice of amitriptyline, duloxetine, gabapentin, or pregabalin as initial treatment for neuropathic pain
- Consider tramadol only if acute rescue therapy is needed
- Consider capsaicin cream for people with localized neuropathic pain who wish to avoid, or who cannot tolerate, oral treatments

For nonpharmacological interventions, TENS and acupuncture, in the hands of experienced practitioners, are safe therapy options with broad anecdotal evidence of efficacy for neuropathic pain.

As mentioned, musculoskeletal pain can be seen in many MS patients due to lack of mobility from muscle weakness, spasticity, and poor posture. It is often exacerbated by loss of musculature due to weight loss and stiffness.

These pains are often chronic, and a comprehensive multidisciplinary assessment is of paramount importance.

Physical therapy and mobilization are extremely beneficial. Nonpharmaceutical interventions, such as heat pads, topical anti-inflammatory treatments, and TENS should be considered. Also, massage therapy has been very popular and anecdotally very helpful for both musculoskeletal symptoms of MS and general well-being.

For pharmacologic approach, some experts recommend that following the same approach of analgesic ladder to cancer pain of (1) nonopioid analgesics, (2) weak opioid analgesics, and (3) morphine and strong opioids, as acceptable management. However, given unfavorable side effects of nausea and constipation, together with concern for opioid epidemic, careful discussion of risks and benefits is warranted.

Use of Cannabis in Symptom Management

Cannabinoid-type drugs have been approved for chemo-induced nausea/vomiting and appetite but remain controversial for efficacy for chronic pain. However, there has been limited but increasing evidence that cannabis might alleviate neuropathic pain in some patients.

For neuropathic pain, randomized studies that have shown statistical significance used either smoked or vaporized cannabis.[12]

Wilsey et al[13] reported cannabis cigarettes (3.5% and 7% THC) significantly reduced pain on the visual analog scale (VAS), compared with placebo (55/100-30/100, p = 0.016), although the number of recruited patients was quite small (n = 38, crossover).

Ware et al[14] reported cannabis smoked in pipe (9.4% THC) significantly reduced pain compared with placebo (0.7 point reduction on average daily pain in VAS 0-10, p < 0.05), with added report of improved ability to fall asleep easier (p = 0.001) and faster (p < 0.001) and were drowsier (p = 0.003). Again, it was a small study with only 23 recruited patients with crossover.

When we focus on MS patients, there is an approved, commercially available cannabinoid-type drug (nabiximols) for treatment of MS, marketed in multiple countries outside of the United States, and there have been rigorous studies to evaluate efficacy of cannabis.

The Cannabinoids in MS (CAMS) study[15] (n = 630) in 2003 was a multicenter, randomized, 15-week, double-blind, placebo-controlled trial, which could not show significant difference in outcomes except for subjective benefits in the measures of spasticity, pain, sleep, and spasms.

A follow-up study[16] was done for all patients who were recruited for the CAMS study showed significant reduction of urge incontinence episodes in both oral cannabinoid extract (OCE) (25%, p = 0.005) and dronabinol (19%, p = 0.039) groups relative to placebo.

Another follow-up to the CAMS study, the MS and Extract of Cannabis trial[17] (n = 279) in 2012, a multicenter, randomized, 12-week, double-blind, placebo-controlled study, was able to show a statistical improvement in "relief of muscle stiffness" in 29.4% of patients on OCE compared with 15.7% of patients on placebo (OR, 2.26; 95% CI, 1.24-4.13; P = .004)

Cannabinoids should be prescribed by licensed, experienced provider and is most effective if patients are proactively involved with dose adjustment of CBD:THC ratio. For example, THC has stronger psychoactive effect, as opposed to CBD may cause drowsiness and lightheadedness in patients.

Although more research is warranted, cannabis may be considered as an alternative option for MS patients in the setting of close monitoring and careful adjustment to maximize efficacy and minimize side effects.

Rehabilitation

MS patients generally scored poorly in physical functioning and vitality when compared with patient with other chronic diseases or healthy controls.

Although rehabilitation is an essential component of management of symptoms and preventing complications, research has not delineated a single modality that is sufficiently effective.

Below is the list of specific modalities that could be used as skilled rehabilitation strategies.

- Range of motion
- Stretching
- Strengthening
- Light pressure stroking
- Heating/cooling

Improving Quality of Life

There have been a number of studies of quality of life among MS patients, and it has been known that MS patients generally report lower in physical functioning and vitality (optimism) compared with patients with other chronic conditions.

Using the communication skills as outlined in the Starting the Conversation section will lead to patient-centered decisions and shared decision-making that promote better end-of-life care that is aligned with patient's values.

Providing adequate symptom relief with multimodal measures, as mentioned in **Symptom Management** section, and proactively providing **Rehabilitation** services, thus preventing secondary conditions, such as urinary tract infections, pneumonia, pressure sores, contractures, are essential to maintaining acceptable quality of life for MS patients.

The goal is to prevent undesirable outcomes, such as frequent ER visits, prolonged hospitalizations, social isolation, loss of employment, institutionalization, and learned helplessness.

Death in MS

There is substantial variability to the natural course of MS. Death in MS patients is often caused by comorbidities, such as infection, cancer, and heart and pulmonary disease. Also, functional decline can lead to skin problems, sometimes resulting in serious skin infection and leading to death. Mortality studies have shown that the lifespan is shorter in MS patients, with mean age at death reported to be about 65 years.[18]

Approximately 10% of the MS are later classified to be primary progressive MS (PPMS). Compared with other types, PPMS progresses without remissions, generally leading to shorter survival time and dying more often as the direct result of complications of MS.

Currently, there are no disease-specific hospice criteria for MS. A Clinical Bulletin from the Professional Resource Center of the National Multiple Sclerosis Society[2] suggests the following as the MS hospice eligibility criteria.

Suggested MS Hospice Eligibility Guidelines

1. Critical nutritional impairment evidenced by
   a. Oral intake of nutrients and fluids insufficient to sustain life and comfort
   b. Continuing weight loss
2. Rapid disease progression in the preceding 12 months evidenced by
   a. Progression from independent ambulation to being confined to a wheelchair or bed
   b. Progression from normal to barely intelligible or unintelligible speech
   c. Progression from normal to pureed diet or feeding tube
   d. Progression from independence in most or all ADLs to the need for major assistance by caretaker in all ADLs
3. Life-threatening complications in the preceding 12 months as evidenced by one or more of the following:
   a. Critically impaired breathing capacity (forced vital capacity less than 30%)
   b. Dyspnea or shallow breathing at rest
   c. BiPAP required for more than 12 hours per day
   d. Patient refusal of artificial ventilation
   e. Recurrent aspiration pneumonia (with or without tube feedings)

4. Other infectious processes (one or more of the following)

    a. Upper urinary tract infection (pyelonephritis)

    b. Recurrent fever after antibiotic therapy

    c. Stage 3 or 4 pressure sores

    d. Sepsis

Combinations of above criteria identify potential eligibility for hospice. It is important that these criteria are documented, shared, and discussed with the organizations that are providing the service to the patients.

References

1. http://www.ihi.org/Topics/WhatMatters/Pages/default.aspx.
2. The National Multiple Sclerosis Society. *Opening Doors: The Palliative Care Continuum in Multiple Sclerosis.* Clinical Bulletin; 2012. Available at https://www.nationalmssociety.org/NationalMSSociety/media/MSNationalFiles/Brochures/Clinical-Bulletin-Palliative-Care-2012-Final.pdf.
3. Kurtzke JF. Neurologic impairment in multiple sclerosis and the disability status scale. *Acta Neurol Scand.* 1970;46(4):493-512. PubMed PMID: 5504332.
4. Kurtzke JF. Rating neurologic impairment in multiple sclerosis: an expanded disability status scale (EDSS). *Neurology.* 1983;33(11):1444-1452. PubMed PMID: 6685237.
5. Iezzoni LI. Make no assumptions: communication between persons with disabilities and clinicians. *Assist Technol.* 2006;18(2):212-219. PubMed PMID: 17236480.
6. Baile WF, Buckman R, Lenzi R, Glober G, Beale EA, Kudelka AP. SPIKES: a six step protocol for delivering bad news: application to the patient with cancer. *Oncologist.* 2000;5:302-311.
7. *Responding to Emotion: Respecting.* VitalTalk; 2017. Accessed August 10, 2018. http://vitaltalk.org/guides/responding-to-emotion-respecting/.
8. Childers JW, Back AL, Tulsky JA, Arnold RM. REMAP: a framework for goals ofCare conversations. *J Oncol Pract.* 2017;13(10):e844-e850. doi:10.1200/JOP.2016.018796. Epub 2017 Apr 26. PubMed PMID: 28445100.
9. National Institute for Health and Care Excellence. *Multiple Sclerosis in Adults: Management (NICE CG186);* 2014. Available at https://www.nice.org.uk/guidance/cg186. Accessed October 22, 2018.
10. Multiple Sclerosis Council for Clinical Practice Guidelines. *Spasticity Management in Multiple Sclerosis (MSC 167-199);* 2005. Available at https://www.sfphysio.fr/docs/2015200854_evidence-based-management-strategies-for-spasticity-treatment-in-multiple-sclerosis-2005.PDF. Accessed October 22, 2018.
11. National Institute for Health and Care Excellence. *Neuropathic Pain in Adults: Pharmacological Management in Non-specialist Settings (NICE CG173);* 2013. Available at https://www.nice.org.uk/guidance/cg173. Accessed October 22, 2018.
12. Noel C. Evidence for the use of "medical marijuana" in psychiatric and neurologic disorders. *Ment Health Clin.* 2018;7(1):29-38. doi:10.9740/mhc.2017.01.029. eCollection 2017 Jan. PubMed PMID: 29955495; PubMed Central PMCID: PMC6007658.

13. Wilsey B, Marcotte T, Tsodikov A, et al. A randomized, placebo-controlled, crossover trial of cannabis cigarettes in neuropathic pain. *J Pain.* 2008; 9(6): 506-521. doi:10.1016/j.jpain.2007.12.010. PubMed PMID: 18403272.
14. Ware MA, Wang T, Shapiro S, et al. Smoked cannabis for chronic neuropathic pain: a randomized controlled trial. *CMAJ.* 2010; 182(14): E694-E701. doi:10.1503/cmaj.091414. PubMed PMID: 20805210.
15. Zajicek J, Fox P, Sanders H, et al. Cannabinoids for treatment of spasticity and other symptoms related to multiple sclerosis (CAMS study): multicentre randomised placebo-controlled trial. *Lancet.* 2003;362(9395): 1517-1526. doi:10.1016/S0140-6736(03)14738-1. PubMed PMID: 14615106.
16. Zajicek JP, Hobart JC, Slade A, Barnes D, Mattison PG. Multiple sclerosis and extract of cannabis: results of the MUSEC trial. *J Neurol Neurosurg Psychiatry.* 2012;83(11): 1125-1132. doi:10.1136/jnnp-2012-302468. PubMed PMID: 22791906.
17. Vaney C, Heinzel-Gutenbrunner M, Jobin P, et al. Efficacy, safety and tolerability of an orally administered cannabis extract in the treatment of spasticity in patients with multiple sclerosis: a randomized, double-blind, placebo-controlled, crossover study. *Mult Scler.* 2004;10(4): 417-424. doi:10.1191/1352458504ms1048oa. PubMed PMID: 15327040.
18. Hirst C, Swingler R, Compston DAS, Ben-Shlomo Y, Robertson NP. Survival and cause of death in multiple sclerosis: a prospective population-based study. *J Neurol Neurosurg Psychiatry.* 2008;79:1016-1021.

Further Reading

MS and Palliative Care. Available at http://www.virtualhospice.ca/Assets/ms_and_palliative_care_-_guide_for_professionals_20081127165937.pdf.
National Multiple Sclerosis Society. Available at https://www.nationalmssociety.org/For-Professionals/Clinical-Care/Managing-MS/Continuum-of-Care/Palliative-Care.

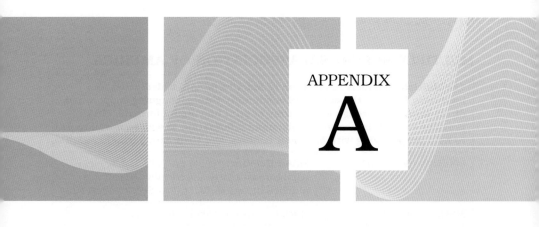

APPENDIX

A

Patient Resources and Support Services

■ ▓ ▒ Andrea Arzt, Lauren Hooper, Dorothy E. Northrop

Introduction to This Chapter

The aim of this chapter is to assist health care providers caring for people with multiple sclerosis (MS) in being informed and comfortable directing patients with MS to a range of agencies and organizations that can provide information, education, and support to people living with MS. Such resources can assure that patients with MS are informed about their disease, prepared to manage their symptoms, and equipped to advocate for themselves with regard to benefits and protections to which they are entitled. Although there are many resources mentioned in this chapter that will be helpful to your patients, we do not claim that this is an exhaustive list. However, hopefully it will provide a place to start and ideas for how to identify other helpful resources, particularly within each individual state and local community.

MS-SPECIFIC ORGANIZATIONS

MS organizations specialize in serving people with MS and have the most comprehensive access to information and resources specifically relevant to this population. Although they are separate organizations with slightly different missions and various services, all work closely together to provide comprehensively for the needs of people living with MS. These organizations should typically be your first resource for information and connection to the many other services and resources noted in this chapter.

MULTIPLE SCLEROSIS ASSOCIATION OF AMERICA

The Multiple Sclerosis Association of America (MSAA) is dedicated to improving lives for the entire MS community through ongoing support and direct services. Through a wide array of print and digital formats, MSAA provides current and easy-to-understand information as well as useful tools to help people living with MS, their families, and their care partners.

800-532-7667, x154	**MSAA Helpline:** People with MS, family members, care partners, and friends can call this number and speak to a Client Services Specialist
MSQuestions@mymsaa.org	Questions can be emailed to MSAA
www.mymsaa.org	Website for MSAA
www.mymsaa.org/chat	Live chat option

MSAA'S PROGRAMS AND SERVICES	
Equipment Distribution Program	Provides free, durable medical items such as shower chairs, grab bars, walkers, and wheelchairs to help improve a person's safety, mobility, and independence
Cooling Distribution Program	Supplies free cooling vests and accessories that provide several hours of cooling relief for individuals who are heat sensitive and who would otherwise experience increased symptoms when in warm temperatures
MRI Access Fund	Assists individuals who are uninsured or underinsured to acquire an MRI examination to help determine a diagnosis of MS or evaluate current MS disease progression
Educational Materials	Publications, videos, and the My MSAA Today e-newsletter
The Motivator	National magazine

LENDING LIBRARY PROGRAM	

Shared management tools including:

- S.E.A.R.C.H. program to assist the MS community with learning about different treatment choices
- Mobile phone app, My MS Manager, which is used to track medications, symptoms, and side effects; measure fatigue; and share progress reports with one's physician
- My MS Resource Locator Resource database

Educational programs	Nationwide
My MSAA Community	Online, peer-to-peer forum for individuals with MS and their care partners

NATIONAL MULTIPLE SCLEROSIS SOCIETY

The National Multiple Sclerosis Society (NMSS) provides a range of patient services and programs to support people with MS and their families, actively engages in advocacy on behalf of people with MS, and facilitates professional education through a variety of modalities and venues. The Society also funds comprehensive research and collaborates with MS organizations around the world in addressing the challenges of MS.

1-800-344-4867	**MS Navigators:** Skilled professionals connect people and families living with MS to the information, resources, and support needed
MSNavigatorCrisisSupport@ nmss.org	Crisis Support (IM is preferred method of communication)
ContactUsNMSS@nmss.org	Email connection to the Society
www.nationalMSsociety.org	Website (live chat available)

NMSS SERVICES AND RESOURCES

- Newly diagnosed support
- Advanced MS support and referrals
- Financial referrals and assistance
- Referrals for MS health care
- Family support symptom and treatment strategies
- Employment and insurance information and guidance
- Assessment for personalized case management
- Crisis intervention (not 24 h)

Publications and videos	Library of booklets, publications, and videos, available digitally and online, focused on education about MS and managing a range of issues facing people with MS
Momentum	National magazine
MSconnection.org	Online community, peer-to-peer connections for individuals with MS and care partners

NMSS PROGRAMS

- **Advocacy:** The Society advocacy program works to advance federal, state, and community policies and programs that benefit people with MS and their families
- **Education programs:** In-person and telelearning on a variety of relevant topics for the newly diagnosed, diverse populations and highlighting current research
- **Wellness:** Self-help groups, aquatics and fitness programs

MULTIPLE SCLEROSIS FOUNDATION

The Multiple Sclerosis Foundation (MS Focus) provides nationally accessible programs and services to those affected by MS to help them maintain their health, safety, self-sufficiency, and personal well-being. They strive to heighten public awareness of MS to elicit financial support while promoting understanding for those diagnosed.	
888-673-6287	Program Services and MS Helpline
Support@msfocus.org	Email questions regarding programs and services
www.msfocus.org	Website for the MS Foundation
MS FOUNDATION PROGRAMS	
• Assistive Technology Program	Connects people with available assistive technology options
• Brighter Tomorrow	Offers one-time financial grants for needed items or services
• Computer Grants	Offers refurbished laptop and desktop computers
• Cooling Program	Provides vests, neck ties/wraps, wrist bands, and hats
• Emergency Assistance Program	Provides full or partial financial assistance for urgent needs, such as rent, utilities, or medication
• Healthcare Assistance Grant	Assists uninsured individuals with the cost of visiting an MS specialist or dentist. The grant may pay for an initial visit and one follow-up visit
• Homecare Assistance Grant	Includes home care, rehabilitation therapy visits, short-term respite care, and one-time aide support upon discharge from the hospital
CAN DO MULTIPLE SCLEROSIS	
CAN DO MS delivers health and wellness education programs to help families living with MS. Programs for individuals living with MS and care partners are offered in-person at locations throughout the country and through webinars.	
www.cando-ms.org	

MS-Specific Resources for Health Care Providers

Professional Resource Center

Website for researchers and MS clinicians hosted by the National MS Society providing information, consultation services, and a wide range of research funding programs, training opportunities and services, and tools and resources to support MS-related work.

www.nationalmssociety.org/For-Professionals/Clinical-Care

Consortium of MS Centers (CMSC)

National organization of MS health care providers focused on improving the lives of those living with MS. Provides a variety of continuing education programs on MS for health care providers through online programs, in-person seminars, and an annual education conference.

www.mscare.org

SUPPORTS AND RESOURCES FREQUENTLY NEEDED BY PEOPLE LIVING WITH MS AND THEIR FAMILIES

MS affects people living with the disease in several areas of their life, such as employment, access to health care, financial security, mobility/accessibility, family relationships, and personal care needs. If you have patients raising any of these concerns, what follows are agencies, organizations, and resources that exist to provide answers and support to them so they can more effectively advocate for themselves and can feel more equipped to navigate systems that can be very daunting and confusing.

Durable Medical Equipment and Assistive Technology

Durable medical equipment and assistive technology enable people with MS to continue to carry out activities of daily living and remain engaged and connected in spite of the limitations they are experiencing.

- **AbleData:** Provides impartial, comprehensive information on products, assistive technology, and equipment. Maintained for the Department of Health and Human Services, National Institute on Disability, Independent Living and Rehabilitation Research

  www.abledata.acl.gov

- **Friends of Man:** Charity organization offering durable medical equipment, home/vehicle modification, and other services

  www.friendsofman.org

- **National Assistive Technology Act Technical and Assistance Training Centers:** Assistive Technology assists those living with disabilities to gain access to and acquisition of assistive technology devices and services

  www.ataporg.org/programs

- **RESNA, the Rehabilitation Engineering and Assistive Technology Society:** Offers a free, online tool to find qualified RESNA-certified assistive technology professionals and manages federally funded programs in most states providing information on devices, borrowing programs, and funding resources for purchasing assistive technology

www.resna.org/about/consumer-and-public-information

■ **United Spinal Association—Disability Products and Services Directory:** Directory provides information and advice on all types of assistive technology, home medical equipment, and other adaptive products

www.unitedspinal.org/disability-products-services

Emotional Support and Domestic Abuse Resources

Variable, unpredictable, and often progressing MS creates considerable anxiety and stress, not only for the person with the disease but for family members as well. Accessing emotional support through various professional and peer support services can be extremely helpful in easing tensions and identifying more effective ways to deal with the significant challenges of MS.

Crisis Hotlines and Websites

Immediate help for emotional crisis situations.

■ **Domestic Shelters.org (for a list of local shelters)**

www.domesticshelters.org/

■ **National Domestic Violence Hotline:** 1-800-799-7233

www.thehotline.org/

Live Chat Services (available daily 7-2 AM CT)

www.thehotline.org (click on CHAT NOW)

■ **National Domestic Violence Hotline—Safe Havens Mapping Project** (Shelter for Pets)

www.thehotline.org/help/pets/

■ **National Organization for Victim Assistance** 1-800-879-6682
■ **National Sexual Assault Hotline** 1-800-656-4673
■ **National Suicide Prevention Lifeline:** 1-800-273-8255 (TALK)

www.suicidepreventionlifeline.org/

■ **Safe Place for Pets** (shelters/options for people and pets)

www.safeplaceforpets.org

■ **Substance Abuse and Mental Health Services Administration**

www.samhsa.gov/

Peer Connections

- National MS Society MSFriends: 1-800-673-7436
- National MS Society: blogs and individual connections

  www.MSconnection.org

- MS Association of America: My MSAA Community forum

  www.healthunlocked.com/mymsaa

- MS Association of America: MS Conversations blog

  www.blog.mymsaa.org

Professional Counseling

- Contact the MS organizations for referrals to professional counselors
- **Mental Health America:** A total of 200 affiliate organizations in 41 states, offers free online mental health screening tools, tools to locate mental health provider, support groups and other mental health resources in the local community

  www.mentalhealthamerica.net/

- **HelpPRO:** Offers an online therapist search to assist in finding a therapist for particular needs

  www.helppro.com

Self-Help and Support Groups

- National MS Society: Self-help groups by location and by phone

  www.nationalmssociety.org/Resources-Support/Find-Support

Resources for Caregiver Support

- **Aging and Disability Resource Centers:** Serves as single points of entry into the long-term services and supports system for older adults, people with disabilities, caregivers, veterans, and families

  www.n4a.org/adrcs

- **American Association of Caregiving Youth:** Information and support for children and adolescents who are 18 years or younger who provide significant or substantial assistance to relatives or household members with physical or mental illness or disability. Connects youth caregivers and their families with health care, education, and resources in their community

  www.aacy.org/

- **ARCH National Respite Network:** Includes a national service to help caregivers locate respite services in their local community

  www.archrespite.org

- **Caregiver Action Network:** Serves a broad spectrum of family caregivers providing education, peer support, and other resources

  www.caregiveraction.org

- **Family Caregiver Alliance:** Offers online information, resources, one-to-one caregiver information and assistance, and a state-by-state online guide to help families locate government, nonprofit, and private caregiver support programs

  www.caregiver.org

- **Well Spouse Association:** Offers peer-to-peer support and education to individuals caring for a chronically ill or disabled spouse or partner. Coordinates a national network of in-person and telephone support groups, online resources, on-line chat forum, and regional respite events

  www.wellspouse.org

Employment

Owing to its age of onset and complex range of symptoms, MS can affect a person's ability to work. There are many resources available to help patients understand their employment rights and explore options available to them for either remaining in the workforce or seeking disability benefits.

Employment Resources

- **Job Accommodation Network (JAN):** Website for employees and employers to educate themselves on workplace accommodations, the Americans with Disabilities Act or Rehabilitation Act, or topics related to disability employment

  www.askjan.org/

- **One-Stop Employment Centers:** Comprehensive job centers offering training referrals, career counseling, job listings, and employment-related services in each community

  www.careeronestop.org

- **Vocational Rehabilitation (VR) Agencies:** Every state has a vocational rehabilitation agency that is designed to help individuals with disabilities meet their employment goals. Vocational rehabilitation agencies assist individuals with disabilities to prepare for, obtain, maintain, or regain employment. To search by state:

  www.askearn.org/state-vocational-rehabilitation-agencies/

Rights and Protections

- **Americans with Disabilities Act (ADA):** Information and technical assistance on the Americans with Disabilities Act and protections under the law for people living with disabilities

  www.ada.gov/

- **National Employment Lawyers Association:** Advances employee rights and provides a listing of attorneys who engage in employment law cases

  www.exchange.nela.org/memberdirectory/findalawyer

- **State Protection and Advocacy Systems (P&A):** The Protection and Advocacy System (P&A) and Client Assistance Program (CAP) comprise the nationwide network of congressionally mandated, legally based disability rights agencies. P&A agencies have the authority to provide legal representation and other advocacy services, under federal laws, to all people with disabilities

  www.acl.gov/programs/aging-and-disability-network/ state-protection-advocacy-systems

- **U.S. Equal Employment Opportunity Commission (EEOC):** Federal agency that is responsible for enforcing federal laws that make it illegal to discriminate against a job applicant or employee because of the person's race, color, religion, sex, national origin, age, disability, or genetic information. EEOC also works to prevent discrimination before it occurs through outreach, education, and technical assistance programs

  www.eeoc.gov/

Benefits

- **Federal Family Medical Leave Act (FMLA):** FMLA allows eligible employees to take up to 12 weeks of leave in any 12-month period, without pay, to care for a close family member or, in some states, themselves. Note individual states may have separate FMLA programs offering different additional benefits
  - ☐ Website that outlines the federal rules and requirements

    www.dol.gov/whd/fmla/employeeguide.pdf

  - ☐ Website to find specific state programs

    www.ncsl.org

Disability Benefits

- **Employer (short term/long term):** Consult with one's human resource department

- **Private (short term/long term):** Benefit will depend on the specifics of the policy. Particularly important to note length of coverage and how it might intersect with any employer or government disability benefit
  - ☐ **Private Disability Insurance Claims: A Guide for People with MS:** Publication offered by National MS Society. Find online at

    www.nationalmssociety.org

- **State (short-term disability):** For specific state information check that state's short-term disability website
- **Federal Long-term Disability Benefits (Social Security Disability Benefits):** The Social Security Administration handles long-term disability claims based on the inability of an individual to engage in any substantial gainful activity (work) by reason of a medically determinable physical or mental impairment expected to remain indefinitely or expected to last at least 12 months
  - ☐ **Social Security Disability Insurance (SSDI)** is based on a work history where the employee has contributed to the Social Security Trust Fund over a number of years of working
  - ☐ **Supplemental Security Insurance (SSI)** are benefits that go primarily to those who are disabled with limited or no work history, income, and resources
    For additional information regarding both programs and to apply:

    www.ssa.gov

  - ☐ Applying for Social Security Disability Benefits: A Guidebook for People with MS and their Healthcare Professionals: Publication offered by National MS Society. Find online at

    www.nationalmssociety.org

Financial Assistance

As income declines and additional costs of living with MS escalate, many people with MS must look to other resources for financial relief. There are organizations and programs offering various kinds of financial assistance to those in need of help, from emergency assistance and one-time grants to ongoing benefits and support. Some organizations listed below offer their own grants; others help locate other appropriate resources.

The MS organizations should be contacted for assistance in locating appropriate financial resources in local communities:

- **MS Association of America:**

  MSQuestions@mymsaa.org or 800-532-7667, x154

- **National Multiple Sclerosis Society:**

  ContactUsNMSS@nmss.org or 1-800-344-4867

- **Multiple Sclerosis Foundation:**

  www.msfocus.org or 888-673-6287

Government Assistance

State and county agencies serve as a gateway to both emergency and on-going financial assistance. Funding of these agencies varies from year to year, so websites need to be checked regularly.

State/county social services: Provides information on a variety of relief programs such as Temporary Assistance for Needy Families (TANF), Head Start, offered in each state and locating providers and facilities as well as complaint or appeal procedures.

For general information

www.hhs.gov/

Describes government benefit eligibility in each state

www.benefits.gov

Nongovernment Assistance

Referral Agencies

- **Aging and Disability Resource Centers:** Serves as single points of entry into the long-term services and supports system for older adults, people with disabilities, caregivers, veterans, and families

  www.n4a.org/

- **Centers for Independent Living:** A consumer-controlled, community-based, cross-disability, nonresidential private nonprofit agency that is designed and operated within a local community by individuals with disabilities. Provides an array of independent living services, including information and referral, independent living skills training, individual and systems advocacy, peer counseling, and transition assistance from nursing homes and other institutions to community-based residences. Programs vary by location

  www.ilru.org/projects/cil-net/cil-center-and-association-directory

Funding Organizations: Potential Resources for Crisis or Short-term Assistance

- **American Red Cross:** Provides shelter to families and individuals after an emergency as well as other temporary assistance. Requirements may vary based on location

  www.redcross.org/

- **Catholic Charities:** Community-based services provided to individuals and families in need, including counseling and mental health, family strengthening programs, food banks/meal delivery for the homebound, housing assistance, limited financial assistance for rent/mortgage, utilities, clothing, and medication

  www.catholiccharitiesusa.org

- **Community Action Partnership:** Lists over a thousand agencies in local communities, as well as state associations and national partners. Locates community agencies by state and county, with focus on helping low-income families

  www.communityactionpartnership.com

- **Food Banks:** Check your local listings for assistance
- **Low Income Home Energy Assistance Program (LIHEAP):** Program assists families with energy costs

  Program information:

  www.acf.hhs.gov/ocs/programs/liheap

  State Listing:

  www.acf.hhs.gov/ocs/liheap-state-and-territory-contact-listing

- **Meals on Wheels:** Delivers meals to individuals whose diminished mobility makes it hard to shop for food, prepare meals, or socialize with others. Typically programs service adults 60 years and over, although age requirement vary by program and areas served

  www.mealsonwheelsamerica.org/

- **Modest Needs:** National nonprofit empowering members of the general public to make small, emergency grants to low-income workers who are at risk of slipping into poverty

  www.modestneeds.org

- **Salvation Army Offices:** Can provide shelter and limited financial assistance to those in emergency need

  www.salvationarmyusa.org/usn/www_usn_2.nsf/vw-local/Home

- **Travelers Aid:** Works with stranded individuals and offers suggestions and limited funding to assist in getting home. In 32 cities, Travelers Aid provides more comprehensive services to prevent homelessness, including housing options, job training, and food assistance. Services vary by area

  www.travelersaid.org

- **United Way:** Provides resources for health, financial assistance, human services, etc. within an area

  www.211.org

Health Insurance

Health insurance coverage is an important factor of one's MS management and care planning. Sources of health insurance for people with MS include employer coverage, the private marketplace, Medicare, Medicaid, and Veteran's services. There are also specific agencies and organizations that provide information on insurance options and advocate on behalf of patients for access to needed medical services.

Sources of Health Insurance

- **Employer or Private Insurance:** Insurance not marketed by government agency; received as an employee benefit or bought through private insurance plan or health insurance agent
- **Affordable Care Act:** This law (sometimes also referred to as Obamacare) provides consumers with subsidies that lower cost for households with incomes between 100% and 400% or federal poverty level. Some states have also expanded their Medicaid program to cover adults with incomes below 138% of poverty level

  www.healthcare.gov

- **Medicare:** Federal health insurance program for people 65 years or older, certain younger people with disabilities, and those with end-stage renal disease

  www.medicare.gov 1-800-Medicare

- **Medicaid:** Health coverage for people with low incomes, administered by states according to federal requirements

  Basic eligibility requirement

  www.medicaid.gov/

  Contact Information

  www.medicaid.gov/about-us/contact-us/index.html

Insurance Rights and Protections

- **Medicare Rights Center:** National nonprofit consumer organization to ensure access to affordable health care for older adults and people with disabilities. Offers counseling, advocacy, educational programs, and public policy activity

  www.medicarerights.org

- **State Departments of Insurance:** National Association of Insurance Commission (NAIC) members are the chief insurance regulators from each of the 50 US states and six territories. Provides information about insurance and regulations. The jurisdiction map locates NAIC members and resources in each state

Map of State Departments of Insurance

www.naic.org/state_web_map.htm

■ **Patient Advocate Foundation:** Patient services provide patients with arbitration, mediation, and negotiation to settle issues with access to care, medical debt, and job retention related to their illness

www.patientadvocate.org

Home Care/Adult Day Programs

Support services are often needed if people with MS require increasingly more assistance while living at home, whether that be for personal care, homemaking help, companionship, or respite for the caregiver. In addition to the following resources, check your local county and state as many offer personal assistance and caregiver respite programs.

■ **Hiring Help at Home-Basic Facts:** Checklists and worksheets for people who need help at home. Forms for a needs assessment, job description, and employment contract. Located on National MS Society website:

www.nationalmssociety.org

■ **Home Care Association of America:** An association of providers of private duty home care, including nonmedical home care services. Organization offers a search tool to find private pay in-home care services across the country

www.hcaoa.org/find-a-provider/advanced/

■ **Home Health Compare:** Compares home health agencies using various survey ratings compiled by Medicare

www.medicare.gov/homehealthcompare/search.html

■ **National Adult Day Services Association:** National association provides information regarding adult day services, comparing services through the different adult day service models, and a tool to find services by state

www.nadsa.org/locator/

Hospice

■ **National Hospice and Palliative Care Organization (NHPCO):** Through their Caring Connections Initiative NHPCO provides an online search tool to find hospice and palliative care programs and resources throughout the nation. It also offers detailed consumer-oriented information on end-of-life issues

www.nhpco.org

Housing

Rental assistance; accessible, affordable housing units; and homeless prevention services are resources that have been developed within communities to assist those for whom market-rate housing is financially impossible. Home modifications and repairs may allow an individual with increasing disability to remain in their home by adding features that create a safe and accessible environment.

Accessible and Affordable Housing

■ **For housing developed specifically for people living with MS in some local areas contact MS Navigator:**

ContactUsNMSS@nmss.org or 1-800-344-4867

■ **Affordable Accessible Housing A Guide for People with MS:** Publication available on the National MS Society website. Access it at:

www.nationalmssociety.org

■ **The ADA Network:** Provides information, guidance, and training on accessibility standards under the Americans with Disabilities Act

www.adata.org

■ **Centers for Independent Living:** Offer housing training and information regarding local housing resources. State listing of independent living centers

www.ilru.org/html/publications/directory/index.html

■ **SocialServe.com:** Provides a toll-free English/Spanish call center helping landlords list and tenants search for affordable properties while monitoring the availability and accuracy of listings. Also search website by state

www.socialserve.com 1-877-428-8844

■ **US Department of Housing and Urban Development (HUD):** Serves people in need of rental, home buying, and homeowner assistance with special programs available to families, the elderly, and persons with disabilities in financial need

Housing Counseling Agency Search

www.hudexchange.info/programs/housing-counseling/customer-service-feedback

HUD Resource Locator

resources.hud.gov

Homeless Assistance

- **Homeless Shelter Directory:** Provides an online directory of homeless resources, including homeless service organizations and shelters by state

  www.homelessshelterdirectory.org

- **National Coalition for the Homeless:** National network of advocates and community-based service providers. Provides referrals to state and local organizations that advocate for the homeless and provide direct services such as emergency shelters, transitional housing, health care, employment counseling, and case management:

  nationalhomeless.org/

- **Homeless Directory**

  www.nationalhomeless.org/directories/directory_local.pdf

Homeless Veterans Assistance

- **HUD VASH:** Combines the Department of Housing and Urban Development (HUD) Housing Choice Voucher (HCV) rental assistance for homeless veterans and their families with case management and clinical services provided by the Department of Veterans Affairs (VA) at its medical centers and in the community

  www.hudexchange.info/programs/hud-vash/hud-vash-eligibility-requirements/

- **Soldier On:** A private nonprofit organization providing homeless veterans with transitional housing and supportive services

  www.wesoldieron.org/

Home Modification and Repairs

- **Global Disability Rights Now:** Offers low-cost solutions for making a home accessible

  www.globaldisabilityrightsnow.org

- **National Home Builders Association:** Information and resource on many topics related to home maintenance and repair, remodeling, and universal design for those aging in place or living with disabilities

  www.nahb.org

- **Rebuilding Together:** Mission to repair homes, revitalize communities, and rebuild lives through building safe homes and communities for everyone; operates through local offices engaging over 100,000 volunteers

  www.rebuildingtogether.org/

Legal Assistance

There are legal rights and protections in place that can protect people with disabilities such as MS from discrimination in many areas of public life, including jobs, school, housing, and transportation. Legal assistance is also an important component of planning for the future in terms of accessing benefits, advance directives, protection of assets, establishment of trusts, etc. In addition to the following resources, visit www.ada.gov for more information related to the Americans with Disabilities Act.

Advance Directives

Advance directives are legal documents that allow individuals to spell out their decisions about end-of-life care ahead of time. They provide a way to tell wishes to family, friends, and health care professionals and to avoid confusion later on.

- **Caring Info** provides free advance directives and instructions for each state

  www.caringinfo.org

Employment

- **Employment Lawyers Association:** National professional organization of attorneys who specialize in employment law and represent employees in such cases

  exchange.nela.org/network/findalawyer

Estate Planning

- **National Academy of Elder Law Attorneys (NAELA):** Provides referrals to elder law and special needs planning attorneys. Offers information to consumers regarding elder law and special needs planning

  www.naela.org

- NAELA in partnership with the National MS Society offers a video series: Legal and Care Planning for People with Multiple Sclerosis

  www.nationalmssociety.org/Living-Well-With-MS/Work-and-Home/Insurance-and-Financial-Information/Financial-Resources/Financial-Planning

- **National Association of Estate Planners & Councils:** Offers an online database of estate planning professionals. Members are credentialed estate planners, including attorneys, accountants, trust officers, and credentialed insurance and financial planner professionals

  www.naepc.org/

- **National Elder Law Foundation (NELF):** Provides referrals for Certified Elder Law Attorneys

  www.nelf.org/find-a-cela/

Financial Counseling and Planning

- **American Association of Daily Money Managers:** Provides personal financial and bookkeeping services to individuals who have difficulty in managing their personal monetary affairs. Services include bill paying, balancing checkbooks, making bank deposits, reviewing medical insurance papers, and organizing tax records

  secure.aadmm.com/find-a-dmm/

- **IRS Volunteer Income Tax Assistance Program:** Provides tax return assistance to individuals of low income, persons with disabilities, or limited English speaking persons

  www.irs.gov/individuals/free-tax-return-preparation-for-you-by-volunteers

- **National Foundation for Credit Counseling (NFCC):** Provides referrals to certified consumer credit counselors. Offers information and counseling to consumers regarding topics such as credit, home buying, and bankruptcy

  www.nfcc.org/

Marital or Child Custody General Legal Assistance

- **Legal Aid: To find legal aid/bar association contact information by state:**

  apps.americanbar.org/legalservices/findlegalhelp/home.cfm

Social Security

- **National Organization of Social Security Claimant's Representatives:** Organization providing referrals to attorneys specializing in Social Security Disability (SSDI) and Supplemental Security Income (SSI) representation

  nosscr.org/

- **Check MS organizations or local bar associations** for specific community attorney referral and other resources

Nursing Facilities/Assisted Living

Nursing home placement is explored when an individual requires 24-hour nursing care and is no longer safe living within the community. Nursing homes operate under both state and federal requirements. Assisted Living is an option for those requiring 24-hour supervision or those who would prefer living in a group environment rather than living alone. Assisted Livings are regulated by the states.

- **Aging and Disability Resource Centers:** Serves as single points of entry into the long-term services and supports system for older adults, people with disabilities, caregivers, veterans, and families

    www.n4a.org/

- **Assisted Living Inspections and Violations by State:** List of states provided so that consumers can research assisted living facilities in that state regarding any publicly available inspections or violation reports from the state licensing bodies

    www.assistedlivingfacilities.org/resources/choosing-an-assist-ed-living-facility/assisted-living-facility-violations/

- **Centers for Independent Living:** Provide information regarding assisted living options and Medicaid waiver in local areas. Search by state/county

    www.ilru.org/html/publications/directory/index.html

- **National Long-Term Care Ombudsman Resource Center:** National source of information, tools, and advocacy for consumers, families, caregivers, and advocates. It refers residents, families, and others to local ombudsman programs

    www.theconsumervoice.org/get_help

- **Nursing Home Compare:** Provides a tool to allow nursing homes and skilled nursing facilities certified by Medicare and Medicaid to be located and compared

    www.medicare.gov/NursingHomeCompare/

Prescription Assistance

Some programs and agencies exist with the primary mission of assisting patients with the prohibitive cost of copays and prescriptions. The nature of the assistance offered, and the eligibility for that assistance, varies from program to program. Many pharmaceutical companies have patient assistance programs. Check with the company.

Referrals for Assistance

- **Healthfinder.gov:** Search for state and corporate prescription programs

    www.healthfinder.gov

- **NeedyMeds:** Provides referrals to prescription assistance programs

  www.needymeds.org

- **The Partnership for Prescription Assistance:** Provides referrals to prescription assistance programs

  www.pparx.org

- **Simplefill:** Program dedicated to offering efficient assistance for patients who are prescribed unaffordable medications, by using the available programs offered through the pharmaceutical companies and foundations that offer grant funding for chronic diseases

  www.simplefill.com

Providers of Assistance

- **The Assistance Fund:** Independent charitable patient assistance foundation that helps patients and families facing high medical out-of-pocket costs by providing financial assistance for their copayments, coinsurance, deductibles, and other health-related expenses

  www.tafcares.org/

- **HealthWell Foundation:** Offers MS copay assistance to those with Medicare insurance

  www.healthwellfoundation.org/

- **Patient Access Network (PAN) Foundation:** Helps underinsured people with life-threatening, chronic, and rare diseases get the medications and treatment they need by paying for their out-of-pocket costs and advocating for improved access and affordability. Copay program available for those with Medicare

  www.panfoundation.org/index.php/en/

Transportation

MS often makes driving a challenge, particularly when dealing with symptoms affecting vision, memory, reflexes, or moving one's arms and legs. There are many options and services available to assist people with MS in remaining mobile and actively engaged in their communities, from modifications to their own automobiles to accessible and flexible public transportation services.

Car Modifications and Driving Evaluations

- **Association for Driver Rehabilitation Specialists (ADED):** Persons seeking driver safety evaluations, vehicle modification/hand control assessments, driver training, and equipment installation. Includes a search tool for resources in local areas

  www.aded.net/

- **Disabled Dealer:** An advertising source where modified vehicles and durable medical equipment are posted for sale

  www.disableddealer.com

- **Mobility Works:** Helps to provide independence to thousands of individuals throughout the country with wheelchair-accessible vans, adaptive equipment, and specialized commercial vehicles

  www.mobilityworks.com

- **National Mobility Equipment Dealers Association (NMED):** A nonprofit trade association of more than 600 mobility equipment dealers and manufacturers and driver rehabilitation specialists. The association hosts a nationwide network of accessible vehicle dealers

  www.nmeda.com

- **National Vehicles/National Highway Traffic Safety Administration:** Provides overview and information regarding driving with a disability

  www.nhtsa.gov/road-safety/adapted-vehicles

Public Transportation for People With Disabilities

- **American Public Transportation Association:** Provides links to find public transportation information in local areas

  www.apta.com/resources/links/Pages/default.aspx

- **National Rural Transit Assistance Program:** Provides information and a toolkit to assist individuals in understanding their rights to equal access to public transportation, including para transit, under the ADA

  www.nationalrtap.org/adatoolkit/

Additionally, check your local state Department of Transportation for accessible transit information.

INDEX ■ ■ ■

Note: Page numbers followed by "t" denotes table, "f" denotes figures and "b" denotes boxes.

RRS1904